Advances in Neurology

Volume 92

ADVANCES IN NEUROLOGY

Volume 92

Ischemic Stroke

Editors

H.J.M. Barnett, O.C., M.D.
John P. Robarts Research Institute
London, Ontario, Canada

Julien Bogousslavsky, M.D.
Department of Neurology
Centre Hospitalier Universitaire Vaudois
Lausanne, Switzerland

Heather Meldrum, B.A.
John P. Robarts Research Institute
London, Ontario, Canada

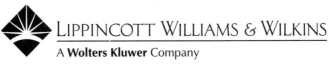

LIPPINCOTT WILLIAMS & WILKINS
A **Wolters Kluwer** Company
Philadelphia · Baltimore · New York · London
Buenos Aires · Hong Kong · Sydney · Tokyo

Acquisitions Editor: Anne M. Sydor
Developmental Editor: Julia Seto
Production Editor: Emily Lerman
Manufacturing Manager: Colin J. Warnock
Cover Designer: Patricia Gast
Compositor: Lippincott Williams & Wilkins Desktop Division
Printer: Maple Press

Printed in the USA

Library of Congress Cataloging-in-Publication Data

Ischemic stroke / editors, H.J.M. Barnett, Julien Bogousslavsky, Heather Meldrum.
    p. ; cm. -- (Advances in neurology ; v. 92)
  Includes bibliographical references and index.
  ISBN 0-7817-3652-8 (alk. paper)
    1. Cerebrovascular disease. I. Barnett, H.J.M. (Henry J.M.) II. Bogousslavsky, Julien.
III. Meldrum, Heather. IV. Series.
    [DNLM: 1. Cerebrovascular Accident. WL 355 I768 2003]
  RC388.5 .I827 2003
  616.8′1--dc21

                                                                    2002043051

Care has been taken to confirm the accuracy of the information presented and to describe generally accepted practices. However, the authors, editors, and publisher are not responsible for errors or omissions or for any consequences from application of the information in this book and make no warranty, expressed or implied, with respect to the currency, completeness, or accuracy of the contents of the publication. Application of this information in a particular situation remains the professional responsibility of the practitioner.

The authors, editors, and publisher have exerted every effort to ensure that drug selection and dosage set forth in this text are in accordance with current recommendations and practice at the time of publication. However, in view of ongoing research, changes in government regulations, and the constant flow of information relating to drug therapy and drug reactions, the reader is urged to check the package insert for each drug for any change in indications and dosage and for added warnings and precautions. This is particularly important when the recommended agent is a new or infrequently employed drug.

Some drugs and medical devices presented in this publication have Food and Drug Administration (FDA) clearance for limited use in restricted research settings. It is the responsibility of the health care provider to ascertain the FDA status of each drug or device planned for use in their clinical practice.

Advances in Neurology Series

Vol. 59: Neural Injury and Regeneration: *F. J. Seil, editor.* 384 pp., 1993.

Vol. 58: Tourette Syndrome: Genetics, Neurobiology, and Treatment: *T. N. Chase, A. J. Friedhoff, and D. J. Cohen, editors.* 400 pp., 1992.

Vol. 57: Frontal Lobe Seizures and Epilepsies: *P. Chauvel, A. V. Delgado-Escueta, E. Halgren, and J. Bancaud, editors.* 752 pp., 1992.

Vol. 56: Amyotrophic Lateral Sclerosis and Other Motor Neuron Diseases: *L. P. Rowland, editor.* 592 pp., 1991.

Vol. 55: Neurobehavioral Problems in Epilepsy: *D. B. Smith, D. Treiman, and M. Trimble, editors.* 512 pp., 1990.

Vol. 54: Magnetoencephalography: *S. Sato, editor.* 284 pp., 1990.

Vol. 53: Parkinson's Disease: Anatomy, Pathology, and Therapy: *M. B. Streifler, A. D. Korczyn, E. Melamed, and M. B. H. Youdim, editors.* 640 pp., 1990.

Vol. 52: Brain Edema: Pathogenesis, Imaging, and Therapy: *D. Long, editor.* 640 pp., 1990.

Vol. 51: Alzheimer's Disease: *R. J. Wurtman, S. Corkin, J. H. Growdon, and E. Ritter-Walker, editors.* 308 pp., 1990.

Vol. 50: Dystonia 2: *S. Fahn, C. D. Marsden, and D. B. Calne, editors.* 688 pp., 1988.

Vol. 49: Facial Dyskinesias: *J. Jankovic and E. Tolosa, editors.* 560 pp., 1988.

Vol. 48: Molecular Genetics of Neurological and Neuromuscular Disease: *S. DiDonato, S. DiMauro, A. Mamoli, and L. P. Rowland, editors.* 288 pp., 1987.

Vol. 47: Functional Recovery in Neurological Disease: *S. G. Waxman, editor.* 640 pp., 1987.

Vol. 46: Intensive Neurodiagnostic Monitoring: *R. J. Gumnit, editor.* 336 pp., 1987.

Vol. 45: Parkinson's Disease: *M. D. Yahr and K. J. Bergmann, editors.* 640 pp., 1987.

Vol. 44: Basic Mechanisms of the Epilepsies: Molecular and Cellular Approaches: *A. V. Delgado-Escueta, A. A. Ward, Jr., D. M. Woodbury, and R. J. Porter, editors.* 1,120 pp., 1986.

Vol. 43: Myoclonus: *S. Fahn, C. D. Marsden, and M. H. VanWoert, editors.* 752 pp., 1986.

Vol. 42: Progress in Aphasiology: *F. C. Rose, editor.* 384 pp., 1984.

Vol. 41: The Olivopontocerebellar Atrophies: *R. C. Duvoisin and A. Plaitakis, editors.* 304 pp., 1984.

Vol. 40: Parkinson-Specific Motor and Mental Disorders, Role of Pallidum: Pathophysiological, Biochemical, and Therapeutic Aspects: *R. G. Hassler and J. F. Christ, editors.* 601 pp., 1984.

Vol. 39: Motor Control Mechanisms in Health and Disease: *J. E. Desmedt, editor.* 1,224 pp., 1983.

Vol. 38: The Dementias: *R. Mayeux and W. G. Rosen, editors.* 288 pp., 1983.

Vol. 37: Experimental Therapeutics of Movement Disorders: *S. Fahn, D. B. Calne, and I. Shoulson, editors.* 339 pp., 1983.

Vol. 36: Human Motor Neuron Diseases: *L. P. Rowland, editor.* 592 pp., 1982.

Vol. 35: Gilles de la Tourette Syndrome: *A. J. Friedhoff and T. N. Chase, editors.* 476 pp., 1982.

Vol. 34: Status Epilepticus: Mechanism of Brain Damage and Treatment: *A. V. Delgado-Escueta, C. G. Wasterlain, D. M. Treiman, and R. J. Porter, editors.* 579 pp., 1983.

Vol. 31: Demyelinating Diseases: Basic and Clinical Electrophysiology: *S. Waxman and J. Murdoch Ritchie, editors.* 544 pp., 1981.

Vol. 30: Diagnosis and Treatment of Brain Ischemia: *A. L. Carney and E. M. Anderson, editors.* 424 pp., 1981.

Vol. 29: Neurofibromatosis: *V. M. Riccardi and J. J. Mulvilhill, editors.* 288 pp., 1981.

Vol. 28: Brain Edema: *J. Cervós-Navarro and R. Ferszt, editors.* 539 pp., 1980.

Vol. 27: Antiepileptic Drugs: Mechanisms of Action: *G. H. Glaser, J. K. Penry, and D. M. Woodbury, editors.* 728 pp.,1980.

Vol. 26: Cerebral Hypoxia and Its Consequences: *S. Fahn, J. N. Davis, and L. P. Rowland, editors.* 454 pp., 1979.

Vol. 25: Cerebrovascular Disorders and Stroke: *M. Goldstein, L. Bolis, C. Fieschi, S. Gorini, and C. H. Millikan, editors.* 412 pp., 1979.

Vol. 24: The Extrapyramidal System and Its Disorders: *L. J. Poirier, T. L. Sourkes, and P. Bédard, editors.* 552 pp., 1979.

Vol. 23: Huntington's Chorea: *T. N. Chase, N. S. Wexler, and A. Barbeau, editors.* 864 pp., 1979.

Vol. 22: Complications of Nervous System Trauma: *R. A. Thompson and J. R. Green, editors.* 454 pp., 1979.

Vol. 21: The Inherited Ataxia: Biochemical, Viral, and Pathological Studies: *R. A. Kark, R. Rosenberg, and L. Schut, editors.* 450 pp., 1978.

Vol. 20: Pathology of Cerebrospinal Microcirculation: *J. Cervós-Navarro, E. Betz, G. Ebhardt, R. Ferszt, and R. Wüllenweber, editors.* 636 pp., 1978.

Vol. 19: Neurological Epidemiology: Principles and Clinical Applications: *B. S. Schoenberg, editor.* 672 pp., 1978.

Contents

The Biochemistry of Ischemic Stroke

Risk Factors in Stroke

Heart and Brain

Brain and Heart

Cerebral Venous and Sinus Disease

The Sequelae of Stroke and Their Treatment

Contributing Authors

Mark J. Alberts, MD
Professor
Department of Neurology
Director, Stroke Program
Northwestern University Medical School
710 North Lake Shore Drive;
Professor
Department of Neurology
Director, Stroke Program
Northwestern Memorial Hospital
251 East Huron Street
Chicago, Illinois 60611
U.S.A.

Ale Algra, MD, PhD
Associate Professor
Departments of Clinical Epidemiology and
    Neurology
Julius Center for Health Sciences and Primary Care
University Medical Center Utrecht
Heidelberglaan 100
3584 CX Utrecht
The Netherlands

Pierre Amarenco, MD
Professor
Department of Neurology
Dennis Diderot University;
Chairman
Department of Neurology and Stroke Centre
Bichat Hospital
46 rue Henri Huchard
Paris 75018
France

Cenk Ayata, MD
Instructor
Department of Radiology
Harvard University;
Graduate Assistant
Department of Neurology
Massachusetts General Hospital
55 Fruit Street
Boston, Massachusetts 02135
U.S.A.

Philip A. Barber, MB, ChB, MRCP
Postdoctoral Fellow
Department of Clinical Neuroscience
University of Calgary;
Neurologist
Department of Clinical Neuroscience
Foothills Medical Centre
1403—29th Street NW
Calgary, Alberta T2N 2T9
Canada

H.J.M. Barnett, OC, MD
Professor Emeritus
University of Western Ontario
London, Ontario N6A 5C1
Canada

Vadim Beletsky, MD, PhD
Senior Stroke Fellow
Department of Clinical Neurosciences
University of Western Ontario
339 Windermere Road;
Consultant
Robarts Imaging Laboratories
100 Perth Drive
London, Ontario N6A 5K8
Canada

Oscar Benavente, MD, FRCP(C)
Associate Professor
Department of Medicine, Division of Neurology
University of Texas Health Science Center
7703 Floyd Curl Drive
San Antonio, Texas 78229-3900
U.S.A.

Eivind Berge, MD, PhD
Department of Internal Medicine
Ullevaal University Hospital
N-0407 Oslo
Norway

Julien Bogousslavsky, MD
Professor and Chair
Department of Neurology
University of Lausanne
rue du Bugnon;
Head, Department of Neurology Services
University Hospital
Centre Hospitalier Universitaire Vaudois
1011 Lausanne
Switzerland

Ruth Bonita, MPH, PhD
Director Surveillance
Noncommunicable Diseases and Mental Health
The World Health Organization
Avenue Appia 20
1121 Geneva 27
Switzerland

Natan M. Bornstein, MD
Professor
Department of Neurology
Tel Aviv University—Sourasky Medical School;
Chief, Department of Neurology and Stroke Unit
Tel Aviv Sourasky Medical Center
6 Weizmann Street
Tel Aviv 64239
Israel

Marie Germaine Bousser, MD
Professor
Department of Neurology
Faculte de Medicine Lariboisière
10 Avenue de Verdun;
Head, Department of Neurology
Hôpital Lariboisière
9 rue Ambroise Paré
75010 Paris
France

Martin M. Brown, MD
Professor
Department of Stroke Medicine
Institute of Neurology
University College of London;
Consultant Neurologist
Acute Brain Injury Service
The National Hospital for Neurology and
* Neurosurgery*
Queen Square
London WCIN 3BG
United Kingdom

Alastair M. Buchan, MD
Professor,
Department of Clinical Neurosciences
University of Calgary;
Head, Stroke Program
Foothills Hospital
1403—29th Street NW
Calgary, Alberta T2N 2T9
Canada

Marco Calabresi, MD
Department of Neurological Sciences
University of Roma "La Sapienza"
Viale dell'Università 30
00185 Rome
Italy

Louis R. Caplan, MD
Professor
Department of Neurology
Harvard Medical School;
Chief, Cerebrovascular Service
Beth Israel Deaconess Medical Center
330 Brookline Avenue
Boston, Massachusetts 02215
U.S.A.

Antonio Carota, MD
Service de Neurologie
Centre Hospitalier Universitaire Vaudois
BH 013
CH-1011 Lausanne
Switzerland

Hugues Chabriat, MD, PhD
Professor
Department of Neurology
Hopital Lariboisière
2 rue Ambroise Paré
75010 Paris
France

Raymond T.F. Cheung, MD, PhD
Associate Professor
Department of Medicine
University of Hong Kong;
Honorary Consultant
Department of Medicine
Queen Mary Hospital
102 Pokfulam Road
Pokfulam, Hong Kong

Marc I. Chimowitz, MB, ChB
Professor
Department of Neurology
Emory University;
Director, Stroke Program
Department of Neurology
Emory University Hospital
1365 Clifton Road
Atlanta, Georgia 30322
U.S.A.

Ariel Cohen, MD
Department of Cardiology
Saint-Antoine Hospital
Pierre and Marie Curie University
Paris
France

George Michael Cuesta, PhD
Clinical Assistant Professor of Neuropsychology
Department of Neurology and Neuroscience
Joan and Sanford I. Weill Medical College of
    Cornell University
525 East 68th Street
New York, New York 10021;
Director of Rehabilitation Psychology and
    Neuropsychology
Burke Rehabilitation Hospital
785 Mamaroneck Avenue
White Plains, New York 10605
U.S.A.

Joseph G. D'Alton, MB
Associate Clinical Professor
Department of Neurology
Tufts Medical School
Boston, Massachusetts;
Active Staff
Department of Medicine (Neurology)
Metrowest Medical Center
Lincoln Street
Framingham, Massachusetts 01701
U.S.A.

Georges Darbellay, MD
Physicist Engineer
Laboratory of Signal Processing
École Polytechnique Fédérale de Lausanne
CH-1011 Lausanne
Switzerland

Thomas J. DeGraba, MD
Director, Clinical Stroke Research Unit
Stroke Branch
National Institute of Neurological Disorders and
    Stroke
Bethesda, Maryland
U.S.A.

Andrew M. Demchuk, MD, FRCPC
Assistant Professor
Faculty of Medicine
Department of Clinical Neurosciences
University of Calgary
3330 Hospital Drive NW;
Neurologist,
Department of Clinical Neurosciences
Foothills Medical Centre
1403—29th Street NW
Calgary, Alberta T2N 2T9
Canada

Paul-André Despland, MD
Associate Professor
Department of Neurology
Centre Hospitalier Universitaire Vaudois
rue du Bugnon 46
CH-1011 Lausanne
Switzerland

Gérald Devuyst, MD
PD and MER and Medecin Associé
Department of Neurology
Centre Hospitalier Universitaire Vaudois
rue du Bugnon 46
CH-1011 Lausanne
Switzerland

Geoffrey A. Donnan, MD
Director, National Stroke Research Institute
Austin & Repatriation Medical Centre
Banksia Street
Heidelberg West, Victoria 3081
Australia

Alexander W. Dromerick, MD
Associate Professor
Department of Neurology
Washington University School of Medicine
4444 Forest Park Avenue;
Attending Physician
Department of Neurology/Rehabilitation
Barnes-Jewish Hospital
One Barnes-Jewish Hospital Plaza
St. Louis, Missouri 63110
U.S.A.

Michael Eliasziw, PhD
Associate Professor
Department of Community Health Sciences and
    Clinical Neurosciences
University of Calgary
3330 Hospital Drive NW
Calgary, Alberta T2N 4N1
Canada

Emad S. Farag, MD
Postdoctoral Fellow
Department of Pathology and Laboratory Medicine
UCLA Medical Center
10833 Le Conte Avenue
Los Angeles, California 90095
U.S.A.

G.G. Ferguson, MD
Department of Clinical Neurological Sciences
University of Western Ontario
London, Ontario
Canada

Marc Fisher, MD
Department of Neurology
University of Massachusetts Medical School
Worcester, Massachusetts
U.S.A.

Anthony J. Furlan, MD
Head, Section of Stroke and Neurological Intensive
   Care
Department of Neurology
Cleveland Clinic
9500 Euclid Avenue
Cleveland, Ohio 44195
U.S.A.

Dimitrios Georgiadis, MD
Department of Neurology
University of Heidelberg
Im Neuenheimer Feld 400
69120 Heidelberg
Germany

Larry B. Goldstein, MD
Professor of Medicine (Neurology)
Director, Center for Cerebrovascular Disease
Duke University Medical Center
Box 3651
Durham, North Carolina 27710
U.S.A.

Philip B. Gorelick, MD, MPH
Jannotta Presidential Professor of Neurology
Department of Neurosciences
Rush Medical College
1645 West Jackson
Chicago, Illinois 60612
U.S.A.

Vladimir Hachinski, MD, FRCPC, DSc
Professor
University of Western Ontario
1151 Richmond Street;
Director, Stroke Program
Department of Clinical Neurological Sciences
London Health Sciences Centre, University Campus
339 Windermere Road
London, Ontario N6A 5A5
Canada

Werner Hacke, MD, PhD
Professor and Chairman
Department of Neurology
University of Heidelberg
Im Neuenheimer Feld 400
D69120 Heidelberg
Germany

Graeme J. Hankey, MD, FRCP, FRACP
Clinical Professor
Department of Medicine
The University of Western Australia
Hackett Drive, Nedlands;
Consultant Neurologist
Stroke Unit
Royal Perth Hospital
197 Wellington Street
Perth 6001
Australia

Robert G. Hart, MD
Professor
Department of Medicine/Neurology
University of Texas Health Science Center
7703 Floyd Curl Drive
San Antonio, Texas 78229-3900
U.S.A.

Robert D. Henderson, FRACP
Senior Lecturer
Department of Medicine
University of Queensland;
Staff Specialist
Department of Neurology
Royal Brisbane Hospital
Herston Road
Brisbane, Queensland 4029
Australia

Stefan Hesse, MD
Department of Neurological Rehabilitation
Free University Berlin;
Consultant
Department of Neurological Rehabilitation
Klinik Berlin
223 Kladower Damm
14089 Berlin
Germany

Lorenz Hirt, MD
Department of Neurology
Centre Hospitalier Universitaire Vaudois
Lausanne
Switzerland

Neville Hogan, PhD
Professor
Mechanical Engineering Department
Massachusetts Institute of Technology
77 Massachusetts Avenue
Cambridge, Massachusetts 02139
U.S.A.

Domenico Inzitari, MD
Full Professor
Department of Neurological and Psychiatric
Sciences
University of Florence;
Chief,
Department of Neurology
Careggi University Hospital
Viale Morgagni, 85
I-50134 Florence
Italy

Reza Jahan, MD
Assistant Professor
Division of Interventional Neuroradiology
UCLA School of Medicine
CHS Room B2-188
10833 LeConte Avenue
Los Angeles, California 90095-1721
U.S.A.

Saran Jonas, MD
Department of Neurology
New York University Medical Center
550 1st Avenue
New York, New York 10016
U.S.A.

Suh-Hang Hank Juo, MD, PhD
Assistant Professor
Head of Genetic Epidemiology/Pharmacogenetics
Genome Center; Department of Epidemiology
Columbia University
1150 St. Nicholas Avenue
New York, New York 10032
U.S.A.

Nadia Kahn, MD
Department of Neurosurgery
University Hospital Zürich
Frauenklinikstrasse 10
8091 Zürich
Switzerland

L.J. Kappelle, MD
Department of Neurology
University Medical Center Utrecht and the Rudolf
Magnus Institute for Neurosciences
C03.228
University Medical Center Utrecht
PO Box 85500
3508 GA Utrecht
The Netherlands

Markku Kaste, MD, PhD
Professor
Department of Neurology
University of Helsinki;
Chairman
Department of Neurology
Helsinki University Central Hospital
Haartmaninkatu 4
FIN-00029 HUS Helsinki
Finland

Syed Ahmed Abdul Khader, MD
Instructor in Clinical Neurology
Department of Neurology
Division of Physical Medicine and Rehabilitation
Washington University School of Medicine
4444 Forest Park Avenue;
Chief Resident
Department of Neurology
Division of Physical Medicine and Rehabilitation
Barnes-Jewish Hospital
One Barnes-Jewish Hospital Plaza
St. Louis, Missouri 63110
U.S.A.

Catharina J.M. Klijn, MD
Neurologist
Department of Neurology
University Medical Center Utrecht
3508 GA Utrecht
The Netherlands

Hermano Igo Krebs, PhD
Principal Research Scientist and Lecturer
Mechanical Engineering Department
Massachusetts Institute of Technology
77 Massachusetts Avenue
Cambridge, Massachusetts 02139;
Adjunct Assistant Research Professor
Burke Medical Research Institute
Weill Medical College of Cornell University
785 Mamaroneck Avenue
White Plains, New York 10605
U.S.A.

Maria Lamassa, MD, PhD
Assistant
Department of Neurological and Psychiatric
  Sciences
University of Florence;
Assistant
Department of Neurology
Careggi University Hospital
Viale Morgagni 85
I-50134 Florence
Italy

Donald H. Lee, MB, BCh, FRCPC
Professor
Department of Radiology and Nuclear Medicine
University of Western Ontario
Faculty of Medicine;
Staff Neuroradiologist
Department of Neurology
London Health Sciences Centre, University Campus
339 Windermere Road
London, Ontario N6A 5A5
Canada

Gian Luigi Lenzi, MD, PhD
Full Professor
Department of Neurological Sciences
University of Roma "La Sapienza"
Viale dell'Università 30;
Chief
Fifth Chair of Neurology
Policlinico Umberto I
Viale Del Policlinico 155
00185 Rome
Italy

Henry Ma, MD
National Stroke Research Institute
Austin & Repatriation Medical Centre
Heidelberg West, Victoria 3081
Australia

Jean-Louis Mas, MD
Professor
Department of Neurology
Paris V University
24 rue du Faubourg St. Jacques;
Chief
Department of Neurology
Sainte-Anne Hospital
1 rue Cabanis
75674 Paris Cedex 14
France

Heather Meldrum, BA
The John P. Robarts Research Institute
100 Perth Drive
London, Ontario N6A 5K8
Canada

Reto Meuli, MD, PhD
Associate Professor
Department of Radiology
Centre Hospitalier Universitaire Vaudois
1011 Lausanne
Switzerland

J.P. Mohr, MS, MD
Director Doris & Stanley Tananbaum Stroke Center
New York Presbyterian;
Sciarra Professor of Clinical Neurology
Department of Neurology
College of Physicians & Surgeons
Columbia University
710 West 168th Street
New York, New York 10032
U.S.A.

John W. Norris, MD
Professor of Neurology
University of Toronto
Sunnybrook Hospital
2075 Bayview Avenue
Toronto, Ontario M4N 3M5
Canada

Aleksandra M. Pavlović, MD, MSc
Specialist in Neurology
Department of Cerebrovascular Diseases
Institute of Neurology
Dr. Subotica 6
Belgrade, Serbia 11000
Yugoslavia

David M. Pelz, MD, FRCPC
Associate Professor
Departments of Diagnostic Radiology and Clinical
  Neurological Sciences
The University of Western Ontario;
Director, Neuroradiology
Department of Diagnostic Radiology
London Health Sciences Centre, University Campus
339 Windermere Road
London, Ontario N6A 5A5
Canada

Fabienne Perren, MD
University of Heidelberg
Neurology Clinic of Mannheim
Theodor-Kutzer-Ufer 1–3
D-68167 Mannheim
Germany

Allan H. Ropper, MD
Department of Neurology
St. Elizabeth's Medical Center,
Tufts University School of Medicine,
736 Cambridge Street
Boston, Massachusetts 02135
U.S.A.

Ralph L. Sacco, MS, MD
Profesor
Department of Neurology and Public Health
(Epidemiology)
Columbia University;
Attending Physician
Department of Neurology
New York Presbyterian Hospital
Neurological Institute
710 West 168th Street
New York, New York 10032
U.S.A.

Stephen D. Samples, MD
Associate Staff
Department of Neurology
Cleveland Clinic Foundation
9500 Euclid Avenue
Cleveland Ohio 44195
U.S.A.

Peter Sandercock, BM, BCh, DM
Professor of Medical Neurology
Department of Clinical Neurosciences
University of Edinburgh;
Honorary Consultant Neurologist
Department of Clinical Neurosciences
Western General Hospital
Crewe Road
Edinburgh EH4 2XU
United Kingdom

Stefan Schwarz, MD
Department of Neurology
University of Heidelberg
Im Neuenheimer Feld 400
69120 Heidelberg
Germany

Juhani Sivenius, MD, PhD
Professor
Department of Neurology
University of Kuopio;
Assistant Chief Physician
Department of Neurology
Kuopio University Hospital
70210 Kuopio
Finland

J. David Spence, MD
Professor
Department of Clinical Neurological Sciences
University of Western Ontario;
Director, Stroke Prevention and Atherosclerosis
Research Centre
Robarts Research Institute
1400 Western Road
London, Ontario N6G 2V2
Canada

Jan Stam, MD, PhD
Professor
Department of Neurology
University of Amsterdam;
Department of Neurology
Academic Medical Centre
1100 DE Amsterdam
The Netherlands

D.J. Thomas, MA, M.D., FRCP
Senior Lecturer
Department of Clinical Neurology
Institute of Neurology
Queen Square;
Senior Consultant Neurologist
Neurosciences Department
St. Mary's Hospital
Praed Street
London W2 1NY
United Kingdom

Thomas Truelsen, MD, PhD
Epidemiologist
Noncommunicable Diseases and Mental Health
The World Health Organization
Avenue Appia 20
1121 Geneva 27
Switzerland

J. van Gijn, MD
Professor and Chairman
Department of Neurology
University Medical Center
Heidelberglaan 100
3504 CX Utrecht
The Netherlands

Harry V. Vinters, MD, FRCP(C), FCAP
Professor
Departments of Pathology, Laboratory Medicine,
and Neurology
University of California, Los Angeles;
Chief of Neuropathology
Department of Pathology and Laboratory Medicine
UCLA Medical Center
10833 Le Conte Avenue
Los Angeles, California 90095
U.S.A.

Fernando Vinuela, MD
Department of Radiological Sciences
UCLA School of Medicine
Box 951721
Los Angeles, California 90095-1721
U.S.A.

Bruce T. Volpe, MD
Professor
Department of Neurology and Neuroscience
Weill Medical College of Cornell University;
The Burke Medical Research Institute
785 Mamaroneck Avenue
White Plains, New York 10605
U.S.A.

Cordula Werner, MD
Junior Researcher
Department of Neurological Rehabilitation
Free University Berlin and Klinik Berlin
Kladower Damm 223
14089 Berlin
Germany

Max Wintermark, MD
Department of Diagnostic and Interventional
  Radiology
University Hospital (CHUV)
1011 Lausanne
Switzerland

Philip A. Wolf, MD
Professor
Department of Neurology
Boston University School of Medicine
715 Albany Street
Boston, Massachusetts 02118
U.S.A.

Yasuhiro Yonekawa, MD
Professor
Department of Neurosurgery
University of Zürich;
Director
Department of Neurosurgery
University Hospital Zürich
Frauenklinikstrasse 10
CH-8091 Zürich
Switzerland

Foreword

It has been ten years since *Advances in Neurology* issued a volume on cerebrovascular disease of any kind.[a] During this decade, there has been an explosion of new, clinically relevant information about stroke and its prevention. This volume on ischemic stroke provides a comprehensive and timely review of prevention and treatment of ischemic cerebrovascular disease. Drs. Barnett and Bogousslavsky are leading clinicians and researchers in North America and Europe, respectively, and have assembled an outstanding group of their colleagues to contribute to this book.

Thirteen sections and 53 chapters compose this book. The first twenty-eight chapters focus on new information about the diagnosis and pathogenesis of stroke. The chapters on epidemiology highlight new insights into the causes of stroke, particularly genetics. Explanations of the advantages and disadvantages of new diagnostic imaging techniques are clear and directly linked to clinical applications. Atherosclerosis and other less common causes of stroke are explored in depth, providing a sound scientific understanding of ischemic stroke for the second half of the book, which focuses on treatment advances. The authors of each chapter are leading researchers whose trials and studies have revolutionized the medical and surgical approach to stroke.

Twenty years ago, stroke management strategies had limited data to support their use. Today, treatments with proven, clinically important benefits are available for patients with stroke and threatened stroke. The result is a larger role for the stroke specialist who can now select among meaningful interventions proven to beneficially alter the course of disease.

While stroke clinicians have spearheaded important clinical trials and epidemiological studies, much is owed to the clinical trial methodologists and biostatisticians who have raised the level of clinical science and have helped to develop better protocols and to analyze and interpret trial results. In a larger sense, every patient is in a clinical trial. While the individual clinician focuses on finding the best treatment for an individual patient, randomized clinical trials provide the necessary framework for treatment decisions. Hypotheses tested prospectively in clinical trials and epidemiological studies have high credibility. Because clinical trials prove them wrong so often, management based on case series, registries, and retrospective exploratory analysis of secondary outcomes must be viewed skeptically. Instead of trying to piece together a patchwork of inference based on biased observations, stroke clinicians now have objective data. While it remains impossible (except in retrospect) to know exactly what an individual patient has to gain or lose from a particular treatment, almost every stroke patient can be considered in the framework of a group that has been evaluated in a randomized clinical trial. For instance, for an individual patient with recent transient ischemic attack, it is not possible to know whether there will be a surgical complication with endarterectomy or whether a stroke will occur if given medical treatment alone. However, the benefit and risks of management options have been defined in clinical trials, and choices can be made based on this invaluable knowledge.

The sections on treatment reflect extensive new information gained from clinical trials and large epidemiological studies in the past 10 years. Progress has been significant. Studies of antiplatelet and anticoagulant drugs and hypertension control have placed the prevention of stroke on a secure foundation that continues to grow and expand. Surgical strategies for stroke prevention offer significant benefits for carefully selected patients. We know treatment of acute stroke is possible, and expanding acute treatment options is crucial to minimizing the burden from stroke.

This is a fine book, summarizing the state of the art for a common and important disease. The challenge remains for clinicians to apply the advances described herein to the treatment of stroke patients. The results will be longer, healthier lives for many. What better way to show our gratitude for the researchers who struggled to advance knowledge and for the patients who volunteered to participate?

John R. Marler, MD
National Institute of Neurological Disorders and Stroke
Bethesda, Maryland

[a]Pullicino P, Caplan LR, Hommel M. *Cerebrovascular Disease. Advances in Neurology, Volume 62.* New York: Raven Press, 1993.

Preface

The 18th century philosopher and historian, David Hume (1711–1776), wrote a critical treatise on miracles. His advice to those who bespoke belief in miraculous phenomena was that "the onus of proof for the improbable rests with the claimant." This was an early call for evidence-based data that after two centuries has become a requirement in the realm of medical science. Evidence-based medicine applied to clinical decision-making has played a major role in the nascence and rapid growth of stroke neurology over the past five decades.

Scrupulous pathological studies of the blood supply to the brain correlated to the clinical pictures were published, especially those of Hultquist and Fisher. At the same time, early confirmatory studies done by vascular and cardiac imaging were appearing. The types and causes of stroke could now be identified. The Framingham study gave us risk profiles, methodologists and statisticians gave us the discipline of clinical trials, surgeons on World War II battlefields learned to operate on arteries, hematologists defined thrombogenesis more accurately, and pharmacologists identified antithrombotic agents. Pioneering imaging methods evolved to the point where the brain, heart, and blood vessels can be studied with awe-inspiring sophistication.

The explosion in stroke diagnosis, prevention, and treatment that resulted from the combined application of all of these advances has borne much fruit. The purpose of this latest volume in the prestigious series *Advances in Neurology* is to give an overview of many of these accomplishments. Collaboration between individuals scattered widely across most continents has been the hallmark of many of the studies that have kept this field active and productive. The editorship and authorship reflect the wide front on which these successful labors have been pursued.

The editors express sincere thanks to all of the authors who took time from active lives to ensure a credible collection of essays. All were selected for their special knowledge of and contributions to the topics appearing under their names. Special thanks and appreciation are due to Anne M. Sydor and Julia Seto of Lippincott Williams &Wilkins. They were a pleasure to work with.

H.J.M. Barnett, OC, MD
Julien Bogousslavsky, MD
Heather Meldrum, BA

Advances in Neurology

Volume 92

Ischemic Stroke: Advances in Neurology, Vol. 92. Edited by
H.J.M. Barnett, Julien Bogousslavsky, and Heather Meldrum.
Lippincott Williams & Wilkins, Philadelphia © 2003.

1

Advances in Ischemic Stroke Epidemiology

Thomas Truelsen and Ruth Bonita

Noncommunicable Diseases and Mental Health, The World Health Organization, Geneva, Switzerland

Stroke is the second leading cause of death world-wide. It accounts for approximately 9.5% of all deaths and is a leading cause of adult disability (1,2). Epidemiologic studies of ischemic stroke occurrence and its risk factors have been essential for understanding how the disease affects different populations and have provided insight into the causes of stroke.

Population studies have provided evidence leading to public health actions in many countries in order to reduce the number of people who develop a stroke and to reduce the sequela in those who already had an attack. During the past few decades, our epidemiologic knowledge about risk factors for stroke has expanded considerably. Studies have shown that stroke rates differ between and within populations. These results have provided evidence contributing to control of stroke occurrence and to management of stroke.

As with other medical sciences, constant development of the discipline of epidemiology is ongoing to meet the new demands for solid epidemiologic data. This chapter presents major advances in ischemic stroke epidemiology that have occurred within the last few decades and outlines challenges for the near future.

STROKE DEFINITION

The most common definition of stroke for epidemiologic studies is "rapidly developing clinical signs of focal (or global) disturbance of cerebral function, with symptoms lasting 24 hours or longer or leading to death, with no apparent cause other than of

vascular origin" (3). This definition by the World Health Organization (WHO) has been accepted for decades as the standard definition of a stroke and has proved to be a valuable tool that can be used regardless of access to diagnostic technologic equipment. Before the establishment of a standard stroke definition, there often was considerable variation among different epidemiologic studies on how stroke was defined (4). These variations hindered comparisons of rates and the interpretation of results of analyses of potential risk factors. A 1976 report comparing stroke statistics from 15 stroke centers in 10 countries established the WHO stroke definition. This clinical definition, which was based on the patient's symptoms and the lack of other known or suspected causes for the attack, has been widely used since then (5). Both ischemic and hemorrhagic strokes are included. Transient ischemic attack, which is defined as an episode lasting less than 24 hours, and patients with stroke symptoms caused by subdural hemorrhage, tumors, poisoning, or trauma are excluded. Consequently, epidemiologic studies using the WHO stroke definition may underestimate the total burden of cerebrovascular disease in the population.

A broad range of other diseases may cause stroke-like symptoms, for example, infections with syphilis, malaria, human immunodeficiency virus, or acquired immunodeficiency syndrome, which may be relatively common in developing countries (6). Despite these limitations, the WHO stroke definition remains the recommended definition for epidemiologic studies of stroke, as will be discussed further later.

STROKE MORTALITY

For decades, routine mortality statistics have provided basic epidemiologic information on rates and

---

Disclaimer: Authors alone are responsible for views expressed in signed articles, which are not necessarily those of the World Health Organization.

trends in stroke. The WHO mortality database has reliable data from 35 developed countries dating from the early 1950s. Routine mortality data currently are available for approximately 80 countries where death certificates are routinely issued, thereby covering one third of the world's population. Sample registration systems in rural and urban China also are available. Analyses based on international comparisons of mortality data have shown vast differences in stroke mortality rates and trends among populations.

In most established market economies in the Western world, stroke is the third leading cause of death after ischemic heart disease and all cancers (7). However, in several Asian countries mortality rates for stroke are higher than rates for ischemic heart disease. For example, in the People's Republic of China more than one million people die of stroke each year, which are approximately three times as many people who die of ischemic heart disease (8). The proportion of cardiovascular disease deaths related to stroke differs among regions, ranging from approximately 20% to 30% in the Americas, Europe, and the Eastern Mediterranean to more than 50% in the Western Pacific (Fig. 1-1).

Some of these findings might be explained by racial variations and different exposures to risk factors, but it is remarkable the degree to which stroke mortality rates differ even among countries with similar cultural characteristics (Fig. 1-2). Western industrialized countries, such as the United States, Canada, Australia, and New Zealand, have relatively low rates, whereas many Eastern European countries have high stroke mortality rates. Further, most Western industrialized countries have experienced a decline in stroke mortality rates since the 1960s, with an acceleration of the decline in the 1970s (9). In contrast, stroke mortality rates are increasing in several Eastern European countries with existing high stroke mortality rates (Fig. 1-3) (10). These trends suggest a widening gap between two groups of nations, namely those with low and declining stroke mortality rates and those with high and increasing mortality rates.

Despite the promising possibilities for using routine mortality data for stroke epidemiology, several limitations hamper their usefulness for detailed analyses. For example, diagnostic patterns change, and early studies suggested that the validity of mortality statistics was doubtful (4,11). Coding practices may differ among countries and over time. New diagnostic technologies change the likelihood that a patient will be correctly identified and classified. In addition, because the quality of data is unknown, routine mortality statistics are inadequate to distinguish with confidence between stroke due to ischemia and that due to hemorrhage. Another major problem is that changes in mortality rates may be the result of changes in rates of incidence, case fatality, or both. For public health policy, it is essential to understand the reason for changing mortality rates and, ideally, whether these changes are related to both ischemic and hemorrhagic stroke.

Despite these limitations, routine mortality statistics on stroke rates in different countries are an easy accessible source of data and provide an important overview of the burden of stroke.

THE "IDEAL" STROKE INCIDENCE STUDY

For a disease such as stroke in which the outcome ranges from complete recovery to death, incidence is a better indicator for the burden of the disease in the population than is mortality. The demand for incidence studies raised questions on how to establish stroke registration systems that ensured inclusion of all stroke patients, that is, those who died directly of the stroke, those who were hospitalized or admitted to some other health facility, and those who were not hospitalized. As with the development of a stroke definition, a common approach for incidence studies was established. In 1987, Malmgren et al. (12) compared stroke incidence studies from around the world using predefined criteria for an ideal stroke incidence study (Table 1-1). They found that only nine of 65 published stroke incidence studies met these criteria.

The paper was a benchmark in the development of stroke epidemiology, providing the basic components for stroke incidence studies. Many studies subsequently adhered to these criteria, contributing to an increase in high-quality, population-based stroke data. However, it is extremely costly to run "ideal" stroke studies, and even countries with a

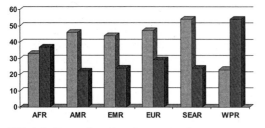

FIG. 1-1. Proportion of cardiovascular disease mortality due to ischemic heart disease and stroke.

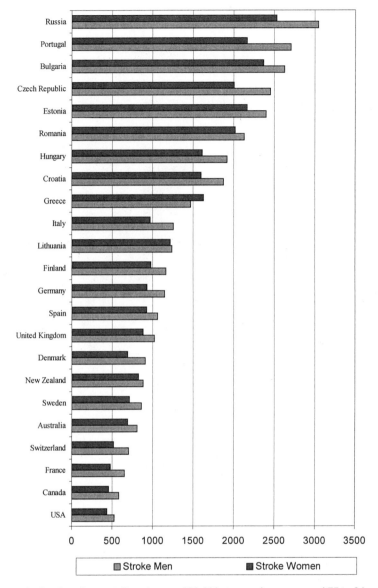

FIG. 1-2. Age-standardized stroke mortality rates per 100,000 men and women aged 75 to 84 years. (Data from Sarti C, Rastenyte D, Cepaitis Z, et al. *Stroke* 2000;31:1588–1601.)

long epidemiologic tradition have experienced difficulties providing stroke data that meet all the criteria listed. It is likely that countries with fewer resources will experience these problems and, as will be described later in this chapter, future stroke studies in developing countries may have to abandon at least some of these recommendations and develop new standards.

THE WHO MONICA PROJECT

The most comparable international stroke incidence data come from the WHO MONICA Project, which used standardized methods to monitor the trends and determinants of cardiovascular disease in 37 defined populations in 21 countries, all of which, except China, are developed countries (13). Strict

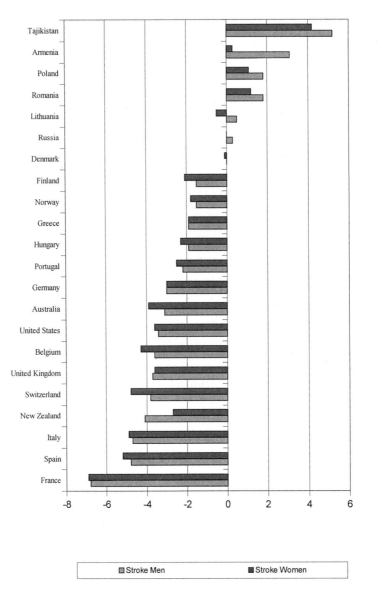

FIG. 1-3. Trends in stroke mortality rates per 100,000 men and women aged 75 to 84 years. (Data from Sarti C, Rastenyte D, Cepaitis Z, et al. *Stroke* 2000;31:1588–1601.)

definitions and tight control of the quality of data collection have permitted detailed analyses of trends over time and comparisons among the populations studied (14,15). As part of the MONICA Project, stroke incidence was monitored in 15 populations in 10 countries in the age group from 35 to 64 years (16). The highest stroke rates, which were found in Russia and Finland, were more than three-fold higher than the lowest rate, which was found in Friuli, Italy. In half the populations studied, the stroke incidence

was twice as high in men as in women (17). For many MONICA populations, good agreement exists between stroke mortality statistics and fatal cases in the stroke register, although this probably is a reflection of approximately equal numbers of "false-positive" and "false-negative" cases in the routine mortality statistics (18). Results of stroke case fatality also indicate large variations among different populations in the WHO MONICA Project, with higher proportions reported from Eastern European than Western

TABLE 1-1. *Criteria for the "ideal" stroke incidence study*

Standard diagnostic criteria
Complete cases ascertainment
Prospective design
First-ever strokes
Classification of pathologic type of stroke if possible
Rates given for all pathologic types of strokes
  combined
Well-defined denominator
Representative population
Large population
Rates calculated for similar periods
Cases collected for whole years
Standard presentation of rates by age, sex, and
  ethnicity

European countries. The reason for this remains uncertain, but it may be related to differences in the treatment of stroke complications and the severity of the events.

Many participating centers included subjects only up to age 65 years, and the remaining studies included subjects only up to age 75 years. These studies omitted the age groups in which the burden of stroke is greatest (16,19,20). However, the WHO MONICA Project has yielded substantial information about the burden of ischemic heart disease and stroke in the communities of the participating centers. Furthermore, the study has markedly increased the knowledge of how differently trends in stroke develop in various populations.

IMPROVED DIAGNOSTIC METHODS

During the late 1970s and 1980s, use of computed tomographic (CT) scanning became increasingly common, especially in the United States and Western European countries. The ability to classify stroke into hemorrhagic and ischemic types in epidemiologic research increased rapidly and promised to improve the understanding of the nature of stroke. Before that time, the distinction between ischemic and hemor-

rhagic stroke was restricted to patients who underwent lumbar puncture or surgical procedures or was made from autopsy reports. Score systems that used clinical signs to distinguish between hemorrhagic and ischemic strokes were developed (21,22), but validation studies showed that the systems lacked validity and could not be used in epidemiologic studies for classification of stroke types (23).

From neuroimaging studies, it became clear that in the patients who fulfilled the clinical stroke definition, approximately 80% of the strokes were due to ischemic infarction, 10% intracerebral hemorrhage, 5% subarachnoid hemorrhage, and 5% other reasons or unknown. These proportions have been reported from many Western countries, whereas a higher proportion of hemorrhages often has been reported in Asian populations. The ability to distinguish between types of stroke has been essential for showing that risk factors have different impacts on risk of hemorrhagic and ischemic stroke, as has been shown for example, for cholesterol (24,25) and alcohol (26–28).

Development and implementation of neuroimaging as a common diagnostic tool has been important for the treatment of stroke patients and the research on new therapies. For stroke epidemiology, it has allowed more detailed studies of the pathologic background for stroke. For example, the data from the Northern Sweden MONICA Study showed the rapid decrease in the late 1980s in the proportion of stroke events of the unknown type (Fig. 1-4). The decrease in the number of autopsies performed is concomitant with increased use of CT scanning (Fig. 1-5). The availability and sensitivity of imaging technology vary with place and time, and because up to one fourth of all stroke events are treated outside of health facilities, differentiation of stroke types has remained difficult.

Neuroimaging has broadened and added to stroke epidemiology, but it also has brought new problems in that it may have caused a shift in coding practices among physicians. An example is the United States, where the decline in stroke rates seems to have lev-

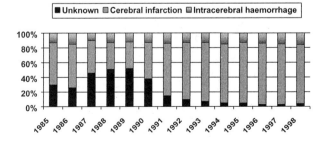

FIG. 1-4. Proportion of stroke subtype (first-ever stroke).

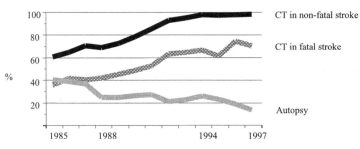

FIG. 1-5. Proportion of stroke events in subjects undergoing computed tomography scanning or autopsy. The Swedish Riks Stroke Study. (Data and figure courtesy of Dr. B. Stegmayr, Umeå, Sweden.)

eled out (29–31). The apparent leveling out in the trends has coincided with the introduction of neuroimaging, and it has been suggested that the findings may be explained in part by identification of a larger number of less severe strokes (29). In analyses of trends in case fatality, increased use of brain CT is likely to lead to increased sensitivity in finding patients with small intracerebral hemorrhages that otherwise would have been classified as ischemic stroke or stroke of undetermined type. Because intracerebral hemorrhages are associated with higher case fatality than ischemic stroke, better detection could account for the apparent decrease in case fatality for ischemic stroke over time (32).

Because of the restrictions in the use of neuroimaging for epidemiologic stroke research, abandoning the clinical definition of stroke for one based on imaging would create spurious variability and further complicate comparisons among studies. Thus, despite the technologic advances, the clinical diagnosis of stroke prevails as the most useful way to identify stroke patients in epidemiologic studies.

STROKE IN DEVELOPING COUNTRIES

Most of the epidemiologic studies on ischemic stroke were conducted in developed countries; however, the majority of the world's population lives in developing countries, where stroke already is a serious public health problem. In 1999 it was estimated that stroke was the cause of death in 5.54 million people worldwide, accounting for approximately 9.5% of all deaths. Two thirds of these deaths occurred in people living in developing countries (Fig. 1-6) (33).

Stroke is not only a lethal disease. Many survivors of stroke will have to adapt to a life with varying degrees of disability. The Global Burden of Disease Study constructed a measure that integrated the sum of life-years lost due to premature mortality and years lived with disability adjusted for severity, creating "disability-adjusted life-years" (DALYs) (1). In 1999 cerebrovascular disease accounted for 50 million DALYs worldwide, representing 3.5% of all DALYs (7). Projections to the year 2020 show that 61 million DALYs are likely to be lost due to cerebrovascular disease each year, with more than four fifths occurring in developing countries (1).

Epidemiologic studies on stroke in developing countries have shown that stroke already is a major health problem (6). In countries such as Taiwan, South Korea, and Singapore, stroke ranks as the second or third leading cause of death. Age-specific stroke mortality rates from population studies in Tanzania were similar or higher than those from England and Wales (34). Prevalence rates for stroke in developing countries were found to be much lower than

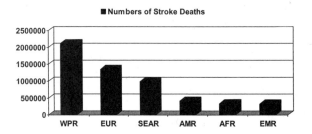

FIG. 1-6. Estimated number of stroke deaths by World Health Organization (WHO) regions in 1999. AFRO, African region; AMRO, American region; EMRO, Eastern Mediterranean region; EURO, European region; SEARO, South East Asian region; WPRO, Western Pacific region. (From World Health Organization. *The World Health Report 2000.* Geneva, Switzerland: World Health Organization, 2000.)

those reported from developed countries (35–37), but the lower prevalence may be explained by high case fatality rather than low incidence. This could be due to either more severe strokes or fewer resources for care of stroke patients, but the information required to interpret these patterns is lacking. Most developing countries have not established studies that allow them to quantify the burden of disease, including stroke (38). For example, the information on stroke occurrence from populous countries such as Thailand, The Philippines, and Indonesia are mainly hospital based. In many developing countries, such as those in South America, Africa, and Asia, the proportion of elderly people is increasing, and this likely will lead to a higher absolute number of stroke patients in the future. The scarcity of epidemiologic data in developing countries is a serious problem because it hampers efficient prevention programs and cost-effective treatment of stroke patients.

RISK FACTORS FOR ISCHEMIC STROKE

Identification and description of risk factors for ischemic stroke have been central in stroke epidemiology. Stroke prevention is of paramount importance given the lack of effective treatment in the acute phase, and application of information about modifiable risk factors is the only way to control the stroke burden.

Many risk factors for ischemic stroke have been described (39). They can be divided into modifiable and nonmodifiable risk factors, and some of the most important factors are listed in Table 1-2.

Increasing age, male gender, and Hispanic or Black ethnicity are associated with increased risk of stroke. Knowledge about the prevalence of nonmodifiable risk factors in a population will permit estimation of future needs for prevention and treatment but offers no possibility for intervention.

At a population level, blood pressure and tobacco use are the two most important modifiable risk factors for stroke because of their strong associations,

TABLE 1-2. *Risk factors for ischemic stroke*

Nonmodifiable	Modifiable
Increasing age	Blood pressure
Male gender	Tobacco use
Race/ethnicity	Diabetes
Family history	Obesity
	Physical inactivity
	Hyperlipidemia
	Atrial fibrillation

high prevalence, and possibility for intervention. Epidemiologic research has shown that increased blood pressure is the single most important risk factor for ischemic stroke, with a population attributable risk of 50% (40). The risk of stroke rises steadily as blood pressure level rises and increases 46% for every 7.5 mm Hg increment in diastolic blood pressure (DBP), with no lower threshold. Treatment with antihypertensive drugs has shown that a DBP reduction of 6 mm Hg is associated with a reduction in stroke incidence of 42% (41). Treatment of isolated hypertension, often seen in elderly people, is associated with a beneficial effect, as shown in the Systolic Hypertension in the Elderly Program (SHEP) in which treatment of isolated systolic hypertension in an elderly population decreased the risk of stroke by 36% (42). Based on these findings, it was expected that stroke occurrence rates would decrease markedly with increasing treatment of hypertensive subjects. However, estimations based on clinical trials and epidemiologic studies have indicated that only between 16% and 25% of the decline in stroke mortality in the United States could be explained by improved treatment of subjects with hypertension (43).

Nevertheless, control of blood pressure remains pivotal in the prevention of stroke. Considering the strong epidemiologic evidence for the potential benefit of controlling blood pressure in the population, it is surprising how much remains to be achieved. Results from the Rotterdam Study, The Netherlands (hypertension defined as DBP ≥95 mmHg and/or systolic blood pressure ≥160 mmHg and/or use of antihypertensive drugs for hypertension) indicated that at the community level among hypertensive subjects aged 20 years or older, only 37% were treated and had a controlled blood pressure, 20% were treated but uncontrolled, and 43% were untreated (44). In the United States, where treatment is more aggressive, results from the third National Health and Nutrition Examination Survey in the United States showed that among stroke and myocardial infarction survivors, the prevalence of uncontrolled hypertension (defined as blood pressure >140/90 mmHg) was 53% among persons with known hypertension, whereas previously undiagnosed hypertension was detected in 11% others (45). The results from these two countries are likely to be of similar magnitude to the rates in other developed countries and indicate the limitations of the high-risk approach to management of increased blood pressure.

Tobacco use increases the risk of ischemic stroke about two-fold (46). There is a dose–response relationship such that heavy smokers are at higher risk for stroke than light smokers. Until recently, studies of tobacco use and stroke focused on the risk to smokers; however, exposure to environmental tobacco smoking also is an independent risk factor for stroke (47). This study suggested that previous analyses based on reference groups that did not differentiate from exposure to nonsmokers might have led to a general underestimation of the risk of stroke in smokers. Smoking cessation in different populations has been shown to lead to a reduction in stroke risk within 2 to 4 years (48,49). The deleterious effects of hypertension and tobacco use have been known for decades, but they still are common risk factors in many populations. Thus, although the epidemiologic research in risk factors for ischemic stroke has produced many results that could prevent stroke occurrence, a major problem may be related to bridging the gap between researchers and public health policy programs.

Most studies of risk factors for ischemic stroke are based on data from populations in developed countries, but there is some evidence from developing countries that many of the risk factors are similar, including high blood pressure, tobacco use, and obesity (50–53). There are an estimated 1.2 billion smokers worldwide, 800 million of whom live in developing countries. In China alone, there are 300 million smokers. A review on obesity in Latin-American countries showed that the prevalence of being overweight, especially in urban areas, may be as high as the prevalence reported in developed nations (54). The concurrent increase in diabetes, which is a major risk factor for stroke, is a worrisome trend. The present knowledge on the prevalence of major risk factors in developing countries is limited and more information is required. If ignored, these countries are

likely to experience an increasing burden of noncommunicable diseases in the near future.

STROKE PREVENTION

Many of the major risk factors are amenable to prevention. The two main preventive strategies are the "high-risk" strategy and the population approach for prevention (Fig. 1-7).

The aim of the high-risk strategy is to identify individuals with markedly elevated risk factors who are at the highest absolute risk of disease. Clinical physicians typically are trained in this method, and the identified individuals are targeted by interventions that aim to reduce the overall risk. If successful, the benefits to the patients can be extensive; however, because the number of persons in this high-risk category is proportionately much smaller than those in the moderate-risk group, the overall benefits to society may be limited in terms of death or disability prevented. The strategy reduces, but does not necessarily minimize, the risk for the individuals concerned. Although a decrease of blood pressure from 160/95 to 150/90 reduces the risk of a stroke, even this attained value poses a greater risk than a lower level of blood pressure. In addition, this strategy, as was shown for hypertension, often is difficult to sustain.

The aim of the population strategy is to reduce the risk factor levels in the population as a whole through community legislative action. Because there is a continuum of risk associated with most risk factors, small widespread changes will result in a large benefit across a wide range of risk. Although individual benefits are relatively small, the cumulative societal benefits are large, the so-called *prevention paradox* (55). Blood pressure provides a good example because it is a key determinant of stroke risk in both developed and devel-

High Risk Approach

Population Approach

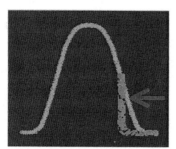 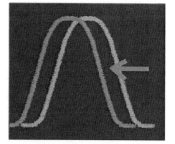

FIG. 1-7. Prevention strategies. High-risk prevention targets individuals with the highest absolute risk of disease. The aim of the population approach for prevention is to reduce the risk factor level in the population as a whole.

oping countries. The Eastern Stroke and Coronary Heart Disease Collaborative Study Group, which analyzed data from 125,000 participants in 18 cohort studies from China and Japan, indicates that population-wide lowering of blood pressure has the potential to produce enormous declines in stroke in Eastern Asia (25). The study demonstrated that a small reduction in average usual DBP (by about 3 mm Hg) averts about one third of all strokes. In the People's Republic of China alone this would result in about 370,000 fewer stroke deaths each year, with most of these averted events occurring in people who were not considered hypertensive. Projections to the year 2020 indicate that a population-wide 2% reduction in DBP in Asian countries would provide a 10% reduction in stroke and coronary heart disease (CHD) deaths (51). If the target group is restricted only to people with an initial DBP ≥95 mmHg, similar reductions in stroke and CHD deaths require an almost 7% decrease in DBP.

The population-based, risk exposure reduction approach is particularly relevant in developing countries, where it is necessary to ensure that communities currently at low risk are protected from acquiring risk factors (sometimes referred to as *primordial prevention*). This is true for adults in rural regions of most developing countries, as well as for children in all populations. Population-wide changes that lower blood pressure, such as decreasing salt intake (56–58), increasing potassium intake (59), more exercise, less obesity (60), and antitobacco legislation, all have the potential to produce large benefits. This approach is eminently applicable to moderate-risk groups in urban areas, where risk modification will help prevent the need for drug therapy with its attendant economic and biologic costs.

STROKE SURVEILLANCE

Studies on stroke occurrence and their risk factors may be conducted either together or separately and the results published as they are generated. This has ensured a rapid contribution to advances in ischemic stroke epidemiology. Sporadic studies providing data at one or a few time periods are of limited value. The aim instead should be to set up stroke surveillance systems. Surveillance refers to the ongoing systematic collection, analysis, interpretation, and dissemination of health information. The primary purpose of establishing and maintaining a system of stroke surveillance is to provide health workers and policy makers with a reliable tool to plan cost-effective strategies to meet the demands for health care and prevention in the population. Surveillance, in general, should be focused on diseases that are, or are likely to become, public health problems (61). Surveillance programs are more likely to be sustained if they address diseases for which effective control or prevention measures are available. Stroke meets many of the criteria for surveillance: it is a major public health problem, it is largely preventable, and it is a disease that has a major impact in all countries. Further, because of its clinical definition, stroke surveillance may be feasible in developing as well as developed countries.

A surveillance system should include not only a capacity for collection and analysis of data and dissemination of information, but also direct links to public health programs, which may improve the likelihood that the results will be used more quickly for prevention. An example where this has been done successfully is California, where knowledge of the adverse effects of tobacco smoking has been backed by public campaigns against tobacco and has been associated with decreasing mortality rates of lung cancer (62).

The WHO currently is developing a stepwise approach to stroke surveillance, the WHO STEPwise approach to Surveillance of stroke (STEPS-Stroke) (Fig. 1-8), which offers a framework for unifying stroke surveillance efforts (63). This strategy encour-

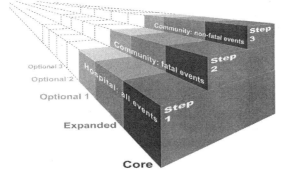

FIG. 1-8. The World Health Organization (WHO) STEPwise approach to stroke surveillance.

ages collection of epidemiologic data on stroke for hospitalized events, fatal events, and nonfatal nonhospitalized events in a population using a stepwise approach. The first level (step 1) includes stroke patients admitted to health facilities. It is a starting point for more sophisticated data collection enabling the education and development of a local team for stroke research. Data from the first level will provide information on how treatment and secondary prevention of stroke patients is managed while in the hospital. It is a selected group of stroke patients, however, and will not be able to produce reliable data on the total stroke occurrence within the population. It is therefore encouraged to advance to the next level, step 2, as soon as resources and capacity are mobilized. Step 2 includes collection of data on fatal stroke events occurring in the population outside of health facilities, which will enable estimation of mortality rates in the source population. To be able to provide incidence and case fatality estimates, step 3, in which nonfatal nonhospitalized stroke events are identified, is necessary.

The WHO STEPS-Stroke is designed to provide the best possible data on stroke, especially from countries with no or only little registration of disease occurrence, and builds on the WHO MONICA project. Better knowledge of the burden of stroke in the population is essential for improving treatment and prevention. However, it is recognized that knowledge about the burden of stroke today says little about future burden, which is related to the demographic composition of the population and the exposure to risk factors for stroke. The WHO STEPS-Stroke can be enhanced with a similar surveillance program for risk factors, the WHO STEPwise Approach to Surveillance of Risk Factors for Noncommunicable Diseases (available at httw://www.who.int/noncommunicable-diseases).

FUTURE OF ISCHEMIC STROKE EPIDEMIOLOGY

Recognition of the global burden of stroke raises new questions on how ischemic stroke epidemiology will continue to develop in the future. Most of the current knowledge is based on studies from developed countries, but more data and results are required from developing countries in order to improve global burden of disease estimates. Malmgren et al. (12) set the standards for incidence studies, and tight data control and validation studies were key components of the WHO MONICA study (13). However, it is unlikely that countries having fewer resources and still facing the double burden of both communicable and noncommunicable diseases will find the current epidemiologic tools sufficient to provide data. As a response, new approaches to conducting epidemiologic studies of ischemic stroke currently are being developed and tested.

Verbal autopsy is a relatively new epidemiologic tool that is being increasingly used to monitor the distribution of age- and gender-specific death rates in areas where medical certification of cause of death is uncommon. The procedure for verbal autopsy is to interview close relatives or caretakers of the deceased and to classify causes of death based on the interview. Until recently verbal autopsy was used predominantly to estimate childhood and maternal deaths, but the development of verbal autopsy questionnaires for adults is ongoing (64). A recent study of stroke mortality in Tanzania serves as an example of a study of adult death where the verbal autopsy methodology was used (34). Difficulties with the validity of verbal autopsy results between and within populations limit its ability to be generalized; however, it is a method that may become important and provide the best possible data from many countries.

The capture–recapture technique also may be developed to become a suitable approach for obtaining data on stroke occurrence (65). Although this technique is promising, only a few investigators have used the capture–recapture technique for stroke (66), and there remain uncertainties about the independence of data sources and correct identification of events (67). Furthermore, this approach assumes public provision of services. In many countries, health reforms have encouraged greater involvement of the private sector in the provision of care, and this makes finding routine cases difficult.

CONCLUSIONS

Epidemiologic studies of stroke have developed considerably during the past few decades. Our knowledge of the substantial differences in stroke rates and trends between populations has increased. Differences in the prevalence of exposure to major risk factors for stroke may largely explain these results. Reducing exposure to major risk factors for stroke, especially high blood pressure and tobacco use, are important tools for preventing an increase in the burden of stroke. Expansion of stroke epidemiology to developing countries is urgently needed and will require the development of new epidemiologic tools if population coverage is to be achieved. In addition, data on population levels of risk factors that predict the future burden of stroke are required.

Stroke is a major health problem in both developed and developing countries, and prevention is of paramount importance.

REFERENCES

1. Murray CJL, Lopez AD. *The global burden of disease,* 1st ed. Cambridge, MA: Harvard School of Public Health, 1996.
2. Murray CJL, Lopez AD. Mortality by cause for eight regions of the world: Global Burden of Disease Study. *Lancet* 1997;349:1269–1276.
3. WHO MONICA Project Investigators. The World Health Organization MONICA Project (monitoring trends and determinants in cardiovascular disease). *J Clin Epidemiol* 1988;41:105–114.
4. Du FC, Senter MG, Acheson RM. A study of the validity of the diagnosis of stroke in mortality data. II. Comparison by computer of autopsy and clinical records with death certificates. *Am J Epidemiol* 1969;89:1524.
5. Hatano S. Experience from a multicentre stroke register: a preliminary report. *Bull WHO* 1976;54:541–553.
6. Poungvarin N. Stroke in the developing world. *Lancet* 1998;352:(SIII)19–22.
7. World Health Organization. *The World Health Report 2000.* Geneva, Switzerland: World Health Organization, 2000.
8. World Health Organization. *World Health Statistics Annual, 1993.* Geneva, Switzerland: World Health Organization, 1993.
9. Bonita R, Alistair S, Beaglehole R. International trends in stroke mortality: 1970–1985. *Stroke* 1990;21:898–992.
10. Sarti C, Rastenyte D, Cepaitis Z, et al. International trends in mortality from stroke, 1968 to 1994. *Stroke* 2000;31:1588–1601.
11. Kuller L, Seltser R. Cerebrovascular disease mortality in Maryland. *Am J Epidemiol* 1967;86:442–450.
12. Malmgren R, Warlow C, Bamford J, et al. Geographical and secular trends in stroke incidence. *Lancet* 1987;2 (8569):1196–1200.
13. Tunstall-Pedoe H, Kuulasmaa K, Amouyel P, et al. Myocardial infarction and coronary deaths in the World Health Organization MONICA Project. *Circulation* 1994;90:583–612.
14. Tunstall-Pedoe H, Vanuzzo D, Hobbs M, et al. Estimation of contribution of changes in coronary care to improving survival, event rates, and coronary heart disease mortality across the WHO MONICA project populations. *Lancet* 2000;355:688–700.
15. Tunstall-Pedoe H, Kuulasmaa K, Mahonen M, et al. Contribution of trends in survival and coronary-event rates to changes in coronary heart disease mortality: 10-year results from 37 WHO MONICA Project populations. Monitoring trends and determinants in cardiovascular disease. *Lancet* 1999;353:1547–1557.
16. Thorvaldsen P, Asplund K, Kuulasmaa K, et al. Stroke incidence, case fatality, and mortality in the WHO MONICA project. *Stroke* 1995;26:361–367.
17. Stegmayr B, Asplund K, Kuulasmaa K, et al. Stroke incidence and mortality correlated to stroke risk factors in the WHO MONICA project. *Stroke* 1997;28:1367–1374.
18. Asplund K, Bonita R, Kuulasmaa K, et al. Multinational comparisons of stroke epidemiology. Evaluation of case ascertainment in the WHO MONICA Stroke Study. World Health Organization Monitoring Trends and Determinants in Cardiovascular Disease. *Stroke* 1995; 26:355–360.
19. Thorvaldsen P, Kuulasmaa K, Rajakangas A, et al. Stroke trends in the WHO MONICA project. *Stroke* 1997;28:500–506.
20. Asplund K, Bonita R, Kuulasmaa K, et al. Multinational comparisons of stroke epidemiology. *Stroke* 1995;26: 355–360.
21. Allen CMC. Clinical diagnosis of the acute stroke syndrome. *Q J Med* 1983;42:515–523.
22. Poungvarin N, Viriyavejakul A, Komontri C. Siriraj stroke score and validation study to distinguish supratentorial intracerebral hemorrhage from infarction. *Br Med J* 1991;302:1565–1567.
23. Hawkins GC, Bonita R, Broad JB, et al. Inadequacy of clinical scoring systems to differentiate stroke subtypes in population-based studies. *Stroke* 1995;26:1338–1342.
24. Prospective Studies Collaboration. Cholesterol, diastolic blood pressure, and stroke. 13,000 strokes in 450,000 people in 45 prospective cohorts. *Lancet* 1995; 346:1647–1653.
25. Eastern Stroke and Coronary Heart Disease Collaborative Group. Blood pressure, cholesterol, and stroke in eastern Asia. *Lancet* 1998;352:1801–1807.
26. Truelsen T, Gronbaek M, Schnohr P, et al. Intake of beer, wine, and spirits and risk of stroke: the Copenhagen City Heart Study. *Stroke* 1998;29:2467–2472.
27. Thrift AG, Donnan GA, McNeil JJ. Epidemiology of intracerebral hemorrhage. *Epidemiol Rev* 1995;17: 361–381.
28. Stampfer MJ, Coldtiz GA, Willett WC, et al. A prospective study of moderate alcohol consumption and the risk of coronary disease and stroke in women. *N Engl J Med* 1988;319:267–273.
29. Broderick JP, Phillips SJ, Whisnant JP, et al. Incidence rates of stroke in the eighties: the end of the decline in stroke? *Stroke* 1989;20:577–582.
30. Cooper R, Cutler J, Desvigne-Nickens P, et al. Trends and disparities in coronary heart disease, stroke, and other cardiovascular diseases in the United States: findings of the National Conference on Cardiovascular Disease Prevention. *Circulation* 2000;102:3137–3147.
31. Gillum RF, Sempos CT. The end of the long-term decline in stroke mortality in the United States? *Stroke* 1997;28:1527–1529.
32. van Straten AF, Reitsma JF, Limburg MF, et al. Impact of stroke type on survival and functional health. *Cerebrovasc Dis* 2001;12:27–33.
33. World Health Organization. *The World Health Report 1998.* Geneva, Switzerland: World Health Organization, 1998.
34. Walker RW, McLarty DG, Kitange HM, et al. Stroke mortality in urban and rural Tanzania. *Lancet* 2000;355: 1684–1687.
35. Bonita R, Solomon N, Broad JB. Prevalence of stroke and stroke-related disability. Estimates from the Auckland stroke studies. *Stroke* 1997;28:1898–1902.
36. Nicoletti A, Sofia V, Giuffrida S, et al. Prevalence of stroke. A door-to-door survey in rural Bolivia. *Stroke* 2000;31:882–885.

37. Abraham J, Rao PSS, Inbara SG, et al. An epidemiological study of hemiplegia due to stroke in South India. *Stroke* 1970;1:477–481.
38. Asian Acute Stroke Advisory Panel. Stroke epidemiological data of nine Asian countries. *J Med Assoc Thai* 2000;83:1–7.
39. Goldstein LB, Adams R, Becker K, et al. Primary prevention of ischemic stroke: a statement for healthcare professionals from the Stroke Council of the American Heart Association. *Stroke* 2001;32:280–299.
40. Dunbabin DW, Sandercock P. Preventing stroke by the modification of risk factors. *Stroke* 1990;21[Suppl IV]:36–39.
41. Collins R, Peto R, MacMahon S, et al. Blood pressure, stroke, and coronary heart disease. Part 2: Short-term reduction in blood pressure: overview of randomised drug trials in their epidemiological context. *Lancet* 1990;335(863):827–838.
42. SHEP Cooperative Research Group. Prevention of stroke by antihypertensive drug treatment in older persons with isolated systolic hypertension: final results of the Systolic Hypertension in the Elderly Program (SHEP). *JAMA* 1991;265:3255–3264.
43. Bonita R, Beaglehole R. Increased treatment of hypertension does not explain the decline in stroke mortality in the United States, 1970–1980. *Hypertension* 1989;13(5 suppl):169–173.
44. Klungel OH, Stricker BHC, Paes AHP, et al. Excess stroke among hypertensive men and women attributable to undertreatment of hypertension. *Stroke* 1999;30:1312–1318.
45. Qureshi AI, Suri FK, Guterman LR, Hopkins LN. Ineffective secondary prevention in survivors of cardiovascular events in the US population. *Arch Intern Med* 2001;161:1621–1628.
46. Shinton R, Beevers G. Meta-analysis of relation between cigarette smoking and stroke. *BMJ* 1989;298:789–795.
47. Bonita R, Jackson RT, Truelsen T, et al. Passive smoking, active smoking, and the risk of stroke. *Tobacco Control* 1999;19:117–125.
48. Wolf PA, D'Agostino RB, Kannel WB, et al. Cigarette smoking as a risk factor for stroke. *JAMA* 1988;259:1025–1029.
49. Kawachi I, Colditz GA, Stampfer MJ, et al. Smoking cessation and decreased risk of stroke in women. *JAMA* 1993;269:232–236.
50. Cooper RS, Rotimi CN, Kaufman JS, et al. Hypertension treatment and control in sub-Saharan Africa: the epidemiological basis for policy. *BMJ* 1998;316:614–617.
51. Singh RB, Suh IL, Singh VP, et al. Hypertension and stroke in Asia: prevalence, control and strategies in developing countries for prevention. *J Hum Hypertens* 2000;14:749–763.
52. Abebe M, Haimanot RT. Cerebrovascular accidents in Ethiopia. *Ethiop Med J* 1990;28:53–61.
53. Yang G, Fan L, Tan J, et al. Smoking in China: findings of the 1996 National Prevalence Survey. *JAMA* 1999;282:1247–1253.
54. Filozof C, Gonzalez C, Sereday M, et al. Obesity prevalence and trends in Latin American countries. *Obes Rev* 2001;2:99–106.
55. Rose G. Strategy of prevention: lessons from cardiovascular disease. *BMJ* 1981;282:1847–1851.
56. Elliott P, Stamler J, Nichols R, et al. Intersalt revisited: further analyses of 24 hour sodium excretion and blood pressure within and across populations. *BMJ* 1996;312:1249–1253.
57. Hooper L, Bartlett C, Smith GD, Ebrahim S. Systematic review of long term effects of advice to reduce dietary salt in adults. *BMJ* 2002;325:628–636.
58. Cutler JA. The effects of reducing sodium and increasing potassium intake for control of hypertension and improving health. *Clin Exp Hypertens* 1999;21:769–783.
59. Whelton PK, He J, Cutler JA, et al. Effects of oral potassium on blood pressure: meta-analysis of randomized controlled clinical trials. *JAMA* 1997;277:1624–1632.
60. Whelton PK, He J, Appel LJ, et al. Primary prevention of hypertension. *JAMA* 2002;288:1882–1888.
61. Berkelman RL, Buehler JW. Surveillance. In: Holland WW, Detels R, Knox G, eds. *Oxford textbook of public health,* 2nd ed. Oxford: Oxford University Press, 1990:161–175.
62. MMWR. Declines in lung cancer rates—California, 1988–1997. *MMWR* 2000;December 1:1066–1069.
63. Truelsen T, Bonita R, Jamrozik K. Surveillance of stroke: a global perspective. *Int J Epidemiol* 2001;30[Suppl 1]:S11–S16.
64. Chandramohan D, Maude GH, Rodrigues LC, et al. Verbal autopsies for adult deaths: their development and validation in a multicentre study. *Trop Med Int Health* 1998;3:436–446.
65. Hook EB, Regal RR. Capture-recapture methods in epidemiology: methods and limitations. *Epidemiol Rev* 1995;17:243–264.
66. Tilling K, Sterne JAC, Wolfe CDA. Estimation of the incidence of stroke using a capture-recapture model including covariates. *Int J Epidemiol* 2001;30:1351–1359.
67. Taub NA, Lemic-Stojcevic N, Wolfe CDA. Capture-recapture methods for precise measurement of the incidence and prevalence of stroke. *J Neurol Neurosurg Psychiatry* 1996;60:696–697.

Ischemic Stroke: Advances in Neurology, Vol. 92. Edited by
H.J.M. Barnett, Julien Bogousslavsky, and Heather Meldrum.
Lippincott Williams & Wilkins, Philadelphia © 2003.

2

Genetic and Molecular Epidemiologic Methods for Stroke

*Suh-Hang Hank Juo and †Ralph L. Sacco

*Genome Center, Columbia University, New York, New York, U.S.A.; †Department of Neurology and
Public Health (Epidemiology), Columbia University and Department of Neurology, New York
Presbyterian Hospital, Neurological Institute, New York, New York, U.S.A.*

Stroke is a complex disease probably related to multiple genetic loci, environmental factors, and gene–environment interactions. Several stroke risk factors, including a family history of stroke, have been identified, although the estimated genetic component of stroke is not well elucidated (1). Genetic factors, however, have been well demonstrated as determinants of several stroke risk factors, such as hypertension, diabetes, hyperlipidemia, and coagulation abnormalities. Presumably, part of the familial aggregation of stroke can be attributed to these known risk factors with well-recognized genetic components.

Although epidemiologic principles help guide the design of genetic stroke studies, there are some important differences that make this area of research more specialized. Terminologies differ, study designs are more complicated, and statistical techniques are more complex. An understanding of genome structure and techniques also is essential. In this chapter, we discuss some of these issues and highlight some of the newer techniques that have led to the development of a whole new field of molecular/genetic epidemiology.

STUDY DESIGNS TO EXPLORE FOR A GENETIC COMPONENT

Familial aggregation is classically viewed as evidence suggesting a possible genetic component in the phenotype of interest; however, familial aggregation can be due to common environmental factors, genetic components, or both. The first step of any genetic study is to estimate the genetic contribution to the phenotype of interest.

Classic case control and cohort studies can assess whether a family history of stroke is an independent risk factor, but they cannot distinguish shared environments from genetic predisposition. Various family study designs, including twin studies, familial correlations, recurrent risk estimation, and complex segregation analysis can be used to assess the importance and magnitude of a genetic effect. Twin studies compare monozygotic twin pairs who have 100% identical genetic component with dizygotic twin pairs who share 50% of the total genetic components. If monozygotic twins have significantly higher concordance in the phenotype of interest than dizygotic twins, the genetic component will be considered the major contributor determining the phenotype of interest. Although the concept of twin studies is straightforward, it is difficult to recruit twin samples.

Familial correlations use the pedigree data to assess the correlations of the phenotype between spouse pairs, sib pairs, and parent–offspring pairs. The correlation between spouse pairs provides the indication of shared environments, and correlations between other biologic relatives are the function of shared genetics and environments. The major weakness of this approach is that the correlation estimation can be biased if the families are not ascertained randomly. Readers can consult the FCOR program in the SAGE software *(http://darwin.cwru.edu/pub/sage. html)* for details.

For discrete traits, the recurrent risk or relative risk (λ) is commonly used by epidemiologists (2). Based on the biologic relationships, several kinds of λs can be calculated. The sibling relative risk (λ_s) is defined as the ratio of risk to individuals who have affected sibs to the population risk. Similarly the parental–offspring relative risk (λ_{po}) is defined as the ratio of risk to individuals who have affected parents to the population risk. The magnitude of λ indicates the degree of genetic component; however, when the population risk is low (~1%), λ can be substantially biased. For example, population risk of 1% or 2% will make λ different by two-fold.

Segregation analysis is statistically complicated. The basic concept is to compare a series of models under various assumptions using the likelihood statistics. The nested models are used to test whether the observed familial aggregation is mainly caused by a genetic or environmental mechanism. These nested models are compared with the full model, which allows all variables to be estimated. The most parsimonious nested model that fits the data as well as the full model is considered the best model to explain familial aggregation. Heritability and penetrance also can be derived from the best fitting model. Readers can consult Khoury et al. (3) for details.

Three parameters are commonly mentioned in the literature to indicate the magnitude of genetic effect: heritability (h^2) for quantitative traits (e.g., serum lipid level); recurrent risk (λ); and penetrance for dichotomized traits (e.g., diabetic or not). Heritability is defined as the ratio of the genetic variance to the total phenotypic variance; however, heritability also can be used for discrete traits. One needs to assume an unobserved continuous variable, liability, underlying the discrete phenotype. When liability crosses a particular threshold, an individual is affected. Several statistical programs are available to estimate heritability, such as SOLAR *(http://www.sfbr.org/sfbr/ public/software/solar)*, SAGE. Penetrance refers to the risk of having a disease for a person who carries a mutant disease gene. h^2 and λ often indicate the overall genetic effect; however, penetrance often is used to indicate a specific gene or mutation.

Readers need to keep in mind that the magnitude of the genetic component in any complex disease can vary in different populations and can be substantially influenced by the environments.

LINKAGE VERSUS ASSOCIATION STUDIES

Identifying a gene conferring susceptibility to a disease is a major task in the postgenome era. Two different approaches can be used in genetic epidemiologic studies: association and linkage studies. Association studies use traditional epidemiologic study designs: the case control, cohort, and cross-sectional studies. The main hypothesis is to test whether a particular allele (or a particular genotype) of a candidate gene is seen more often among those with the disease compared to controls. The more expensive cohort approach would test whether the risk of developing the disease is greater among those with the particular allele (or genotype) of a candidate gene compared to those without the allele or genotype. Association cross-sectional studies also can be done, such as comparing the mean of low-density lipoprotein (LDL) cholesterol levels among different genotypes of a candidate gene among all study participants. With all of these designs, it is difficult to determine if the candidate allele (or genotype) is the cause of the disease or may be in linkage disequilibrium (LD) (see Glossary) with the true, but unmeasured, disease causing allele.

Linkage studies use a different approach in terms of study subjects, study design, statistical analysis, and result interpretation. The hypothesis of linkage analysis is to see whether the phenotype of interest segregates along with a particular genetic markers in a family regardless of any common allele across all participating families. If so, the disease gene is located in the vicinity of the marker. In order to conduct a linkage study, researchers need to recruit families with multiple cases if the phenotype of interest is a discrete trait. If the phenotype is a continuous trait, then the recruitment can be relatively easier because every family member has phenotypic data for analysis. The design of family recruitment can be generally divided into two types: extended pedigrees and affected sib pair approach. Extended pedigrees provide better statistical power; however, they are more time consuming and costly for such a study design. In addition, the distant relatives may be less enthusiastic about participating in a study, so the data quality can be another concern. The affected sib pair approach, on the other hand, focuses on nuclear families where two or more affected sibs exist. Although it avoids the shortcoming of recruiting extended families, it has low statistical power.

Table 2-1 summarizes the key differences between association and linkage studies. Comparing these two different approaches, association studies are technically simple; however, they have a long track record of false-positive results. Linkage analysis followed by positional cloning, which relies on molecular mapping techniques to locate a gene at a specific region identified by linkage analysis, is extremely successful in mendelian diseases where there is one-to-one correspondence between genotypes and phenotypes, but

TABLE 2-1. *Comparison between linkage and association studies*

	Linkage	Association
Hypothesis	Phenotype is linked to a particular chromosomal region	Phenotype is associated with a particular allele of a candidate gene
Subjects	Family data	Unrelated individuals
Genotype	Anonymous markers or polymorphisms of candidate genes	Polymorphisms of candidate genes
Statistics	Likelihood-based or shared IBD-based approach	Regression-based approach
Result interpretation	Disease gene is located in the vicinity of the tested marker	Allele is related to the phenotype
Strengths	Test for the causation and avoid the spurious association	Technically simple, less expensive, less time-consuming, easy to recruit the data
Weaknesses	Lower statistical power, time-consuming, costly, technically complicated	May have spurious association, cannot test for causation

IBD, identical by descent.

its application in complex diseases is not as promising as expected. From an epidemiologic perspective, the high false-positive rate in association studies has been attributed mainly to confounding factors due to population stratification (see Glossary) and the lack of good candidate genetic polymorphisms. The reasons for the lack of positive results from linkage studies in complex diseases include inappropriate phenotyping, locus heterogeneity, phenocopies, low statistical power, and lack of appropriate tests for gene–environmental interactions. Depending on the availability of samples, in our opinion either study design has its pros and cons. Readers can consult the section "Candidate Gene versus Genome-Wide Screen" and "Detecting Population Stratification" in the section "Future Genetic Epidemiologic Studies" when conducting a genetic epidemiologic study.

LINKAGE ANALYSIS

Before conducting a linkage study, family recruitment and the statistical approach need to be thoroughly planned. Linkage analysis is a statistical technology that does not require the knowledge of any underlying biochemical mechanism of a disease. It has become a key step in the disease gene-mapping task. Two linkage methods are commonly mentioned in the context of linkage analysis: parametric (or model-based) and nonparametric (or model-free) analysis. Parametric analysis requires the assumptions of the underlying genetic model (i.e., dominant, recessive, or codominant inheritance), the population frequency of the disease-causing allele, penetrance in disease allele carriers, and phenocopy rate; therefore, it also is called model-based analysis. Because log of

odds (LOD) is used in the statistical results of parametric analysis, sometimes it also is called LOD score analysis. The LOD score statistics use the likelihood method to test whether a marker is linked or unlinked to the unobserved disease locus. The traditional cutoff point for mendelian diseases is an LOD score ≥ 3 for linkage, and ≤ -2 against linkage.

Although parametric analysis has been shown to map mendelian disorders, the nonparametric method has gained popularity as research in complex diseases has intensified. The major advantage of using the nonparametric method in complex diseases is that it does not require the assumption of the genetic model or parameters, which often are unknown for complex diseases. Several statistical tests have been proposed as nonparametric approaches, such as sib pair analysis, variance component, and nonparametric linkage. These nonparametric methods are based on a general principle: to test whether there is excess sharing of a marker allele identical by descent (IBD) among affected family members. The concept of sib pair analysis is straightforward: for a quantitative trait, the closer the trait data between two sibs, the higher the possibility of more IBD sharing, when there is linkage. If there is no linkage, the IBD sharing will follow the null distribution: sharing 0, 1, or 2 IBD with probabilities of 25%, 50%, and 25%, respectively. Similarly, for discrete traits, concordant affected sib pairs have a higher possibility of more IBD sharing than discordant affected–unaffected sib pairs, when there is linkage. In other words, the more similar the phenotype, the higher the possibility of a same genotype. Readers can consult the various articles for the variance component (4–6) and nonparametric linkage (7) approaches.

SELECTING APPROPRIATE PHENOTYPES FOR GENETIC STUDIES

Stroke is a heterogeneous clinical outcome that includes several subtypes, and each subtype can have several etiologies. A careful study design to select less heterogeneous study subjects and to refine the phenotype will largely increase the odds of success. In addition to finding families segregating in a mendelian fashion of stroke, one can carefully select a subtype of stroke as the phenotype of interest. Based on the successful examples in previous genetic studies on breast cancer, epilepsy, and migraine, several associated clinical features can be used to construct inclusion criteria aimed at reducing the phenotypic heterogeneity. Commonly used characteristics include more severe symptoms, early-onset form of stroke, stroke accompanied by a constellation of other symptoms such as familial hemiplegic migraine, and white matter hyperintensities.

In studying more specific stroke phenotypes, it is generally believed that one could discover disease genes that have a strong effect but are relatively less common in the general population. Genes discovered by this approach, however, also may have mild and common mutations conferring relatively lower risk in the general population. A good example is the mutations in the ABC1 gene that cause both Tangier disease (TD) and familial high-density lipoprotein (HDL) deficiency (FHD). TD is an extremely rare disease and is associated with almost complete absence of HDL cholesterol (HDL-C) levels. FHD, which is more common than TD, has inherited low HDL-C levels, usually below the fifth percentile, but an absence of the clinical manifestations of TD. TD was mapped to chromosome 9q31 (8), and then mutations in the ABC1 gene were found to cause TD. Interestingly, other mutations in the ABC1 gene were found to be involved in the etiology of FHD (9). This example shows how genetic studies on mendelian diseases may help research on complex diseases.

Another approach is to reduce the disease complexity and increase the cost-effectiveness by studying intermediate phenotypes, such as lipids, hypertension, diabetes, homocysteine, or intima-media thickness of the carotid artery. This approach may increase the likelihood of finding important genes regulating these intermediate phenotypes and eventually facilitate the understanding of the genetic susceptibility to stroke. The basic rationale of using intermediate phenotypes is illustrated in Figure 2-1. Each of these intermediate or precursor phenotypes, in essence, is a complex trait influenced by both genetic and environmental factors. When we study an individual intermediate phenotype, the number of genes can be reduced. Compared with stroke, each intermediate phenotype is closer to the underlying susceptibility genes; the genetic effect is supposed to be stronger and detected more easily in these phenotypes than in stroke.

There are additional advantages if the intermediate phenotypes are quantitative traits rather than the discrete outcome of stroke or no stroke. From the data collection point of view, it is easier to collect quantitative traits because every person has such data. When one conducts a family study, each family member offers both phenotype and genotype for linkage analysis regardless of whether or not they have stroke; thus, the cost and efforts can be significantly reduced. From the analytic point of view, a quantitative trait can be adjusted for confounding factors, and the residual values can be used in genetic analysis to increase the power to detect a genetic effect. Finally, from the public health point of view, these intermediate phenotypes can be used as screening tests for early detection and prevention.

Focusing on intermediate quantitative phenotypes with a significant hereditary component may be an efficient method to establish the genetic determinants of complex diseases such as stroke. For example, cholesterol, particularly a low level of HDL-C, is a risk factor for stroke (10,11). The hepatic lipase gene

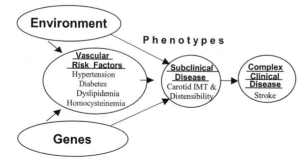

FIG. 2-1. A hypothetic pathway of genetic effects on stroke.

(LIPC) is an ideal candidate gene because it encodes hepatic lipase, which has an important role in the metabolism of lipids. LIPC was reported to be linked to HDL-C levels (12), and then a promoter polymorphism (-514 C/T) at LIPC was found to be associated with HDL-C levels (13). Although several independent studies replicated the positive results, some failed to show association [for review, see reference (14)]. The conflicting results are likely to be caused by using HDL-C as the phenotype of interest rather than its subfractions HDL$_2$-C and HDL$_3$-C. Based on the molecular studies, hepatic lipase promotes the conversion of buoyant HDL$_2$ particles to small HDL$_3$ particles by remodeling triglycerides and phospholipids (15). When HDL subfraction data were analyzed (14,16), the results showed that this polymorphism had an effect only on HDL$_2$-C and not HDL$_3$-C, and the TT genotype was associated with high HDL$_2$-C levels. Clinical intervention by lipid-lowering medication also shows that only HDL$_2$-C and not HDL$_3$-C significantly increased after treatment, and the CC genotype has greater response than the TT genotype (17). Similarly, the improvement in coronary artery stenosis is significantly greater in the CC genotype than the CT or TT genotype (17). Although coronary heart disease cannot be demonstrated to be associated with this polymorphism (17–19), both the lipid profile and angiographic studies show the association with this polymorphism, which indirectly suggests the role of this polymorphism in cardiovascular or cerebrovascular disease. This example underscores the importance of choosing an appropriate phenotype based on our knowledge of the pathophysiology of the disease and highlights the difficulty of using a clinical outcome as the phenotype of interest.

CANDIDATE GENE VERSUS GENOME-WIDE SCREEN

Regardless of whether the study design is a linkage or association study, two methods can be used to investigate genotypes: candidate gene approach and genome-wide screen (GWS). For a laboratory without a high-throughput genotyping facility, choosing the candidate gene approach is a more realistic and economic way to conduct a study. Several guidelines can be used to choose promising candidate genes. (a) Are the candidate genes biologically reasonable? We can judge this point by the function of the encoded protein from a candidate gene. Similarly, we can analyze the physiologic pathway of the trait of interest and pick up the candidate genes encoding the key

enzymes in the pathway. (b) Have the candidate genes been shown to be important in animal studies or in vitro studies such as gene expression studies? (c) Is the polymorphism of the candidate gene common and functional? An uncommon polymorphism (<10% of the population) is unlikely to be important for common complex diseases. A nonfunctional polymorphism will not have any biologic meaning despite the finding of a significant statistical association with the disease of interest. A common and functional polymorphism is the best candidate for studies of complex diseases. (d) If the plan is to conduct an association study, one may need to ask whether the potential candidate gene has been linked to the phenotype in linkage studies, and vise versa. One major limitation of the candidate gene approach is that the study is restricted to the current limited number of potential candidate genes and cannot lead to the discovery of new genes (see "DNA Microarray" and "Bioinformatics" in the "Future Genetic Epidemiologic Studies" for more information).

Instead of focusing on the limited number of known candidate genes, using GWS can allow us to explore the whole genome. As a result of the development of high-throughput facilities and the rapidly declining costs for genotyping, many linkage studies have chosen to use the genome-wide approach. Due to limitations in current molecular technologies and statistics, GWS has been used only in linkage studies and not in association studies. The basic idea of this approach is to use a large number of equally spaced polymorphic microsatellite markers to cover the whole genome. Currently, most studies choose to genotype approximately 350 to 400 markers with an average marker density of ~10 cM in the GWS. Although this approach seems to avoid the problem of having a limited number of potential candidate genes, this approach has several statistical concerns in multiple testing (20). The two approaches, however, are not mutually exclusive. Once evidence of linkage is found through GWS, one may need to look for potential candidate genes in the linked chromosomal region for further studies.

FUTURE GENETIC EPIDEMIOLOGIC STUDIES: INCORPORATING NEW GENOMIC TECHNOLOGIES

Astounding data and technologies have been developed since the worldwide efforts to sequence the human genome. The study of the genetic determinants of complex diseases will be refined with the development of molecular, statistical, and bioinformatic technologies. Successful future studies will need to incorporate these new technologies. Here, we briefly mention several major issues, and readers can consult the cited references for further details.

Single Nucleotide Polymorphisms for Linkage Disequilibrium Mapping

Linkage disequilibrium (LD) mapping has gained more attention because a large number of single nucleotide polymorphisms (SNPs) can be used in SNP-based association studies. SNPs in noncoding regions that have no functional consequences can be used to track disease causing polymorphisms through the LD mechanism, whereas SNPs with functional consequences can be tested for either direct association or LD. The success of SNP-based association studies depends on the degree of LD when the tested SNP per se is not the trait causing polymorphism. Recent studies have shown that LD might not be as complicated as originally thought (21,22). If so, the pattern of LD will influence the number of genotypings and the strategies for analysis. Readers can consult the review paper for further information (23,24).

Haplotype Analysis

Haplotype data are extremely useful in studies of LD, particularly in tracking chromosomal segments harboring disease susceptibility genes. A haplotype may have higher LD than a single SNP and be a surrogate for an unobserved susceptibility locus. Using haplotypes composed of a relatively small number of SNPs to represent all the functional polymorphisms of a candidate gene may become a more powerful strategy for future LD mapping. Constructing haplotypes could be difficult when there are no DNA samples from additional family members. Recent developments from both the statistical and molecular methods have made this task possible using data from unrelated individuals (25,26), which will facilitate research in disease gene mapping.

High-Throughput and Low-Cost Genotyping

The cost of microsatellite genotyping has decreased significantly in the past few years, which makes GWS studies affordable and popular. However, increasingly more studies propose to genotype a large number of candidate genes using SNP-based association studies. The newly developed pyrosequencing technique allows us to pool DNA samples together (27). Using this method, we will be able to

compare the allele frequencies between cases and controls and rapidly screen many potential genes at a relatively low cost.

DNA Microarray

One main purpose of the DNA microarray is to measure levels of gene expression for tens of thousands of genes simultaneously. This powerful technology will provide us the tool to investigate both known and newly identified genes. For example, one can compare the gene expression patterns in neurons before and after stroke to understand the genetic response to stroke. The genes with significant changes in expression levels may indicate that they play a critical role in determining the clinical outcome and may indicate good targets for gene mapping studies and therapeutic intervention. Readers can consult the recent studies of this kind (28,29).

Bioinformatics

Bioinformatics has emerged as one of the fastest growing fields in the genomic research because of the need to handle large amounts of genetic and biochemical data. Using bioinformatic technologies, researchers are able to quickly annotate the DNA sequence data into biologic sense. A large proportion of genes currently are annotated, and their functions are predicted. A recent study comparing the human and mouse DNA sequences around the APOAI/CIII/AIV gene complex incidentally found an unknown gene in the vicinity of the APOAI/CIII/AIV gene complex (30). The more exciting finding is that this previously unknown gene was annotated to be in the APO gene family and was named APOAV. Using the transgenic mouse study and SNP-based association study, the researchers showed that APOAV is an important determinant of triglyceride levels in both the mouse and human. This study provides a paradigm of a multidisciplinary genetic epidemiologic study (30).

Detecting Population Stratification

In the past decade, genetic epidemiologic studies have focused primarily on the family-based approach because association studies are subject to problems from population stratification leading to spurious associations. However, association studies can be more powerful when there is no population stratification (24). Recently, several studies tried to solve the issue of population stratification by genotyping multiple markers across the whole genome (31–33). These markers are chosen to be unlikely to link to the phenotype of interest; thus, they can serve as a control to adjust the degree of false-positive associations due to population stratification. This new approach may make association studies more attractive because they are simple and less costly.

Pharmacogenetics

Pharmacogenetics can substantially influence future medicine. Individual variations to medication have long been recognized, and the variation can be due to differences of drug absorption, metabolism, and excretion among individuals. All of these factors can be related to individual genetic makeup. Pharmacogenetics is aimed at investigating drug response according to different genotypes. The development of pharmacogenetics will lead to the era of personalized medication. In the future, physicians may be able to select a better medication and to reduce the chance of side effects for patients based on the results of genetic tests. Readers can consult several review papers for details (34,35)

CONCLUSIONS AND PROSPECTS

Human genetic studies of stroke or other complex diseases will lead to a substantial impact on prevention, diagnosis, and treatment. To conduct a successful genetic study, an investigator needs to use the new tools of molecular/genetic epidemiology, which include careful design of the study protocol, selection of a highly heritable phenotype, choosing the appropriate study design (association or linkage study), focusing on a genome-wide scan or reasonable candidate genes and their polymorphisms, and using the most sophisticated statistical tools. A multidisciplinary research team that includes experts from genetics, epidemiology, and statistics will be able to take full advantage of the new technologies that will greatly increase the chance of successfully elucidating the genetic determinants of complex diseases such as stroke.

GLOSSARY

Microsatellite marker A kind of DNA variation due to the different length of tandem repetition of a short DNA sequence (often two to four nucleotide repeats).

Single nucleotide polymorphism (SNP) A kind of DNA variation due to change in a single nucleotide in the sequence.

Haplotype Two or more alleles on the same strand of DNA comprise a haplotype. For example, Aa and Bb are two genotypes at two distinct loci, and they constitute four possible haplotypes: AB, Ab, aB, and ab.

Linkage disequilibrium (LD) Two alleles coexist more often than by chance. Taking the above haplotype example, if we can only find AB and ab, but not Ab or aB, the two loci are in LD.

Population stratification When two populations have distinct genetic backgrounds, the populations have stratification. For example, the rare T allele at -514 C/T polymorphism of the hepatic lipase gene has a frequency ~20% in whites but ~50% in blacks. When cases are from one population and controls from the other, a case control study will create a spurious association.

REFERENCES

1. Kiely DK, Wolf PA, Cupples LA, et al. Familial aggregation of stroke. The Framingham Study. *Stroke* 1993;24:1366–1371.
2. Risch N. Linkage strategies for genetically complex traits. I. Multilocus models. *Am J Hum Genet* 1990;46:222–228.
3. Khoury M, Beaty TH, Cohen B. *Fundamentals of genetic epidemiology.* Oxford University Press, 1993:233–283.
4. Amos CI, Krushkal J, Thiel TJ, et al. Comparison of model-free linkage mapping strategies for the study of a complex trait. *Genet Epidemiol* 1997;14:743–748.
5. Amos CI. Robust variance-components approach for assessing genetic linkage in pedigrees. *Am J Hum Genet* 1994;54:535–543.
6. Schork NJ. Extended pedigree patterned covariance matrix mixed models for quantitative phenotype analysis. *Genet Epidemiol* 1992;9:73–86.
7. Kruglyak L, Daly MJ, Reeve-Daly MP, et al. Parametric and nonparametric linkage analysis: a unified multipoint approach. *Am J Hum Genet* 1996;58:1347–1363.
8. Rust S, Walter M, Funke H, et al. Assignment of Tangier disease to chromosome 9q31 by a graphical linkage exclusion strategy. *Nat Genet* 1998;20:96–98.
9. Brooks-Wilson A, Marcil M, Clee SM, et al. Mutations in ABC1 in Tangier disease and familial high-density lipoprotein deficiency. *Nat Genet* 1999;22:336–345.
10. Aronow WS, Ahn C. Correlation of serum lipids with the presence or absence of atherothrombotic brain infarction and peripheral arterial disease in 1,834 men and women aged > or = 62 years. *Am J Cardiol* 1994;73:995–997.
11. Sacco RL, Benson RT, Kargman DE, et al. High-density lipoprotein cholesterol and ischemic stroke in the elderly: the Northern Manhattan Stroke Study. *JAMA* 2001;285:2729–2735.

12. Cohen JC, Wang Z, Grundy SM, et al. Variation at the hepatic lipase and apolipoprotein AI/CIII/AIV loci is a major cause of genetically determined variation in plasma HDL cholesterol levels. *J Clin Invest* 1994; 94:2377–2384.

13. Guerra R, Wang J, Grundy SM, et al. A hepatic lipase (LIPC) allele associated with high plasma concentrations of high density lipoprotein cholesterol. *Proc Natl Acad Sci U S A* 1997;94:4532–4537.

14. Juo SH, Han Z, Smith JD, et al. Promoter polymorphisms of hepatic lipase gene influence HDL(2) but not HDL(3) in African American men: CARDIA study. *J Lipid Res* 2001;42:258–264.

15. Kuusi T, Saarinen P, Nikkila EA. Evidence for the role of hepatic endothelial lipase in the metabolism of plasma high density lipoprotein2 in man. *Atherosclerosis* 1980;36:589–593.

16. Zambon A, Deeb SS, Hokanson JE, et al. Common variants in the promoter of the hepatic lipase gene are associated with lower levels of hepatic lipase activity, buoyant LDL, and higher HDL2 cholesterol. *Arterioscler Thromb Vasc Biol* 1998;18:1723–1729.

17. Zambon A, Deeb SS, Brown BG, et al. Common hepatic lipase gene promoter variant determines clinical response to intensive lipid-lowering treatment. *Circulation* 2001;103:792–798.

18. Tahvanainen E, Syvanne M, Frick MH, et al. Association of variation in hepatic lipase activity with promoter variation in the hepatic lipase gene. The LOCAT Study Investigators. *J Clin Invest* 1998;101:956–960.

19. Hong SH, Song J, Kim JQ. Genetic variations of the hepatic lipase gene in Korean patients with coronary artery disease. *Clin Biochem* 2000;33:291–296.

20. Lander E, Kruglyak L. Genetic dissection of complex traits: guidelines for interpreting and reporting linkage results. *Nat Genet* 1995;11:241–247.

21. Daly MJ, Rioux JD, Schaffner SF, et al. High-resolution haplotype structure in the human genome. *Nat Genet* 2001;29:229–232.

22. Jeffreys AJ, Kauppi L, Neumann R. Intensely punctate meiotic recombination in the class II region of the major histocompatibility complex. *Nat Genet* 2001;29: 217–222.

23. Risch NJ. Searching for genetic determinants in the new millennium. *Nature* 2000;405:847–856.

24. Risch N, Merikangas K. The future of genetic studies of complex human diseases. *Science* 1996;273:1516–1517.

25. Stephens M, Smith NJ, Donnelly P. A new statistical method for haplotype reconstruction from population data. *Am J Hum Genet* 2001;68:978–989.

26. Douglas JA, Boehnke M, Gillanders E, et al. Experimentally-derived haplotypes substantially increase the efficiency of linkage disequilibrium studies. *Nat Genet* 2001;28:361–364.

27. Fakhrai-Rad H, Pourmand N, Ronaghi M. Pyrosequencing: an accurate detection platform for single nucleotide polymorphisms. *Hum Mutat* 2002;479–485.

28. Trapp T, Olah L, Holker I, et al. GTPase RhoB: an early predictor of neuronal death after transient focal ischemia in mice. *Mol Cell Neurosci* 2001;17:883–894.

29. Jin K, Mao XO, Eshoo MW, et al. Microarray analysis of hippocampal gene expression in global cerebral ischemia. *Ann Neurol* 2001;50:93–103.

30. Pennacchio LA, Olivier M, Hubacek JA, et al. An apolipoprotein influencing triglycerides in humans and mice revealed by comparative sequencing. *Science* 2001;294:169–173.

31. Pritchard JK, Rosenberg NA. Use of unlinked genetic markers to detect population stratification in association studies. *Am J Hum Genet* 1999;65:220–228.

32. Pritchard JK, Stephens M, Rosenberg NA, et al. Association mapping in structured populations. *Am J Hum Genet* 2000;67:170–181.

33. Bacanu SA, Devlin B, Roeder K. The power of genomic control. *Am J Hum Genet* 2000;66:1933–1944.

34. Roses AD. Pharmacogenetics and the practice of medicine. *Nature* 2000;405:857–865.

35. Wieczorek SJ, Tsongalis GJ. Pharmacogenomics: will it change the field of medicine? *Clin Chim Acta* 2001; 308:1–8.

Ischemic Stroke: Advances in Neurology, Vol. 92. Edited by
H.J.M. Barnett, Julien Bogousslavsky, and Heather Meldrum.
Lippincott Williams & Wilkins, Philadelphia © 2003.

3

Genetic Epidemiology of Ischemic Stroke

Mark J. Alberts

*Department of Neurology, Northwestern University Medical School and Stroke Program,
Northwestern Memorial Hospital, Chicago, Illinois, U.S.A.*

The genetics of ischemic stroke is a complex and evolving field of study. It is complicated by many factors, including the heterogeneous mechanisms that can lead to an ischemic stroke and the genetic factors that may contribute to many of the well-known risk factors associated with strokes. With rare exceptions, ischemic stroke is likely to be more of a synthetic trait or a complex genetic trait, not a simple monogenic disorder (1–4). All of these factors make it challenging to clearly define genetic aspects of ischemic stroke. This chapter reviews different approaches that can be used to study the genetics of stroke, as well as some of the important genetic epidemiologic studies of ischemic stroke that have been published.

GENETIC EPIDEMIOLOGIC STUDIES OF ISCHEMIC STROKE

The past 10 years has seen a significant increase in the number of studies that have examined in detail the genetic epidemiology of stroke. These studies vary in terms of design, number of patients, and results. A summary of these studies is given in Table 3-1.

One of the best studied cohorts for vascular disease is the Framingham Study. In a study of almost 5,000 individuals, the Framingham group did not detect an association for stroke or transient ischemic attack (TIA) between cohort members and a parental death from stroke (5). However, paternal or maternal history of stroke was associated with an increased risk of stroke among offspring (relative risk 2.4 and 1.4, respectively). Sibling history of stroke or TIA was not associated with an increased risk of stroke or TIA among cohort members. The authors conclude that parental history of stroke may be a risk factor for stroke.

Another important study was the Family Heart Study funded by National Heart Lung and Blood Institute. This study consisted of 3,168 probands and 29,325 first-degree relatives. After adjusting for differences in age, race, and gender, they found a statistically significant increased risk [odds ratio (OR) 2.0] for paternal stroke history but not maternal stroke history (6). The increased risk persisted after controlling for common stroke risk factors, such as hypertension, diabetes, smoking, and coronary artery disease.

The Atherosclerosis Risk in Communities (ARIC) Study also examined the influence of family stroke history on clinical and subclinical stroke. They identified 261 patients with a clinical stroke and 202 individuals with subclinical strokes (detected by magnetic resonance imaging (7). A weak association was found between parental history of stroke and subclinical strokes (OR 1.64) after controlling for the usual stroke risk factors; however, no association was found for clinical strokes in this same cohort.

A useful study design for determining the influence of genetic factors is a twin cohort. Brass et al. (8) performed a large twin study for cerebrovascular disease. The study used the National Academy of Sciences Veteran Twin Registry and a mailed health survey. This study found that the overall rate of stroke (all types) was similar between monozygotic twins (131/4,200) and dizygotic twins (143/4,585). The rates did not differ appreciably between the twins and other populations; however, the concordance rate for monozygotic pairs was 17.7% compared to 3.6% for dizygotic pairs ($p < 0.05$). These results suggest that there is a significant genetic contribution to the development of stroke. This study did not report separate results for ischemic and hemorrhagic types of stroke.

Another large twin study was reported from Denmark using the Danish Twin Registry. Using a sample

TABLE 3-1. *Family studies of ischemic stroke*

Study	Prospective	No. of patients	Controls	Stroke subtypes	Multivariate analysis	Genetic/familial factors for stroke
Gifford 1966 (31)	Yes	255	Yes	No	No	Yes
Alter 1967 (32)	Yes	239	Yes	No	No	Yes
Heyden 1969 et al. 1969 (33)	Yes	120	Yes	No	No	Yes (risk factors)
Marshall 1971 (34)	Yes	1,307	Yes	Yes	No	Yes
Alter and Kluznik 1972 (35)	Yes	544	Yes	No	No	No
Herman et al. 1983 (36)	Yes	371	Yes	No	Yes	No
Diaz et al. 1986 (37)	Yes	131	Yes	No	No	Yes (risk factors)
Khaw and Barrett-Connor 1986 (38)	Yes	3,415	No	No	Yes	Yes (women)
Welin et al. 1987 (39)	Yes	92	No	Yes	Yes	Yes
Boysen et al. 1988 (40)	Yes	295	Yes	Yes	Yes	No
Thompson et al. 1989 (41)	Yes	603	Yes	No	Yes	No (yes for MI)
Howard et al. 1990 (42)	Yes	55	No	Yes	Yes	Yes
Brass and Shaker 1991 (43)	No	117	No	Yes	No	No (yes for > 70 yr)
Brass et al. 1992 (8)	No	292	Yes	No	No	Yes
Kiely et al. 1993 (44)	Yes	34	Yes	Yes	Yes	Yes
Rotimi et al. 1994 (10)	No	1,420	Yes	No	No	Yes (risk factors)
Carrieri et al. 1994 (45)	Yes	164	Yes	Yes	Yes	Yes (young patients)
Vitullo el al. 1996 (46)	Yes	237	Yes	Yes	Yes	Yes
Bogousslavsky et al. 1996 (47)	Yes	822	No	Yes	Yes	Yes
Brass et al. 1996 (48)	Yes	545	Yes	No	No	Yes (not older patients)
Kubota et al. 1997 (49)	Yes	502	Yes	Yes	Yes	Yes (SAH)
Liao et al. 1997 (6)	Yes	105	Yes	Yes	Yes	Yes
Jousilahti et al. 1997 (50)	Yes	754	Yes	Yes	Yes	Yes
Morrison et al. 2000 (51)	Yes	463	Yes	Yes	Yes	Yes
Nicolaou et al. 2000 (17)	No	354	Yes	No	Yes	Yes
Decode Research Group 2002 (12)	No	476	Yes	Yes	Yes	Genetic linkage chromosome 5q12

MI, myocardial infarction; SAH, subarachnoid hemorrhage.

of 351 monozygotic twins and 639 dizygotic twins, the investigators found a concordance rate for stroke death of 10% for monozygotic twins versus 5% for dizygotic twins (9). The study also found an 11% monozygotic pair concordance rate for stroke hospitalization or stroke death versus 7% in dizygotic twin pairs. These results yielded a heritability estimate of 0.32 for stroke death and 0.17 for stroke hospitalization or death (9). This study did not distinguish between ischemic and hemorrhagic strokes.

Most of the studies cited focused on mainly Caucasian populations. A large study of familial stroke risk was reported in 1994 by Rotimi et al. (10). This study included 232 African-American pedigrees with 1,420 individuals. They found an increased disease risk for stroke among relatives of affected probands compared to relatives of unaffected probands of 3.24 for stroke, which was statistically significant. It is unclear whether this association was independent of classic stroke risk factors such as hypertension and diabetes.

Genetic epidemiologic studies are subject to biases from multiple sources, including ascertainment, disease confirmation, disease misclassification, and early mortality. Another potential source of bias is gender and age. A large survey study by Saito et al. (11) found that males were more likely to have a stroke than females (OR 2.5), and the risk of stroke increased with age. Although the gender differences reported are higher than those reported in other studies, the increasing risk of stroke with age has been well described. These factors could bias genetic epidemiologic studies of stroke, but the bias may not be straightforward. Ascertaining a cohort with an average age of 50 years certainly will produce fewer individuals with stroke than if an older cohort were studied. However, one could argue that the influence of a potent genetic factor would be most pronounced or apparent in the younger cohort, before other stroke risk factors (e.g., hypertension, diabetes) exert their full influence on the disease pathogenesis. This is true if one assumes that the active genetic factor is working independently of other risk factors. However, the genetic stroke risk factor may be working in concert with other classic risk factors and may produce the stroke phenotype at a later age. This certainly is the case with some types of inherited, late-onset Alzheimer's disease. Until we fully understand the nature and impact of the presumed genetic risk factors, it is premature to assume that they are only important in a young versus an older population.

GENETIC LINKAGE STUDIES AND POLYMORPHISMS

One of the most potentially significant developments in the genetic epidemiology of stroke was reported recently by the Decode Research Group from Iceland. This study included 476 patients with strokes (95% ischemic) in 179 families and 438 of their relatives (12). The whole genome scan consisted of 1,000 microsatellite markers. The linkage study produced a maximum LOD score of 4.40 on chromosome 5q12 at marker D5S1474. Further analyses using additional markers were able to narrow the region of linkage to about 6 cM between D5S1474 and D5S398. When the small number of patients with hemorrhagic stroke was excluded, the LOD score increased to 4.86 at marker D5S2080. The authors report that this locus does not appear to function through any well-known stroke risk factors such as hypertension and diabetes. Candidate genes within this region are being analyzed for their role in the pathogenesis of stroke.

If these results are confirmed in other populations, it may suggest that one or more specific genetic risk factors exist for the common types of ischemic stroke. Such a genetic risk factor may function through a variety of mechanisms, including coagulation pathways, vascular endothelium, vessel morphology, and others. This new discovery certainly supports the concept of the importance of genetic factors in the pathogenesis of at least some cases of ischemic stroke.

Genetic linkage studies have identified two loci for the rare familial form of moyamoya disease. Moyamoya is defined by bilateral narrowing of the distal intracranial internal carotid arteries and proximal portions of the middle cerebral arteries. It can lead to ischemic as well as hemorrhagic strokes. Studies have established genetic linkage to loci on chromosome 17q25 and chromosome 6 (13,14). The locus on chromosome 17 is near the locus for neurofibromatosis type 1.

Specific polymorphisms have been found to be associated with stroke. There have been several studies looking at the role of apolipoprotein E (apoE) and the risk of stroke. In a meta-analysis of over 1,800 patients and controls with ischemic stroke, McCarron et al. (15) found a small but significant association between the apoE ε4 allele and ischemic stroke (OR 1.68, $p < 0.001$). Among stroke patients, 27% were carriers of the ε4 allele versus 18% of controls who had the ε4 allele ($p < 0.001$). A Japanese study of 322 stroke patients (201 ischemic) found a significant association of atherothrombotic stroke with the apoE ε2 and ε4 alleles (OR 3.9 and 2.1, respectively) (16). These results were published after the meta-analysis cited earlier. These results may indicate that the influence of the apoE genotype as a risk factor for stroke differs with race and ethnicity of the population under study.

There are dozens of genetic polymorphisms that have been associated with stroke. The vast majority of these polymorphisms do not appear to produce significant changes in the expression or function of a gene; therefore, their role as a causative factor in producing strokes remains unclear and unproved at this time.

GENETICS OF STROKE RISK FACTORS

One of the major issues when discussing the genetic epidemiology of stroke is that we may really be studying the genetics of some well-known stroke risk factors such as hypertension and diabetes, which themselves have a significant genetic component. This aspect of stroke genetics was studied by Nicolaou et al. (17). They obtained medical and family histories from 354 hypertensive probands, 1,427 first-degree relatives, and 239 spouses, and examined for the risk of stroke using a logistic model adjusting for age and gender. They found a statistically significant increased risk for hypertension among relatives of the hypertensive probands, with an OR of 2.4. The risk of stroke among parents of the probands was increased with an OR of 7.3, using the spouses of the reference group. The risk among siblings was not significantly elevated (OR 1.6). When hypertension, obesity, smoking, diabetes, cholesterol, and coronary artery disease were controlled for, the parents still had an increased risk of stroke (OR 5.4). These results suggest that in some cases, the increased risk of stroke in families with hypertension is not due solely to the hypertension, thereby indicating that other factors (presumably genetic) are influencing stroke risk.

Other studies of the genetic influence in the pathogenesis of essential hypertension have led to mixed results. Overall, it appears that most forms of hypertension are either polygenic or have a relatively small genetic component (18). There are rare forms of monogenic hypertension, but they account for only a few cases. Attempts to map genes for the common form of essential hypertension suggest that there may be many quantitative trait loci that each contributes a small genetic influence (19). Some specific genes have been the focus on more intense study, including renin and angiotensinogen (20–22). In both cases, there appears to be a small genetic influence for both genes. Other studies using genome wide scans have identified several promising loci and genetic regions (23,24).

Diabetes is another common and important risk factor for stroke that appears to have a genetic contribution to its etiology. Type I diabetes is influenced by genes that control the immune system and immunologic responses. Type II diabetes is due to defects in insulin secretion and insulin sensitivity, some aspects of which are also under genetic control (25). Several dozen mutations in the glucokinase gene have been described in patients with maturity-onset diabetes of the young (26). A rare form of diabetes (sometimes associated with hearing loss) is due to specific mutations in mitochondrial DNA (27). This mutation is at position 3243 and involves the transfer RNA for leucine. It is the same mutation that

is responsible for the most common form of mitochondrial encephalomyopathy, lactic acidosis, and strokelike episode (MELAS) (28–30). Diabetes due to the mutation typically is maternally inherited, which is typical for mitochondrial disorders. Obesity and lipid metabolism may share some common genetic traits with adult-onset diabetes.

CONCEPTUAL ASPECTS OF GENETICS AND STROKE

From the studies and data reviewed, it seems likely that there is some genetic contribution to stroke through its risk factors and possibly in a more direct manner based on the Icelandic study. Clearly, stroke is not a monogenic disorder in the vast majority of cases. Perhaps it is most correct to envision possible genetic effects at various points along the pathway for the development of cerebrovascular disease (Fig. 3-1); however, such effects may not be present in all people. Another reasonable framework for understanding stroke genetics is as a continuum of effects based on two parameters: the prevalence of genetic factors and the magnitude of their effects (Fig. 3-2). Such a matrix can be used to understand the importance of genetic effects on a population of patients, as well as for a particular patient. Once we better understand the importance and prevalence of genetic factors, our ability to use such a matrix will be enhanced. The effects of environmental factors (e.g., diet, smok-

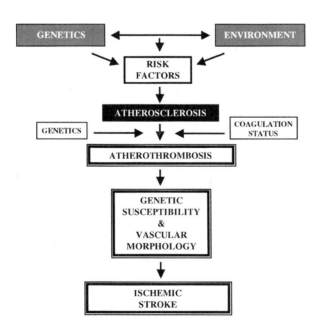

FIG. 3-1. Role of genetic factors along the pathway in the development of atherosclerosis, atherothrombosis, and ischemic stroke.

Importance of Genetic Factors in the Etiology of Ischemic Stroke

		PREVALENCE OF GENETIC FACTORS	
MAGNITUDE OF GENETIC EFFECT		LOW	HIGH
	WEAK	+	++
	MODERATE	++	+++
	STRONG	++	++++

+   Little or no genetic influence
++   Modest genetic influence in some cases
+++   Important genetic influence in many cases
++++ Genetic factors are key in disease etiology

FIG. 3-2. Interaction between the prevalence of genetic factors and the magnitude of the genetic effect in the pathogenesis of ischemic stroke.

ing, alcohol intake, exercise) are of obvious importance for all of these paradigms.

Another consideration is the "snapshot" effect. When we ascertain a patient or individual for a genetic study, we typically only assess their current and past clinical status using routine tools of clinical examination, supplemented by some tests such as neuroimaging studies. One can certainly envision an "unaffected" individual with a 95% stenosis of a small cerebral artery that has not yet thrombosed or caused a clinical deficit. Although such a person might be considered "unaffected" from a stroke point of view, they certainly could become affected if the lesion were to change slightly. In the future, we will need more sensitive and noninvasive methods to assess the status of a person's cerebral vessels, along with longitudinal clinical follow-up to determine if an unaffected person is truly unaffected and if an asymptomatic individual remains symptom-free. Only then will we be able to accurately match genotypes and phenotypes for cerebrovascular disease.

remain unclear. There may be a small number of very potent and common "stroke genes" that are involved in producing the stroke phenotype. Conversely, the stroke phenotype may be determined by the interaction among dozens or hundreds of genes and/or polymorphisms that have varying influences in different patient populations. Another possibility is that there are as yet unidentified stroke risk factors (such as derangements in lipid metabolism, coagulation, or endothelial reactivity) under environmental control that are important in disease pathogenesis but may only seem to be inherited because we cannot currently control for them. This is clearly an area in need of more extensive research. It likely will require sophisticated studies that ascertain in-depth family histories and follow large cohorts prospectively to determine stroke risk in a well-characterized but diverse patient population. The hope is that by identifying and understanding genetic factors for stroke we will be able to intervene early and prevent strokes in many cases.

CONCLUSIONS

There is a growing body of evidence suggesting that for ischemic stroke there is a genetic component that contributes to its occurrence and pathogenesis. The nature and magnitude of these genetic factors

REFERENCES

1. Rastenyte D, Tuomilehto J, Sarti C. Genetics of stroke—a review. *J Neurol Sci* 1998;153:132–145.
2. Hademenos GJ, Alberts MJ, Awad I, et al. Advances in the genetics of cerebrovascular disease and stroke. *Neurology* 2001;56:997–1008.

3. Hassan A, Markus HS. Genetics and ischaemic stroke. *Brain* 2000;123:1784–1812.
4. Brass L, Alberts M. Genetic epidemiology and family studies of stroke. In: Alberts M, ed. *Genetics of cerebrovascular disease.* Armonk, NY: Futura Publishing Co., 1999:159–182.
5. Kiely DK, Wolf PA, Cupples LA, et al. Familial aggregation of stroke: The Framingham Study. *Stroke* 1993; 24:1366–1371.
6. Liao D, Myers R, Hunt S, et al. Familial history of stroke and stroke risk. The Family Heart Study. *Stroke* 1997;28:1908–1912.
7. Morrison AC, Fornage M, Liao D, et al. Parental history of stroke predicts subclinical but not clinical stroke: the Atherosclerosis Risk in Communities Study. *Stroke (Online)* 2000;31:2098–2102.
8. Brass LM, Isaacsohn JL, Merikangas KR, et al. A study of twins and stroke. *Stroke* 1992;23:221–223.
9. Bak S, Gaist D, Sindrup SH, et al. Genetic liability in stroke: a long-term follow-up study of Danish twins. *Stroke* 2002;33:769–774.
10. Rotimi C, Cooper R, Cao G, et al. Familial aggregation of cardiovascular diseases in African-American pedigrees. *Genet Epidemiol* 1994;11:397–407.
11. Saito T, Nanri S, Saito I, et al. Importance of sex and age factor in assessing family history of stroke. *J Epidemiol* 2000;10:328–334.
12. Gretarsdottir S, Sveinbjorndottir S, Jonsson H, et al. Localization of a susceptibility gene for common forms of stroke to 5q12. *Am J Hum Genet* 2002;70:593–603.
13. Yamauchi T, Tada M, Houkin K, et al. Linkage of familial moyamoya disease (spontaneous occlusion of the circle of Willis) to chromosome 17q25. *Stroke* 2000;31: 930–935.
14. Inoue TK, Ikezaki K, Sasazuki T, et al. Linkage analysis of moyamoya disease on chromosome 6. *J Child Neurol* 2000;15:179–182.
15. McCarron MO, Delong D, Alberts MJ. APOE genotype as a risk factor for ischemic cerebrovascular disease: a meta-analysis. *Neurology* 1999;53:1308–1311.
16. Kokubo Y, Chowdhury AH, Date C, et al. Age-dependent association of apolipoprotein E genotypes with stroke subtypes in a Japanese rural population. [erratum appears in *Stroke* 2000;31:2279]. *Stroke* 2000;31: 1299–1306.
17. Nicolaou M, DeStefano AL, Gavras I, et al. Genetic predisposition to stroke in relatives of hypertensives. *Stroke* 2000;31:487–492.
18. Crook ED. The genetics of human hypertension. *Semin Nephrol* 2002;22:27–34.
19. Dominiczak AF, Negrin DC, Clark JS, et al. Genes and hypertension: from gene mapping in experimental models to vascular gene transfer strategies. *Hypertension* 2000;35:164–172.
20. Frossard PM, Malloy MJ, Lestringant GG, et al. Haplotypes of the human renin gene associated with essential hypertension and stroke. *J Hum Hypertens* 2001;15: 49–55.
21. Lalouel JM, Rohrwasser A, Terreros D, et al. Angiotensinogen in essential hypertension: from genetics to nephrology. *J Am Soc Nephrol* 2001;12:606–615.
22. O'Shaughnessy KM. The genetics of essential hypertension. *Br J Clin Pharmacol* 2001;51:5–11.
23. Hsueh WC, Mitchell BD, Schneider JL, et al. QTL influencing blood pressure maps to the region of PPH1 on chromosome 2q31-34 in Old Order Amish. *Circulation* 2000;101:2810–2816.
24. Timberlake DS, O'Connor DT, Parmer RJ. Molecular genetics of essential hypertension: recent results and emerging strategies. *Curr Opin Nephrol Hypertens* 2001;10:71–79.
25. Marklova E. Genetic aspects of diabetes mellitus. *Acta Med (Hradec Kralove)* 2001;44:3–6.
26. Bell GI, Pilkis SJ, Weber IT, et al. Glucokinase mutations, insulin secretion, and diabetes mellitus. *Annu Rev Physiol* 1996;58:171–186.
27. Liou CW, Huang CC, Wei YH. Molecular analysis of diabetes mellitus-associated A3243G mitochondrial DNA mutation in Taiwanese cases. *Diabetes Res Clin Pract* 2001;54[Suppl]:S39–S43.
28. Maassen JA, van Essen E, van den Ouweland JM, et al. Molecular and clinical aspects of mitochondrial diabetes mellitus. *Exp Clin Endocrinol Diabetes* 2001;109: 127–134.
29. Iwasaki N, Babazono T, Tsuchiya K, et al. Prevalence of A-to-G mutation at nucleotide 3243 of the mitochondrial tRNA(Leu(UUR)) gene in Japanese patients with diabetes mellitus and end stage renal disease. *J Hum Genet* 2001;46:330–334.
30. Janssen GM, Maassen JA, van Den Ouweland JM. The diabetes-associated 3243 mutation in the mitochondrial tRNA(Leu(UUR)) gene causes severe mitochondrial dysfunction without a strong decrease in protein synthesis rate. *J Biol Chem* 1999;274: 29744–29748.
31. Gifford AJ. An epidemiological study of cerebrovascular disease. *Am J Public Health* 1966;56:452–461.
32. Alter M. Genetic factors in cerebrovascular disease. *Trans Am Neurol Assoc* 1967;92:205–208.
33. Heyden S, Heyman A, Camplong L. Mortality patterns among parents of patients with atherosclerotic cerebrovascular disease. *J Chronic Dis* 1969;22:105–110.
34. Marshall J. Familial incidence of cerebrovascular disease. *J Med Genet* 1971;8:84–89.
35. Alter M, Kluznik J. Genetics of cerebrovascular accidents. *Stroke* 1972;3:41–48.
36. Herman B, Schmitz PIM, Leyten ACM. Multivariate logistic analysis of risk factors for stroke in Tiburg, the Netherlands. *Am J Epidemiol* 1983;118:514–525.
37. Diaz JF, Hachinski VC, Pederson LL, et al. Aggregation of multiple risk factors for stroke in siblings of patients with brain infarction and transient ischemic attacks. *Stroke* 1986;17:1239–1242.
38. Khaw K, Barrett-Connor EB. Family history of stroke as an independent predictor of ischemic heart disease in men and stroke in women. *Am J Epidemiol* 1986;123: 59–66.
39. Welin I, Svardsudd K, Wilhelmsen L, et al. Analysis of risk factors for stroke in a cohort of men born in 1913. *N Engl J Med* 1987;317:521–526.
40. Boysen G, Nyboe J, Appleyard M, et al. Stroke incidence and risk factors for stroke in Copenhagen, Denmark. *Stroke* 1988;19:1345–1353.
41. Thompson SG, Greenberg G, Meade T. Risk factors for stroke and myocardial infarction in women in the United Kingdom as assessed in general practice: a case-control study. *Br Heart J* 1989;61:403–409.
42. Howard G, Evans GW, Toole JF, et al. Characteristics of

stroke victims associated with early cardiovascular mortality in their children. *J Clin Epidemiol* 1990;43: 49–54.

43. Brass LM, Shaker LA. Family history in patients with transient ischemic attacks. *Stroke* 1991;22:837–841.

44. Kiely DK, Wolf PA, Cupples LA, et al. Familial aggregation of stroke. The Framingham Study. *Stroke* 1993; 24:1366–1371.

45. Carrieri PB, Orefice G, Maiorino A, et al. Age-related risk factors for ischemic stroke in Italian men. *Neuroepidemiology* 1994;13:28–33.

46. Vitullo F, Marchioli R, Di Mascio R, et al. Family history and socioeconomic factors as predictors of myocardial infarction, unstable angina and stroke in an Italian population. PROGETTO 3A Investigators. *Eur J Epidemiol* 1996;12:177–185.

47. Bogousslavsky J, Castillo V, Kumral E, et al. Stroke subtypes and hypertension. Primary hemorrhage vs infarction, large- vs small-artery disease. *Arch Neurol* 1996; 53:265–269.

48. Brass LM, Carrano D, Hartigan PM, et al. Genetic risk for stroke: a follow-up study of the NAS/VA twin registry. *Neurology* 1996;46:A212(abst).

49. Kubota M, Yamaura A, Ono J, et al. Is family history an independent risk factor for stroke? *J Neurol Neurosurg Psychiatry* 1997;62:66–70.

50. Jousilahti P, Rastenyte D, Tuomilehto J, et al. Parental history of cardiovascular disease and risk of stroke. A prospective follow-up of 14371 middle-aged men and women in Finland. *Stroke* 1997;28:1361–1366.

51. Morrison AC, Fornage M, Liao D, et al. Parental history of stroke predicts subclinical but not clinical stroke: the Atherosclerosis Risk in Communities Study. *Stroke* 2000;31:2098–2102.

Ischemic Stroke: Advances in Neurology, Vol. 92. Edited by
H.J.M. Barnett, Julien Bogousslavsky, and Heather Meldrum.
Lippincott Williams & Wilkins, Philadelphia © 2003.

4

The Role of Inflammation in Atherosclerosis

Thomas J. DeGraba

Stroke Branch, National Institute of Neurological Disorders and Stroke, Bethesda, Maryland, U.S.A.

Atherosclerosis treatment strategies focused on lowering low-density lipoprotein (LDL) levels, reducing hypertension, treating diabetes, and smoking cessation as endpoints for reduction of stroke and heart attack have achieved some success from the 1960s through the mid-1990s; however, 750,000 strokes and more than 1.4 million heart attacks still occur annually, with a majority resulting from uncontrolled atherosclerotic disease (1). Accumulating data indicate that atherosclerosis is not just a "cholesterol disease" and that activation of inflammatory pathways is central to the development of "unstable" or "vulnerable" plaque, which is believed to be linked to acute coronary syndromes and thromboembolic stroke.

This chapter reviews the role of inflammation in the pathophysiology of atherosclerosis; discusses conventional risk factors and the inflammatory state and the "antiinflammatory" effect of available medications; examines the role of putative inflammatory factors believed to increase the risk of stroke; and briefly discusses the role of genetic factors that affect the inflammatory pathways.

INFLAMMATION: CELLULAR AND MOLECULAR MECHANISMS

Response to Injury

The initiation and formation of atherosclerotic plaques represents a complex interplay of environmental factors and genetic susceptibility that results in a chronic inflammatory process eventually leading to stroke [and myocardial infarction (MI)]. Evidence indicates that exposure of endothelial surfaces to a variety of stimuli, such as shear stress forces of hypertension, hyperglycemia, oxidized LDL, toxins from cigarette smoke, infections, and other inflammatory compounds, results in the deposition and accumulation of lipids in the subintimal ground space

of large arteries. This process results in the expression of surface adhesion molecules such as intercellular adhesion molecule-1 (ICAM-1), vascular cell adhesion molecule-1 (VCAM-1), and P-selectin. Expression of these adhesion molecules results in the migration of circulating monocytes and T-lymphocytes into the wall of the vessel. The monocyte-derived macrophages become filled with lipid (foam cell formation) and contribute to the release of a number of inflammatory mediators that perpetuate the inflammatory and chemotactic state of the growing atherosclerotic plaque. The atherogenic process also results in the production of transforming growth factor-β (TGF-β) and platelet-derived growth factor (PDGF), which results in proliferation of smooth muscle cells and fibroblasts that leads to the deposition of an interstitial fibrous matrix. The extracellular matrix of collagen, elastin, proteoglycans, and other proteins, including fibronectin and thrombospondin, serves to form a fibrous cap that constitutes the key to plaque stabilization of the underlying inflammatory and necrotic lipid core (Fig. 4-1).

Mechanism of Intraluminal Thrombosis

There are two major mechanisms by which intraluminal thrombus formation are hypothesized to occur that result in thromboembolic stroke (and MI).

First, the release of proinflammatory cytokines, such as tumor necrosis factor-α (TNF-α) and interleukin-1β (IL-1β), from activated macrophages results in the conversion of the endothelium over the plaque to a prothrombotic state (2–7). This conversion is characterized by a reduction of tissue plasminogen activator and protein S synthesis, along with an increased production of plasminogen activator inhibitor-1, platelet-activating factor (PAF), leukocyte adhesion molecules such as ICAM-1, VCAM-1,

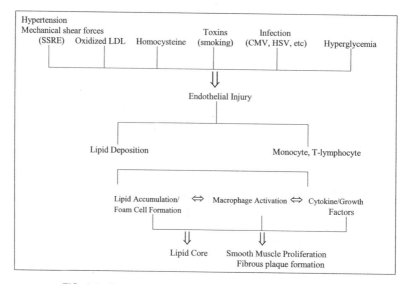

FIG. 4-1. Endothelial injury model of atherosclerosis initiation.

P-selectin, and E-selectin, chemotactic factors such as interleukin-8 (IL-8) and monocyte chemotactic protein-1 (MCP-1), and endothelin-1 (ET-1, a potent vasospastic agent). These changes are brought about by activation of transcription factors such as nuclear factor-κB (NFκB). In addition, T-cell interaction of CD40L with CD40 receptors on macrophages results in the release of tissue factor, a key initiating cofactor in the coagulation pathway. These events promote platelet aggregation and clot formation. Recent studies support the concept that a proinflammatory, prothrombotic state is associated with symptomatic carotid disease. Studies in human carotid atherosclerotic plaque reveal a significant elevation in endothelial surface ICAM-1 expression, VCAM-1 expression, tissue factor expression, and HLA-DR2 antigen in symptomatic individuals (8–10).

Second, plaque instability is enhanced by a thinning of the fibrous matrix that maintains a "cover" over the necrotic lipid core. Breakdown of the fibrous matrix-by-matrix metalloproteinases released from activated macrophages via CD40 exposure and exposure to soluble cytokines such as IL-1 and TNF-α cause the degradation of the collagen and elastin fibers. T-lymphocyte activation of the macrophages resulting in the production of collagenases, gelatinase-B (MMP-9), stromelysin (MMP-3), and gelatinase-A (MMP-2) causes degradation of the matrix. In addition, when T-lymphocytes are activated, they produce interferon-γ (IFN-γ), which reduces the synthesis of collagen material normally produced by smooth muscle cells. IFN-γ also can result in the apoptosis of

smooth muscle cells, thus reducing both the cellular component and the constituents of stabilization by the extracellular matrix. This phenomenon results in the potential for plaque rupture and extrusion of lipid and collagen material into the lumen of the vessel, leading to fibrin clot formation and either arterial occlusion at the site or thromboembolic events.

RISK FACTORS, MARKERS, AND MANAGEMENT

Exposure to vascular endothelium to the conventional risk factors for atherosclerosis results not only in the development of vascular disease but also in an emerging pattern of inflammatory markers that, in part, characterize the injury imparted by these factors. A better understanding of these pathophysiologic changes may allow for future modification of therapeutic intervention targeted at specific inflammatory profile markers in individual patients.

Hypertension

Mechanical forces, such as those caused by hypertension, result in endothelial changes and injury that promote the formation of atherosclerosis. In addition to increased vascular lipid deposition in the setting of endothelial cell injury, hypertension activates shear stress response elements in endothelial cells that result in the up-regulation of genes for leukocyte adhesion molecules such as ICAM-1 and VCAM-1 (11). In addition, hypertension reduces factors such as thrombomodulin, which is essential for the normal anticoagulant state of the endothelium (12).

Angiotensin-Converting Enzyme Inhibitors

Recent studies demonstrated that angiotensin-converting enzyme (ACE) inhibitors reduce the risk of heart attack and stroke in patients with atherosclerosis (13). Although used as an "antihypertensive agent," the beneficial effects of ACE inhibitors on risk reduction, in part, may be independent of their effects on hypertension. The Heart Outcome Prevention Evaluation (HOPE) Study revealed that ACE inhibitors were associated with a reduction in stroke even in patients who did not have appreciable reduction in blood pressure. The effects of ACE blockade (14) on the development of atherosclerosis is thought to be related to both its antihypertensive effect and its reduction in inflammatory mediators. The blockade of angiotensin-II results in the reduction of oxygen free radicals, transcription factors, adhesion molecule expression, inflammatory cytokines, and smooth muscle proliferation (15). The emerging understanding of the antiinflammatory pathophysiologic effects of ACE inhibitors suggests a future role for monitoring inflammatory markers, such as C-reactive protein (CRP) and leukocyte adhesion molecules, in patients with atherosclerosis (16). Levels of these markers may provide endpoint targets for individualization of therapy with ACE inhibitors, as well as other agents that affect the inflammatory pathways.

β-Blockers

β-Blockers clearly have been shown to reduce the incidence of sudden death after MI and may have a positive beneficial effect on the reduction of inflammation by reducing adrenergic effects in the blood vessels (17).

Oxidized Low-Density Lipoprotein

Vessel exposure to oxidized LDL results in increased development of atherosclerosis (18). In addition to lipid deposition in the subintimal ground space of large vessels, oxidized LDL results in increased expression of leukocyte adhesion molecules, increased permeability of lipids, monocyte migration into the vessel wall, and development of lipid-laden macrophages (foam cells) that further increase the inflammatory characteristics of atherosclerotic plaques. Furthermore, oxidized LDL can be presented by macrophages as a foreign antigen to T-lymphocytes within the plaque, causing a potential increase in T-cell proliferation and inflammatory profile (19).

βHydroxy-βMethylglutaryl Coenzyme-A Reductase Inhibitors (Statins)

The use of statins [βhydroxy-βmethylglutaryl coenzyme-A (HMG-CoA) reductase inhibitors] has been extensively reported to reduce the incidence of cardiovascular and cerebrovascular ischemic events. In addition to the clinically beneficial effects of LDL reduction (20), statins are reported to have antiinflammatory effects (21), which may account for long-term reduction in plaque development and the short-term effect on plaque stabilization. Clinical and preclinical studies have demonstrated that statins reduce levels of CRP (22), adhesion molecules, and expression of cytokines and chemokines such as TNF-α, IL-1β, MCP-1, and IL-8 (23–25). In addition, statins reduce the oxidation of LDL and improve vasoreactivity by increased endothelial nitric oxide synthase (eNOS) (26).

To examine clinical relevance, Crisby et al. (27) studied atherosclerotic plaque in 24 symptomatic patients undergoing carotid endarterectomy. They reported that 13 patients treated with pravastatin 40 mg/day for 3 months had a less "inflammatory profile" than 11 patients taking placebo. Morphologic analysis of plaque in patients treated with statins had significantly lower LDL content and matrix metalloproteinases, 50% fewer macrophages, 40% fewer lymphocytes, and an increase in collagen and tissue inhibitors of metalloproteinases compared to placebo-treated patients (27). These data suggest not only a long-term benefit of statins with respect to plaque progression but also more immediate effects of plaque destabilization.

Because of the recognized benefit in vascular event reduction, as well as the evolving understanding of the antiinflammatory effects of the statins, the National Cholesterol Education Program recommends the use of statins in the setting of atherosclerotic disease even when LDL levels are within a "normal" (less than 130 mg/dL) range. This position is supported by data from studies such as the Cholesterol and Recurrent Events (CARE) Trial, which demonstrated benefit in patients with coronary artery disease and normal cholesterol levels. Further, studies indicate that markers of inflammation, such as CRP, TNF-α, IL-6, and IL-8, may be used to demonstrate target efficacy for the antiinflammatory effects of statins in individual patients (28,29).

Cigarette Smoking

Cigarette smoking has been strongly associated with a proatherogenic and prothrombotic condition (30–35). Active compounds from cigarette smoke, including nicotine, carbon monoxide, and other active agents, result in an adverse effect on endothelial function, vascular tone, hemostasis, lipid profile, and inflammatory cells (36,37). The actions of oxidizing and toxic glycation products present in cigarette smoke are believed to be the principal mediators. Smoking also is associated with increased platelet aggregation (due to increased thromboxane A_2) and fibrinogen levels when cigarette smoke is inhaled (38). The effect of platelet hypercoagulability resulting from smoking appears to be a nicotine-independent affect. Studies reveal that nicotine patches used during cessation of smoking do not result in increased activation of the glycoprotein IIb/IIIa receptor (fibrinogen receptor). This suggests that immediate benefits are gained by smoking cessation, in addition to the long-term reduction of stroke and MI.

Diabetes

Hyperglycemia, secondary to diabetes, potentiates atherosclerosis by resulting in endothelial injury and glucose-mediated cross-linking causing the retention of proatherogenic triglyceride-rich lipoprotein within the vessel wall. Elevated lipid levels enhance inflammatory pathways, as previously described. Further, hyperglycemia has been associated with a proinflammatory profile as previously characterized by patients with non–insulin-dependent diabetes mellitus who have a significant increase in circulating activated monocytes compared to nondiabetics (39). Elevated plasma glucose levels also are associated with a rise in plasma ICAM-1 levels. Although conventional wisdom has recommended close control of glucose levels in the setting of diabetes, studies now reveal the pathophysiologic benefit of the antiinflammatory affects of insulin therapy with an association of ICAM-1 level reduction (40).

Hyperhomocystinemia

Elevated plasma homocysteine levels have been identified as an independent risk factor for atherosclerotic vascular disease, including coronary artery, cerebrovascular, and peripheral arterial occlusive disease. Homocysteine is a highly reactive amino acid that is toxic to the vascular endothelium and is believed to have both proatherogenic and prothrombotic effects on vessels. The proatherogenic effects are believed to be mediated through a number of pathophysiologic mechanisms, including the formation of reactive oxygen species during auto-oxidation of homocysteine in the plasma, decreased production of nitric oxide, proliferation of vascular smooth muscle cells, and promotion of LDL oxidation. In addition, prothrombotic effects of plasma homocysteine are postulated to be due to homocysteine-induced vascular endothelial cell injury, which results in increased coagulation factor V, inhibition of thrombomodulin, and a decrease in protein C.

Although unconfirmed by definitive prospective studies, interest in identifying individual patient levels and risk is fostered by the potential beneficial therapeutic effects of antioxidant vitamins in the setting of homocysteine. Given that the adjusted odds ratio for MI and stroke is 2.4 (95% confidence interval 1.0–1.5) in men as reported in the National Health and Nutrition Examination Survey III (NHANES III), elevated homocysteine levels represent fertile ground for potential impact as a modifiable risk factor for stroke (41).

Antioxidant Vitamins

Use of the B vitamin complex (B_{12}, B_6, and folate) has been positively associated with reduction of homocysteine levels (42) and carotid atherosclerotic plaque progression (43). The effects of the B vitamins are related to their ability to serve as cofactors or substrates for homocysteine metabolism. Studies suggest that treatment of levels as low as 9 μM may be beneficial in patients with atherosclerotic disease. In a study conducted by Hackam et al. (43), treatment with B vitamin complex of folic acid 2.5 mg, pyridoxine 25 mg, and cyanocobalamin 250 μg/day demonstrated regression of carotid atherosclerotic plaque as measured by two-dimensional B-mode ultrasound. The greatest benefit in reduction of atherosclerotic plaque progression was seen in patients with levels greater than 14 μmol/L, although benefit was seen as low as 9 μmol/L (43).

Although studies have demonstrated reduction of homocysteine levels and plaque regression with use of the B vitamin complex, reduction in stroke event rate with the therapy has not yet been proved.

Studies that may demonstrate significant benefit in stroke reduction with the use of the B vitamin complex are ongoing. The Vitamin Intervention in Stroke Prevention (VISP) Trial currently is enrolling 3,600 subjects with recent cerebral ischemic event(s) and elevated homocysteine levels (men >9.5 mg/dL;

women >8.5 mg/dL). Subjects will be randomized to a high-dose or low-dose B complex vitamin regimen. Analysis of the primary endpoint of cerebral ischemic event and the secondary endpoint of MI or fatal coronary heart disease will help identify a potential therapeutic dose (44).

Homocysteine levels and their effects on the development of atherosclerosis are known to be related with specific disease states and medication use. Elevated homocysteine levels in chronic renal failure, diabetes, and increased lipoprotein (a) all can accentuate the development of atherosclerotic disease. Elevated homocysteine levels have been associated with isolated systolic hypertension. Use of estrogen-containing oral contraceptives may increase plasma homocysteine concentrations, as will anticonvulsants such as phenytoin and carbamazepine, which interfere with folate metabolism. Excessive intake of alcohol, which interferes with folate utilization, may raise homocysteine concentrations. Cigarette smoking has been associated with plasma folate levels and higher levels of homocysteine.

Despite the lack of evidence showing that reducing plasma homocysteine, in turn, reduces the risk of cardiovascular and cerebrovascular disease, it is reasonable to identify and treat elevated levels given that the B vitamin complex is relatively safe and inexpensive. Optimal therapeutic doses have not been identified, although a minimal supplement of folic acid intake of 400 µg/day or greater is recommended to reduce homocysteine levels (45).

Other Antioxidant Vitamins

The case for use of other antioxidant vitamins, such as vitamins E and C, are still unclear. Data suggest that the beneficial antioxidant effect of vitamin E therapy is enhanced by concomitant use of vitamin C (46,47). The doses of these vitamins necessary for clinically relevant effects on atherosclerosis remain to be determined.

C-Reactive Protein and Other Biologic Markers

Numerous systemic markers have been associated with active atherosclerotic disease, including elevated levels of CRP (48), IL-6, ICAM-1 (8,49), TNF-α, VCAM-1, and fibrinogen (21,50,51). These markers represent a purported increase in the inflammatory profile of carotid and coronary disease, which is associated with thromboembolic stroke and acute coronary syndromes, respectively. Numerous studies have demonstrated that elevated CRP levels predict future cardiovascular events. CRP may be more than just a nonspecific marker of inflammation, and evidence indicates that CRP plays a direct role in the pathogenesis of inflammation in atherosclerosis. CRP has been reported to induce expression of leukocyte adhesion molecules, tissue factor, monocyte recruitment to the arterial wall with enhancement of MCP-1 production, and the ability to activate complement.

Studies demonstrate that elevated CRP levels are associated with vascular disease in both men and women (52). Further, Ridker (52) reported that a strong interactive effect exists between total cholesterol/high-density lipoprotein ratios and high-sensitivity CRP. Analysis of quintile grouped data of both parameters revealed a very high risk for cardiovascular disease in men with high-sensitivity CRP levels and total cholesterol/high-density lipoprotein ratio in the highest quintile. In addition, high-sensitivity CRP had an additive predictive value to all cholesterol levels and demonstrated increased risk even at the lowest lipid levels, conventionally thought to impart a low risk (Fig. 4-2). Although the predictive value of CRP has been associated most commonly with cardiovascular disease, a clear increase in relative risk of ischemic stroke also is associated with elevated CRP levels (53).

Although use of CRP as a marker and potentially as a general indicator of inflammatory vascular disease, the strength of its predictive value is increased by data that reveal treatment associated with these levels imparts significant benefit in the reduction of vascular events. In a randomized clinical trial of acetylsalicylic acid, the highest relative risk reduction of cardiovascular events were seen among patients with the highest baseline level of high-sensitivity CRP in the upper quartile, with a correspondingly declining benefit with lower quartiles (53). The Air Force/Texas Coronary Atherosclerosis Prevention Study (AFCAPS/TexCAPS) revealed a significant reduction of primary cardiovascular events with the use of lovastatin in patients with elevated LDL and CRP levels (54). Significant reductions in vascular events were noted in the lovastatin-treated group, which had high CRP but low LDL levels. The association among inflammation, thrombotic vascular events, and antiinflammatory therapy is supported by the basic literature demonstrating that CRP is a direct stimulant of inflammatory mediators such as MCP-1, an effect blocked by statins (55).

These studies suggest that CRP levels can be used as both a predictive indicator of vascular risk and a marker of efficacy in individual patient therapy (56,57). The specificity of target levels remains to be determined.

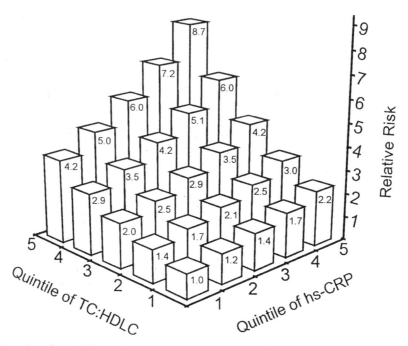

FIG. 4-2. Interactive effects of C-reactive protein and lipid testing as determinants of cardiovascular risk. Hs-CRP, high-sensitivity C-reactive protein assay; TC, total cholesterol. (From Libby P, Ridker PM, Maseri A. Inflammation and atherosclerosis. *Circulation* 2002;105:1135–1143, with permission.)

Drug Interactions: Aspirin, Antiinflammatory Drugs, and Angiotensin-Converting Enzyme Inhibitors

The emerging complexities of the role of inflammation in atherosclerotic plaques prompt a reevaluation of the drug interactions that affect these pathways. Recent reports suggest a potential negative interaction between aspirin and the nonsteroidal antiinflammatory drugs (NSAIDs), as well as between aspirin and the ACE inhibitors.

Interaction Between Aspirin and Angiotensin-Converting Enzyme Inhibitors

ACE inhibitors are known to be effective in the reducing the risk of MI, stroke, and vascular death in patients with congestive heart failure and vascular disease. Because antiplatelet agents, such as aspirin, are routinely prescribed in patients with atherosclerotic disease, the use of the ACE inhibitors and aspirin is a common combination in a large patient population.

ACE is responsible for converting angiotensin-1 into angiotensin-2, which is an agent that has potent vasoconstrictor effects and the potential for increasing inflammatory components such as oxygen-free

radicals, leukocyte adhesion molecules, inflammatory cytokines, and transcription factors. The vasodilatory effects of ACE inhibitors are believed to be mediated by three mechanisms: prevention of increased angiotensin-2 levels; inhibition of breakdown of bradykinin (a vasodilator) (58); and increased breakdown of arachidonic acid into vasodilatory prostaglandins I$_2$ (PGI$_2$) and E$_2$ (PGE$_2$). The specific percentage by which each of these mechanisms has an effect on vasodilation is unclear. Acetylsalicylic acid is believed to have a potentially negative counter effect on ACE inhibitors. Aspirin irreversibly blocks cyclooxygenase, which blocks platelet thromboxane A$_2$, a vasoconstrictor and platelet activator. Aspirin also reduces the production of PGG$_2$ from arachidonic acid, thereby decreasing the vasodilatory prostaglandins PGE$_2$ and PGI$_2$. It is the blockade of these prostaglandins that is believed to be the negative interactive effect of aspirin on a potential beneficial effect of ACE inhibitors.

Studies suggest that the beneficial effects of preserving bradykinin and increasing PGI$_2$ and PGE$_2$ by ACE inhibitors are only a loading effect of ACE inhibitor dosing and that these factors play a much less important role in chronic dosing of this class of drugs (59,60). Further, studies have reported that only high doses of aspirin have a significant negative effect on levels of prostaglandins, with lower doses having a less profound effect (61).

Conflicting data exist as to the actual clinical consequences of the combination of ACE inhibitors and aspirin. Studies by Katz et al. (62) using ACE inhibitors and aspirin revealed no difference in mean arterial pressure, forearm blood flow, and forearm vascular resistance in patients who were randomized to placebo and enalapril compared to patients randomized to aspirin 325 mg and enalapril 10 mg/day.

Although the interaction between ACE inhibitors and aspirin has theoretical complications, use of the combination in patients with congestive heart failure and atherosclerosis is generally recommended. Large randomized trials currently are underway to study the endpoint effects of MI, stroke, and vascular death in patients randomized to this combination and should provide definitive information with respect to clinically relevant recommendations.

Interaction of Aspirin and Cyclooxygenase Inhibitors

The mechanism by which aspirin reduces the risk of heart attack and stroke through the inhibition of platelet aggregation centers around the irreversible inhibition of cyclooxygenase-1 (COX-1). Recent studies raise the concern that NSAIDs can impede the antiplatelet activity of aspirin by preventing the irreversible acetylation of the serine residue in the hydrophobic channel of platelet COX-1 (63,64). COX-1 inhibitors, such as ibuprofen, are believed to have the greatest effect on the inhibition of aspirin's activity. COX-2 selective drugs, such as rofecoxib and celecoxib, have a much lower affinity for the COX-1 enzyme. These drugs, which are geared to specifically reduce inflammation, also decrease vascular prostacyclin (PGI_2) production, thereby decreasing vasodilation and the antiaggregate properties of blood vessels. These features of COX-2 inhibition theoretically could shift the in vivo state to a more prothrombotic setting. Further, meta-analysis of the COX-2 inhibitor studies performed predominantly in patients with arthritis suggests that prospective studies examining the effects of COX-2 inhibition on cardiovascular and cerebrovascular risk may be warranted (65).

A randomized crossover study of combination dosing of aspirin with COX-1 and COX-2 inhibitors revealed that use of ibuprofen, given either 30 minutes before aspirin dosing or multiple times per day, antagonized the irreversible platelet inhibition induced by aspirin. Assessment of the mean inhibition of platelet COX-1 activity and platelet aggregation revealed significant reduction in aspirin efficiency in combination with COX-1 but not with COX-2 inhibitors (63). Further studies have revealed no evidence that COX-2 inhibitors increase the risk of cardiovascular thromboembolic events compared to conventional COX-1 NSAIDs (66).

In summary, the data suggest that ibuprofen could limit the cardioprotective effects of aspirin in the "at risk" population, depending on dosing regimen. COX-2 inhibitors do not evoke the same caution with respect to the antiplatelet effects of aspirin; however, studies remain to be performed that would examine any clinically relevant effects of vascular prostacyclin blockade on the incidence of stroke and heart attack.

THE ROLE OF INFECTION IN ATHEROSCLEROSIS

Infection has been strongly associated with the formation, progression, and activation of atherosclerotic disease (67–69). Injury to the vessel wall resulting in the migration of inflammatory cells, and the release of proinflammatory cytokines [T_h1 (helper T-cell) cytokines] and growth factors, has been attributed to infectious agents. In addition, memory T-lymphocytes for specific infectious agents, with or without the presence of the organism, have been identified in atherosclerotic plaques of all ages. This suggests that infection may play a role in the initiation of plaque formation, which may progress without the infection necessarily being chronic. Further, resting or "inactive" memory T-cells may be activated by reinfection or endogenous antigens that mimic prior sensitizing organisms. This event could promote rapid proliferation of T-lymphocytes, resulting in plaque destabilization, rupture, and clot formation leading to heart attack and stroke.

Several specific types of infectious agents have been proposed to be causally related to atherosclerosis on the basis of epidemiologic and pathologic studies. These agents include cytomegalovirus and other herpes viruses (70,71), *Helicobacter pylori* (72–74), chronic periodontal disease with Gram-negative organisms (75), and *Chlamydia pneumoniae.* The causal relationship between any of these infections and atherosclerosis remains unproved, but the accumulated data regarding the plausible role of *C. pneumoniae* in common forms of chronic vascular disease are the most convincing. The following sections review the data on each of these organisms and the pathogenetic mechanisms and potential clinical implications of the data for each.

Herpes Viruses

Data have long been available that support the premise that a viral infection initiates atherogenesis (76). Herpes viruses were demonstrated many years ago to induce atherosclerosis-like changes in animal models (77,78). An avian herpes virus was found to cause atherosclerosis similar to that seen in humans in both normal and hypercholesterolemic chickens. In addition, herpes simplex virus has been found in early aortic atherosclerotic lesions (79).

Cytomegalovirus

Human serologic evidence of cytomegalovirus (CMV) infection is more common in patients with coronary artery disease than in normal controls (80). A cross-sectional study of serologies in patients showed a higher proportion of CMV seropositivity in patients with angiographically documented stenosis (81). Results of other studies have been less definitive about the role of CMV in atherosclerosis (82–84). In the Intermountain Heart Study, however, both CRP and CMV seropositivity were associated with long-term mortality in patients with angiographically verified coronary artery disease. Restenosis after coronary angioplasty also occurs more frequently in patients positive for CMV (85,86). CMV has been detected by polymerase chain reaction (PCR) techniques in atherosclerotic plaques in patients with coronary disease more frequently than in patients without atherosclerosis (87). These findings represent associations only. An attempt to demonstrate causality has led to experiments of CMV infection in animals and in vitro human tissue. The results of these studies reveal that CMV increases the expression of PDGF and transforming growth factor (88) and regulates proinflammatory cytokines and transcription factors (89,90). CMV promotes human vascular smooth muscle cell proliferation and the coagulation cascade (91–93), and it facilitates adherence of leukocytes to endothelial cells (94–96).

Chlamydia Pneumoniae

Chlamydia pneumoniae has been widely reported to be identified in coronary and carotid atherosclerotic plaque. In addition, elevated immunoglobulin A levels have been strongly associated with symptomatic atherosclerotic disease (97). A number of factors make *C. pneumoniae* an attractive candidate as a potential mediator of plaque activation. *Chlamydia pneumoniae* is an obligate intracellular parasite that commonly infects mononuclear phagocytes. Macrophages derived from monocytes are characteristically localized in human atherosclerotic plaque and provide a mechanism for entry of the organism into the vessel wall (98). Infection with chlamydia may create a persistent nonlethal infection that can lead to a chronic inflammatory state (99).

There are multiple mechanisms by which chronic infection can contribute to an inflammatory state in atherosclerosis. Endotoxin release and heat shock protein-60 (HSP-60) from chlamydia have been associated with an increase of TNF-α and matrix metalloproteinase from macrophages (100,101). Chlamydia HSP-60 causes oxidation of LDL, which alters LDL to its highly atherogenic form (102) and converts macrophages into foam cells (103). *Chlamydia pneumoniae* increases CRP (104) and tissue factor, and it can cause a hypersensitivity reaction upon reexposure to organism (105,106). Animal studies have demonstrated an association with inoculation of *C. pneumoniae* and the development of atherosclerotic disease in New Zealand white rabbits (107,108) and in apoE-deficient mice (109). Despite the association, no definitive proof exists that the presence of chlamydia or other infectious agents can cause the initiation or progression of the atherosclerotic plaque in humans.

Even with the lack of proof, antibiotic therapy has been used in the population at risk for cardiac events. These studies have met with mixed results. Theoretically, reduction of inflammatory effects due to the eradication of infectious organisms holds some promise. Reduction of MI has been associated with a history of prior use of tetracycline antibiotics (110). Among 3,315 patients aged 75 years or older with MI and 13,139 matched controls, the patients were significantly less likely to have taken tetracycline or quinolone antibiotics, although no beneficial effect was found for macrolides, sulfonamides, penicillins, or cephalosporins (110). Conflicting prospective studies reveal that a reduction of cardiovascular events was not observed with antibiotic use in a 2-year follow-up study (111).

The data currently do not support the use of antibiotic therapy for patients with symptomatic atherosclerotic disease. Accurate identification of infected plaque, duration of antibiotic therapy, and need for recurrent antibiotic therapy remain to be delineated for testing this potential therapy.

Helicobacter Pylori

Helicobacter pylori is another organism postulated to initiate or affect the pathophysiology of atherosclerosis. Identification of *H. pylori* (chronic infectious state) as an etiologic factor for gastritis and peptic ulcer disease (112–114) has sparked interest in the involvement of this organism in other potentially chronic inflammatory disease processes such as atherosclerosis. Several retrospective epidemiologic studies have suggested an association between the presence of *H. pylori* and coronary disease by identifying a higher antibody titer in patients who experienced a coronary event. Most of these studies were small and were unable to confirm the association when correcting for other risk factors (72,115–120). In addition, studies to date have been unable to identify *H. pylori* in atherosclerotic plaques, in contrast to positive studies with other organisms such as chlamydia (121).

It has been suggested that virulence factors among subtypes of *H. pylori* may have led to inconsistency of the data. The *H. pylori* strain carrying the virulence factor cytotoxin-associated gene A and producing cytotoxin-associated protein A was found to be associated with an increase in cytokine expression (122,123). This finding has not been confirmed in subsequent studies (115). Because of the nature of *H. pylori* and its association with chronic inflammatory process, *H. pylori* will continue to be studied as a potential factor in causing atherosclerosis.

Periodontal Disease

Periodontal disease is a chronic progressive infection of the gingiva, connective tissue, and alveolar bone that could contribute to atherosclerosis by the mechanism of chronic systemic inflammation. The prevalence of advanced periodontitis has been estimated to be approximately 15% in patients aged 60 to 64 years (124), and as high as 45% in patients older than 65 years (125). There is an increased prevalence of periodontitis among African-Americans (126,127), Mexican-Americans, and other Hispanic groups, each of which has an increased risk of stroke compared with whites. In addition, periodontal disease is expected to increase with the aging of the population. Given the high prevalence of periodontal disease, any increased association in risk of atherosclerosis with periodontal disease could have a substantial adverse clinical impact on health in the United States.

The National Health and Nutrition Examination Survey I (NHANES I) demonstrated that periodontitis was associated with a 25% increased risk of coronary heart disease. The association was particularly strong in patients younger than 50 years. More recent study with rigorous adjustment for other confounding factors demonstrated an association between periodontal disease and stroke (128) but not heart disease (129), suggesting that stroke (relative risk of 2.1) and coronary artery disease may differ in their relationship to periodontal disease.

More than 300 types of bacteria may live in the oral cavity, but only a minority cause periodontal disease. Gram-positive organisms commonly colonize healthy teeth, whereas Gram-negative organisms are associated with gingivitis and periodontitis. These Gram-negative organisms may induce pathogenic effects that contribute to atherosclerosis and up-regulate coagulation factors that cause plaque to be prothrombotic.

Research continues to determine specific relationships between infection and inflammatory processes that may lead to the development of an active or "unstable" atherosclerotic plaque.

GENETIC CONTRIBUTION TO INFLAMMATION AND ATHEROSCLEROSIS

The pathophysiology involved in the initiation, progression, and activation of atherosclerotic plaques is a complex interplay of environmental risk factor exposure and genetic condition with intermediate phenotypes (130). Individual genetic profiles can affect pathophysiologic mediators of plaque development, and several large-scale epidemiologic studies have shown that family history is associated with increased risk of stroke (131,132). Although few doubt that there is a hereditary contribution to cerebrovascular risk, the quantification of genetic factors remains elusive. Clearly genes have been identified that influence traditional vascular risk factors such as hypertension and diabetes. Single gene disorders that manifest primarily as cerebrovascular disease have been recognized, including cerebral autosomal dominant arteriopathy with subcortical infarcts and leukoencephalopathy (CADASIL) (133); however, the majority of ischemic strokes likely are multigenic and reflect complex interactions of genes and environment. Along that line, many of the genes that regulate inflammatory cytokines and adhesion molecules have been found to be polymorphic in nature. Specific alleles for cytokines, such as TNF-α and IL-1β, have been associated with increased frequency in other inflammatory diseases such as lupus, chronic inflammatory bowel disease, and multiple sclerosis (134–136). Later studies demonstrated that these polymorphisms of the inflammatory cytokine pathways are associated with coronary and carotid atherosclerosis (137,138). The emergence and identification of susceptibility factors can enhance the ability to predict in advance who is at greatest risk for developing vascular disease.

Host genetic susceptibility may include a predisposition for infectious organisms that can interact with overall individual risk (139,140). A recent study revealed that IL-1 gene variance, which is associated with an increased risk of coronary artery disease, imparted a greater than 25% increase of coronary vascular disease prevalence in the presence of seropositivity for *C. pneumoniae*. Further, the combination of *C. pneumonia* positivity and the presence of an IL-1 gene variant was associated with a two-fold increase in MI compared to patients with either seropositivity or the gene variance alone (141). These data serve to highlight not only the multiple gene influence in susceptibility for disease but also the interplay of genetic and environmental factors that are potential targets for risk factor modification.

Understanding genetic susceptibility has implications for therapeutic intervention in the future. Theoretically, gene therapy could deliver wild-type proteins to atherosclerotic lesions to prevent progression, promote regression, stimulate collateral vascular formation, and stabilize plaque. Preliminary studies generated enthusiasm with the discovery of vascular endothelial-derived growth factor, which showed potential for therapeutic gene intervention in coronary atherosclerotic disease (142). Although it has fallen short of its desired goals (143), gene modification is an expanding field of study, and care must be taken to derive consensus guidelines (144) so as to promote both good science and adequate patient safeguards.

REFERENCES

1. Gillum RF, Sempas CT. The end of the long-term decline in stroke mortality in the United States? *Stroke* 1997;28:1527–1529.
2. Benveniste EN. Inflammatory cytokines within the central nervous system: source, function, and mechanism of action. *Am J Physiol* 1992;263:C1–C16.
3. Hallenbeck JM. Inflammatory reactions at the blood-endothelial interface in acute stroke. *Adv Neurol* 1996; 71:281–300.
4. Rothwell NJ, Loddick SA, Stroemer P. Interleukins and cerebral ischemia. *Int Rev Neurobiol* 1997;40: 281–298.
5. Bevilacqua MP, Pober JS, Majeau GR, et al. Interleukin-1 (IL-1) induces biosynthesis and cell surface expression of pro-coagulant activity in human vascular endothelial cells. *J Exp Med* 1984;160:618–623.
6. Nawroth PP, Handley DA, Esmon CT, et al. Interleukin-1 induces endothelial cell procoagulant while suppressing cell-surface anticoagulant activity. *Proc Natl Acad Sci U S A* 1986;83:3460–3464.
7. Nawroth PP, Stern DM. Modulation of endothelial cell hemostatic properties by tumor necrosis factor. *J Exp Med* 1986;163:740–745.
8. DeGraba TJ, Sirén A-L, Penix L, et al. Increased endothelial expression of intercellular adhesion molecule-1 (ICAM-1) in symptomatic vs asymptomatic human atherosclerotic plaque. *Stroke* 1998;29: 1405–1410.
9. Jander S, Sitzer M, Schumann R, et al. Inflammation in high-grade carotid stenosis: a possible role for macrophages and t cells in plaque destabilization. *Stroke* 1998;29:1625–1630.
10. van der Wal AC, Becker AE, van de Loos CM, et al. Site of intimal rupture or erosion of thrombosed coronary atherosclerotic plaques is characterized by an inflammatory process irrespective of the dominant plaque morphology. *Circulation* 1994;89:36–44.
11. Morigi M, Zoja C, Figliuzzi M, et al. Fluid shear stress modulates surface expression of adhesion molecules by endothelial cells. *Blood* 1995;85:1696–1703.
12. Malek AM, Jackman R, Rosenberg RD, et al. Endothelial expression of thrombomodulin is reversibly regulated by fluid shear stress. *Circ Res* 1994;74:852–860.
13. The Heart Outcomes Prevention Evaluation Study Investigators. Effects of an angiotensin-converting-enzyme inhibitor, ramipril, on cardiovascular events in high-risk patients. *N Engl J Med* 2000;342:145–153.
14. Fukuhara M, Geary RL, Diz DI, et al. Angiotensin-converting enzyme expression in human carotid artery atherosclerosis. *Hypertension* 2000;35[Pt 2]:353–359.
15. Dzau VJ. Mechanism of protective effects of ACE inhibition on coronary artery disease. *Eur Heart J* 1998;19[Suppl J]:J2–J6.
16. Andersen S, Schalkwijk CG, Stehouwer RCD, et al. Angiotensin-II blockade is associated with decreased plasma leukocyte adhesion molecule levels in diabetic nephropathy. *Diabetes Care* 2000;23:1031–1032.
17. Fitzgerald JD. By what means might beta-blockers prolong life after acute myocardial infarction? *Eur Heart J* 1987;3:945–951.
18. Steinberg D, Parthasarathy S, Carew TE, et al. Beyond cholesterol: modifications of low-density lipoprotein that increase its atherogenicity. *N Engl J Med* 1989; 320:915–924.
19. Stemme S, Faber B, Holm J, et al. T-lymphocytes from human atherosclerotic plaques recognize oxidized low density lipoprotein. *Proc Natl Acad Sci U S A* 1995;92: 3893–3897.
20. Scandinavian Simvastatin Study Group. Randomised trial of cholesterol lowering in 4444 patients with coronary heart disease: the Scandinavian Simvastatin Survival Study (4S). *Lancet* 1994;344:1383–1389.
21. Sacks FM, Pfeffer MA, Moye LA, et al., for the Recurrent Events Trial Investigators. The effect of pravastatin on coronary events after myocardial infarction in patients with average cholesterol levels. *N Engl J Med* 1996;335:1001–1009.
22. Ridker PM, Rifai N, Pfeffer MA, et al. Inflammation, pravastatin, and the risk of coronary events after myocardial infarction in patients with average cholesterol levels. For the Cholesterol and Recurrent Events (CARE) Investigators. *Circulation* 1998;98:839–844.

23. Romano M, Diomede L, Sironi M, et al. Inhibition of monocyte chemotactic protein-1 synthesis by statins. *Lab Invest* 2000;80:1095–1100.

24. Bustos C, Hernandez-Presa MA, Orgego M, et al. HMG-CoA reductase inhibition by atorvastatin reduces neointimal inflammation in a rabbit model of atherosclerosis. *J Am Coll Cardiol* 1998;32: 2057–2064.

25. Kothe H, Dalhoff K, Rupp J, et al. Hydroxymethylglutaryl coenzyme A reductase inhibitors modify the inflammatory response of human macrophages and endothelial cells infected with *Chlamydia pneumoniae*. *Circulation* 2000;101:1760–1763.

26. Vaughan CJ, Gotto AM Jr, Basson CT. The evolving role of statins in the management of atherosclerosis. *J Am Coll Cardiol* 2000;35:1–10.

27. Crisby J, Nordin-Fredriksson G, Shah PK, et al. Pravastatin treatment increases collagen content and decreases lipid content, inflammation, metalloproteinases, and cell death in human carotid plaques. *Circulation* 2001;103:926–933.

28. Ridker PM, Rifai N, Pfeffer MA, et al., for the Cholesterol and Recurrent Events (CARE) Investigators. Long-term effects of pravastatin on plasma concentration of C-reactive protein. The Cholesterol and Recurrent Events (CARE) Investigators. *Circulation* 1999; 100:230–235.

29. Musial J, Undas A, Gajewski P, et al. Anti-inflammatory effects of simvastatin in subjects with hypercholesterolemia. *Int J Cardiol* 2001;77:247–253.

30. Zhu B, Sun Y, Sievers RE, et al. Passive smoking increases experimental atherosclerosis in cholesterol-fed rabbits. *J Am Coll Cardiol* 1993;21:225–232.

31. Miller GJ, Bauer KA, Cooper JA, et al. Activation of the coagulant pathway in cigarette smokers. *Thromb Haemost* 1998;79:549–553.

32. Newby DE, Wright RA, Labinjoh C, et al. Endothelial dysfunction, impaired endogenous fibrinolysis, and cigarette smoking. *Circulation* 1999;99:1411–1415.

33. Zidovetzki R, Chen P, Fisher M, et al. Nicotine increases plasminogen activator inhibitor-1 production by human brain endothelial cells via protein kinase C-associated pathway. *Stroke* 1999;30:651–655.

34. Markovitz JH, Tolbert L, Winders SE. Increased serotonin receptor density and platelet GPIIb/IIIa activation among smokers. *Arterioscler Thromb Vasc Biol* 1999;19:762–766.

35. Matetzky S, Tani S, Kangavari S, et al. Smoking increases tissue factor expression in atherosclerotic plaques: implications for plaque thrombogenicity. *Circulation* 2000;102:602–604.

36. Celermajer DS, Adams MR, Clarkson P, et al. Passive smoking and impaired endothelium-dependent arterial dilatation in healthy young adults. *N Engl J Med* 1996: 334:150–154.

37. Hutchison SJ, Sudhir K, Sievers RE, et al. Effects of L-arginine on atherogenesis and endothelial dysfunction due to secondhand smoke. *Hypertension* 1999;34: 44–50.

38. Benowitz NL, Fitzgerald GA, Wilson M, et al. Nicotine effects on eicosanoid formation and hemostatic function: comparison of transdermal nicotine and cigarette smoking. *J Am Coll Cardiol* 1993;22: 1159–1167.

39. Patiño R, Ibarra J, Rodriguez A, et al. Circulating monocytes in patients with diabetes mellitus, arterial disease, and increased CD14 expression. *Am J Cardiol* 2000;85:1288–1291.

40. Marfella R, Esposito K, Giunta R, et al. Circulating adhesion molecules in humans: role of hyperglycemia and hyperinsulinemia. *Circulation* 2000;101: 2247–2251.

41. Morris MS, Jacques PF, Rosenberg IH, et al. Serum total homocysteine concentration is related to self-reported heart attack or stroke history among men and women in the NHANES III. *J Nutr* 2000;130: 3073–3076.

42. Woodside JV, Yarnell JW, McMaster D, et al. Effect of B-group vitamins and antioxidant vitamins on hyperhomocystinemia: a double-blind, randomized, factorial-design, controlled trial. *Am J Clin Nutr* 1998;67: 858–866.

43. Hackam DG, Peterson JC, Spence JD. What level of plasma homocyst(e)ine should be treated?: effects of vitamin therapy on progression of carotid atherosclerosis in patients with homocyst(e)ine levels above and below 14 µmol/L. *Am J Hypertens* 2000;13:105–110.

44. Spence JD, Howard VJ, Chambless LE, et al. Vitamin Intervention for Stroke Prevention (VISP) trial: rationale and design. *Neuroepidemiology* 2001;20:16–25.

45. Gerhard GT, Duell PB. Homocysteine and atherosclerosis. *Curr Opin Lipidol* 1999;10:417–428.

46. Liao K, Yin M. Individual and combined antioxidant effects of seven phenolic agents in human erythrocyte membrane ghosts and phosphatidylcholine liposome systems: importance of the partition coefficient. *J Agric Food Chem* 2000;48:2266–2270.

47. Hamilton IMJ, Gilmore WS, Benzie IFF, et al. Interactions between vitamins C and E in human subjects. *Br J Nutr* 2000;84:261–267.

48. Tataru MC, Heinrich J, Junker R, et al. C-reactive protein and the severity of atherosclerosis in myocardial infarction patients with stable angina pectoris. *Eur Heart J* 2000;21:1000–1008.

49. Rohde LE, Lee RT, Rivero J, et al. Circulating cell adhesion molecules are correlated with ultrasound-based assessment of carotid atherosclerosis. *Arterioscler Thromb Vasc Biol* 1998;18:1765–1770.

50. Ridker PM, Rifai N, Pfeffer M, et al. Elevation of tumor necrosis factor-alpha and increased risk of recurrent coronary events after myocardial infarction. *Circulation* 2000;101:2149–2153.

51. Hwang SJ, Ballantyne CM, Sharrett AR, et al. Circulating adhesion molecules VCAM-1, ICAM-1 and E-selectin in carotid atherosclerosis and incident coronary heart disease cases: the atherosclerosis risk in communities (ARIC) study. *Circulation* 1997;96: 4219–4225.

52. Ridker, PM. High sensitivity C-reactive protein. *Circulation* 2001;103:1813–1818.

53. Ridker PM, Cushman M, Stanpfer MJ, et al. Inflammation, aspirin, and the risk of cardiovascular disease in apparently healthy men. *N Engl J Med* 1997;336: 973–979.

54. Downs JR, Clearfield M, Weis S, et al. Primary prevention of acute coronary events with lovastatin in men and women with average cholesterol levels: results of AFCAPS/TexCAPS. Air Force/Texas Coro-

nary Atherosclerosis Prevention Study. *JAMA* 1998; 279:1615–1622.

55. Pasceri V, Chang J, Willerson JT, et al. Modulation of C-reactive protein-mediated monocyte chemoattractant protein-1 induction in human endothelial cells by anti-atherosclerosis drugs. *Circulation* 2001;103: 2531–2534.

56. Ridker PM, Rifai N, Pfeffer MA, et al., for the Cholesterol and Recurrent Events (CARE) Investigators. Long-term effects of pravastatin on plasma concentration of C-reactive protein. The Cholesterol and Recurrent Events (CARE) Investigators. *Circulation* 1999; 100:230–235.

57. Ridker PM, Cushman M, Stampfer MJ, et al. Inflammation, aspirin, and the risk of cardiovascular disease in apparently healthy men. *N Engl J Med* 1997;336: 973–979.

57a. Libby P, Ridker PM, Maseri A. Inflammation and atherosclerosis. *Circulation* 2002;105:1135–1143.

58. Carretro OA, Miyazaki S, Scidli AG. Role of kinins in the acute anti-hypertensive effect of converting enzyme inhibitor, captopril. *Hypertension* 1985;3: 8–22.

59. Baur LH, Schipperheyn JJ, van der Laarse A, et al. Combining salicylate and enalapril in patients with coronary artery disease and heart failure. *Br Heart J* 1995;73:227–236.

60. van Wijngaarden J, Smit AJ, de Graeff PA, et al. Effects of acetylsalicylic acid on peripheral hemodynamics in patients with chronic heart failure treated with angiotensin-converting enzyme inhibitors. *J Cardiovasc Pharmacol* 1994;23:240–245.

61. Weksler BB, Pett SB, Alonso D, et al. Differential inhibition by aspirin of vascular and platelet prostaglandin synthesis in atherosclerotic patients. *N Engl J Med* 1983;308:800–805.

62. Katz SD, Radin M, Graves T, et al. Effect of aspirin and ifetroban on skeletal muscle blood flow in patients with congestive heart failure treated with Enalapril. Ifetroban Study Group. *J Am Coll Cardiol* 1999;34: 170–176.

63. Catella-Lawson F, Reilly MP, Kapoor SC, et al. Cyclooxygenase inhibitors and the antiplatelet effects of aspirin. *N Engl J Med* 2001;345:1809–1817.

64. Ouellet M, Riendeau D, Percival MD. A high level of cyclooxygenase-2 inhibitor selectivity is associated with a reduced interference of platelet cyclooxygenase-1 inactivation by aspirin. *Proc Natl Acad Sci U S A* 2001;98:14583–14588.

65. Mukherjee D, Nissen SE, Topol EEJ. Risk of cardiovascular events associated with selective COX-2 inhibitors. *JAMA* 2001;286:954–959.

66. White WB, Faich G, Whelton A, et al. Comparison of thromboembolic events in patients treated with celecoxib, a cyclooxygenase-2 specific inhibitor, versus ibuprofen or diclofenac. *Am J Cardiol* 2002;89: 425–430.

67. Libby P, Egan D, Skarlatos S. Roles of infectious agents in atherosclerosis and re-stenosis: an assessment of the evidence and need for future research. *Circulation* 1997;96:4095–4103.

68. Epstein SE, Zhou YF, Zhu J. Infection and atherosclerosis: emerging mechanistic paradigms. *Circulation* 1999;100:E20–E28.

69. Vercellotti G. Infectious agents that play a role in atherosclerosis and vasculopathies. What are they? What do we do about them? *Can J Cardiol* 1999;15[Suppl B]:13B–15B.

70. Nieto FJ, Adam E, Sorlie P, et al. Cohort study of cytomegalovirus infection as a risk factor for carotid intimal-medial thickening, a measure of subclinical atherosclerosis. *Circulation* 1996;94:922–927.

71. Sorlie PD, Adam E, Melnick SL, et al. Cytomegalovirus/herpes virus and carotid atherosclerosis: the ARIC Study. *J Med Virol* 1994;42:33–37.

72. Whincup PH, Mendall MA, Perry IJ, et al. Prospective relations between *Helicobacter pylori* infection, coronary heart disease, and stroke in middle-aged men. *Heart* 1996;75:568–572.

73. Patel P, Mendall MA, Carrington D, et al. Association of Helicobacter pylori and Chlamydia pneumoniae infections with coronary heart disease and cardiovascular risk factors. *BMJ* 1995;311:711–714.

74. Ponzetto A, La Rovere MT, Sanseverino P, et al. Association of Helicobacter pylori with coronary heart disease. Study confirms previous findings. *BMJ* 1996; 312:251.

75. Beck J, Garcia R, Heiss G, et al. Periodontal disease and cardiovascular disease. *J Periodontol* 1996;67: 1123–1137.

76. Span AH, vam Dam-Mieras MC, Mullers W, et al. The effect of virus infection on the adherence of leukocytes or platelets to endothelial cells. *Eur J Clin Invest* 1991; 21:331–338.

77. Hajjar DP. Viral pathogenesis of atherosclerosis. *Am J Pathol* 1991;139:1195–1211.

78. Minick CR, Fabricant CG, Fabricant J, et al. Atheroarteriosclerosis induced by infection with a herpes virus. *Am J Pathol* 1979;96:673–700.

79. Benditt EP, Barrett T, McDougall JK. Viruses in the etiology of atherosclerosis. *Proc Natl Acad Sci U S A* 1983;80:6386–6389.

80. Melnick JL, Adam E, Debakey ME. Possible role of cytomegalovirus in atherogenesis. *JAMA* 1990;263: 2204–2207.

81. Zhu J, Quyyumi AA, Norman JE, et al. Cytomegalovirus in the pathogenesis of atherosclerosis: the role of inflammation as reflected by elevated C-reactive protein levels. *J Am Coll Cardiol* 1999;34:1738–1743.

82. Ridker PM, Hennekens CH, Stampfer MJ, et al. Prospective study of herpes simplex virus, cytomegalovirus, and the risk of future myocardial infarction and stroke. *Circulation* 1998;98:2796–2799.

83. Ridker PM, Hennekens CH, Roitman-Johnson B, et al. Plasma concentration of soluble ICAM-1 and risk of future myocardial infarction in apparently healthy men. *Lancet* 1998;351:88–92.

84. Fagerberg B, Gnarpe J, Gnarpe H, et al. *Chlamydia pneumoniae* but not cytomegalovirus antibodies are associated with future risk of stroke and cardiovascular disease. *Stroke* 1999;30:299–305.

85. Speir E, Modali R, Huang ES, et al. Potential role of human cytomegalovirus and p53 interaction in coronary restenosis. *Science* 1994;265:391–394.

86. Zhou YF, Leon MB, Waclawiw MA, et al. Association between prior cytomegalovirus infection and the risk of restenosis after coronary atherectomy. *N Engl J Med* 1996;335:624–630.

87. Hendricks MG, Salimans MM, van Boven CP, et al. High prevalence of latently present cytomegalovirus in arterial walls of patients suffering from grade III atherosclerosis. *Am J Pathol* 1990;136:23–28.

88. Lemstrom KB, Aho PT, Bruggeman CA, et al. Cytomegalovirus infection enhances mRNA expression of platelet-derived growth factor-BB and transforming growth factor-beta 1 in rat aortic allografts: possible mechanism for cytomegalovirus-enhanced graft arteriosclerosis. *Arterioscler Thromb* 1994;14:2043–2052.

89. Geist LJ, Monick MM, Stinski MF, et al. The immediate early genes of human cytomegalovirus upregulate tumor necrosis factor-alpha gene expression. *J Clin Invest* 1994;93:474–478.

90. Kowalik TF, Wing B, Haskill JS, et al. Multiple mechanisms are implicated in the regulation of NF-B activity during human cytomegalovirus infection. *Proc Natl Acad Sci U S A* 1993;90:1107–1111.

91. Van Dam-Mieras MCE, Muller AD, van Hinsbergh VWM, et al. The procoagulant response of cytomegalovirus infected endothelial cells. *Thromb Haemost* 1992;68:364–370.

92. Eingen OR, Silverstein RL, Friedman HM, et al. Viral activation of the coagulation cascade: molecular interactions at the surface of infected endothelial cells. *Cell* 1990;61:657–662.

93. Pryzdial ELG, Wright JF. Prothrombinase assembly on an enveloped virus: evidence that the cytomegalovirus surface contains procoagulant phospholipid. *Blood* 1994;84:3749–3757.

94. Span AH, vam Dam-Mieras MC, Mullers W, et al. The effect of virus infection on the adherence of leukocytes or platelets to endothelial cells. *Eur J Clin Invest* 1991; 21:331–338.

95. Grundy JE, Downes KL. Up-regulation of LFA-3 and ICAM-1 of the surface of fibroblasts infected with cytomegalovirus. *Immunology* 1993;78:405–412.

96. Span AH, Mullers W, Miltenberg AM, et al. Cytomegalovirus induced PMN adherence in relation to an ELAM-1 antigen present on infected endothelial cell monolayers. *Immunology* 1991;72:355–360.

97. LaBiche R, Koziol D, Quinn T, et al. Presence of *Chlamydia pneumoniae* in human symptomatic and asymptomatic carotid atherosclerotic plaque. *Stroke* 2001;32:855–860.

98. Gaydos CA, Summersgill JT, Sahne NN, et al. Replication of Chlamydia pneumoniae in vitro in human macrophages, endothelial cells, and aortic artery smooth muscle cells. *Infect Immun* 1996;64: 1614–1620.

99. Beatty WL, Byrne GI, Morrison RP. Repeated and persistent infection with Chlamydia and the development of chronic inflammation and disease. *Trends Microbiol* 1994;2:94–98.

100. Kol A, Sukhova GK, Lichtman AH, et al. Chlamydial heat shock protein 60 localizes in human atheroma and regulates macrophage tumor necrosis factor-α and matrix metalloproteinase expression. *Circulation* 1998;98:300–307.

101. Rothermel CD, Schachter J, Lavrich P, et al. *Chlamydia trachomatis*-induced production of interleukin-1 by human monocytes. *Infect Immun* 1989;57: 2705–2711.

102. Kalayoglu MV, Hoerneman B, LaVerda D, et al. Cellular oxidation of low density lipoprotein by Chlamydia pneumoniae. *J Infect Dis* 1999;180:780–790.

103. Kalayoglu MV, Byrne BI. Induction of macrophage foam cell formation by Chlamydia pneumoniae. *J Infect Dis* 1998;177:725–729.

104. Papanicolaou DA, Wilder RL, Manolagas SC, et al. The pathophysiologic roles of interleukin-6 in human disease. *Ann Intern Med* 1998;128:127–137.

105. Watkins NG, Hadlow WJ, Moos AB, et al. Ocular delayed hypersensitivity: a pathogenetic mechanism of chlamydial conjunctivitis in guinea pigs. *Proc Natl Acad Sci U S A* 1986;83:7480–7487.

106. Morrison RP, Belland RJ, Lyng K, et al. Chlamydial disease pathogenesis. The 57-kD chlamydial hypersensitivity antigen is a stress response protein. *J Exp Med* 1989;170:1271–1283.

107. Laitinen K, Aluria A, Pyhala L, et al. Chlamydia pneumoniae infection induces inflammatory changes in the aortas of rabbits. *Infect Immun* 1997;65:4832–4835.

108. Fong IW, Chiu B, Viira E, et al. Rabbit model for Chlamydia pneumoniae infection. *J Clin Microbiol* 1997;35:48–52.

109. Moazed TC, Campbell LA, Rosenfeld ME, et al. Chlamydia pneumoniae accelerates the progression of atherosclerosis in apolipoprotein E deficient mice. *J Infect Dis* 1999;180:238–241.

110. Meier CR, Derby LE, Jick SS, et al. Antibiotics and risk of subsequent first-time acute myocardial infarction. *JAMA* 1999;281:427–431.

111. Anderson JL, Muhlestein JB, Carlquist J, et al. Randomized secondary prevention trial of azithromycin in patients with coronary artery disease and serological evidence for Chlamydia pneumoniae infection: the Azithromycin in Coronary Artery Disease: Elimination of Myocardial Infection with Chlamydia (ACADEMIC) study. *Circulation* 1999;99:1540–1547.

112. Veldhyuzen van Zanten SJO, Sherman PM. *Helicobacter pylori* infection as a cause of gastritis, duodenal ulcer, gastric cancer and nonulcer dyspepsia: a systemic overview. *Can Med Assoc J* 1994;150: 177–185.

113. Sipponen P, Seppala K, Aarynen M, et al. Chronic gastritis and gastroduodenal ulcer: a case control study on risk of coexisting duodenal or gastric ulcer in patients with gastritis. *Gut* 1989;30:922–929.

114. Cullen DJE, Collins BJ, Christiansen KJ, et al. Long term risk of peptic ulcer disease in people with Helicobacter pylori infection—a community based study. *Gastroenterology* 1993;104:A60.

115. Koenig W, Rothenbacher D, Hoffmeister A, et al. Infection with *Helicobacter pylori* is not a major independent risk factor for stable coronary heart disease. *Circulation* 1999;100:2326–2331.

116. Strandberg TE, Tilvis RS, Vuoristo M, et al. Prospective study of *Helicobacter pylori* seropositivity and cardiovascular diseases in a general elderly population. *BMJ* 1997;314:317–318.

117. Wald NJ, Law MR, Morris JK, et al. *Helicobacter pylori* infection and mortality from ischaemic heart disease: negative result from a large, prospective study. *BMJ* 1997;315:1199–1201.

118. Folsom AR, Nieto JF, Sorlie P, et al., for the Atherosclerosis Risk in Communities (ARIC) Study Investigators. *Helicobacter pylori* seropositivity and coro-

nary heart disease incidence. *Circulation* 1998;98: 845–850.

119. Strachan DP, Mendall MA, Carrington D, et al. Relation of *Helicobacter pylori* infection to 13-year mortality and incident ischemic heart disease in the Caerphilly Prospective Heart Disease Study. *Circulation* 1998;98:1286–1290.

120. Danesh J, Peto R. Risk factors for coronary heart disease and infection with *Helicobacter pylori*: meta-analysis of 18 studies. *BMJ* 1998;316:1130–1132.

121. Blasi F, Denti F, Erba M, et al. Detection of *Chlamydia pneumoniae* but not *Helicobacter pylori* in atherosclerotic plaques of aortic aneurysms. *J Clin Microbiol* 1996;34:2766–2769.

122. Pasceri V, Cammarota G, Patti G, et al. Association of virulent *Helicobacter pylori* strains with ischemic heart disease. *Circulation* 1998;97:1675–1679.

123. Peek RM, Miller G, Tham KT, et al. Heightened inflammatory response and cytokine expression in vivo to CagA+ *Helicobacter pylori* strains. *Lab Invest* 1995;71:760–770.

124. Williams RC. Periodontal disease. *N Engl J Med* 1990; 322:373–382.

125. Brown LJ, Brunelle JA, Kingman A. Periodontal status in the United States, 1988–9: prevalence, extent, and demographic variation. *J Dent Res* 1996;75:672.

126. Beck JD, Koch GG, Rozier RG, et al. Prevalence and risk indicators for periodontal attachment loss in a population of old community-dwelling blacks and whites. *J Periodontol* 1991;61:520.

127. Alpagot T, Smith QT, Tran SD. Risk indicators for periodontal disease in a racially diverse urban population. *J Clin Periodontol* 1996;23:982.

128. Wu T, Trevisan M, Genco RJ, et al. Periodontal disease and risk of cerebrovascular disease: the first National Health and Nutrition Examination Survey and its follow-up study. *Arch Intern Med* 2000;160:2749–2755.

129. Hujoel PP, Drangsholt M, Spiekerman C, et al. Periodontal disease and coronary heart disease risk. *JAMA* 2000;284:1406–1410.

130. Worrall BB, DeGraba TJ. The genetics of cerebrovascular atherosclerosis. *Semin Cerebrovasc Dis Stroke* 2002;2:14–23.

131. Liao D, Myers R, Hunt S, et al. Family history of stroke and stroke risk. The Family Heart Study. *Stroke* 1997;28:1908–1912.

132. Kiely DK, Wolf PA, Cupples LA, et al. Familial aggregation of stroke: the Framingham Study. *Stroke* 1993; 24:1366–1371.

133. Joutel A, Corpechot C, Ducros A, et al. Notch 3 mutation in cerebral autosomal dominant arteriopathy with subcortical infarcts and leukoencephalopathy (CADASIL), a mendelian condition causing stroke and vascular dementia. *Ann N Y Acad Sci* 1997;826: 213–217.

134. Tjernstrom F, Hellmer G, Nived O, et al. Synergetic effect between interleukin-1 receptor antagonist allele (IL1RN*2) and MHC class II (DR17,DQ2) in determining susceptibility to systemic lupus erythematosus. *Lupus* 1999;8:103–108.

135. Schrijver HM, Crusius JB, Uitdehaag BM, et al. Association of interleukin-1beta and interleukin-1 receptor antagonist genes with disease severity in MS. *Neurology* 1999;52:595–599.

136. Bioque G, Crusius JB, Koutroubakis I, et al. Allelic polymorphism in IL-1 beta and IL-1 receptor antagonist (IL-1Ra) genes in inflammatory bowel disease. *Clin Exp Immunol* 1995;102:379–283.

137. Francis SE, Camp NJ, Dewberry RM, et al. Interleukin-1 receptor antagonist gene polymorphism and coronary artery disease. *Circulation* 1999;99:861–866.

138. Iacoviello L, Donati MB, Gattone M. Possible different involvement of interleukin-1 receptor antagonist gene polymorphism in coronary single vessel disease and myocardial infarction [Letter]. *Circulation* 2000; 101:E193.

139. Kokkotou E, Philippon V, Gueye-Ndiaye A, et al. Role of the CCR5 delta 32 allele in resistance to HIV-1 infection in West Africa. *J Hum Virol* 1998;1:469–474.

140. Taylor ML, Perez-Mejia A, Yamamoto-Furusho JK, et al. Immunologic, genetic and social human risk factors associated to histoplasmosis: studies in the state of Guerrero, Mexico. *Mycopathologia* 1997;138:137–142.

141. Momiyama Y, Hirano R, Taniguchi H, et al. The effects of interleukin-1 gene polymorphisms on the development of coronary artery disease associated with *Chlamydia pneumoniae* infection. *J Am Coll Cardiol* 2001;38:712–717.

142. Inoue M, Itoh H, Ueda M, et al. Vascular endothelial growth factor (VEGF) expression in human coronary atherosclerotic lesions: possible pathophysiological significance in VEGF in progression of atherosclerosis. *Circulation* 1998;98:2108–2116.

143. Schaper W, Buschmann I. VEGF and therapeutic opportunities in cardiovascular disease. *Curr Opin Biotechnol* 1999;10:541–543.

144. Simons M, Bonow RO, Chronos NA, et al. Clinical trials in coronary angiogenesis: issues, problems, consensus: an expert panel summary. *Circulation* 2000; 102:E73–E86.

Ischemic Stroke: Advances in Neurology, Vol. 92. Edited by
H.J.M. Barnett, Julien Bogousslavsky, and Heather Meldrum.
Lippincott Williams & Wilkins, Philadelphia © 2003.

5

Magnetic Resonance Angiography

Donald H. Lee

*Departments of Radiology and Nuclear Medicine, University of Western Ontario and Department of
Neurology, London Health Sciences Centre, London, Ontario, Canada*

Magnetic resonance angiography (MRA) is the result of the flow-sensitive nature of magnetic resonance imaging (MRI). The early literature on MRI, using spin-echo image acquisition, described different types of flow effects and the use of MRI for flow measurement. The MRI flow effects described included flow void, with loss of signal in the lumen; even-echo rephasing, with high signal in the lumen; diastolic pseudogating, producing high signal in the vessel lumen; pulsatile cerebrospinal fluid (CSF) flow, producing CSF signal loss; and entry slice phenomena, producing high signal in the vessel lumen or CSF space. Gradient-echo imaging added another dimension to MRI of flow. Because of its rapid acquisition times compared to spin-echo imaging, MRA became feasible. This chapter briefly outlines the modalities used for MRA, their advantages and disadvantages, and current clinical applications of MRA. More complete reviews of MRA techniques are provided in various articles (1–6) and in book chapters on neuroradiology and MRI texts. Techniques of MRA continue to evolve, not only because of hardware development, with high-speed gradients, but also because of surface (receiver) coil and computer development. In addition, clinical MRA now is being performed at higher magnetic fields [3 Tesla (T)] (7,8).

Currently, MRA allows sensitive noninvasive evaluation of both the intracranial and extracranial circulation and can be combined with other MR sequences, such as diffusion imaging and perfusion, to allow comprehensive evaluation of the patient with stroke, all in clinically reasonable scan times, even within the time limitations imposed for administration of tissue plasminogen activator.

Like all MRIs, however, these techniques cannot be used on patients with known contraindications to MRI. Because some of the newer techniques are very rapid (<1 minute for scan acquisition), the effects of patient motion are less. Claustrophobia, especially with smaller magnet bore sizes at high field, remains a problem (7).

TECHNIQUES

There are two types of MRA techniques: time-of-flight (TOF) and phase contrast (PC).

Time-of-Flight Imaging

TOF MRA techniques are subdivided into two types: "bright blood" and "black blood" (Figs. 5-1 and 5-2). "Bright blood" techniques have high signal in the vessel, due to either inflow of fully magnetized blood, which has very high signal, or injected contrast agent. Because the slice has been saturated (it received some form of radiofrequency energy) its signal is lower, so the high signal blood or contrast-containing blood is easily identified. In black blood techniques, flow is of lower signal than the surrounding tissue, the typical "flow void" seen in vessels on conventional spin-echo images.

Both types of MRA techniques can be acquired using two-dimensional (2D) or three-dimensional (3D) scanning. Two-dimensional scanning acquires each slice separately to produce a contiguous or overlapping dataset. Three-dimensional scanning acquires data from a block (or volume) of tissue, which is divided into individual slices (termed partitions) in different phase steps through the volume.

In general, 2D TOF techniques are quicker (because each slice is completely acquired) and more sensitive to slow flow. The 2D TOF technique is, however, limited by gradient coil design, so only rela-

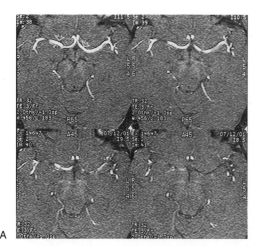

A

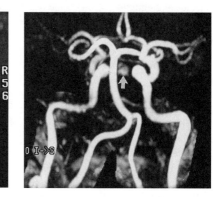

FIG. 5-1. Time-of-flight magnetic resonance angiography (TOF MRA). **A:** Source dataset for TOF MRA (multiple overlapping thin-slab angiography). Note high signal of arteries compared to background *(open arrows)*. **B:** Reprojected image in the coronal view [anterior-posterior (AP)]: normal appearance of arteries. **C:** Reprojected image in the oblique view: normal arteries. Posterior pituitary hyperintensity appears in both images *(arrow)*.

B   C

tively thick slices can be obtained (1.5–2 mm thick). It also has lower signal-to-noise ratios. The 3D TOF techniques are capable of very thin slice partitions (>0.5 mm, typically between 0.7 and 1.0 mm) and usually have higher signal-to-noise ratios. Because flow in the 3D slab is subjected to multiple radiofrequency pulses in the course of acquiring all the data, there may be more saturation (signal suppression) of flow through the slice. Several strategies have been developed to reduce this effect: TONE (tilted optimized nonsaturating excitation) (9) and MOTSA (multiple overlapping thin-slab angiography) (10). TONE uses a different flip angle as the volume is sequentially excited to reduce saturation effects. MOTSA uses multiple overlapping thin slabs, which improve entry slice phenomena, while maintaining the high resolution of 3D MRA. Magnetization transfer further suppresses the background signal of the slice, enhancing the high signal in the vessel. It is mainly used in intracranial MRA; it does not work well in the neck. Contrast-enhanced MRA (CE-MRA) uses 3D acquisitions and very short acquisi-

tion times (<1 minute). In this technique, the blood signal is increased by addition of gadolinium contrast agent. Using high-speed acquisitions, arterial or later phases in the angiographic sequence, as needed, can be obtained. One form of CE-MRA uses pump injection to produce a uniform bolus and some form of triggering to start the acquisition at the time of maximum intensity of contrast in the vessel. Another form, time-resolved imaging of contrast kinetics (TRICKS) (11), uses keyhole imaging, rapidly sampling the contrast part of the MR image. No pump is needed for contrast injection. TRICKS is significantly more computer intensive, but it can provide information on multiple phases of the angiographic sequence in one acquisition. Clinical experience, and correlation with conventional digital subtraction angiography (DSA), shows that these contrast-enhanced sequences are very similar to conventional DSA, although they still suffer, albeit to a lesser degree, from occasional underestimation and overestimation of stenosis when North American Symptomatic Carotid Endarterectomy Trial (NASCET) measurements are attempted.

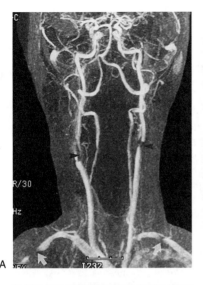

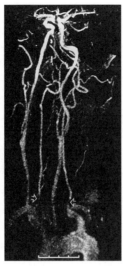

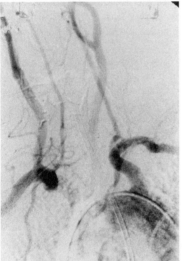

FIG. 5-2. Contrast-enhanced magnetic resonance angiography (MRA). **A:** Severe stenosis of the right and left carotid arteries *(arrowheads)*, as well as stenosis of both subclavian arteries distal to vertebral artery origins *(arrows)*. **B:** Contrast-enhanced MRA showing apparent stenosis of both vertebral arteries in the neck *(arrows)*. **C:** Arch angiogram shows no stenosis of either vertebral artery.

Although black blood imaging may not be as good for depiction of stenosis, it is reemerging as a promising technique for evaluation of the arterial wall. Different types of plaques are seen, and enhancement can be seen in the plaques. This technique shows promise for better characterization of plaque and demonstration of unstable plaque, although this still remains to be shown.

Phase-Contrast Imaging

In PC MRA, bipolar (balanced) gradients are applied in specific directions (three or more) during gradient-echo acquisition (Figs. 5-3 and 5-4). These additional gradients induce phase shifts in nonstatic tissue (flow/motion). The images with additional gradients applied are combined mathematically with images without gradients to generate images that show only flow. This technique results in better background suppression compared to TOF techniques because the static tissue has been removed. It also allows characterization of flow, both its direction and speed. The strength of the gradient (low gradient— rapid flow, high gradient— slow flow) determines the flow detected within the vessel (or CSF space). Images can be acquired as either 2D or 3D datasets. Computer processing of the images yields magnitude images (showing the background with superimposed

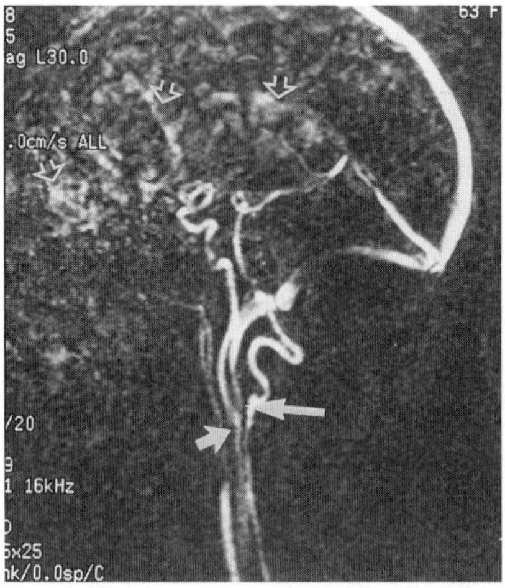

FIG. 5-3. Phase-contrast magnetic resonance angiography. Sagittal 50-mm thick slab to left of midline (1:30-minute acquisition time). There is motion artifact from minor head movement *(open arrows)*, but recognizable arterial and venous detail. Overlap of jugular vein *(long arrow)* and internal carotid artery *(short arrow)* can be seen.

flow), speed images (which show flow only as high signal), or directional images (flow in one direction, depending on the applied gradient, is shown as either white or black). The speed images are used for MRA image production. Because this technique is sensitive to all flow, PC images depict both arterial and venous flow. If gradient sensitization is for extremely low flow, then even CSF flow can be visualized.

Postprocessing

All TOF or 3D PC MRA images are post-processed to yield images that look like conventional arterial angiograms, venograms, or both. New workstations use maximum intensity pixel (MIP) detection (or minimum intensity pixel for black blood) to isolate vessels. Sophisticated programs, including connectivity algorithms, then produce rotational images of the vessels. Most radiologists use the individual image slices (partitions or source images), which show the vessels, as well as the reprojected dataset, to evaluate the arteries. Surrounding tissue can be cropped out to produce images that look similar to intraarterial DSA.

Limitations of Magnetic Resonance Angiography

1. *Lower resolution.* Compared to DSA, MRA (even the more recent CE-MRA) has lower resolution. This difference is at least half. It becomes progressively more noticeable as the size of the vessel decreases.

2. *Artifacts.* Slow flow, turbulent flow, and in-plane flow all can cause loss of signal, leading to overestimation of degree of stenosis and even nonvisualization of the vessel or aneurysm. Postprocessing artifacts in TOF MRA may be due to a normally hyperintense posterior pituitary, blood in the vessel wall or in a thrombosed vascular structures, or an aneurysm, producing apparent lumina or unusual-appearing arteries. Black blood MRA suffers from potential overestimation of lumen size or stenosis,

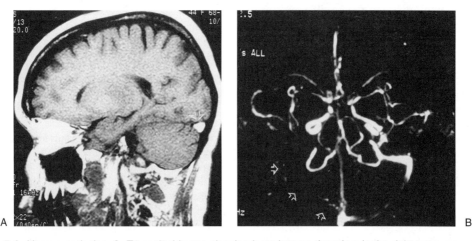

FIG. 5-4. Venous occlusion. **A:** T1 sagittal image showing hyperintense thrombus in the right transverse sinus *(open arrow)*. **B:** Axial phase-contrast image showing absence of flow in the right transverse sinus *(open arrows* along expected course of sinus).

especially when the vessel lies close to a naturally dark structure such as the air-containing sphenoid sinus. Turbulence in black blood MRA—swirling—generates higher signal and apparent worsening of stenosis. Because TOF techniques (except black blood MRA) and PC techniques use gradient-echo acquisitions, items that reduce or destroy the local signal may significantly affect the image, e.g., aneurysm clip(s), dental work, dental appliance, or local metal present for another reason. This may lead to nonvisualization of the vessel.

3. *Limited area of coverage.* Most studies routinely image either the carotid bifurcation or the intracranial vascular structures. Larger coverage is possible with multiple coils (phased-array coils). CE-MRA is advantageous because the signal in the vessel is from the contrast and is not as dependent on direction of flow. Using a multiple coil, the acquisition can be done coronally, using smaller volumes to cover the area of interest, compared to TOF imaging, which requires slices to be perpendicular to flow as much as possible (hence, most acquisitions are axial).

4. *Patient motion.* Except for CE-MRA, MRA sequences take between 2 and 10 minutes to cover the area of interest. Motion can produce minor to major degradation of image quality. Longer imaging times have a higher chance of poorer qualities of study. Because of its short imaging times, CE-MRA offers significant benefits in this regard.

CLINICAL APPLICATIONS

Vascular Stenosis

Extracranial

For depiction of extracranial arterial stenosis, non-contrast 2D and 3D TOF techniques have sensitivities and specificities similar to those of duplex sonography (Figs. 5-2 and 5-5). However, all show overestimation of degree of stenosis. Sensitivity is high (>85%), but specificity is lower (74%–95%; lower with 2D than 3D techniques, and around 88% when NASCET-type measurement is made) (12). False-positive results are due to kinking or overestimation of stenosis. False-negative results are due to nonimaging of the stenosis or artifact. Comparison of CE-MRA at 1.5 T with conventional DSA has shown that it is more sensitive than either of the other TOF techniques. Sensitivities range from 83% and 93% (for source or MIP image, respectively), specificities 85% to 97% (for MIP or source image, respectively) up to 100%, and accuracy 87% to 92% (for MIP or source image, respectively) (13–16). Although there was overestimation of disease in the moderate NASCET category (30%–69%) in all studies, arterial occlusion or near occlusion was well demonstrated by CE-MRA.

Intracranial

Three-dimensional techniques are mostly used to demonstrate intracranial vascular stenosis, although

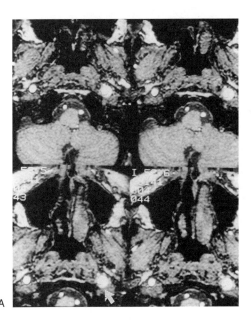

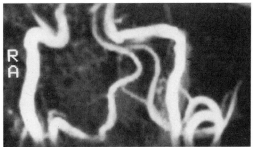

FIG. 5-5. Carotid dissection. **A:** Source image: hyperintensity in arterial wall due to methemoglobin *(arrow).* **B:** Reprojected image: narrowed lumen of internal carotid artery *(arrowhead)* due to blood in the arterial wall.

A

B

quick screening for large arterial patency can be done in the acute stroke setting in less than 2 minutes using 2D PC MRA. Compared with conventional angiography for showing stenosis of the arteries at the base of the brain, 3D TOF MRA has accuracy of 80% to 90%, with sensitivity and specificity between 70% and 90% (17). Use of CE-MRA for detection of intracranial arterial stenosis is still being evaluated. MRA is of little value for detection of arterial stenosis of very small arteries (<1 mm). The resolution needed to demonstrate small arteries is beyond what is currently achievable with MRA (18). MR depiction of small veins at 3 T suggests that this field strength may be promising to improve resolution of small vessels (19).

Venous Occlusion

MR and MRA are highly sensitive for detection of venous sinus or deep cerebral vein thrombosis (Fig.

5-4). Various MRA techniques, mostly TOF MRA (20) but including CE-MRA, can be used.

Aneurysms

In small numbers of patients, CE-MRA is very sensitive for detection of aneurysms (100% sensitive, 94% specific) compared to conventional 3D TOF MRA (sensitivity 96%, specificity 100%) or PC MRA (7/23 aneurysms missed) (Fig. 5-6) (21–24). The smallest size of aneurysm detected remains around 4 mm. In acute subarachnoid hemorrhage, MRA has limitations (in one of the studies, only 49% of patients could be scanned); despite this limitation, sensitivity was reasonable (81%–90%). MRA and DSA may be complementary in the assessment of patients with acute subarachnoid hemorrhage, especially in anatomically complex areas or in areas where there is intraaneurysmal thrombus (22,23).

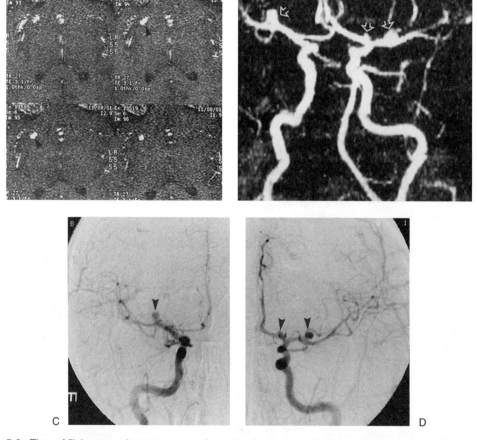

FIG. 5-6. Time-of-flight magnetic resonance angiography of aneurysm. **A:** Source images: right middle cerebral artery (MCA) aneurysm *(arrowheads)*. **B:** Reprojection image: right-sided and left-sided aneurysms *(open arrows)*. **C:** Digital subtraction angiography (DSA) of right carotid: MCA aneurysm *(arrowhead)*. **D:** DSA of left carotid: multiple aneurysms *(arrowheads)*

Problems include limited coverage (important for mycotic aneurysms or more distal aneurysms), clip artifact [two studies document the inability of postoperative MRA to reveal the neck or adjacent artery after clipping (24,25)], and hyperintensity of subacute hemorrhage (methemoglobin) simulating aneurysm. The latter is less important on CE-MRA. Even the more recent titanium clips have surrounding artifact, although in lesser amounts (25,26).

Neither MRI nor MRA can image ferromagnetic aneurysm clips. There is at least one report of a fatal outcome. MRA is less affected by intraaneurysmal coils (27) and may prove to be better for noninvasive follow-up of patients than computed tomographic angiography. Conventional invasive DSA remains the only effective diagnostic modality for evaluating the post coil appearance of the aneurysm lumen.

MRA is used relatively infrequently in vasospasm. Narrowing of vessels in six of eight arteries showing vasospasm, in three patients (28), and reversible vasospasm in preeclampsia (29) has been described.

Carotid Dissection

MRA findings in carotid or vertebral arterial dissection have been described (Fig. 5-5) (30,31). Most reports in the literature provide findings in one or two patients. The characteristic finding is arterial luminal narrowing and eccentric intramural hematoma. The hematoma is visualized because of methemoglobin in the wall; this can persist for up to 10 months after symptom onset. Hematoma is best detected with fat-suppressed sequences.

Moyamoya

Moyamoya can be shown with MRA, based on bilateral stenosis or occlusion of the distal internal carotid artery and the proximal anterior and middle cerebral arteries, as well as bilateral abnormal moyamoya vessels (Fig. 5-7). MRA has been shown to have high sensitivity (98%) and specificity (100%) for diagnosis (32). The only vessels poorly demonstrated by MRA in moyamoya are leptomeningeal and transdural collaterals.

Arterial Wall Imaging

In addition to imaging of stenosis, newer applications of MRA include imaging of the actual plaque (Fig. 5-8). The absence of artifact from calcification and the soft tissue resolution of MR indicate that it potentially is a powerful tool in the evaluation of the unstable plaque. On MOTSA, a thick fibrous cap appears as a dark band between the white lumen and the gray wall, a thin fibrous cap appears as no band between them, and recent cap rupture appears as no band between them, a bright gray region near the lumen, or a smooth or irregular luminal surface depending on the extent of plaque rupture (33). Plaque imaging has been reviewed (34,35). Based on the weighting of the image (T1, T2, or proton density), calcium usually is hypointense on all sequences; lipid is very hyperintense on T1 and proton-density sequences and becomes hypointense on T2 images; and fibrous plaque is isointense to slightly hyperintense on T1, proton-density, and T2 images. Blood has variable characteristics on the

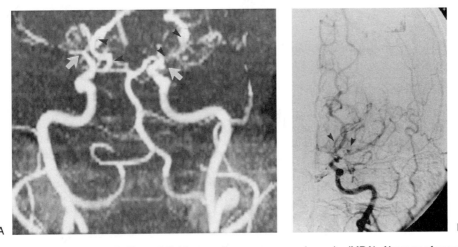

A   B

FIG. 5-7. Moyamoya disease. **A:** Time-of-flight magnetic resonance angiography (MRA). Absence of normal distal internal carotid artery (ICA) and carotid bifurcations *(arrows)* and absence of normal middle or anterior cerebral arteries *(arrowheads* indicate posterior cerebral arteries). **B:** Left carotid digital subtraction angiography. Similar findings to MRA but better delineation of lenticulostriate collaterals *(arrowheads).*

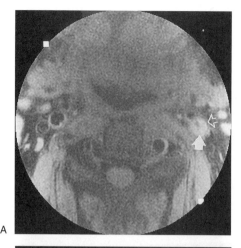

A

FIG. 5-8. Arterial wall imaging showing internal carotid near occlusion. **A:** Axial double inversion sequence (T2, with both fat and blood low signal) shows different components of the arterial wall: hyperintense plaque *(arrow)* and hypointense plaque (calcification; *open arrow*). **B:** Multiple overlapping thin-slab angiography (MOTSA) before contrast: tiny lumen through plaque *(open arrow)*. **C:** MOTSA after contrast: enhancing plaque *(open arrow)* and marked arterial wall enhancement *(long arrows)*.

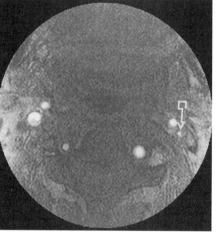

B

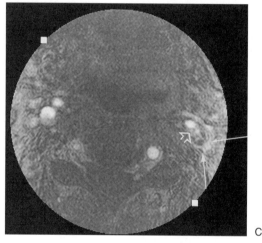

C

sequences, ranging from hyperintense to hypo-intense.

Miscellaneous: Arteriovenous Malformations

The role of MRA in the evaluation of vascular malformations has been reviewed (36). MRI can show moderate-to-large arteriovenous malformations (AVMs) well. MRA can do the same, providing information about the AVM (large local feeders and draining veins, and nidus size) (37), as well as temporal sequencing (for large vessels) (38,39). It is useful for radiosurgical planning (40) and follow-up. Very small AVMs, especially dural AVMs, can be missed on MRA and require angiography for detection.

Both PC and TOF MRA are good screening modalities for showing the large veins of spinal AVMs. Resolution is a problem; usually, only the draining vein is visualized. CE-MRA in limited numbers of patients

(41,42) appears to be better than noncontrast techniques, potentially showing both the feeding artery and the draining vein from the fistula in the intervertebral foramen.

SUMMARY

MRA is a robust technique that still is undergoing modifications and improvements. As a noninvasive, or minimally invasive, technique using intravenous contrast injection, it offers complementary assessment of intracranial and extracranial arteries at the time of MRI, using similar coils and sequences. Images are similar to, but of lower resolution than, those of conventional angiography.

REFERENCES

1. Clifton AG. MR angiography. *Br Med Bull* 2000;56: 367–377.

2. Leclerc X, Pruvo J-P. Recent advances in magnetic resonance angiography of carotid and vertebral arteries. *Curr Opin Neurol* 2000;13:75–82.
3. Wetzel S, Bongartz G. MR angiography: supra-aortic vessels. *Eur Radiol* 1999;9:1277–1284.
4. Jara H, Barish MA. Black-blood MR Angiography. *Magn Reson Imaging Clin N Am* 1999;7:303–317.
5. Laub G. Principles of contrast-enhanced MR angiography. Basic and clinical applications. *Magn Reson Imaging Clin N Am* 1999;7:783–795.
6. Wilms G, Bosmans H, Demaerel P, et al. Magnetic resonance angiography of the intracranial vessels. *Eur J Radiol* 2001;38:10–18.
7. Campeau NG, Huston J 3rd, Bernstein MA, et al. Magnetic resonance angiography at 3.0 Tesla: initial clinical experience. *Topics Magn Reson Imaging* 2001;12:183–204.
8. Bernstein MA, Huston J 3rd, Lin C, et al. High resolution intracranial and cervical MRA at 3.0T: technical considerations and initial experience. *Magn Reson Med* 2001;46:955–962.
9. Tkach JA, Masaryk TJ, Ruggieri PM, et al. The use of tilted optimized nonsaturating excitation (TONE) RF pulses and MTC to improve the quality of MR angiograms of the carotid bifurcation. Presented at 11th annual scientific meeting of the SMRM, August 8–14, 1992, Berlin, P3905.
10. Blatter DD, Parker DJ, Robinson RO. Cerebral MR angiography with multiple overlapping thin slabs acquisition: part 1. Quantitative analysis of vessel visibility. *Radiology* 1991;179:805–811.
11. Korosec FR, Frayne R, Grist TM, et al. Time-resolved contrast-enhanced 3D MR angiography. *Magn Reson Med* 1996;36:345–351.
12. Rosokovsky MA, Litt AW. MR angiography of the extracranial carotid arteries. *Magn Reson Imaging Clin N Am* 1995;3:439–454.
13. Huston J 3rd, Fain SB, Wald JT, et al. Carotid artery: elliptic centric contrast-enhanced MR angiography compared with conventional angiography. *Radiology* 2001;218:138–143.
14. Scarabino T, Carriero A, Giannatempo GM, et al. Contrast enhanced MR angiography (CEMRA) in the study of the carotid stenosis: comparison with digital subtraction angiography (DSA). *J Neuroradiol* 1999;26:87–91.
15. Remoda L, Heid O, Schroth G. Carotid artery stenosis, occlusion and pseudo-occlusion: first-pass, gadolinium-enhanced three-dimensional MR angiography- preliminary study. *Radiology* 1998;209:95–102.
16. Phan T, Huston J 3rd, Bernstein MA, et al. Contrast-enhanced magnetic resonance angiography of the cervical vessels: experience with 422 patients. *Stroke* 2001;32:2282–2286.
17. Stock KW, Radue EW, Jacob AL, et al. Intracranial arteries: prospective blinded comparative study of MR angiography and DSA in 50 patients. *Radiology* 1995;159:451–456.
18. Stock KW, Wetzel S, Kirsch E, et al. Anatomic evaluation of the circle of Willis: MR angiography versus intraarterial digital subtraction angiography. *Am J Neuroradiol* 1996;17:1495–1499.
19. Reichenbach JR, Barth M, Haacke EM, et al. High-resolution MR venography at 3.0 Tesla. *J Comput Assist Tomogr* 2000;24:949–957.
20. Finn JP, Zisk JHS, Edelman RR, et al. Central venous occlusion: MR angiography. *Radiology* 1993;33:165–167.
21. Metens T, Rio F, Baleriaux D, et al. Intracranial aneurysms: detection with gadolinium-enhanced dynamic three-dimensional MR angiography—initial results. *Radiology* 2000;216:39–46.
22. Jager HR, Mansmann U, Hausmann O, et al. MRA versus digital subtraction angiography in acute subarachnoid hemorrhage: a blinded multireader study of prospectively recruited patients. *Neuroradiology* 2000;42:313–326.
23. Adams WM, Laitt RD, Jackson A. The role of MR angiography in the pre-treatment assessment of intracranial aneurysms: a comparative study. *Am J Neuroradiol* 2000;21:1618–1628.
24. Schmieder K, Falk A, Hardenack M, et al. Clinical utility of magnetic resonance angiography in the evaluation of aneurysms from a neurosurgical point of view. *Zentralbl Neurochir* 1999;60:61–67.
25. Grieve JP, Stacey R, Moore E, et al. Artefact on MRA following aneurysm clipping: an in vitro study and prospective comparison with conventional angiography. *Neuroradiology* 1999;41:680–686.
26. Lawton MR, Heiserman JE, Prendergast VC, et al. Titanium aneurysm clips: part III—clinical application in 16 patients with subarachnoid hemorrhage. *Neurosurgery* 1996;38:1170–1175.
27. Gonner F, Heid O, Remonda L, et al. MR angiography with ultrashort echo time in cerebral aneurysms treated with Guglielmi detachable coils. *Am J Neuroradiol* 1998;19:1324–1328.
28. Horikoshi T, Fukamachi A, Nishi H, et al. Observation of vasospasm after subarachnoid hemorrhage by magnetic resonance angiography. A preliminary study. *Neurol Med Chir (Tokyo)* 1993;35:298–304.
29. Ito T, Sakai T, Inagawa S, et al. MR angiography of cerebral vasospasm in preeclampsia. *Am J Neuroradiol* 1995;16:1344–1346.
30. Kirsch E, Kaim A, Engelter S, et al. MR angiography in internal carotid artery dissection: improvement of diagnosis by selective demonstration of the intramural hematoma. *Neuroradiology* 1998;40:704–709.
31. Oelerich M, Stogbauer F, Kurlemann G, et al. Craniocervical artery dissection: MR imaging and MR angiographic findings. *Eur Radiol* 1999;9:1385–1391.
32. Yamada I, Nakagawa T, Matsushima Y, et al. High-resolution turbo magnetic resonance angiography for diagnosis of moyamoya disease. *Stroke* 2001;32:1825–1831.
33. Hatsukami TS, Ross R, Polissar NL, et al. Visualization of fibrous cap thickness and rupture in human atherosclerotic carotid plaque in vivo with high-resolution magnetic resonance imaging. *Circulation* 2000;102:959–964.
34. De Marco JK, Rutt BK, Clarke SE. Carotid plaque characterization by magnetic resonance imaging: review of the literature. *Topics Magn Reson Imaging* 2001;12:205–217.
35. Fayuad ZA, Fuster V. Clinical imaging of the high-risk or vulnerable atherosclerotic plaque. *Circ Res* 2001;89:305–316.
36. Kesava PP, Turski PA. MR angiography of vascular malformations. *Neuroimaging Clin N Am* 1998;8:349–370.
37. Warren DJ, Hoggard N, Walton L, et al. Cerebral arteriovenous malformations: comparison of novel magnetic

resonance angiographic techniques and conventional catheter angiography. *Neurosurgery* 2001;48:973–982.

38. Tsuchiya K, Katase S, Yoshino A, et al. MR digital subtraction angiography of cerebral arteriovenous malformations. *Am J Neuroradiol* 2000;21:707–711.

39. Griffiths PD, Hoggard N, Warren DJ, et al. Brain arteriovenous malformations: assessment with dynamic MR digital subtraction angiography. *Am J Neuroradiol* 2000;21:1892–1899.

40. Bednarz G, Downes B, Werner-Wasik M, et al. Combining stereotactic angiography and 3D time-of-flight magnetic resonance angiography in treatment planning for arteriovenous malformation radiosurgery. *Int J Radiat Oncol Biol Phys* 2000;46:1149–1154.

41. Binkert CA, Kollias SS, Valavanis A. Spinal cord vascular disease: characterization with fast three-dimensional contrast-enhanced MR angiography. *Am J Neuroradiol* 1999;20:1773–1774.

42. Masalchi M, Cosottini M, Ferrito G, et al. Contrast-enhanced time-resolved MR angiography of spinal vascular malformations. *J Comput Assist Tomogr* 1999;23:341–345.

Ischemic Stroke: Advances in Neurology, Vol. 92. Edited by
H.J.M. Barnett, Julien Bogousslavsky, and Heather Meldrum.
Lippincott Williams & Wilkins, Philadelphia © 2003.

6

Invasive Angiography for Arterial Lesions of Stroke

David M. Pelz

Departments of Diagnostic Radiology and Clinical Neurological Sciences, The University of Western Ontario and Department of Diagnostic Radiology, London Health Sciences Centre, London, Ontario, Canada

Despite the widespread use of ultrasound, computed tomographic angiography, and magnetic resonance angiography, conventional invasive angiography using digital subtraction (DSA) remains the gold standard for investigation of both intracranial and extracranial vascular disease. Although the techniques and technology have evolved, the clarity of vascular imaging has remained unmatched since the pioneering work of the Portuguese neurologist Egas Moniz (Fig. 6-1A) in the 1930s. Using strontium bromide in cadavers and then sodium iodide and surgical neck incisions in humans, he revolutionized the diagnosis and treatment of cerebrovascular disease. The

first catheter arteriogram was performed in 1947, followed by Seldinger's description of the transfemoral catheter technique in 1953 (Fig. 6-1B) (1). Safer contrast agents appeared in the 1950s, and the non-ionic, low osmolar agents became available in the 1980s. High-resolution DSA, recently augmented with three-dimensional rotational capability (computerized rotational angiography), now is the standard for modern neuroangiography.

This chapter briefly reviews the techniques, risks, and complications of current neuroangiography, followed by the angiography of common arterial lesions associated with stroke.

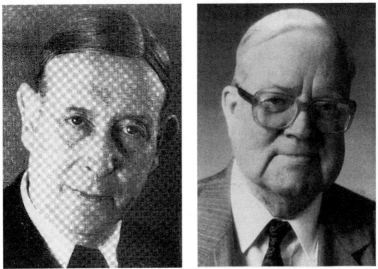

FIG. 6-1. A: Egas Moniz. **B:** Sven Seldinger.

TECHNIQUES

Patient Preparation

Proper patient education and preparation are essential before any invasive procedure. Cardiac and renal status must be evaluated, and blood work should include complete blood count, platelets, clotting factors, and creatinine. Informed consent is mandatory, and the patient must be well hydrated on the day of the procedure. Electrocardiographic and oxygen saturation monitoring must be available in the angiography suite. Intravenous access must be secured. Sedation with sublingual lorazepam or intravenous fentanyl/midazolam usually is adequate.

Transfemoral Technique

Surprisingly little has changed since Seldinger's original description of this technique, which still is the most common method for performing nearly all forms of angiography. After femoral arterial puncture with an 18- or 19-gauge needle, many operators will insert a 5- or 6-Fr sheath, to minimize arterial trauma if catheter changes are anticipated. Many centers use systemic heparinization in atherosclerosis cases, with 2,000 IU given upon placement of the sheath and 3,000 IU per 500-mL saline catheter flushing solution. A multitude of guidewires and catheters are available for selective cerebrovascular catheterization. The catheters are 4 to 6 Fr in size, with many preformed shapes and hydrophilic coatings. The use of non-ionic, low osmolar contrast agents now is standard to maximize patient safety and comfort. Biplane DSA units with $1,024 \times 1,024$ matrix size optimize spatial resolution and decrease the number of contrast runs. Computerized rotational angiography is becoming commercially available, allowing three-dimensional imaging of complex vascular lesions.

The vessel of most clinical interest should be studied first. Selective injections of 8 to 12 mL of contrast for the common carotid artery (CCA) and 6 to 9 mL for vertebral studies are standard. At least two views of each carotid bifurcation and the intracranial vessels are required; oblique projections often are necessary. Selective vertebral injections should only be done if clinically indicated. If a vascular occlusion is revealed, collateral channels should be demonstrated. Despite the low yield for significant disease (2), most operators will administer an aortic arch injection (45–55 mL) or obtain views showing the origins of the great vessels.

After the procedure, the femoral sheath is removed and compression of the puncture site is performed, preferably manually. Mechanical compression devices are available, as are expensive arterial closure devices that are more appropriate for interventional procedures using large-bore catheters. The patient should be observed for a minimum of 1 hour in a supervised nursing unit and must remain supine for 4 to 6 hours.

Transbrachial and Transradial Techniques

The transbrachial approach, using 4-Fr catheters, has been popularized as an outpatient procedure (3) and as an alternative when femoral access is poor. Success and complication rates are similar to those of the transfemoral method. A transradial approach has been described (4).

COMPLICATIONS

Neurologic

Strokes are the most common and most feared complications of cerebral angiography. They result from the formation of blood clot on catheters and guidewires, dislodgment of plaque and clot from vessel walls, and iatrogenic dissection. The end result of each is embolus formation and distal branch occlusion. Many studies have been performed over the years, estimating the risk of transient neurologic deficit from 0.5% to 4.0% (5,6) and permanent deficit from 0.09% to 1.0% (7,8). Recent studies using transcranial Doppler monitoring during, and diffusion-weighted imaging immediately after, cerebral DSA have shown an alarmingly high incidence of cerebral emboli, most of which were clinically silent (9).

Two prospective studies best reflect current practice. Dion et al. (7) showed a stroke rate of 0.4% in 1,002 procedures, with a higher rate (0.7%) in patients with atherosclerotic disease. Factors increasing the risk were longer procedure time, hypertension, diabetes, and higher contrast dosages. In a series of 1517 patients, Earnest et al. (8) found a 0.3% stroke rate (0.6% in atherosclerosis patients) and higher risk with increasing age, higher creatinine, and number of catheter changes. Other studies have shown that operator inexperience and the degree of carotid stenosis can influence complication rates.

Headaches can occur in up to 33% of patients undergoing cerebral DSA (10). Transient global amnesia can occur immediately after vertebral artery injections and may last up to 24 hours (11). Although the etiology is uncertain, it may be due to emboli in the posterior circulation or neurotoxic effects of transiently flooding of the mesial temporal lobes with contrast material.

Hematoma at Puncture Site

There is an approximately 5% to 11% risk of significant hematoma formation at femoral puncture sites, 0.3% to 1.5% of which may require transfusion or surgical evacuation (7,12). Femoral pseudoaneurysms may be seen in 0.05% to 0.55% of patients undergoing angiography (13). The incidence of major hematoma after brachial punctures has been reported to be as high as 2% to 4% (3).

Contrast Reactions

Although initially controversial, most centers performing high volumes of angiography now use nonionic, low osmolar contrast agents. The cost differential with older high osmolar agents has decreased, and the advantages in safety and patient comfort are clear (14,15). The actual mechanism of anaphylactic reactions to contrast is still uncertain but is thought to be mediated by immunoglobulin E (16). The incidence of life-threatening reactions is rare, 0.04% in the largest reported series (14). There is a higher risk in patients with a history of asthma, renal disease, or prior reaction (17%–35%). Pretreatment with corticosteroids and antihistamines has been shown to decrease the risk in those with prior anaphylactic reaction (17). Pretesting with small doses of contrast has no predictive value for subsequent reaction (18).

Vasovagal Reactions

Vasovagal reactions are very common, likely related to patient anxiety, and often are seen at the conclusion of the procedure, during groin compression. They are easily and effectively treated with intravenous atropine.

PATHOLOGY

Atherosclerotic Disease

Carotid Bulb

Atherosclerotic disease at or near the carotid bulb is the underlying cause of greater than 90% of all thromboembolic strokes. The unique anatomy of the bulb, in which a parent vessel bifurcates into a branch

initially larger than itself, subjects it to shear stresses, flow, and stasis patterns that combine to make it the most common place for cerebral atherosclerosis (19). Despite the popularity of less invasive imaging modalities, DSA remains the gold standard for measuring the degree of stenosis, identifying tandem lesions, evaluating collateral channels, and detecting coexistent pathology.

Angiography most commonly reveals wall irregularity and luminal stenosis by plaque, usually on the posterior wall of the bulb and in the first 2 to 3 cm of the internal carotid artery (ICA) (Fig. 6-2). Distal cervical ICA atherosclerotic stenosis is rare. The stenosis may be smooth or irregular, and it must be seen in at least two orthogonal views. Oblique views may be necessary to avoid the pitfalls of external carotid artery (ECA) overlap, tortuosity with foreshortening, weblike stenosis, and overhanging plaque margins (Fig. 6-3A–B).

Ulceration with friable atheromatous material and platelet thrombus may be the most common cause of microemboli (20) and is revealed angiographically as a classic niche in the vessel wall (Fig. 6-4A–B) or double density if viewed en face. An ulcer may be simulated by a normal vessel, surrounded by plaque, in which case the neck is broader than the base of the

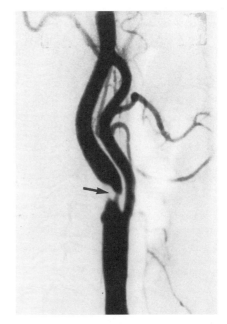

FIG. 6-2. Common carotid artery digital substraction angiography, lateral view. Severe atherosclerotic stenosis of the proximal internal carotid artery *(arrow)*, which measures 75% by North American Symptomatic Carotid Endarterectomy Trial (NASCET) criteria.

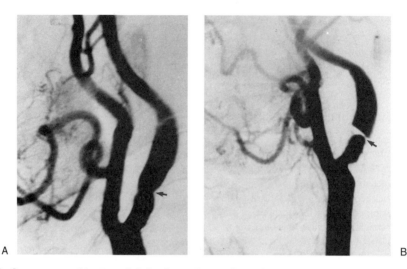

FIG. 6-3. A: Common carotid artery digital substraction angiography, lateral view. There is an apparent mild stenosis of the internal carotid artery *(arrow)*. **B:** Anteroposterior oblique view of the same vessel. There is a very severe internal carotid artery stenosis, with overhanging edges *(arrow)*.

defect (Fig. 6-5). Angiography may be relatively insensitive for detection of ulceration, showing characteristic features in 53% to 86% of patients with pathologically proven ulceration in postoperative specimens (21). Intraluminal thrombus, although not common, is seen as a polypoid or linear filling defect, surrounded on three sides by contrast (Fig. 6-6).

As the degree of stenosis increases, ICA diameter eventually decreases, and near occlusion produces the classic "string" sign (Fig. 6-7). As flow drops, it may be necessary to prolong filming runs to show slow distal filling of the ICA and continuity with intracranial vessels. A more recently coined term, "approaching" near occlusion, is used to describe a severe stenosis that decreases cervical ICA diameter below normal, but not yet to a string, thus invalidating most commonly used measurement schemes. Angiographic features of this condition, arbitrarily

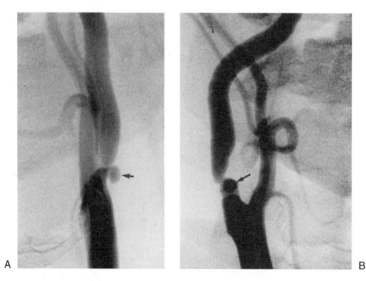

FIG. 6-4. A: Common carotid artery digital substraction angiography, lateral oblique view. Classic ulcer niche is seen in the proximal internal carotid artery *(arrow)*. **B:** Anteroposterior oblique view of the same vessel shows the double density of the ulcer viewed en face *(arrow)*.

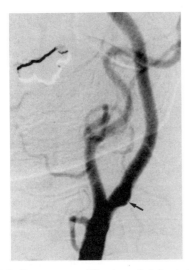

FIG. 6-5. Common carotid artery digital substraction angiography, lateral view. A remnant of the carotid bulb *(arrow)* is seen just distal to atherosclerotic plaque in the bulb, simulating ulceration.

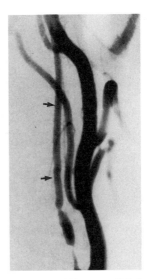

FIG. 6-7. Common carotid artery digital substraction angiography, lateral view. Near occlusion of the internal carotid artery, with a "string" sign *(arrows)*.

assigned a severity of 95%, include cervical ICA diameter less than or equal to the adjacent ECA, filling of terminal ECA branches before the appearance of pial cerebral vessels, and spontaneous filling of ipsilateral hemispheric collateral vessels (Fig. 6-8) (22). Occlusion of the bulb may be blunt, rounded, or pointed. A cone shape can occur with distal occlusion, but it may be indistinguishable from dissection or tapered thrombus (Fig. 6-9). Complete embolic occlusion may show a smooth edge or meniscus, as opposed to the irregular convex edge of plaque.

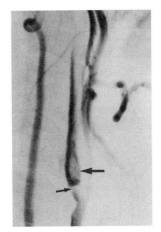

FIG. 6-6. Common carotid artery digital substraction angiography, lateral view. Intraluminal thrombus *(large arrow)* distal to a severe atherosclerotic stenosis *(small arrow)* with a tapered occlusion of the internal carotid artery.

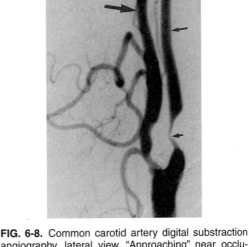

FIG. 6-8. Common carotid artery digital substraction angiography, lateral view. "Approaching" near occlusion. The internal carotid artery is decreased in caliber *(small arrow)* beyond a severe stenosis *(arrowhead)* and is smaller than the adjacent internal maxillary artery *(large arrow)*.

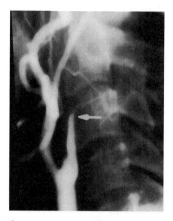

FIG. 6-9. Common carotid artery arteriogram, lateral view. Complete occlusion of the internal carotid artery *(arrow)*.

Measurement of Carotid Stenosis

Measurement of carotid stenosis is shown in Fig. 6-10.

NASCET (North American Symptomatic Carotid Endarterectomy Trial) Method

This method uses the linear measurement of the minimal residual lumen (MRL) on the angiographic projection that shows the narrowest stenosis diameter and compares it to the cervical ICA diameter beyond the bulb, where the vessel walls are parallel. This method also was used in ACAS (Asymptomatic Carotid Atherosclerosis Study) and the Veterans Affairs Trial.

ECST (European Carotid Surgery Trial) Method

This method compares the MRL to a subjectively estimated normal diameter of the carotid bulb.

CSI (Carotid Stenosis Index or Common Carotid) Method

This method compares the MRL to the diameter of the disease-free CCA.

There are problems with each of these measurement schemes. Although probably most commonly used worldwide, the NASCET scheme tends to overestimate stenosis severity by comparing a bulb stenosis to the more distal ICA, not to the bulb itself. The ECST method is theoretically more valid, yet the bulb measurement used is entirely subjective and this method produces smaller values, i.e., a 50% ECST stenosis is equal to a 70% NASCET lesion, the cutoff for surgical intervention. The CSI method may be the most accurate overall, but it is not commonly used. Most new DSA units come equipped with electronic measurement programs, but these may be inaccurate when compared with strict measurement criteria (23).

Other Extracranial Sites of Atherosclerotic Disease

The other sites of extracranial disease, in decreasing order of frequency, are the vertebral artery origins, the distal CCA, and the origins of the subclavian and innominate arteries from the aortic arch.

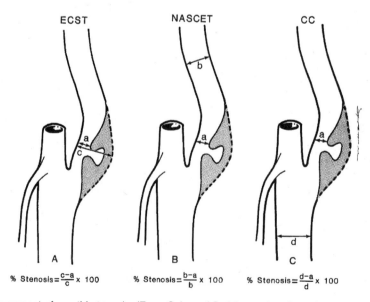

$$\% \text{ Stenosis} = \frac{c-a}{c} \times 100 \qquad \% \text{ Stenosis} = \frac{b-a}{b} \times 100 \qquad \% \text{ Stenosis} = \frac{d-a}{d} \times 100$$

FIG. 6-10. Measurement of carotid stenosis. (From Osborn AG. Atherosclerosis and carotid stenosis. In: *Diagnostic cerebral angiography.* Philadelphia: Lippincott Williams & Wilkins, 1999:73.)

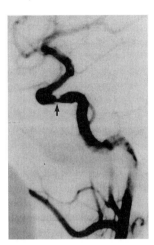

FIG. 6-11. Common carotid artery digital substraction angiography, lateral view. A focal, notchlike atherosclerotic lesion is seen in the cavernous internal carotid artery *(arrowhead)*.

Intracranial Atherosclerosis

The cavernous and supraclinoid segments of the ICA are the most common sites for intracranial disease, followed by the small vessels, which more likely are involved in hypertensive or diabetic patients. Angiographic features include irregular circumferential or asymmetric narrowing and notchlike filling defects (Fig. 6-11). The differential diagnosis includes vasospasm and vasculitis, but atherosclerosis is the most common cause of diffuse small vessel disease (Fig. 6-12).

Stroke

Angiography in the acute stroke setting usually is performed before intraarterial thrombolysis or to rule out an underlying vascular lesion in hemorrhagic stroke. The most common findings are vessel occlusion and intraluminal thrombus. The occlusion may be tapered or sharp, or it may show the meniscal-filling defect of thrombus. The middle cerebral artery (MCA), just beyond the first major anterior temporal branch, often is involved (Fig. 6-13), followed by the posterior cerebral artery (PCA), basilar artery, and anterior cerebral artery (ACA). Vessels occluded by clot may recanalize within minutes, and 50% will reopen within 1 week (24).

Other angiographic findings in acute stroke are slow antegrade flow in a branch with prolonged circulation time (Fig. 6-14), avascular or "bare areas," local mass effect, retrograde filling of a proximally occluded branch by leptomeningeal collaterals, arteriovenous shunting with early venous filling, and "luxury" perfusion or a prominent vascular blush in a newly infarcted zone (Fig. 6-15A–B). This latter condition, possibly related to loss of autoregulation, often is gyriform in appearance and may persist for up to 3 weeks.

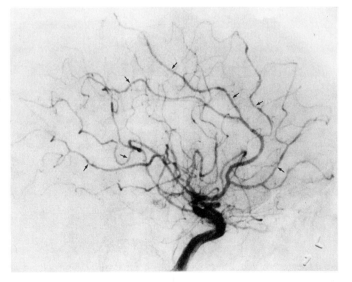

FIG. 6-12. Common carotid artery digital substraction angiography, lateral view. Numerous small, focal irregularities are seen in the middle and anterior cerebral artery branches *(small arrows)*, representing diffuse, small-vessel atherosclerotic disease.

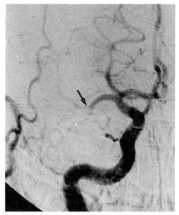

FIG. 6-13. Common carotid artery, digital substraction angiography, anteroposterior view. There is near complete occlusion of the proximal middle cerebral artery by thrombus with a meniscal filling defect *(arrow)*.

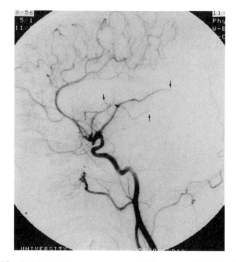

FIG. 6-14. Left common carotid artery digital substraction angiography, lateral view. There is delayed filling of middle cerebral artery branches due to distal embolic branch occlusions *(small arrows)*.

Collaterals

The circle of Willis is the most commonly used collateral network in occlusive ICA disease, but only 25% of the population has a "complete" circle. ECA to ICA connections are the next most frequently observed collaterals in ICA occlusion, including internal maxillary artery to cavernous ICA via the ophthalmic artery (Fig. 6-16) and via cavernous dural branches. Dural and transosseous ECA collaterals can form to pial vessels, although these are seen more commonly in slowly progressive obliterative processes such as moyamoya disease. A suboccipital arcade can link the occipital and vertebral arteries via muscular collateral vessels, and flow may be seen in either direction (Fig. 6-17). Other pathways include ECA to contralateral ECA and the ascending pharyngeal artery to the ipsilateral ICA and vertebral artery.

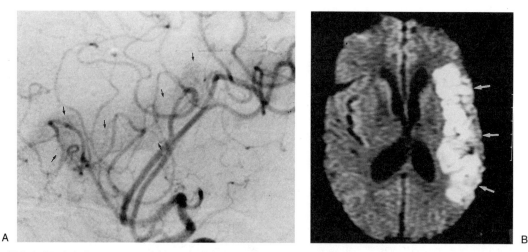

FIG. 6-15. A: Left common carotid artery digital substraction angiography, lateral oblique view. An early capillary blush is seen in the sylvian cortex *(small arrows)*. **B:** Diffusion weighted magnetic resonance imaging. The acute middle cerebral artery infarct is well seen *(arrows)*.

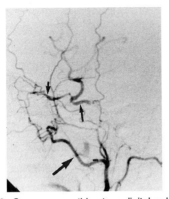

FIG. 6-16. Common carotid artery digital substraction angiography, lateral view. The internal carotid artery (ICA) is occluded. Exuberant external carotid artery to ICA collaterals are seen from the internal maxillary artery *(large arrow)* to the cavernous ICA *(small arrow)* via ethmoidal collaterals to the ophthalmic artery *(arrowhead)*.

Steal Syndrome

The term steal syndrome usually is applied to describe a proximal subclavian artery occlusion, with reversal of flow in the ipsilateral vertebral artery to supply the arm, resulting in symptoms of posterior fossa ischemia. It is actually an unusual phenomenon and may be overrated as a cause of neurologic findings, with up to 64% of patients showing reversal of vertebral artery flow being asymptomatic (25).

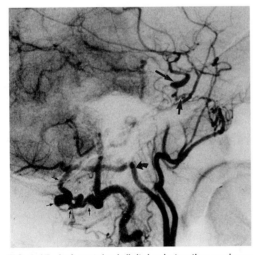

FIG. 6-17. Left vertebral digital substraction angiography, lateral view. The left common carotid artery is occluded. A suboccipital arcade *(small arrows)* links the vertebral artery to the occipital artery *(curved arrow)* and internal maxillary artery, which eventually reaches the cavernous internal carotid artery *(large arrow)* via cavernous dural collaterals *(arrowhead)*.

Fibromuscular Dysplasia

The ICA is involved in 75% of patients with this disorder, the vertebral arteries in 15% to 25%. Angiographic detection may be incidental, as 50% of patients may be asymptomatic (26). There are three histologic forms of this disease, with the medial form representing the vast majority (90%–95%). The classic angiographic appearance is the "string of beads," a series of multifocal stenoses alternating with focal dilations, usually in the cervical ICA, centered at C2-3 (Fig. 6-18A). The

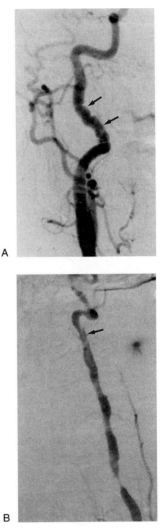

A

B

FIG. 6-18. A: Right common carotid artery digital substraction angiography, anteroposterior (AP) oblique view. Fibromuscular dysplasia of the cervical internal carotid artery *(arrows)*. **B:** Left vertebral digital substraction angiography, AP view. Fibromuscular dysplasia of the vertebral artery, with a focal dissection *(arrow)*.

proximal 2 to 5 cm of the ICA is rarely involved. Other features include septa, diverticula, pseudoaneurysms, and dissections (Fig. 6-18B). A smooth tubular stenosis can occur in the intimal form of fibromuscular dysplasia. The differential diagnosis includes several conditions. Standing waves are small regular serrations in the vessel wall related to either catheter spasm or local reaction to contrast material. Atherosclerosis and dissection can resemble the intimal form, but the bulb usually is involved with atherosclerotic disease and the degree of stenosis tends to be worse with dissection.

Moyamoya Disease

This condition was first described in 1968, and the term was coined by Suzuki and Takahu (27) to describe its angiographic hallmark, the basal arterial collateral network, which resembles a hazy puff of cigarette smoke (Fig. 6-19A–B). The initial stage of this obliterative process involves progressive smooth stenosis of the supraclinoid ICA. Subsequent development of collaterals to the MCA and ACA occurs through lenticulostriate perforating vessels. Leptomeningeal and posterior choroidal artery collaterals are prominent from the PCA to the anterior circulation (Fig. 6-19B). These perforating networks intensify as the MCA and ACA occlude, followed by development of a "rete mirabile" from ECA anasto-moses to dural and pial cortical branches. As the ICA disease worsens, the basal collateral network diminishes and the transdural and transosseous pathways predominate.

The pattern of basal perforating collaterals is not unique to this disease, as any process causing progressive occlusion of the distal ICA and origins of the MCA or ACA can produce a moyamoya-like appearance.

Dissection

These can be classified as intracranial or extracranial, traumatic or spontaneous. The spontaneous extracranial variety is characterized angiographically by an irregular, eccentric, tapered stenosis of the ICA, anywhere from the bulb to the skull base, although the proximal 2 to 3 cm often is spared. Vertebral artery involvement usually begins near C2 and may extend intracranially. Another common finding is the "pearl and string" sign of a segmental stenosis with pseudoaneurysm (Fig. 6-20), which often presents with subarachnoid hemorrhage when the distal vertebral artery is involved. Less commonly, a string sign, double lumen, or complete occlusion can be seen. Spontaneous resolution occurs in up to 60% of cases (28).

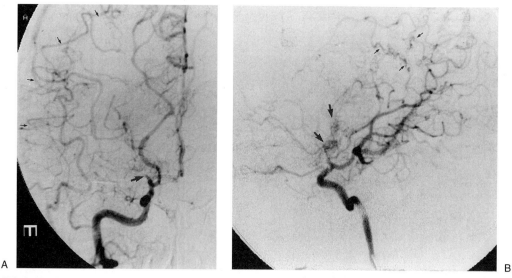

A   B

FIG. 6-19. A: Right common carotid artery digital substraction angiography, anteroposterior view. Moyamoya disease, with complete occlusion of the internal carotid artery *(arrowhead)* just beyond the posterior cerebral artery origin. There is leptomeningeal filling of middle cerebral artery branches from the anterior and posterior cerebral arteries *(small arrows)*. **B:** Common carotid artery digital substraction angiography, lateral view. Moyamoya disease with the "puff of smoke" basal collateral network *(arrowheads)*. Extensive leptomeningeal collateral channels from the posterior cerebral artery to anterior cerebral artery are seen *(small arrows)*.

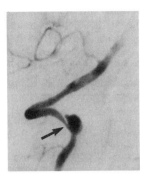

FIG. 6-20. Left vertebral digital substraction angiography, lateral view. The classic "pearl and string" of spontaneous vertebral artery dissection with pseudoaneurysm is seen *(arrow)*.

Vasculitis/Arteritis

The vasculitides can be classified as primary angiitis of the central nervous system or secondary to a multitude of systemic conditions including systemic lupus erythematosus; polyarteritis nodosa; neurofibromatosis; radiation; and drugs such as cocaine, methamphetamines, and other sympathomimetics. The angiographic appearance of all these conditions is identical, characterized by multifocal, circumferential, small-vessel narrowing, with intervening normal or dilated segments (Fig. 6-21). This "beaded" appearance supposedly is typical for vasculitis, but it also may be seen in small-vessel atherosclerotic disease, in which the affected segments may be more focal. The differential diagnosis includes infection, in which arterial walls are shaggier, and vasospasm after subarachnoid hemorrhage.

Fusiform Aneurysms/Dolichoectasia

Dilated, tortuous intracranial vessels are not uncommonly seen angiographically in elderly patients, a sequela of atherosclerosis. They may become symptomatic from mass effect, particularly in the posterior circulation. Occlusion of perforating vessels and emboli caused by stasis of flow can result in ischemic symptoms, which can be aggravated by angiography (29).

ACKNOWLEDGMENTS

The author thanks Dr. Allan J. Fox, Dr. Stephen P. Lownie, and Cathy Lockhart.

REFERENCES

1. Seldinger SI. Catheter replacement of the needle in percutaneous arteriography: a new technique. *Acta Radiol* 1953;39:368.
2. Akers DL, Markowitz IA, Kerstein MD. The value of aortic arch study in the evaluation of cerebrovascular insufficiency. *Am J Surg* 1987;154:230.
3. Barnett FJ, Lecky DM, Freiman DB, et al. Cerebrovascular disease: outpatient evaluation with selective

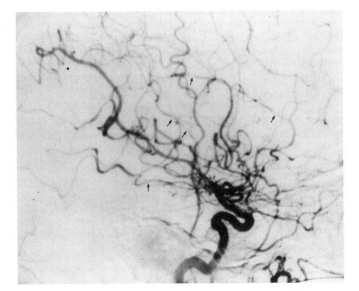

FIG. 6-21. Common carotid artery digital substraction angiography, lateral view. Primary central nervous system angiitis showing multifocal arterial stenoses and irregularities *(small arrows)* in the middle and anterior cerebral arteries.

carotid DSA performed via a transbrachial approach. *Radiology* 1989;170:535–539.

4. Matsumoto Y, Hongo K, Toriyama T, et al. Transradial approach for diagnostic selective cerebral angiography: results of a consecutive series of 166 cases. *AJNR Am J Neuroradiol* 2001;22:704–708.

5. Heiserman JE, Dean BL, Hodak JA, et al. Neurologic complications of cerebral angiography. *AJNR Am J Neuroradiol* 1994;15:1401–1407.

6. Hankey GJ, Warlow CP, Sellar RJ. Cerebral angiographic risk in mild cerebrovascular disease. *Stroke* 1990;21:209–222.

7. Dion JE, Gates PC, Fox AJ, et al. Clinical events following neuroangiography: a prospective study. *Stroke* 1987;18:997–1004.

8. Earnest F, Forbes G, Sandok BA, et al. Complications of cerebral angiography: prospective assessment of risk. *AJR Am J Roentgenol* 1984;142:247–253.

9. Bendszus M, Koltzenburg M, Burger R, et al. Silent embolism in diagnostic cerebral angiography and neurointerventional procedures: a prospective study. *Lancet* 1999;354:1594–1597.

10. Ramadan NM, Gilkey SJ, Mitchell M, et al. Postangiographic headache. *Headache* 1995;35:21–24.

11. Pexman JHW, Coates RK. Amnesia after femorocerebral angiography. *AJNR Am J Neuroradiol* 1983;4:979–983.

12. Mani RL, Eisenberg RL. Complications of catheter cerebral angiography: analysis of 5000 procedures. *AJR Am J Roentgenol* 1978;131:871–874.

13. Coley BD, Roberts AC, Fellmeth BD, et al. Postangiographic femoral artery pseudo- aneurysms: further experience with US-guided compression repair. *Radiology* 1995;194:307–311.

14. Katayama H, Yamaguchi K, Kozuka T, et al. Adverse reactions to ionic and nonionic contrast media. *Radiology* 1990;175:621–628.

15. Kido DK, Potts DG, Bryan RN, et al. Iohexol cerebral angiography. Multicenter clinical trial. *Invest Radiol* 1985;20:S55–S57.

16. Laroche DL, Aimone-Gastin I, Dubois F, et al. Mechanisms of severe, immediate reactions to iodinated contrast material. *Radiology* 1998;209:183–190.

17. Lasser EC. Pretreatment with corticosteroids to prevent reactions to IV contrast material: overview and implications. *AJR Am J Roentgenol* 1988;150:257–259.

18. Yamaguchi K, Katayoma H, Takashima T, et al. Prediction of severe adverse reactions to ionic and nonionic contrast media in Japan: evaluation of pretesting. *Radiology* 1991;178:363–367.

19. Fox AJ. The role of angiography in the assessment of atherosclerotic disease: assessment of the carotid bifurcation. *Neuroimaging Clin N Am* 1996;6:645–649.

20. Sitzer M, Muller W, Siebler M, et al. Plaque ulceration and lumen thrombus are the main sources of cerebral microemboli in high-grade internal carotid artery stenosis. *Stroke* 1995;26:1231–1233.

21. Streifler JY, Eliasziw M, Fox AJ, et al. Angiographic detection of carotid plaque ulceration. *Stroke* 1994;25:1130–1132.

22. Fox AJ, Sharpe BL, Wortzman G, et al. The art of carotid stenosis measurement: recognition of "approaching" near occlusion (a). ASNR Proceedings, Chicago, April 23, 1995, p. 20.

23. Pelz DM, Fox AJ, Eliasziw M, et al. Stenosis of the carotid bifurcation: subjective assessment compared with strict measurement guidelines. *Can Assoc Radiol J* 1993;44:247–252.

24. Irino T, Taneda M, Minami T. Angiographic manifestations in postrecanalized cerebral infarction. *Neurology* 1977;27:471.

25. Hennerici M, Klemm C, Rautenberg W. The subclavian steal phenomenon: a common vascular disorder with rare neurological deficits. *Neurology* 1988;38:669.

26. Houser OW, Baker HL, Sandok BA, et al. Cephalic arterial fibromuscular dysplasia. *Radiology* 1971;101:605.

27. Suzuki J, Takahu A. Cerebrovascular "moya-moya" disease. *Arch Neurol* 1969;20:288.

28. Houser OW, Mohri V, Sundt TM, et al. Spontaneous cervical cephalic arterial dissection and its residuum: angiographic spectrum. *AJNR Am J Neuroradiol* 1984;5:27.

29. Lownie SP. Cerebral angiography. In: Barnett HJM, Mohr JP, Stein BM, et al., eds. *Stroke,* 3rd ed. New York: Churchill-Livingstone, 1998:257–283.

Ischemic Stroke: Advances in Neurology, Vol. 92. Edited by
H.J.M. Barnett, Julien Bogousslavsky, and Heather Meldrum.
Lippincott Williams & Wilkins, Philadelphia © 2003.

7

Intracranial Atherosclerosis

L. J. Kappelle

*Department of Neurology, University Medical Center Utrecht and the Rudolf Magnus Institute
for Neurosciences, Utrecht, The Netherlands*

Stenosis of an intracranial artery frequently occurs in the setting of widespread atherosclerotic vascular disease, particularly in black, Hispanic, and Asian people (1–4). In the Northern Manhattan Stroke Study, 1% of white patients, 6% of black patients, and 11% of Hispanic patients suffered from a stroke that was caused by an intracranial atherosclerotic lesion (2). Among 387 Caucasian patients with an acute ischemic stroke or transient ischemic attack (TIA) studied in Spain, 5% had a symptomatic middle cerebral artery (MCA) stenosis (5). In another hospital-based study of 166 black and 108 white patients with acute ischemic stroke or TIA, intracranial stenosis was the only possible etiology in 8% (4).

Half of the intracranial atherosclerotic stenoses occur in the distal part of the internal carotid artery (ICA), 20% in the proximal part of the MCA, 10% in the anterior cerebral artery, 10% in the posterior cerebral artery, and 10% in the distal vertebral or basilar arteries (6). Ischemic events distal to such a stenosis can occur because of hemodynamic insufficiency or by artery-to-artery embolism. An alternative, more rare, etiology is occlusion of the origin of one or more small side branches by an atherosclerotic plaque in a large artery, resulting in small infarcts in the deep regions of the brain (7).

The fact that stroke recurrence in patients with intracranial atherosclerotic stenosis is not reduced by extracranial/intracranial (EC/IC) bypass surgery and the suggestion that anticoagulation may be the best medical treatment to prevent subsequent strokes may indicate that embolism is a more frequent cause of cerebral ischemia in these patients than hemodynamic impairment. However, microembolic signals were not detected with transcranial Doppler sonography (TCD) in patients with chronic MCA stenosis, suggesting that hemodynamic impairment is the most common cause of ischemic stroke or TIA in patients with persisting intracranial arterial stenosis (8).

DIAGNOSIS

Intracranial atherosclerotic stenosis should be considered in patients with an ischemic stroke that is characterized by cortical symptoms such as aphasia or neglect, particularly if there is no source of embolism in the heart, aorta, or extracranial carotid artery. In a series of 33 patients with ischemia in the territory of the MCA in whom no extracranial source of embolism could be found, five patients had a stenosis of more than 50% of this artery (9). In patients without cortical symptoms, atherosclerotic plaques that block the origin of one or more small penetrating branches usually cause subcortical infarcts. This etiology probably has been the major cause of ischemic events in 15% of the patients with MCA stenosis or occlusion who participated in the EC/IC Bypass Trial and who presented with pure motor hemiparesis (10).

Intracranial occlusive disease may present with either transient or permanent neurologic deficit, independent of the degree of the stenosis. In 352 patients with MCA stenosis or occlusion who participated in the EC/IC Bypass Study, isolated TIAs occurred in 28% of patients with moderate stenosis, 36% of patients with severe stenosis, and 12% of patients with MCA occlusion (10). Warning TIAs before a stroke occurred in one third of patients (10). In this cohort, onset of stroke was smoothly progressive in about 20% and stepwise in about 10%.

Conventional angiography or digital subtraction angiography (DSA) is associated with significant hazards and, therefore, has not been used on a routine basis for diagnosis of intracranial stenosis. With recent advances in noninvasive investigations, it has become more feasible to diagnose intracranial stenosis and perform follow-up studies. Noninvasive imaging methods that now are available include TCD, magnetic resonance angiography (MRA), and computed tomographic angiography (CTA).

TCD is accurate for detection of MCA stenosis (5,8,11), especially in moderate- and high-grade stenosis (12). Narrowing of the posterior cerebral artery can also be detected by TCD (13). Advantages of the TCD method are its low price, the possibility to use it at the bedside in the stroke unit, and its potential to search for microembolic signals in order to establish whether the stenosis itself is the source of emboli (14,15). Another advantage of TCD is the possibility to obtain information about vasomotor reactivity during the same procedure. A drawback of TCD for diagnosis of MCA stenosis is insufficient ultrasound penetration through the temporal window in a small percentage of the patients, although this has been reported in up to 35% of patients with stroke (16). Other problems are the operator dependency and the lack of commonly accepted diagnostic criteria, especially with respect to the level at which Doppler flow velocities should be considered significantly elevated (8,12).

MRA is a promising method to study intracranial vessels and is becoming more available (17). A disadvantage may be that it tends to overestimate the degree of stenosis (18). The sensitivity of the combination of TCD and MRA has been reported to be very high and may even be better than that of routine DSA alone (12).

CTA is useful for diagnosis of MCA stenosis or occlusion (19). It probably is as reliable as MRA for grading MCA stenosis (20,21). An advantage of CTA is that it can be performed directly after routine computed tomographic scanning of patients with acute stroke and requires only a short period of extra time. This may be important if local intraarterial thrombolysis is considered in the acute stage. Obviously, a disadvantage of CTA is the need for intravenous contrast. Another drawback in comparison with DSA and MRA is that only a limited segment of the intracranial vasculature can be imaged.

RISK FACTORS

Intracranial atherosclerotic lesions occur more commonly in nonwhite people, but information on whether race is an independent factor for these lesions is controversial. In the cohort of the EC/IC Study, race was the only factor that was independently associated with the location of atherosclerosis. Black and Asian patients more often had occlusive disease of the MCA than white patients (22); however, in the Northern Manhattan Stroke Study, nonwhite race was not an independent risk factor (odds ratio: 4.4; 95% confidence interval: 0.6–35) (2). Intracranial atherosclerosis was found in about one fourth of both black and white patients in another series, but isolated intracranial disease was more common in black patients (4).

Patients with intracranial atherosclerosis tend to be older than patients with normal intracranial vessels (22) but younger than patients with extracranial atherosclerosis (2). Whether gender is an independent risk factor for intracranial atherosclerotic disease is unclear. Intracranial atherosclerotic lesions may be more common in men than in women (4). In the cohort of the EC/IC Study, 79% of patients with MCA stenosis were male. In contrast, in the Stroke Data Bank, only 10 of 23 patients with intracranial atherosclerotic stenosis were men (1), and gender was not an independent risk factor for the presence of intracranial ICA stenosis in other studies (2,23).

Hypertension is a common finding among patients with intracranial atherosclerotic disease (1,2). This may be influenced by the fact that hypertension has a relative high prevalence in black people. It was reported as an independent risk factor for the presence of an intracranial atherosclerotic stenosis in patients who underwent angiography between 1983 and 1986 at the Mayo Clinic (23), but this could not be confirmed in patients studied in Northern Manhattan (2).

Insulin-dependent diabetes mellitus is independently associated with intracranial atherosclerosis (2). Among the patients randomized in the EC/IC Bypass Study, 15% had diabetes mellitus (22), which is twice as common as in the Northern Manhattan Stroke Study and in the Stroke Data Bank (1,2). The duration of cigarette smoking was the most significant independent predictor of the presence of intracranial stenosis of the ICA in the cohort of the Mayo Clinic (23). The Northern Manhattan Stroke Study is the only study that reported an association between hypercholesterolemia and stroke caused by intracranial atherosclerosis (2).

The presence of intracranial atherosclerotic disease doubled the risk of complications after coronary artery bypass graft surgery (24). It also is a risk factor for subsequent stroke in patients with symptomatic extracranial ICA stenosis (25).

PROGNOSIS

In general, prognosis of chronic intracranial arterial disease is unfavorable. Mortality has been reported to be as high as 50% in patients with symptomatic distal ICA stenosis during a mean follow-up of 5 years (26). About one fourth of patients with a 50% to 99% symptomatic intracranial atherosclerotic stenosis suffered from a subsequent stroke during a mean follow-up of 19 months. (27). In the medically treated arm of the EC/IC Bypass Trial, 36% of patients with high-grade distal ICA stenosis and 24% of patients with MCA stenosis had a subsequent stroke during a mean follow-up of 55.8 months (28).

During a mean follow-up of 6.1 years, a stroke rate of only 18% was found in a series of 44 patients with intracranial disease of the vertebrobasilar arteries, of whom 73% were symptomatic at baseline (29). The Warfarin-Aspirin Symptomatic Intracranial Disease (WASID) Investigators, however, found a stroke rate of 22% during a mean follow-up of 13.8 months in a series of 68 patients with arterial stenosis in the posterior fossa (30).

Rapid acceleration of atherosclerosis in intracranial arteries has been reported in elderly people, whereas progression of atherosclerosis in extracranial arteries usually is more equal over all ages (31). In a series of 49 patients, after 2 years the degree of symptomatic intracranial atherosclerotic stenosis had progressed in about one third (32). Improvement of the stenosis has been reported after EC/IC bypass surgery (33). In a series of 21 patients with intracranial atherosclerotic stenosis, repeat angiography after a mean follow-up of 26.7 months showed progression of the stenosis in 40%, regression in 20%, and a stable lesion in 40% (6).

TREATMENT

In the acute stage of an intracranial occlusion, systemic thrombolysis should be considered if the treatment can be given within 3 hours after onset of the clinical features (34). Intraarterial thrombolysis administered within 6 hours after onset of the neurologic deficit has been demonstrated to be beneficial in patients with MCA occlusion (35).

For secondary prevention, management of risk factors deserves primary priority. Medical treatment has not yet been sufficiently investigated in patients with intracranial atherosclerosis. Aspirin is used frequently based on the results of studies showing a benefit for preventing stroke in patients with noncardioembolic stroke. Aspirin also was prescribed in the medical arm of the EC/IC Bypass Study. In a retrospective study, the relative risk of a major vascular event in patients treated with warfarin was about half that of patients who took aspirin (27), and a recent meta-analysis also suggested a protective effect of warfarin, but not for aspirin, in patients with extracranial carotid occlusion or intracranial occlusive disease (36). The use of antiplatelet agents rather than warfarin was associated with therapeutic failure in a retrospective series of 52 patients with symptomatic intracranial arterial stenosis (37). For definite conclusions, the results of the current WASID trial are awaited (38). In this trial, the secondary protective values of warfarin (international normalized ratio 2:3) and 1,300 mg of aspirin daily are being compared in patients with 50% to 99% symptomatic intracranial arterial stenosis (38).

Currently, there are no surgical options for intracranial atherosclerotic stenosis. EC/IC bypass did not confer any additional benefit to aspirin (28). Endovascular treatment has been advocated (39) but is still in its infancy (40). Preliminary results from small retrospective series are promising (41,42), but more prospectively collected data are needed to determine the role of angioplasty or stenting. The Stenting of Symptomatic Atherosclerotic Lesions in the Vertebral or Intracranial Arteries (SSYLVIA) trial will provide data about the safety of extracranial vertebral or intracranial arterial stenosis (40). If the results of this trial are promising, further randomized clinical trials are needed to obtain a definite answer as to whether endovascular treatment should be performed in patients with intracranial atherosclerotic stenosis.

Coexistence of mild or moderate intracranial stenosis in patients with symptomatic high-grade stenosis of the extracranial ICA is not a reason to preclude carotid endarterectomy (25). Only three patients with intracranial atherosclerotic disease need to undergo carotid endarterectomy for a symptomatic extracranial ICA stenosis between 85% and 99% to prevent one ipsilateral stroke in the next 3 years (25). In the absence of intracranial atherosclerotic lesions, this number is six (25).

REFERENCES

1. Caplan LR, Gorelick PB, Hier DB. Race, sex and occlusive cerebrovascular diseases: a review. *Stroke* 1986;17: 648–655.
2. Sacco RL, Kargman DE, Gub Q, et al. Race-ethnicity and determinants of intracranial atherosclerotic cerebral infarction. The Northern Manhattan Stroke Study. *Stroke* 1995;26:14–20.
3. Leung SY, Ng THK, Yuen ST, et al. Pattern of cerebral atherosclerosis in Hong Kong Chinese. Severity in

intracranial and extracranial vessels. *Stroke* 1993:24: 779–786.

4. Wityk RJ, Lehman D, Klag M, et al. Race and sex differences in the distribution of cerebral atherosclerosis. *Stroke* 1996;27:1974–1980.

5. Segura T, Serena J, Castellanos M, et al. Embolism in acute middle cerebral artery stenosis. *Neurology* 2001; 56:497–501.

6. Akins PT, Pilgram TK, Cross DT, et al. Natural history of stenosis from intracranial atherosclerosis by serial angiography. *Stroke* 1998;29:433–438.

7. Caplan LR. Intracranial branch atheromatous disease: a neglected understudied, and underused concept. *Neurology* 1989;39:1246–1250.

8. Sliwka U, Klötzsch C, Popescu O, et al. Do chronic middle cerebral artery stenoses represent an embolic focus? A multirange transcranial Doppler study. *Stroke* 1997;28:1324–1327.

9. Lutsep HL, Clark WM. Association of intracranial stenosis with cortical symptoms or signs. *Neurology* 2000;55:716–718.

10. Bogousslavsky J, Barnett HJM, Fox AJ, et al., for the EC/IC Bypass Study Group. Atherosclerotic disease of the middle cerebral artery. *Stroke* 1986;17:1112–1120.

11. Ley-Pozo J, Ringelstein EB. Noninvasive detection of occlusive disease of the carotid siphon and middle cerebral artery. *Ann Neurol* 1990;28:640–647.

12. Röther J, Schwartz A, Wentz KU, et al. Middle cerebral artery stenoses: assessment by magnetic resonance angiography and transcranial Doppler ultrasound. *Cerebrovasc Dis* 1994;4:273–279.

13. Diehl RR, Sliwka U, Rautenberg W, et al. Evidence for embolization from a posterior cerebral artery thrombus by transcranial Doppler monitoring. *Stroke* 1993;24: 606–608.

14. Nabavi DG, Georgoadis D, Mumme T, et al. Detection of microembolic signals in patients with middle cerebral artery stenosis by means of a bigate probe. *Stroke* 1996;27:1347–1349.

15. Wong KS, Gao S, Lam WW, et al. A pilot study of microembolic signals in patients with middle cerebral artery stenosis. *J Neuroimaging* 2001;11:137–140.

16. Laps M, Teschendorf U, Dorndorf W. Haemodynamic studies in early stroke. *J Neurol* 1992;239:138–142.

17. Wilms G, Bosmans H, Demaerel P, et al. Magnetic resonance angiography of the intracranial vessels. *Eur J Radiol* 2001;38:10–18.

18. Stock KW, Radue EW, Jacob AL, et al. Intracranial arteries: prospective blinded comparative study of MR-angiography and DSA in 50 patients. *Radiology* 1995;195:451–456.

19. Wong KS, Liang EY, Lam WWM, et al. Spiral computed tomography angiography in the assessment of middle cerebral artery occlusive disease. *J Neurol Neurosurg Psychiatry* 1995;59:537–539.

20. Wong KS, Lam WWM, Liang E, et al. Variability of magnetic resonance angiography and computed angiography in grading middle cerebral artery stenosis. *Stroke* 1996;27:1084–1087.

21. Lavados P, Oppenheimer S, Enger C. Variability of magnetic resonance angiography and computed angiography in grading middle cerebral artery stenosis using the unweighted kappa statistic. *Stroke* 1996;27:2340.

22. Inzitari D, Hachinski VC, Taylor DW, et al. Racial differences in the anterior circulation in cerebrovascular disease. How much can be explained by risk factors? *Arch Neurol* 1990;47:1080–1084.

23. Ingall TJ, Homer D, Baker HL, et al. Predictors of intracranial carotid artery atherosclerosis. Duration of cigarette smoking and hypertension are more powerful than serum lipid levels. *Arch Neurol* 1991;48:687–691.

24. Yoon BW, Bae HJ, Kang DW, et al. Intracranial cerebral artery disease as a risk factor for central nervous system complications of coronary artery bypass graft surgery. *Stroke* 2001;32:94–99.

25. Kappelle LJ, Eliasziw M, Fox AJ, et al., for the North American Symptomatic Carotid Endarterectomy Trial (NASCET) Group. Importance of intracranial atherosclerotic disease in patients with symptomatic stenosis of the internal carotid artery. *Stroke* 1999;30:282–286.

26. Marzewski DJ, Furlan AJ, St. Louis P, et al. Intracranial internal carotid artery stenosis: long-term prognosis. *Stroke* 1982;13:821–824.

27. Chimowitz MI, Kokkinos P, Strong J, et al., for the Warfarin-Aspirin Symptomatic Intracranial Disease Study Group. The warfarin-aspirin symptomatic intracranial disease study. *Neurology* 1995;45:1488–1493.

28. The EC/IC Bypass Study Group. Failure of extracranial-intracranial arterial bypass to reduce the risk of ischemic stroke: results of an international randomized trial. *N Engl J Med* 1985;313:1191–2000.

29. Mouifarrij NA, Little JR, Furlan AJ, et al. Basilar and distal vertebral artery stenosis: long-term follow-up. *Stroke* 1986;17:938–942.

30. The Warfarin Aspirin Symptomatic Intracranial Disease (WASID) Study Group. Prognosis of patients with symptomatic vertebral or basilar artery stenosis. *Stroke* 1998;29:1389–1392.

31. D'Armiento FP, Bianchi A, de Nigris F, et al. Age-related effects on atherogenesis and scavenger enzymes of intracranial and extracranial arteries in men without classic risk factors for atherosclerosis. *Stroke* 2001;32: 2472–2480.

32. Bauer RB, Boulos RS, Meyer JS. Natural history and surgical treatment of occlusive cerebrovascular disease evaluated by serial arteriography. *Am J Roentgenol Radium Ther Nucl Med* 1968;104:1–17.

33. Awad I, Furlan AJ, Little JR. Changes in intracranial stenotic lesions after extracranial-intracranial bypass surgery. *J Neurosurg* 1984;60:771–776.

34. The National Institute of Neurological Disorders and Stroke rt-PA Stroke Study Group. Tissue plasminogen activator for acute ischemic stroke. *N Engl J Med* 1995; 333:1581–1587.

35. Furlan A, Higashida R, Wechsler, et al. Intra-arterial prourokinase for acute ischemic stroke. The PROACT II Study: a randomized controlled trial. *JAMA* 1999:282: 2003–2011.

36. Klijn CJM, Kappelle LJ, Algra A, et al. Outcome in patients with symptomatic occlusion of the internal carotid artery or intracranial arterial lesions: a meta-analysis of the role of baseline characteristics and type of antithrombotic treatment. *Cerebrovasc Dis* 2001;12:228–234.

37. Thijs VT, Albers GW. Symptomatic intracranial atherosclerosis. Outcome of patients who fail antithrombotic therapy. *Neurology* 2000;55:490–497.

38. Benesch CG, Chimowitz MI, for the WASID Investigators. Best treatment for intracranial arterial stenosis? 50 years of uncertainty. *Neurology* 2000;55:465–466.

39. Gomez CR, Orr SC. Angioplasty and stenting for pri-

mary treatment of intracranial arterial stenoses. *Arch Neurol* 2001;58:1687–1690.

40. Chimowitz MI. Angioplasty or stenting is not appropriate as first-line treatment of intracranial stenosis. *Arch Neurol* 2001;58:1690–1692.

41. Clark WM, Barnwell SL, Nesbit G, et al. Safety and efficacy of percutaneous transluminal angioplasty for intracranial atherosclerotic stenosis. *Stroke* 1995;26:1200–1204.

42. Marks MP, Marcellus M, Norbash AM, et al. Outcome of angioplasty for atherosclerotic intracranial stenosis. *Stroke* 1999;30:1065–1069.

Ischemic Stroke: Advances in Neurology, Vol. 92. Edited by
H.J.M. Barnett, Julien Bogousslavsky, and Heather Meldrum.
Lippincott Williams & Wilkins, Philadelphia © 2003.

8

Collateral Circulation Imaging for Arterial Lesions of Stroke

Robert D. Henderson

*Department of Medicine, University of Queensland and Department of Neurology,
Royal Brisbane Hospital, Brisbane, Queensland, Australia*

The brain requires approximately 20% of the oxygen used by the body, with the primary blood supply supplied via the internal carotid artery (ICA) (~75%–80%) and the vertebrobasilar system (~20%–25%) (1,2). The term *collateral circulation* is used for the connections between these major arterial pathways that form the circle of Willis, the anterior communicating artery (AcoA) and posterior communicating arteries (PcoA), and the terminal connections of the anterior, middle, and posterior cerebral arteries (usually called leptomeningeal pathways). Collateral circulation also is used for other pathways that can supply blood flow to the brain, predominantly the branches of the external carotid artery (ECA) that connect with the ophthalmic artery (OA), although other connections also exist (3). Rare connections may exist between the ECA and vertebral arteries, and pial to dural connections. The term *primary collaterals* is useful to designate the pathways of the circle of Willis, the AcoA, and the PcoA that may provide cerebral blood flow in normal physiologic circumstances. The term *secondary collaterals* is useful for those pathways that usually provide significant flow only in situations of pathologic or iatrogenic obstruction to the ICA or its major branches. Some consider that functionally significant flow only occurs through the secondary pathways with ICA obstruction and poor primary collateral pathways (4).

A number of factors influence the ability of imaging modalities to identify collateral pathways, and the heterogeneity of patient populations are important when comparing different imaging techniques. Normal variation in the anatomic presence and size of collateral pathways from autopsy data occurs with age and gender differences (5). From anatomic and angiographic studies in the normal and atherosclerotic population, fewer than 5% lack the anatomic presence of the AcoA; higher percentages lack the PcoA (5). In the normal and nonstenotic atherosclerotic population, a hypofunctional (hypoplastic) AcoA may occur in up to one third and the PcoA in up to half of those studied based on imaging and anatomic investigations (5–7). However, when occlusion or near occlusion of the ICA occurs, primary collateral pathways that previously were poorly imaged (hypoplastic) become functional and can be visualized as shown by increased vessel diameters with ICA occlusion (5). There is increased visualization of collaterals with increasing degrees of severe ICA stenosis (8,9). With moderate ICA stenosis, flow through primary collateral pathways often is not demonstrable (8). The increased flow through primary collateral pathways is assumed to occur soon after an ICA occlusion and may not change over time (10), although it can be argued that collateral flow develops slowly over months with increasing degrees of ICA stenosis. Atherosclerotic vascular risk factors, particularly hypertension, may limit the formation of collateral pathways (11).

The importance of the cerebral collateral circulation remains an area of investigation. Without significant obstruction, the absence of components of the primary collateral pathways (the normal variants of the circle of Willis) or secondary collateral pathways has not been shown to play a pathophysiologic role. In the setting of ICA stenosis or occlusion, the collateral circulation may affect ischemic events and determine cerebral perfusion. In the large North American Symptomatic Carotid Endarterectomy Trial (NASCET) study of symptomatic ICA stenosis, the

presence of angiographic collateral flow through
either of the primary collateral pathways was associated with a reduced risk of hemispheric stroke or
transient ischemic attack in medically treated patients
and a reduced perioperative risk of stroke in surgically treated patients (8). Others have shown that
patients with no collateral filling of the middle cerebral artery and an ICA occlusion are more likely to
have watershed or full infarct on CT (12). The likely
mechanism is the protective effect of collateral pathways to enhance washout of emboli and to improve
delivery of nutrients to ischemic regions (13). It is
likely that a relatively small subset of stroke patients
have recurrent events due to perfusion failure. In situations of decreased cerebral perfusion, there have
been conflicting reports on the importance of collateral pathways to cerebral hemodynamics. Clearly,
cerebral perfusion is likely to be reduced in the
absence of both the AcoA and the PcoA on the side
of an occlusion (9). Blood flow then is dependent on
the ECA. Similarly, cerebral perfusion is reduced
when there are poor primary collateral pathways in
the setting of bilateral occlusion (9). In the setting of
unilateral ICA occlusion combined with the absence
of only one primary collateral pathway, most studies
have been unable to show a reduction in cerebral perfusion as shown by hemodynamic events or perfusion
studies (14). The relative clinical importance of the
primary and secondary collateral pathways is debated
in the literature. Some studies support the concept
that the AcoA is the more important pathway for supply of the anterior and middle cerebral arteries when
there is ICA occlusion (1,8,9). The absence of the
AcoA alone increases the risk of stroke (8) but probably not perfusion failure (4,14). One small study that
showed fewer infarcts in the presence of a PcoA of
large diameter (15) was not replicated by work from
the Dutch group (14). The presence of leptomeningeal
collaterals has been associated with poor cerebral
hemodynamics and recurrent symptoms after occlusion, suggesting that the presence of leptomeningeal
collaterals is a marker of poor cerebral perfusion (4).
Significant cerebral flow through the OA is reported
to occur in the presence of poor primary collateral
pathways (16).

Conventional angiography has been the gold standard of imaging modalities for the collateral pathways and is consistent with anatomic studies (1).
More information is provided than by noninvasive
techniques. Collateral pathways are an important feature of angiographic near occlusion (Fig. 8-1) (17).
Angiography provides evidence of anatomic collateral pathways and may provide evidence regarding

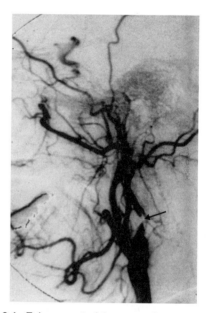

FIG. 8-1. Enlargement of the external cerebral artery
pathways in an internal carotid artery near occlusion
(arrow).

flow. Grading systems have been used to quantify
flow through the AcoA (8). With injection of the common carotid artery, flow can be visualized through the
AcoA filling the contralateral anterior and middle
cerebral arteries (Figs. 8-2 and 8-3). Flow in the OAs

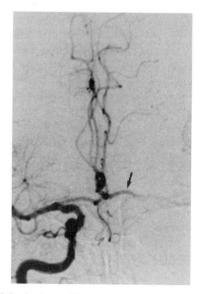

FIG. 8-2. Angiographic anterior communicating artery
with filling of the anterior cerebral artery and slight filling of the middle cerebral artery *(arrow)* from the contralateral internal cerebral artery.

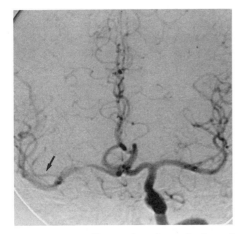

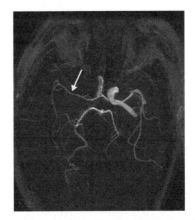

FIG. 8-3. Angiographic anterior communicating artery with more extensive filling of the middle cerebral artery branches *(arrow)* from the contralateral internal cerebral artery.

FIG. 8-4. Magnetic resonance angiography showing filling of the right middle cerebral artery *(arrow)* via the anterior communicating artery in a patient with a right internal cerebral artery occlusion.

can be visualized from the ECA, and with delayed sequences flow through leptomeningeal pathways can be seen. Filling via the PcoA can be seen in the presence of carotid artery obstruction, but ipsilateral flow requires a vertebral artery injection to demonstrate filling of the middle cerebral artery, and in some clinical studies data are not available from vertebral injections. Angiography is particularly useful in assessing collateral pathways such as the patterns seen in moyamoya disease or unusual connections between the ICA and ECA.

Magnetic resonance imaging is noninvasive and provides anatomic and physiologic evidence of flow through the major collateral pathways (5). Two- and three-dimensional magnetic resonance angiography (MRA) can provide morphologic information and assess velocities with phase contrast visualizing the direction of flow. Time-of-flight MRA allows the arteries of the circle of Willis to be visualized through the endogenous contrast of flow-related spin enhancement (Figs. 8-4 and 8-5). The addition of gadolinium can improve visualization but the suppression of venous pathways is important. Flow through small-caliber arteries may not be well visualized because of the lower sensitivity of three-dimensional time-of-flight MRA to detect either low or turbulent flow, and the presence of the AcoA and PcoA is variably less than that reported with angiography (5,14). It can be debated whether arteries that do not show blood flow on MRA are functionally significant in contributing to cerebral perfusion. MRA is less useful for visualizing other collateral pathways such as the ophthalmic and leptomeningeal pathways, but

it can be used to assess other collateral pathways at the base of the brain, such as those seen with moyamoya disease.

Computed tomographic angiography is being performed as an alternative to angiography or MRA for depiction of the collateral pathways of the circle of Willis (18). The generally perceived lower resolution has meant that its main indication for assessment of collateral pathways has occurred when angiography or MRA are contraindicated, but this may change.

Ultrasonography using transcranial Doppler (TCD) provides another noninvasive means of assessing flow

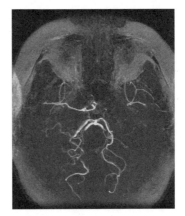

FIG. 8-5. Magnetic resonance angiography in a patient with bilateral internal cerebral artery occlusion. Serial sequences show that the right middle cerebral artery was primarily reconstituted by the right posterior communicating artery with the left middle cerebral artery probably formed from left middle meningeal artery collaterals.

through collateral pathways and is particularly useful for detection of reversed flow through the OA. Reversed flow through the OA has been used to increase the noninvasive identification of severity of an ICA stenosis; however, significant flow through the OA probably requires poor primary collateral flow in addition to a near occlusive stenosis. Detection of reversed flow in the AcoA and first part of the anterior cerebral artery ipsilateral to the occluded ICA stenosis is feasible with TCD techniques (7,19). TCD can be useful before carotid endarterectomy to indicate patients who may not require shunting during the operation (20). Flow through the PcoA can be assessed but is technically limited by the temporal bone. Additional maneuvers, such as compression or refinements including the use of color-coding and echo or contrast enhancement, probably improve the sensitivity of TCD to detect the PcoA (21). Arteries with low flow (hypoplastic) are not well depicted with standard TCD (22).

REFERENCES

1. Mount LA, Taveras JM. Arteriographic demonstration of the collateral circulation of the cerebral hemispheres. *AMA Arch Neurol Psych* 1957;78:235–253.
2. Van Everdingen KJ, Klijn CJM, Kapelle LJ, et al., for the Dutch EC-IC Bypass Study Group. MRA flow quantification in patients with a symptomatic internal carotid artery occlusion. *Stroke* 1997;28:1595–1600.
3. Gillilan LA. Potential collateral circulation to the human cortex. *Neurology* 1974;24:941–948.
4. Powers WJ. Cerebral hemodynamics in ischemic cerebrovascular disease. *Ann Neurol* 1991;29:231–240.
5. Hartkamp MJ, van der Grond J, van Everdingen KJ, et al. Circle of Willis collateral flow investigated by magnetic resonance angiography. *Stroke* 1999;30:2671–2678.
6. Hoksbergen AW, Fulesdi B, Legemate DA, et al. Collateral configuration of the circle of Willis: transcranial color-coded duplex ultrasonography and comparison with postmortem anatomy. *Stroke* 2000;31:1346–1351.
7. Ringelstein EB, Zunker P. Low-flow infarction. In: Ginsberg MD, Bogousslavsky J, eds. *Cerebrovascular disease.* Boston: Blackwell Science, 1998:1084
8. Henderson RD, Eliasziw M, Fox AJ, et al. Angiographically defined collateral circulation and risk of stroke in patients with sever carotid artery stenosis. *Stroke* 2000;31:128–132.
9. Klutymans M, van der Grond J, van Everdingen KJ, et al. Cerebral hemodynamics in relation to patterns of collateral flow. *Stroke* 1999;30:1432–1429.
10. Rutgers DR, Klijn CJM, Kapelle LJ, et al. A longitudinal study of collateral flow patterns in the circle of Willis and the ophthalmic artery in patients with a symptomatic internal carotid artery occlusion. *Stroke* 2000;1:1913–1920.
11. Hedera P, Bujdakova J, Traubner P, et al. Stroke risk factors and development of collateral flow in carotid occlusive disease. *Acta Neurol Scand.* 1998;98:182–186.
12. Harrison MJG, Marshall J. The variable clinical and CT findings after carotid occlusion: the role of collateral blood supply. *J Neurol Neurosurg Psychiatry* 1988;51: 269–272.
13. Caplan LR, Hennerici M. Impaired clearance of emboli (washout) is an important link between hypoperfusion, embolism and ischemic stroke. *Arch Neurol* 1998;55: 1475–1482.
14. Van Everdingen KJ, Visser GH, Klijn CJ, et al. Role of collateral flow on cerebral hemodynamics in patients with unilateral internal artery occlusion. *Ann Neurol* 1998;44:167–176.
15. Schomer DF, Marks MP, Steinberg GK, et al. The anatomy of the posterior communicating artery as a risk factor for ischemic cerebral infarction. *N Engl J Med* 1994;330:165–170.
16. Tatemichi TK, Chamorro A, Petty GW, et al. Hemodynamic role of ophthalmic artery collateral in internal carotid artery occlusion. *Neurology* 1990;40:461–464.
17. Morgenstern LB, Fox AJ, Sharpe BL, et al. The risks and benefits of carotid endarterectomy in patients with near occlusion of the carotid artery. *Neurology* 1997;48: 911–915.
18. Shrier DA, Tanaka H, Numaguchi Y, et al. CT angiography in the evaluation of acute stroke. *AJNR Am J Neuroradiol* 1997;18:1011–1020.
19. Baumgartner RW, Baumgartner I, Mattle HP, et al. Transcranial color-coded duplex sonography in the evaluation of collateral flow through the circle of Willis. *AJNR Am J Neuroradiol* 1997;18:127–133.
20. Visser GH, Wieneke GH, van Huffelen AC, et al. The use of preoperative transcranial Doppler variables to predict which patients do not need a shunt during carotid endarterectomy. *Eur J Vasc Endovasc Surg* 2000;19:226–232.
21. Droste DW, Jurgens R, Weber S, et al. Benefit of echocontrast-enhanced transcranial color-coded duplex ultrasound in the assessment of intracranial collateral pathways. *Stroke* 2000;31:920–923.
22. Klötsch C, Popescu O, Berlit P. Assessment of the posterior communicating artery by transcranial color-coded duplex sonography. *Stroke* 1996;27:486–489.

Ischemic Stroke: Advances in Neurology, Vol. 92. Edited by
H.J.M. Barnett, Julien Bogousslavsky, and Heather Meldrum.
Lippincott Williams & Wilkins, Philadelphia © 2003.

9

Update on Imaging Aortic Atherosclerosis

Pierre Amarenco and *Ariel Cohen

*Department of Neurology, Denis Diderot University, and
Department of Neurology and Stroke Centre, Bichat Hospital, Paris France, and *Department of
Cardiology, Saint-Antoine Hospital, Pierre and Marie Curie University, Paris, France*

In the past few years, evidence has accumulated that atherosclerotic disease of the aortic arch probably is an underestimated source of emboli, particularly moving thrombi in the lumen because the aortic arch is actually a precerebral artery. Pathologic studies and more recently transesophageal echocardiography (TEE) studies have shown that atherosclerotic disease of the aortic arch is an independent risk factor for ischemic stroke and carries a high risk of recurrent vascular events. It could account for a more or less important portion of brain infarcts of unknown cause, with no carotid or cardiac source of emboli detected (1). Atherosclerosis in the aortic arch is a strong marker of generalized atherosclerosis, particularly coronary, carotid, and peripheral artery disease. A causal link is generally accepted between brain infarcts and complicated plaques with highly mobile thrombus in the lumen of the aortic arch (2), particularly in patients with otherwise unexplained stroke or stroke occurring after aortography (3) or aortic cannulation for cardiopulmonary bypass (4–7).

Several studies reinforced the notion that plaques in the aortic arch are independent risk factors for brain ischemia. The questions are as follows: how to image aortic plaques in 2002; how can vulnerable plaques be recognized and which morphologic parameter is relevant in terms of predicting risk; are aortic plaques good predictors of coronary, carotid, and peripheral artery disease; how frequent is cholesterol embolization versus thromboembolic complication of moving thrombi floating into the lumen of the aortic arch; and finally which treatment can be reasonably recommended in the absence of a specific randomized controlled trial?

IMAGING THE AORTIC ARCH PLAQUES

Although it is limited by its semi-invasive nature and by a blinded portion of the ascending aorta, TEE is still the gold standard in daily practice to detect protruding plaques and mobile thrombi in the thoracic aorta. Correlations between TEE images and pathology, or between endarterectomy material and intraoperative epiaortic ultrasonography, have shown good concordance (7–9). TEE can nicely demonstrate large plaques or floating and moving thrombi in the lumen. Vaduganathan et al. (10) had 73% agreement between intraoperative TEE of the thoracic aorta and histology performed thereafter. TEE was unable to detect ulcerations, but complex atheroma and mobile debris were detected in 100% of cases. Thrombus was detected with a sensitivity of 91% and a specificity of 90%.

Magnetic resonance angiography (MRA) compares well with TEE and may be superior in showing culprit lesions in the ascending aorta; however, the sensitivity of detection of plaques greater than 5 mm is 54% with MRA versus 92% with TEE (11). Supraclavicular approach with ultrasound examination may image the ascending aorta well, but it requires training with use of the method (12).

A new noninvasive techniques is transthoracic echocardiography by suprasternal harmonic imaging, which allows a positive predictive value of 91% and a negative predictive value of 98% for large protruding plaques; however adequate image quality could be obtained in only 89% of patients (13). The most promising tool and next gold standard probably is high-resolution magnetic resonance imaging (MRI).

IMAGING VULNERABLE PLAQUES

Several works have established a statistical link between the presence of atherosclerotic disease in the aortic arch and ischemic stroke (13–22). The main morphologic parameters that were studied to identify vulnerable plaques were ulcerations at autopsy and plaque thickness at TEE, as well as surface irregularities, calcifications, hypoechoic plaques (suggestive of thrombus), and mobile thrombus floating in the lumen of the aortic arch.

Plaque Thickness

The most important parameter that has been related to the risk for complication and clinical events is the thickness of the aortic plaque.

Case Control Studies

In 1991, Tunick et al. (14) reported a retrospective study based on recruitment of patients to their echocardiography laboratory. They compared the frequency of plaques ≥5 mm thickness in the thoracic aorta in 12 patients referred for determination of the source of emboli and in 12 patients referred for other cardiologic reasons (Table 9-1). They found these large plaques in 27% of patients who had an embolic event and in 9% of those who had no emboli. After adjustment for principal risk factors, the odds ratio

(OR) was 3.2 [95% confidence interval (CI), 1.6–6.5] (14). This study was retrospective, and the results were not adjusted for the presence of other potential causes of brain infarct or peripheral emboli.

A prospective case control study using TEE in 250 consecutively admitted patients older than 60 years with brain infarcts found a frequency of plaques in the aortic arch significantly different from that of controls (16). In this study, we looked at the risk according to plaque thickness and found that the risk of brain infarct attached to aortic arch plaques located proximal to the left subclavian artery ostium increased with the thickness of the plaques (Table 9-2).

This large increase was observed only for lesions of ≥4 mm located proximal to the left subclavian artery ostium in the ascending aorta or proximal arch, not for lesions distal to the left subclavian artery ostium in the distal arch or descending aorta. The increase in risk for ischemic stroke associated with plaques ≥4 mm in the proximal arch was independent of the presence of the two major risk factors for stroke in the elderly, which are carotid stenosis and atrial fibrillation. The frequency of plaques ≥4 mm in the proximal arch did not differ according to the degree of carotid stenosis, and the frequency of such plaques was lower in patients with atrial fibrillation than in those without atrial fibrillation. Plaques ≥4 mm in thickness located proximal to the left subclavian artery ostium also are associated with an abrupt increase in the risk for stroke among patients who had ischemic strokes with no apparent

TABLE 9-1. *Prevalence and risk of ischemic stroke in the presence of large protruding plaques in the aortic arch in case control studies*

Case control studies	Plaque thickness	N	Patients	Controls	Adjusted odds ratio
Autopsy					
Amarenco et al. (15)	UP	239	28%	5%	4.0 (95% CI, 2.1–7.8)
Khathibzadeh et al. (24)	UP, thrombi, debris	40	68%	34%	5.8 (95% CI, 1.1–31.7)
Transesophageal echocardiography					
Tunick et al. (14)	≥5mm	122	27%	9%	3.2 (95% CI, 1.6–6.5)
Amarenco et al. (16)	≥4mm	250	14.4%	2.0%	9.1 (95% CI, 3.3–25.2)
Jones et al. (17)	≥5mm	215	21.4%	3.5%	8.2 (95% CI, 3.0–22.4)
Nihoyannopoulos et al. (18)	Not measured	42	48%	22%	Not done
Stone et al. (19)	≥5mm	49	32.7%	7%	Not done
Di Tullio el al. (20)	≥5mm	106	26%	13%	2.6 (95% CI, 1.1–5.9)
Intraoperative epiaortic echocardiography					
Dávilla-Román et al. (7)	≥3mm	158	26.6%	18.1%[a]	1.65 (95% CI, 1.1–2.4)

CI, confidence interval; UP, ulcerated plaques.

[a]88.3% of patients in this study underwent coronary artery bypass grafting, thus explaining this high rate of aortic plaques in the control group.

TABLE 9-2. Risk of cerebral infarct as a function of thickness of atherosclerotic plaques in the ascending aorta and proximal arch

Wall thickness (mm)	Patients [% (no.)]	Controls [% (no.)]	Crude OR (95% CI)	Adjusted OR[a] (95% CI)	p Value
<1[b]	39.6 (99)	75.6 (189)	1	1	/
1–1.9[c]	11.2 (28)	6.4 (16)	3.3 (1.7; 6.5)	4.4 (2.1–8.9)	<0.001
2–2.9[c]	22.4 (56)	10.4 (26)	4.1 (2.4; 7.0)	5.0 (2.7–9.0)	<0.001
3–3.9[c]	12.4 (31)	5.6 (14)	4.2 (2.2; 8.3)	3.4 (1.5–7.4)	<0.001
≥4	14.4 (36)	2.0 (5)	13.8 (5.2; 36.1)	9.1 (3.3–25.2)	<0.001

CI, confidence interval; OR, odds ratio.
[a]After controlling for age, sex, hypertension, cigarette smoking, high serum cholesterol, diabetes, past myocardial infarction, and atrial fibrillation.
[b]Reference category.
[c]Adjusted risk of plaques 1.3–9 mm is 4.4 (95% CI, 2.8–6.8).
From Amarenco R, Cohen A, Tzourio C, et al. Atherosclerotic disease of the aortic arch and the risk of ischemic stroke. N Engl J Med 1994;1474–1479.

cause. Furthermore, the presence of a mobile component of the plaque was associated with an OR of 14 among patients with ischemic stroke of unknown cause.

These results were strengthened by another case control study performed the same year in Australia by Jones et al. (17), who found a 7.1-fold increase in the risk for ischemic stroke in the presence of "complex atheroma" in the aortic arch. The singularity of this study was that the authors compared patients with brain infarcts or transient ischemic attacks (TIAs) with a population-based control group that included only healthy volunteers. From among 304 consecutive patients with a first-ever ischemic stroke, they included 215 patients (20 of whom had only TIAs) and in addition 202 healthy volunteers for TEE examination; 94% of patients with ischemic stroke and 78% of control subjects also had carotid imaging. They found "simple" plaques that were <5 mm thick and smoothes in the ascending aorta and aortic arch in 33% of patients and 22% of controls. They found "complex" plaques that were >5 mm thick or plaques with an irregular surface or a mobile component in 22% of patients and 4% of controls. In a further analysis using a more objective measure of atheroma severity comparing patients and controls with plaques ≥5 mm thick or <5 mm thick rather than "simple" and "complex" plaques, they found an adjusted OR of 8.2 (95% CI, 3.0–22.4) for plaques ≥5 mm thick and 2.2 (95% CI, 1.2–4.1) for plaques <5 mm. They also found mobile protruding atheroma in the aortic arch in 11 patients and in only one control subject (crude OR = 10.8; 95% CI, 1.4–84.7). They did not confirm a significant asso-

ciation between complex aortic arch plaques and ischemic stroke of unknown origin (20% in patients with stroke of unknown origin and 23% in patients with ischemic stroke with a known cause) (17).

Dávila-Román et al. (7) studied a consecutive series of 1,334 cardiac patients 50 years or older who were undergoing open heart surgery. This study was important because the investigators used an intraoperative epiaortic ultrasonography device (not TEE), which allows assessment of the entire length of the ascending aorta from the root of the aorta to the level of the proximal arch, a region that is difficult to image with TEE (which shows mainly the aortic arch). The ascending aorta is more likely to be a donor site for brain embolism than more distal regions of the aorta. Among 1,200 patients who underwent epiaortic ultrasonography, 158 had a previous embolic event and 1,042 were free of embolic events. They found plaques ≥3 mm in the ascending aorta in 26.6% of patients who had a previous neurologic event and in 18.1% of "control" subjects who were free of neurologic events. Most of these patients (88.3%) were undergoing coronary artery bypass grafting, which easily explains the high rate of protruding plaques in the control group. Multivariate analysis showed that significant predictors of previous neurologic ischemic events were hypertension (OR = 1.81), ascending aorta atherosclerosis (OR = 1.65), atrial fibrillation (OR = 1.54), and in the subset of 789 patients who were evaluated for carotid artery disease with ultrasound, severe carotid stenosis (OR = 2.7).

Nihoyannopoulos et al. (18) prospectively studied the aorta of 152 consecutive patients older than 40 years referred for detection of atherosclerosis of the thoracic aorta. Lesions in the aorta were classified into fixed atherosclerotic lesions and mobile lesions. Duplex ultrasound of the carotid arteries was performed in all patients with distinction between obstructive lesion (stenosis >50%) and nonobstructive lesion (stenosis <50%). Among the group of 152 patients, 44 (29%) had at least one major atheromatous lesion in the thoracic aorta. In these 44 patients, atherosclerotic plaques were located in the horizontal portion of the aortic arch in 20 (45%), in the ascending aorta in 7 (16%), and in the descending aorta in 17 (39%). All but two patients with major atherosclerotic lesions in the descending aorta had other smaller lesions at the horizontal portion. Only 3 (8%) of the 44 patients had mobile lesions. Atherosclerotic plaques in the thoracic aorta were present in 20 (48%) of 42 patients with an embolic event and in 24 (22%) of 110 patients without embolic events ($p < 0.001$). Among the 152 patients, 26 had atherosclerotic lesions in the carotid arteries, including 7 with >50% stenosis, all associated with extensive atherosclerotic disease in the thoracic aorta; and 19 with <50% stenosis, 16 of them with plaques in the aorta and 3 without plaque.

Using TEE, Stone et al. (19) studied 49 consecutive patients 40 years or older with ischemic stroke and 57 age-matched control subjects without stroke. They found protruding plaque ≥5 mm in 16 (32.7%) patients and 4 (7%) control subjects.

Di Tullio et al. (20) studied 106 patients and 114 stroke-free control subjects and more frequently found large (≥0.5 cm) protruding atheroma in the proximal aortic arch in the stroke patients than in controls (26% vs 13%), particularly in patients 60 years or older with unexplained stroke than in controls (22% vs 8%). After multivariate analysis, proximal aortic atheroma was found to be independently associated with stroke (adjusted OR = 2.6, 95% CI, 1.1–5.9).

Prospective Studies

Plaque thickness was the most studied morphologic parameter prospectively (Table 9-3). Tunick et al. (21) found an annual event rate of 33% in patients who had protruding plaques ≥5 mm in the thoracic aorta compared with 7% in matched controls. This study did not focus on plaques that were located in the aortic arch but rather in the entire thoracic aorta. The difference between the two groups was not significant with regard to brain and retinal emboli only (7 events in patients vs. 3 events in controls) (21). In studying 33 patients at 1 year, Montgomery et al. (22) found that 24% had died. At follow-up TEE examination they found that severe lesions were dynamic, with formation of new mobile components in 61% of cases, whereas there was resolution of specific previously documented mobile lesions in up to 70% of cases (22).

TABLE 9-3. *Risk of new vascular events in patients with large protruding plaques compared with control subjects*

Follow-up study	N	Patients	Controls	Relative risk
Tunick et al. (2)	42	PI ≥5 mm	No atheroma	
Mean follow-up 14 mo				
Stroke + MI + peripheral emboli		33% at 2 yr	7% at 2 yr	4.3 (95% CI, 1.2–15.0)
Stroke + retina		16% at 2 yr	7% at 2 yr	
FAPS study (23)[a]	331	PI ≥4 mm	No atheroma	
788 p-y of follow-up				
Stroke + MI + peripheral emboli		26 per 100 p-y	5.9 per 100 p-y	3.5 (95% CI, 2.1–5.9)
Stroke		11.9 per 100 p-y	2.8 per 100 p-y	3.8 (95% CI, 1.8–7.8)
Mitusch et al. (62)	183			
241 p-y of follow-up		PI ≥5 mm or mobile thrombi	PI <5 mm	
Stroke + peripheral emboli		13.8 per 100 p-y	4.1 per 100 p-y	4.3 (95% CI, 1.5–12.0)
Previously symptomatic patients: stroke + peripheral emboli		15.9 per 100 p-y	7.1 per 100 p-y	
Dávila-Ráman et al. (67)	1,800	PI ≥5 mm	No atheroma	
All events		30% at 1 yr	9% at 1 yr	1.7 (95% CI, 1.4–2.0)
Neurologic events		11% at 1 yr	3% at 1 yr	1.6 (95% CI, 1.2–3.2)

CI, confidence interval; MI, myocardial infarction; PI, plaque thickness; p-y; patient-year.
[a]For the estimated risk at 1, 2, 3, and 4 years, see the Kaplan-Meier curve and make projections on axix (Figs. 9-1 and 9-2).

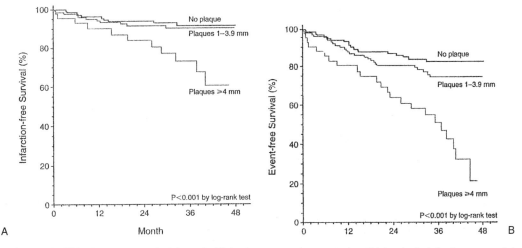

FIG. 9-1. A: Risk of recurrent brain infarct. **B:** Risk of new vascular events (combining brain infarcts, myocardial infarctions, peripheral events, and vascular deaths). (From The French Study of Aortic Plaques in Stroke Group. Atherosclerotic disease of the aortic arch as a risk factor for recurrent ischemic stroke. *N Engl J Med* 1996;334:1216–1221, with permission.)

The French Study of Aortic Plaques in Stroke (FAPS) Study followed 331 consecutive patients admitted to the hospital for brain infarct for 2 to 4 years (23). All patients had TEE at presentation. The annual incidence of recurrent brain infarcts was 11.9 per 100 patient-years of follow-up in patients with aortic arch plaques ≥4 mm compared with an incidence of 3.5 in patients with plaques from 1 to 3.9 mm and an incidence of 2.8 in patients with no plaque. The incidence of all vascular events (combining stroke, myocardial infarction, peripheral emboli, and vascular death) was 26 compared with 9.1 and 5.9 per 100 patient-years of follow-up, respectively (Fig. 9-1). In patients with cryptogenic brain infarcts at entry and with plaques ≥4 mm thick, the event rates

per 100 patients-years of follow-up were 16 for recurrent brain infarct and 26 for all vascular events.

Multivariate analysis showed that aortic arch plaques ≥4 mm thickness were significant predictors of new brain infarcts, independent of the presence of carotid stenosis, atrial fibrillation and peripheral artery disease, with a relative risk of 3.8 (95% CI, 1.8–7.8; *p* < 0.002). The significant difference observed among the three Kaplan-Meier curves (Figs. 9-1 and 9-2) according to aortic plaque thickness is a further strong argument for a causality link between plaques ≥4 mm thick and brain infarcts in some of these patients. However, this study also showed that the presence of plaques ≥4 mm thick in the aortic arch is a strong and independent predictor of all vascular events, with a rel-

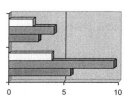

Odds ratio

FIG. 9-2. Risk of new vascular events (brain infarction, myocardial infarction, peripheral emboli, or vascular death) in patients with plaques ≥4 mm in the aortic arch proximal to the takeoff of the left subclavian artery, according to the presence or lack of calcification of plaques (From Cohen A, Tzourio C, Bertrand B, et al., on behalf of the FAPS Investigators. Aortic plaque morphology and vascular events. A follow-up study in patients with ischemic stroke. *Circulation* 1997;96:3838–3841).

ative risk of 3.5 (95% CI, 2.1–5.9; $p < 0.001$] (23). These observations led to the conclusion that the presence of plaques ≥4 mm in the aortic arch is a good marker for generalized atherosclerosis that could be used to select patients at high vascular risk in therapeutic trials. Clearly, the thickness of plaques in the aortic arch identifies vulnerable plaques.

Ulcerated Plaques

Ulcerations may be difficult to diagnose or is overdiagnosed with TEE, which was shown to be not highly sensitive by Vaduganathan et al. (10).

In our autopsy study of 500 consecutive patients performed in the laboratory of Neuropathology at La Salpêtrière hospital, we and others found ulcerated plaques in the aortic arch in 28% of patients with cerebrovascular disease and in only 5% of patients with other neurologic disease (15). This difference was very significant. After adjustment for age, gender, and hypertension, we found an OR of 4.0 (95% CI, 2.1–7.8). When the frequency of ulcerated plaques in the aortic arch in patients with brain infarct of unknown cause was compared with the frequency in patients who suffered infarcts of known etiology, we also found a very significant difference (61% vs. 28%, adjusted OR = 5.7; 95% CI, 2.4–13.6). The presence of ulcerated plaques in the aortic arch was not correlated to the presence of internal carotid artery stenosis or atrial fibrillation (15). These two last points suggest that ulcerated plaques in this autopsy series may have been causally related to brain infarction of unknown etiology. Another important point of this study was the observation that among the 75 patients who had ulcerated plaques in the aortic arch, only two were younger than 60 years and 73 (97%) were 60 years or older (15).

Khathibzadeh et al. (24) studied 120 consecutive autopsies, 40 of whom had cerebral, visceral, or lower limb embolisms noted on pathologic examination. They were able to confirm an association between ulcerated plaques, mural thrombi, or both in the aortic arch and arterial embolism. Ulcerated plaques, mural thrombi, or both in the aortic arch or descending aorta were found in 25 patients (69%) with cerebral infarction. Interestingly, 9 patients among the 12 with cerebral infarction that had not been diagnosed clinically had ulcerated plaques in the aortic arch, and 28 patients with cerebral infarction had silent visceral embolisms noted on pathologic examination.

Stone et al. (19) attempted to distinguish ulceration within plaques and adherent mobile debris by using video calipers. Ulcers were defined using multiplane transducer as craters ≥2 mm deep and wide. The 49 patients were divided into two groups: 23 with unexplained ischemic stroke and 26 with a known cause. Ulcerated plaques were seen significantly more frequently in patients with unexplained ischemic stroke (39%) than in patients with a known cause (8%) and in control subjects (7%) with $p < 0.001$ (19). This was an important study because it was the first attempt to determine the clinical importance of what can be interpreted as ulceration on TEE examination. Although the numbers were small, the authors believe that the results concur with what has been found at autopsy with ulcerated plaques in the same groups of patients with brain infarcts of unknown cause (15).

Di Tullio et al. (20) also noted that ulcerated (using the same definition for ulceration) and mobile atherosclerotic lesions were seen more frequently in patients than in controls (12% vs. 5%; $p < 0.06$). They also found that differences were entirely attributable to patients 60 years or older and concluded that the absence of carotid stenosis does not exclude aortic atheromas as a potential cause for ischemic stroke (20). The same group recorded asymptomatic microembolisms to the brain [high-intensity transient signals (HITS)] in the middle cerebral artery using transcranial Doppler. Microembolisms are bright signals in the spectrum and are likely to be released by ulcerations or superimposed thrombi. They found that HITS occurred significantly more frequently in patients with plaques <4 mm, and the difference was even more important when there were no TEE findings other than plaques in the thoracic aorta. Finally, HITS were present in 100% of cases of what were called ulcerated or mobile lesions (25).

Other Morphologic Parameters: Calcification, Plaque Surface Irregularities, Hypoechoic Plaque, and Mobile Thrombi

In the FAPS Study (23), case control analysis showed that calcifications and surface irregularities suggestive of ulcerations were independently associated with brain infarction, but plaque thickness still had the strongest association (Table 9-4). When we combined plaque thickness and calcification, plaque thickness and surface irregularities, and plaque thickness and no calcification, the strongest association was found in patients with plaques <4 mm and no calcification.

In the prospective follow-up of the FAPS Study, we found that among morphologic parameters such as plaque thickness, surface irregularities, calcifications, and hypoechoic plaques suggestive of thrombus, plaque thickness <4 mm still had the highest event rate. When we combined plaque thickness and hypoechoic plaques

TABLE 9-4. *Risk of brain infarction as a function of morphologic characteristics of atherosclerotic plaques in the ascending aorta and proximal arch in 338 patients compared with 357 controls*

Wall thickness	Crude OR (95% CI)	p Value	Adjusted OR[a] (95% CI)	p Value
Calcifications	2.9 (2.1; 4.2)	<0.001	2.3 (1.6; 3.3)	<0.001
Irregular surface	4.3 (2.5; 7.1)	<0.001	3.4 (2.0; 5.7)	<0.001
Thickness ≥4 mm	7.6 (3.4; 17.2)	<0.001	5.4 (2.3; 12.4)	<0.001
Thickness ≥4 with calcifications	6.9	<0.001	2.2	= 0.095
Thickness ≥4 mm with irregular surface	11.3 (4.0; 32.2)	<0.001	7.4 (2.6; 21.8)	<0.001
Thickness ≥4 mm without calcifications	8 (7.0; 8)	<0.001		

CI, confidence interval; OR, odds ratio.
[a]Adjusted for sex, peripheral vascular diseases, tobacco consumption, and hypertension.
Data from the FAPS Study (23).

or surface irregularities, we found no additive prognostic value compared with only plaque thickness <4 mm. However, we found a very significant prognostic additive value when we compared plaques <4 mm with no calcification to plaques <4 mm (Fig. 9-2) (26).

Plaques in the aortic arch ≥4 mm as detected by TEE are markers for a high risk of recurrent brain infarcts and mainly for other vascular events. Surface irregularities, hypoechoic appearance of plaques, and presence of calcification have little or no additive prognostic value, but plaques ≥4 mm with no calcifications are much more predictive of new vascular events than plaques ≥4 mm with calcification. These noncalcified hypoechoic plaques, probably the youngest, lipid-laden

plaques, are likely to be the most vulnerable and perhaps the most accessible to preventative treatment. The relative benefits and risks of therapeutic interventions need to be evaluated in these patients.

Mobile thrombi, floating into the lumen of the thoracic aorta, are highly independently associated with brain infarction, and obviously they predict new events (27). They are found in 8% of patients with otherwise negative workup, and a mobile component adds to the risk of a 4-mm-thick plaque (16). Mobile thrombi are very rare in young patients; Laperche et al. (28) found such a lesion in one of 1,000 TEE examinations. However, in older patients, mobile thrombi represent 6% to 8% of unexplained embolic events (Table 9-5).

TABLE 9-5. *Prevalence of mobile thrombi in the lumen of the aortic arch in consecutive series*

Origin of series	Sample size	Mobile thrombi	Percentage of mobile thrombi
Consecutive ischemic stroke patients			
Toyoda et al. 1992 (8) (embolic stroke)	62	3	4.8%
Nihoyannopoulos et al. 1993 (18)	152	3	2%
Jones et al. 1994 (17) (unselected patients)	202	11	5.4%
Amarenco et al. 1994 (16) (unselected patients)	250	7	2.8%
Stone et al. 1995 (19) (unselected patients)	49	2	4.1%
Consecutive TEE performed in an echocardiography laboratory			
Tunick et al. 1991 (14)	122	11	9.0%
Karalis et al. 1991 (68)	556	11	2.0%
Mitchell et al. 1992 (69)	600	5	0.8%
Mitusch et al. 1995 (70)	335	8	2.4%
Embolic events or unexplained brain infarction			
Tunick et al. 1991 (14) (embolic events)	122	11	9.0%
Karalis et al. 1991 (68) (embolic events)	44	11	25.0%
Horowitz et al. 1992 (71) (embolic stroke)	183	7	4%
Nihoyannopoulos et al. 1993 (18) (embolic events)	42	3	7.1%
Amarenco et al. 1994 (16) (unexplained brain infarct)	78	6	7.7%
Stone et al. 1995 (19) (unexplained brain infarct)	23	2	8.7%
Mitusch et al. 1995 (70) (embolic events)	80	5	6.3%

TEE, transesophageal echocardiography.

ETIOLOGIC BURDEN OF AORTIC ARCH PLAQUES AT LEAST FOUR MILLIMETERS THICK IN ISCHEMIC STROKE

The presence of aortic arch plaques ≥4 mm thick is a new, strong, independent risk factor for brain infarcts with a possible causal link. Plaques ≥4 mm are present in one third of patients with cryptogenic stroke, who themselves account for one third of the total ischemic stroke population aged 60 years or older (16). Some of these patients have complicated plaques with pedunculated and mobile thrombotic components, which constitute a permanent threat for brain emboli. This can be expected in 1 of 10 patients with cryptogenic stroke (Table 9-5) (16). The attributable risk of plaques ≥4 mm is 12.6% with a CI 7.6% to 17.6%. This indicates that the etiologic part of plaques ≥4 mm could be as high as that of nonvalvular atrial fibrillation or severe stenosis of internal carotid artery origin.

AORTIC ARCH PLAQUES AS RISK MARKERS

Aortic Arch Plaques as Markers for Coronary Artery Disease

In 1988, Tobler and Edwards (29) studied at autopsy 97 specimens of the ascending aorta from adults who had clinically symptomatic coronary heart disease. All of the patients had myocardial infarction, and most of them had undergone coronary artery bypass grafting. They found that 38% of these patients had atherosclerotic plaques >8 mm thick in the ascending aorta. This result showed that the association between plaques in the ascending aorta and symptomatic coronary artery plaques may be stronger than that observed between ulcerated plaques in the aortic arch and ischemic stroke in another pathologic study in which only 26% of patients with ischemic stroke had ulcerated plaques in the aortic arch (3).

Later, in the Framingham cohort, Witteman et al. (30) found that the presence of calcified thoracic aortic plaques on chest x-ray film was associated with an increased risk for cardiovascular death. Using TEE for detection of aortic plaques in 600 consecutive examinations of patients seen in their echocardiography laboratory or in the operating room, Fazio et al. (31) selected 61 patients who previously had coronary angiography for various cardiologic reasons within 1 year of TEE examination. They found a coronary artery obstruction in at least one vessel in 41 patients and atherosclerotic plaques of the aorta in

39 patients. Atherosclerotic plaques in the thoracic aorta were present in 37 (90%) of the 41 patients with coronary artery obstruction compared with 2 (10%) of the 20 patients without coronary artery obstruction, with a sensitivity of 90% and a specificity of 90% for angiographically proved obstructive coronary artery disease. The positive predictive value for obstructive coronary artery disease was 95% and the negative predictive value was 82%. In a study with a similar design, Tribouilloy et al. (32) found that thoracic aortic plaques had a negative predictive value of 99% for significant coronary obstructive disease. Despite evident bias of recruitment, these studies convincingly showed that atherosclerotic aortic plaques appear to be sensitive and specific predictors of obstructive coronary artery disease.

The FAPS Investigators followed 331 consecutive patients with a previous ischemic stroke during 788 person-years (23). The incidence of myocardial infarction and sudden death was 9 per 100 person-years of follow-up in patients with plaques in the proximal aortic arch ≥4 mm thick, 4.2 per 100 person-years in patients with plaques 1 to 3.9 mm thick, and 1.4 per 100 person-years in patients with no plaques in the aortic arch. These results clearly show that aortic arch plaques are good markers for future coronary artery events, at least in patients with previous ischemic stroke.

Aortic Arch Plaques and Other Markers for Atherosclerosis

Among risk factors such as hypertension, diabetes mellitus, hypercholesterolemia, and cigarette smoking, cigarette smoking seems to be the strongest risk factor associated with severe aortic arch atherosclerosis in case control studies (Table 9-6). Hypertension (15) and diabetes mellitus (17) occasionally have been found associated with aortic arch plaques, particularly those ulcerated at autopsy.

Hypercholesterolemia has been found to be associated with severe aortic arch plaques in only one case control study with a mean total cholesterol level of 218 ± 48 mg/dL versus 210 ± 47 mg/dL ($p < 0.030$) (7). This case control study included patients with coronary artery disease. It is well known that the main risk factor for carotid stenosis is hypertension, the main risk factor for coronary artery disease is hypercholesterolemia, and the main risk factor for peripheral arterial disease is smoking. From the data currently available, it seems that the main risk factor associated with aortic arch atherosclerotic disease is smoking. In these studies, peripheral arterial disease

TABLE 9-6. *High-resolution magnetic resonance imaging: aortic atherosclerotic plaques versus risk factors in an asymptomatic population (318 subjects) in the Framingham Heart Study*

Risk factors	Contemporaneous		25-year longitudinal	
	OR	95% CI	OR	95% CI
Smoking (yes/no)	2.74	1.23–6.16	5.85	2.54–13.47
Systolic blood pressure (per 1 SD)	1.04	0.79–1.37	1.09	0.83–1.43
Total cholesterol (per 1 SD)	1.10	0.85–1.43	1.46	1.11–1.92
Risk score (per 1 SD)	1.31	1.01–1.72	1.59	1.21–2.09

CI, confidence interval; OR, odds ratio.

also was strongly associated with aortic arch disease (Table 9-7).

High-resolution MRI used in 318 asymptomatic subjects of the Framingham cohort allowed evaluation of risk factors according to the presence of aortic plaques (Table 9-6), confirming that smoking status was the most important risk factor associated with aortic plaques, but also total cholesterol, in the 25-year longitudinal follow-up (33).

The relationship between aortic arch and carotid atherosclerosis have been more debated. In our autopsy study there was a proportion of carotid stenosis ≥75% as frequent in patients with as in patients without ulcerated plaques in the aortic arch. Similarly, carotid stenoses <75% or normal carotid artery were as frequent in patients with as in patients without ulcerated plaques in the aortic arch (15). In our case control study using TEE in living patients, there was a significant relation between the severity of carotid stenosis and aortic arch plaques 1 to 3.9 mm thick, but we confirmed the lack of association between carotid stenosis and plaques ≥4 mm thick. We found plaques ≥4 mm thick in 14% of patients with no carotid stenosis, 15% of patients with moderate (<70%) carotid stenosis, and 15% of patients with

severe (≥70%) carotid stenosis (16). Dávila-Román et al. (7) had similar findings. They reported the presence of severe carotid stenosis in 4% of patients with no atheroma and in 6.5% of patients with atherosclerosis of the ascending aorta. In another study of 100 patients undergoing cardiac surgery using epiaortic ultrasonography and carotid ultrasound, Dávila-Román et al. (34) found that the 10 patients with severe atherosclerosis in the ascending aorta were well distributed in the group of patients with mild carotid stenosis <50% (4 patients), moderate carotid stenosis 50% to 79% (3 patients), and severe carotid stenosis 80% to 99% (3 patients).

In contrast, Di Tullio et al. (20) found that the frequency of large atheromas in the aortic arch increased with the degree of carotid stenosis: 6% in patients with no carotid stenosis, 29% in patients with <60% carotid stenosis, and 40% in patients with ≥60% carotid stenosis. However, the positive predictive value of ≥60% carotid stenosis was only 16% for large aortic atheroma. Moreover, 36% of patients with mild or no carotid stenosis had large or complex aortic arch atherosclerosis (20). Jones et al. (17) reported similar results. There was a significant association between the severity of aortic arch atheroscle-

TABLE 9-7. *Association among smoking, peripheral arterial disease, and severe aortic arch atherosclerosis*

	No aortic arch atheroma	Large aortic arch plaques[a]	p Value
FAPS Study (23)			
Smoking	39.9%	57.8%	0.03
Peripheral vascular disease	7%	24.4%	0.003
Dávila-Román et al. (7)			
Smoking	46.4%	61.3%	<0.001
Peripheral vascular disease	6.8%	19.5%	<0.001
Jones et al. (17)			
Smoking	11%	24%	0.01
SPARC Study (Olmsted) (73)			
Smoking	43.1%	63.6%	<0.001

[a]Correspond to plaques ≥4 mm thick in the FAPS Study, ≥3 mm thick in the Dávila-Román et al. study, and ≥5 mm thick in the Jones et al. study.

TABLE 9-8. *Distribution of TEE findings in the SPAF-III TEE substudy population and associated risk of embolic events*

TEE findings	Percentage of the total population	Risk per year
Isolated atrial fibrillation	35%	1.2%
Atrial fibrillation and thrombus or spontaneous echocontrast	28%	7.5%
Atrial fibrillation and aortic arch plaques ≥4 mm	17%	12%
Atrial fibrillation and both thrombus and aortic arch plaques ≥4 mm	20%	20.5%

SPAF, Stroke Prevention in Atrial Fibrillation; TEE, transesophageal echocardiography.

rosis and the severity of carotid stenosis; however, as in the study by Di Tullio et al. (20), Jones et al. (17) found that the presence of carotid disease was not a reliable predictor of aortic atherosclerosis (positive predictive value 57%; negative predictive value 73%).

Demopoulos et al. (35) compared the frequency of protruding aortic arch atheroma in 45 patients with carotid stenosis ≥50% and ischemic stroke and in 45 patients with ischemic stroke without carotid stenosis. Aortic plaques were found in 17 (38%) and 7 (16%) patients, respectively. Mobile lesions were found almost exclusively in patients with carotid stenosis (13% vs. 2%). However, in selecting as "control" group 45 patients without carotid stenosis, the authors likely selected patients referred to them for detection of a cardiac source of emboli, which is mainly those with atrial fibrillation or embolic brain infarct of unknown source. In this manner, they biased their study toward patients with atherosclerotic disease in one group and without atherosclerotic disease in the second group. In the FAPS study (23), which included consecutive patients with ischemic stroke, 13.3% of patients with carotid stenosis ≥70% and 11.8% of patients with carotid stenosis ≥ 30% had plaques ≥4 mm.

Data from the SPAF-III TEE substudy showed that 17% of patients with atrial fibrillation included in the study had large plaques in the thoracic aorta, and this greatly increased the risk of developing a brain or systemic emboli (Table 9-8) (36).

AORTIC ARCH PLAQUES AS CAUSAL FACTORS FOR BRAIN INFARCTION

Atheroemboli (Cholesterol Crystal Emboli) to the Brain

Cholesterol Emboli to the Brain

Ulcerated plaques in the aortic arch were first recognized pathologically as potential donor sites of cholesterol crystal emboli (atheroemboli) to the brain, retina, peripheral organs such as kidneys, and distal lower limb arteries with blue toe syndrome (Figs. 9-3 and 9-4). These crystals only block distal arteriolar vessels and may only cause very small cortical or subcortical infarctions. Most frequently they are asymptomatic, as routinely found in retinal arteries (37), in muscle biopsy when performed (38), or in small arteries of abdominal viscera at autopsy (39). Panum (40) is generally acknowledged as the first to propose, as early as 1862, that ulcerated atherosclerotic plaques could give rise to artery-to-artery emboli. In 1945, Flory (41) pointed out that embolization of the systemic arterial system from atherosclerotic plaques of the aorta probably is more frequent than generally realized. Winter (42) reported in 1957 two observations of patients with multiple cerebral infarctions due to cholesterol emboli from eroded atheromata of the ascending segment of the aorta.

In 1964, Saloway and Aronson (43) found 16 cases of atheromatous embolism to the brain among 6,685 consecutive adult autopsies performed during 5 years in their institution, and they found 14 previously published cases in the literature. The presence of aortic atherosclerosis was noted in each of the 16 cases. The majority of the supratentorial malacic lesions were located in the lateral cortical and subcortical cerebral tissues, as well as in the basal ganglia. The infarcts often varied in age, suggesting an intermittent release of emboli. Atheromatous emboli were of small size

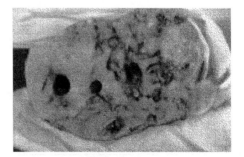

FIG. 9-3. Ulcerated plaques in the aortic arch at autopsy.

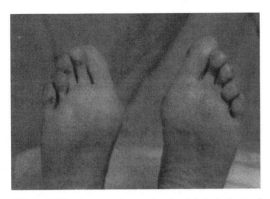

FIG. 9-4. Blue toe syndrome due to distal cholesterol embolization.

and arrested in vessels with diameters <200 μm. In their discussion, the authors emphasized that any trauma, surgical manipulation of aortic aneurysm, carotid angiography, or carotid thromboendarterectomy significantly increased the hazard of atheroembolism to the kidneys or brain.

Beal et al. (44) reported the unique observation of one patient who had innumerable TIAs lasting 3 to 8 minutes during a 3-year-period; the patient then developed progressive left arm weakness. At that time he underwent right carotid endarterectomy, but postoperatively his left leg gradually became paralyzed,

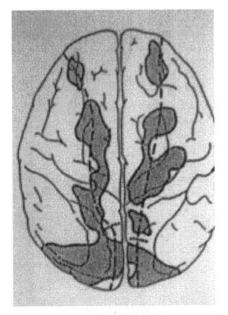

FIG. 9-5. Border zone infarcts in the distal fields of the territory of the middle cerebral, anterior cerebral, and posterior cerebral arteries.

with lateral gaze palsy to the left. He remained drowsy and disoriented, and he died of renal failure, gastrointestinal bleeding, and empyema. At pathologic examination, the patient was noted to have severe ulcerative atherosclerosis of the thoracic aorta, with multiple infarcts in the adrenal glands, spleen, pancreas, kidneys, and brain. Brain infarctions were mainly distributed to the cortical border zone areas on each side (Fig. 9-5). Many small (15 to 120 μm) arteries adjacent to the infarcts were occluded by cholesterol crystals (44).

A frequent feature is the occurrence of several focal ischemic episodes involving the retina and brain, then the development of progressive encephalopathy with confusional state and astasia. Skin and muscle biopsies may show typical cholesterol crystals (45). Rare clinical presentations may be falsely diagnosed as panarteritis nodosa (39,46).

Cholesterol Emboli to the Retinal Artery

Another frequent feature of atheromatous cholesterol emboli is retinal infarction, amaurosis fugax, or asymptomatic bright plaques discovered at funduscopy (37,47,48). Bruno et al. (49) studied 70 consecutive men with asymptomatic retinal cholesterol emboli seen in an eye clinic and 21 men without cholesterol emboli randomly selected from the same clinic. They found carotid stenosis ipsilateral to embolus in 13% of patients and in none of the control subjects ($p = 0.18$). Heterogeneous or echolucent plaque on either side was present in 95% of patients and 60% of controls ($p < 0.001$). The authors concluded that cholesterol emboli indicate systemic atherosclerosis rather than ipsilateral carotid artery stenosis (49). One can suggest that the source of embolism, if not in the carotid, should be located further down in the aortic arch. Bruno et al. (50) followed these 70 patients and 70 controls during a mean of 3.4 years. The annual event rate of ischemic stroke was 8.5% in patients compared with 0.8% in controls (relative risk 9.9; 95% CI, 2.3–43.1). Myocardial infarction or vascular death occurred with at an annual event rate of 7.7% compared with 4.9% in controls. This study showed that retinal cholesterol emboli are an important risk factor for brain infarction independent of common vascular risk factors.

Atheroemboli and Cardiac Surgery

Atheromatous emboli from the aortic arch has been recognized the cause of brain infarction in patients undergoing cardiac surgery. Price and Harris (48) in

1970 and then McKibbin et al. (5) in 1976 each reported the clinical and necropsy findings of one patient who had atheroemboli during cardiac surgery under retrograde aortic perfusion. In the case reported by Price and Harris, the aorta was studded with calcified atherosclerotic plaques. Embolic arterial occlusions were found in the heart, kidney, spleen, pancreas, and brain. The majority of occluded vessels had inner diameter less than 200 μm (range 54–384 μm). In these vessels, there was the biconvex, needle-shaped crystals characteristic of atheromatous embolism. The cerebral arteries were moderately atherosclerotic. The distribution of infarction was mostly in border zone areas (Fig. 9-5) (48). In the case reported by McKibbin et al. (5), postmortem examination showed multiple infarcts in the brain, eyes, and spleen due to emboli of cholesterol crystals and other atheromatous debris from a ruptured plaque in the ascending aorta at the site of the aortotomy.

In 1985, Gardner et al. (4) identified risk factors for perioperative strokes in 3,279 consecutive patients undergoing coronary artery bypass grafting. They made a case control study in 56 patients who had perioperative stroke and 112 control patients. They identified increased age, preexisting stroke (20% vs. 8%), protracted cardiopulmonary bypass time, and severe perioperative hypotension (23% vs. 4%) as significant risk factors for perioperative stroke. Severe atherosclerotic disease of the ascending aorta (14% vs. 3%) also was found to be a very significant predictor of perioperative stroke.

The landmark autopsy study reported in 1992 by Blauth et al. (51) showed a close relationship between severe atherosclerosis of the ascending aorta, atheroembolism, and age in patients who died after cardiac surgery for myocardial revascularization or valve operations. Among 221 patients who died, embolic disease was identified in 69 patients and atheroemboli in 48 patients. Of these 48 patients, 46 (95.8%) had severe atherosclerosis of the ascending aorta at autopsy. Conversely, among 123 patients who had severe atherosclerosis in the ascending aorta, 46 (37.4%) had pathologic evidence of atheroembolic events versus only 2 (2%) of the 98 patients without significant atherosclerosis in the ascending aorta.

Cholesterol Embolization and Antithrombotic Treatments

Treatment of this condition has been controversial because anticoagulants can accelerate cholesterol emboli. There has been a temporal association of cho-

lesterol emboli with both warfarin and streptokinase therapy (52–54). Cholesterol emboli may occur because antithrombotic effects prevent thrombosis over an ulcerated plaque (55). Bruns et al. (56) reported a patient who developed livedo reticularis, confusion, transient monocular blindness, pancreatitis, and renal failure while taking warfarin for phlebitis. Renal biopsy showed cholesterol emboli. After discontinuation of anticoagulant, the patient was asymptomatic and renal function improved. Only antiplatelet therapy seems reasonable in these cases.

Thromboemboli to the Brain

Various circumstances have suggested that thromboemboli to the brain can originate from the aortic arch, resulting in territorial brain infarction (Fig. 9-6). Tunick et al. (2) reported in 1990 the first observations of large protruding plaques in the thoracic aorta diagnosed by TEE in three patients who had recurrent brain and peripheral emboli and no other source of emboli.

In 1991 and 1992, Tunick et al. (57,58) reported two patients with recurrent systemic emboli despite adequate antithrombotic therapy and large protruding and moving plaques in the aortic arch. After endarterectomy to remove these plaques with superimposed thrombi, the patients no longer had recurrent emboli.

Hausmann et al. (59) reported successful thrombolysis of an aortic arch thrombus in a patient who had a mesenteric embolism with no further emboli after the procedure. There is a growing body of anatomic (pathologic and echographic), clinical, and even preliminary therapeutic evidence pointing to atherosclerotic plaques with superimposed thrombi in the aortic arch moving into the lumen as potential sources of brain and systemic emboli.

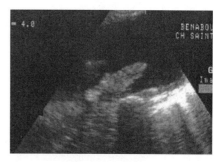

FIG. 9-6. Protruding plaque in the aortic arch with superimposed mobile thrombus.

Treatment

No randomized trials have been conducted to evaluate the role of any antithrombotic therapy in patients with aortic atheroma. Two studies showed a benefit of an oral anticoagulant over aspirin in patients with mobile thrombi in the aortic arch, but the studies were retrospective and nonrandomized, and hemorrhagic complications possibly outweighed the benefits of the anticoagulants. Concerns also exist regarding the possibility of anticoagulation increasing the risk of cholesterol embolism in these patients (56). Koren et al. (60) followed a cohort of 78 patients with protruding plaques ≥5 mm thick for an average of 29 weeks. The patients were treated with anticoagulant or antiplatelet agents. Among 38 patients taking heparin or warfarin, four subsequently had a blue toe syndrome associated with progressive renal insufficiency, an increased frequency of TIAs, or both. On the other hand, there was no blue toe syndrome among the 40 patients on antiplatelet agents. The two groups of patients were similar with regard to age and vascular risk factors. The blue toe syndrome may represent accelerated embolization of cholesterol. The hypothesis is that anticoagulation prevents thrombus formation on ulcerated plaques, allowing the release of atheromatous material contained in the plaques. However, there are suggestions that the risk of anticoagulation-induced embolization probably is not that great. In our autopsy study we found that 28% of unselected consecutive patients with ischemic stroke had ulcerated plaques in the aortic arch (15). If these figures are extrapolated to everyday practice, high rates of cholesterol embolization would be expected, given the extensive use of anticoagulants. This does not seem to be the case and has not been reported in large trials of warfarin in patients with atrial fibrillation and previous stroke (61). In the future, however, well-designed trials should evaluate the frequency of such adverse events.

In the FAPS cohort (23) as well as in the follow-up study of Mitusch et al. (62), no difference in event rates was found in patients treated with anticoagulant or antiplatelet agents. However, in the subset of patients with mobile thrombus in the lumen of the aortic arch, anticoagulant therapy seems logical although this awaits confirmation in a randomized study. In our opinion, in the presence of thrombi in the aortic arch (especially mobile thrombi in the lumen), a short-term anticoagulant therapy should be considered. In other cases, only antiplatelet therapy seems to be needed.

Because of the high risk of larger plaques in the aortic arch, the new possibilities of intraarterial therapy as well as surgery have been considered (63,64). Surgery potentially has a high morbidity in patients with severe aortic arch atherosclerosis who frequently are older than 75 years (64). In this study, among the 268 patients who underwent coronary artery bypass grafting, the rate of intraoperative stroke was 11.6% in patients who did not have an arch endarterectomy (225 patients) and 34.9% in those who had an arch endarterectomy (43 patients).

Thrombolysis proved to be successful in one case, but again an anecdotal report is of limited clinical use (59), and thrombolysis has been suspected as the cause of cholesterol embolization (65).

Currently available data are inadequate to generate a treatment recommendation for patients with ischemic stroke thought to be caused by embolization of aortic atheroma (66).

Because aortic arch atheroma is a strong marker for recurrent vascular events, the risks and benefits of different therapeutic options should be evaluated in randomized trials. In the meantime, either antiplatelet therapy or oral anticoagulation is considered an acceptable option. Occasionally, surgical endarterectomy can be performed in well-selected patients.

REFERENCES

1. Sacco RL, Ellenberg JH, Mohr JP, et al. Infarcts of undetermined cause: the NINCDS stroke data bank. *Ann Neurol* 1989;25:382–390.
2. Tunick PA, Kronzon I. Protruding atherosclerotic plaque in the aortic arch of patients with systemic embolism: a new finding seen by TEE. *Am Heart J* 1990;120:658–660.
3. Ramirez G, O'Neill WM, Lambert R, et al. Cholesterol embolization, a complication of angiography. *Arch Intern Med* 1978;138:1430–1432.
4. Gardner TJ, Horneffer PJ, Manolio TA, et al. Stroke following coronary artery bypass grafting: a ten-year study. *Ann Thorac Surg* 1985;40:574–580.
5. McKibbin DW, Bukley BH, Green WR, et al. Fatal cerebral atheromatous embolization after cardiopulmonary bypass. *J Thorac Cardiovasc Surg* 1976;71:741–745.
6. Katz ES, Tunick PA, Rusinek H, et al. Protruding aortic atheromas predict stroke in elderly patients undergoing cardiopulmonary bypass: experience with intraoperative transesophageal echocardiography. *J Am Coll Cardiol* 1992;20:70–77.
7. Dávila-Román VG, Barzilai B, Wareing TH, et al. Atherosclerosis of the ascending aorta. Prevalence and role as independent predictor of cerebrovascular events in cardiac patients. *Stroke* 1994;25:2010–2016.
8. Toyoda K, Yasaka M, Nagata S, et al. Aortogenic embolic stroke: a transesophageal echocardiographic approach. *Stroke* 1992;23:1056–1061.
9. Wareing TH, Dávila-Román VG, Daily BB, et al. Strat-

egy for the reduction of stroke incidence in cardiac surgical patients. *Ann Thorac Surg* 1993;55:1400–1408.

10. Vaduganathan V, Ewton A, Nagueh SF, et al. Pathologic correlates of aortic plaques, thrombi and mobile "aortic debris" imaged in vivo with transesophageal echocardiography. *J Am Coll Cardiol,* 1997;30:357–363.

11. Kutz SM, Lee VS, Tunick PA, et al. Atheromas of the thoracic aorta: a comparison of transesophageal echocardiography and breath-hold gadolinium-enhanced 3-dimensional magnetic resonance angiography. *J Am Soc Echocardiogr* 1999;12:853–858.

12. Weinberger J, Azhar S, Danisi F, et al. A new noninvasive technique for imaging atherosclerotic plaque in the aortic arch of stroke patients by transcutaneous real-time B-mode ultrasonography: an initial report. *Stroke* 1998;29:673–676.

13. Schwammenthal A, Schwammenthal Y, Tanne D, et al. Transcutaneous detection of aortic arch atheromas by suprasternal harmonic imaging. *J Am Coll Cardiol* 2002;39:1127–1132.

14. Tunick PA, Perez JL, Kronzon I. Protruding atheromas in the thoracic aorta and systemic embolization. *Ann Intern Med* 1991;115:423–427.

15. Amarenco P, Duyckaerts C, Tzourio C, et al. The prevalence of ulcerated plaques in the aortic arch in patients with stroke. *N Engl J Med* 1992;326:221–225.

16. Amarenco P, Cohen A, Tzourio C, et al. Atherosclerotic disease of the aortic arch and the risk of ischemic stroke. *N Engl J Med* 1994;331:1474–1479.

17. Jones EF, Kalman JM, Calafiore P, et al. Proximal aortic atheroma. An independent risk factor for cerebral ischemia. *Stroke* 1995;26:218–224.

18. Nihoyannopoulos P, Joshi J, Athanasopoulos G, et al. Detection of atherosclerotic lesions in the aorta by transesophageal echography. *Am J Cardiol* 1993;71:1208–1212.

19. Stone DA, Hawke MW, LaMonte M, et al. Ulcerated atherosclerotic plaques in the thoracic aorta are associated with cryptogenic stroke: a multiplane transesophageal echocardiographic study. *Am Heart J* 1995;130:105–108.

20. Di Tullio MR, Sacco RL, Gersony D, et al. Aortic atheromas and acute ischemic stroke: a transesophageal echocardiographic study in an ethnically mixed population. *Neurology* 1996;46:1560–1566.

21. Tunick PA, Rosenzweig BP, Katz ES, et al. High risk for vascular events in patients with protruding aortic atheromas: a prospective study. *J Am Coll Cardiol* 1994;23:1085–1090.

22. Montgomery DH, Ververis JJ, McGorisk G, et al. Natural history of severe atheromatous disease of the thoracic aorta: a transesophageal echocardiographic study. *J Am Coll Cardiol* 1996;27:95–101.

23. The French Study of Aortic Plaques in Stroke Group. Atherosclerotic disease of the aortic arch as a risk factor for recurrent ischemic stroke. *N Engl J Med* 1996;334:1216–1221.

24. Khathibzadeh M, Mitusch R, Stierle U, et al. Aortic atherosclerotic plaques as a source of systemic embolism. *J Am Coll Cardiol* 1996;27:664–669.

25. Rundek T, Di Tullio MR, Sciacca RR, et al. Association between large aortic arch atheromas and high-intensity transient signals in elderly stroke patients. *Stroke* 1999;30:2683–2686.

26. Cohen A, Tzourio C, Bertrand B, et al., on behalf of the FAPS Investigators. Aortic plaque morphology and vascular events. A follow-up study in patients with ischemic stroke. *Circulation* 1997;96:3838–3841.

27. Arko F, Buckley C, Baisden C, et al. Mobile atheroma of the aortic arch is an underestimated source of embolization. *Am J Surg* 1999;174:737–740.

28. Laperche T, Laurian C, Roudaut R, et al. Mobile thromboses of the aortic arch without aortic debris. A transesophageal echocardiographic finding associated with unexplained arterial embolism. The Filiale Echocardiographie de la Societe Francaise de Cardiologie. *Circulation* 1997;96:288–294.

29. Tobler HG, Edwards JE. Frequency and location of atherosclerotic plaques in the ascending aorta. *J Thorac Cardiovasc Surg* 1988;96:304–306.

30. Witteman JCM, Kannel WB, Wolf PA, et al. Aortic calcified plaques and cardiovascular disease (Framingham Study). *Am J Cardiol* 1990;66:1060–1064.

31. Fazio GP, Redberg RF, Winslow T, et al. Transesophageal echocardiographically detected atherosclerotic aortic plaques is a marker for coronary artery disease. *J Am Coll Cardiol* 1993;21:144–150.

32. Tribouilloy C, Shen WF, Peltier M, et al. Noninvasive prediction of coronary artery disease by transesophageal echocardiographic detection of thoracic aortic plaque in valvular heart disease. *Am J Cardiol* 1994;74:258–260.

33. O'Donnell CJ, Larson MG, Jaffer FA, et al. Aortic Atherosclerosis detected by MRI is associated with contemporaneous and longitudinal risk factors: the Framingham Heart Study. (4019)AHA Nov 2000.

34. Dávila-Román VG, Barzilai B, Wareing TH, et al. Intraoperative ultrasonographic evaluation of the ascending aorta in 100 consecutive patients undergoing cardiac surgery. *Circulation* 1991;83[Suppl III]:III-47–III-53.

35. Demopoulos LA, Tunick PA, Bernstein NE, et al. Protruding atheromas of the aortic arch in symptomatic patients with carotid stenosis. *Am Heart J* 1995;129:40–44.

36. Blackshear JL, Pearce LA, Hart RG, et al., for the Stroke Prevention in Atrial Fibrillation Investigators Committee on Echocardiography. Aortic plaque in atrial fibrillation. Prevalence, predictors, and thromboembolic implications. *Stroke* 1999;30:834–840.

37. Pfaffenbach DD, Hollenhorst RW. Morbidity and survivorship of patients with embolic cholesterol crystals in the ocular fundus. *Am J Ophthalmol* 1973;75:66–72.

38. Amarenco P, Cohen A, Baudrimont M, et al. Transesophageal echocardiographic detection of aortic arch disease in patients with cerebral infarction. *Stroke* 1992;23:1005–1009.

39. Chomette G, Auriol M, Tranbaloc P, et al. Les embolies cholestéroliques. Incidence anatomique et expressions cliniques. *Ann Med Intern* 1980;131:17–21.

40. Panum LP. Experimentelle beiträge zur lehre von der embolie. *Virchows Arch Pathol Anat* 1862;25:308–310.

41. Flory CM. Arterial occlusions produced by emboli from eroded aortic atheromatous plaques. *Am J Pathol* 1945;21:549–565.

42. Winter WJ. Atheromatous emboli: a cause of cerebral infarction. *Arch Pathol* 1957;64:137–142.

43. Soloway HB, Aronson SM. Atheromatous embolism to central nervous system. *Arch Neurol* 1964;11:657–667.

44. Beal MF, Williams RS, Richardson EP, et al. Cholesterol embolism as a cause of transient ischemic attacks and cerebral infarction. *Neurology* 1981;31:860–865.

45. Buge A, Vincent D, Rancurel G, et al. Embolies rétiniennes, musculaires et cutanées de cholestérol. Encéphalopathie progressive. *Rev Neurol (Paris)* 1985; 142:577–581.

46. Richards AM, Eliot RS, Kanjuh VI, et al. Cholesterol embolism: a multisystem disease masquerading as polyarteritis nodosa. *Am J Cardiol* 1965;15:696–707.

47. Hollenhorst RW. Vascular status of patients who have cholesterol emboli in the retina. *Am J Ophthalmol* 1966; 61:1159.

48. Price DL, Harris J. Cholesterol emboli in cerebral arteries as a complication of retrograde aortic perfusion during cardiac surgery. *Neurology* 1970;20:1209–1214.

49. Bruno A, Russell PW, Jones WL, et al. Concomitants of asymptomatic retinal cholesterol emboli. *Stroke* 1992; 23:900–902.

50. Bruno A, Jones WL, Austin JK, et al. Vascular outcome in men with asymptomatic retinal cholesterol emboli. A cohort study. *Ann Intern Med* 1995;122:249–253.

51. Blauth CI, Cosgrove DM, Webb BW, et al. Atheroembolism from the ascending aorta. An emerging problem in cardiac surgery. *J Thorac Cardiovasc Surg* 1992;103: 1104–1112.

52. Feder W, Auerbach R. "Purple toes": an uncommon sequela of oral coumadin drug therapy. *Ann Intern Med* 1961;55:911–917.

53. Mendia R, Cavaliere G, Sparacio F, et al. Does thrombolysis produce cholesterol embolisation? *Lancet* 1992; 339:562.

54. Oster P, Rieben FW, Waldherr R, et al. Blood clotting and cholesterol crystal embolization. *JAMA* 1979;242: 2070–2071.

55. Moldveen-Geronimus M, Merriam JC. Cholesterol embolization, from pathological curiosity to clinical entity. *Circulation* 1967;35:946–953.

56. Bruns FJ, Segel DP, Adler S. Control of cholesterol embolization by discontinuation of anticoagulant therapy. *Am J Med Sci* 1978;275:105–108.

57. Tunick PA, Lackner H, Katz ES, et al. Multiple emboli from a large aortic arch thrombus in a patient with thrombotic diathesis. *Am Heart J* 1992;124:239–241.

58. Tunick PA, Culliford AT, Lamparello PJ, et al. Atheromatosis of the aortic arch as an occult source of multiple systemic emboli. *Ann Intern Med* 1991;114: 391–392.

59. Hausmann D, Gulba D, Bargheer K, et al. Successful thrombolysis of an aortic arch thrombus in a patient after mesenteric embolism. *N Engl J Med* 1992;327: 500–501.

60. Koren MJ, Bryant B, Hilton TC. Atherosclerotic disease of the aortic arch and the risk of ischemic stroke [Letter]. *N Engl J Med* 1994;332:1237.

61. EAFT (European Atrial Fibrillation Trial) Study Group. Secondary prevention in non-rheumatic atrial fibrillation after transient ischaemic attack or minor stroke. *Lancet* 1993;342:1255–1262.

62. Mitusch R, Doherty C, Wucherpfennig H, et al. Vascular events during follow-up in patients with aortic arch atherosclerosis. *Stroke* 1997;28:36–39.

63. Belden JR, Caplan LR, Bojar RM, et al. Treatment of multiple cerebral emboli from a ulcerated, thrombogenic ascending aorta with aortectomy and graft replacement. *Neurology* 1997;49:621–622.

64. Stern A, Tunick PA, Culliford AT, et al. Protruding aortic arch atheromas: risk of stroke during heart surgery with and without aortic arch endarterectomy. *Am Heart J* 1999;138[4 Pt 1]:746–752.

65. Mendia R, Cavaliere G, Sparacio F, et al. Does thrombolysis produce cholesterol embolisation? *Lancet* 1992; 339:562.

66. Albers GW, Amarenco P, Easton JD, et al. Antithrombotic and thrombolytic therapy for ischemic stroke. *Chest* 2001;119:300S–320S.

67. Dávila-Román V, Murphy SF, Nickerson NJ, et al. Atherosclerosis of the ascending aorta is an independent predictor of long-term neurologic events and mortality. *J Am Coll Cardiol* 1999;33:1308–1316.

68. Karalis DG, Chandrasekaran K, Victor MF, et al. Recognition and embolic potential of intraaortic atherosclerotic debris. *J Am Coll Cardiol* 1991;17:73–78.

69. Mitchell MM, Frankville DD, Weinger MB, et al. Detection of thoracic atheroma with transesophageal echocardiography in patients without symptoms of embolism. *Am Heart J* 1991;122:1768–1771.

70. Mitusch R, Stierle U, Kummer-Kloess D, et al. Systemic embolism in aortic arch atheromatosis. *Eur Heart J* 1994;15:1373–1380.

71. Horowitz D, Tuhrim S, Budd J, et al. Aortic plaque in patients with brain ischemia: diagnosis by transesophageal echocardiography. *Neurology* 1992;42: 1602–1604.

72. Russell RWR. Atheromatous retinal embolism. *Lancet* 1963;ii:1354–1356.

73. Agmon Y, Khandheria BK, Meissner I, et al. Independent association of high blood pressure and aortic atherosclerosis: a population-based study. *Circulation* 2000;102:2087–2093.

Ischemic Stroke: Advances in Neurology, Vol. 92. Edited by
H.J.M. Barnett, Julien Bogousslavsky, and Heather Meldrum.
Lippincott Williams & Wilkins, Philadelphia © 2003.

10

Advances in Cerebrovascular Ultrasound

Fabienne Perren, *Georges Darbellay, Julien Bogousslavsky, Paul-André
Despland, and Gérald Devuyst

*Department of Neurology, Centre Hospitalier Universitaire Vaudois, Lausanne, Switzerland;
Laboratory of Signal Processing, Écol Polytechnique Fédérale de Lausanne, Lausanne, Switzerland

Over the last decade, considerable progress has been made in neurosonology, providing more sensitivity and specificity when diagnosing extracranial and intracranial arterial disease. Thus, ultrasound plays an increasingly important role in morphologic and functional evaluation of cerebrovascular diseases. New ultrasound equipment and neurosonologic methods, including three-dimensional (3D) sonography, transcranial Doppler microembolism detection, and harmonic and echo-contrast imaging, improve identification of morphologic characteristic of precerebral and intracranial arteries and allow assessment of the embolic origin of stroke or observation of disease progression.

PREDICTIVE PARAMETERS OF INTERNAL CAROTID ARTERY STENOSIS

Since the North American Symptomatic Carotid Endarterectomy Trial (NASCET) Study demonstrated a benefit of carotid endarterectomy for symptomatic patients with $\geq 70\%$ internal carotid artery (ICA) stenosis, most researchers have been interested in defining the Doppler cut points that identify patients with $\geq 70\%$ ICA stenosis as determined by arteriography. Traditional duplex categories (50%–79%, 80%–99%) are not directly applicable to NASCET, and there is some controversy about the Doppler parameter(s) that is most predictive of $\geq 70\%$ ICA stenosis (1). From recent studies, it seems that ICA peak systolic velocity (PSV_{ICA}) is the sole best Doppler parameter that distinguishes severe from less severe carotid stenosis (2–4).

The criteria chosen for depiction of $\geq 70\%$ ICA stenosis were as follows:

$$PSV_{ICA} > 210 \text{ cm/s or} \geq 250 \text{ cm/s (4).}$$

PSV_{ICA} appears as the best single predictor of $\geq 70\%$ ICA stenosis, whereas other parameters, such as

- Internal carotid artery end-diastolic velocity (EDV_{ICA}),
- Common carotid artery PSV (PSV_{CCA}),
- Common carotid artery end-diastolic velocity (EDV_{CCA}),
- Ratios of PSV_{ICA}/PSV_{CCA},
- EDV_{ICA}/EDV_{CCA}, and
- PSV_{ICA}/EDV_{CCA}

do not notably improve predictive ability (3) and must be locally validated in each Doppler laboratory (4).

However:

$$EDV_{ICA} > 70 \text{ cm/s criterion (2)}$$

is a useful index for high-grade stenoses when aliasing is problematic for measurements of PSV_{ICA}, whereas

$$PSV_{ICA}/PSV_{CCA} > 3 \text{ and } EDV_{ICA}/EDV_{CCA} > 3.3$$

ratios are useful for overcoming variability in interval determination of PSV and EDV from examination to examination (2).

To continue increasing the noninvasive depiction of $\geq 70\%$ ICA stenosis, a battery of transcranial Doppler (TCD) findings is suggested: (a) ophthalmic flow reversal; (b) anterior cerebral artery (ACA) flow reversal, low middle cerebral artery (MCA) flow acceleration, and pulsatility were associated ($p < 0.001$) with $\geq 70\%$ carotid stenosis on cerebral arteriography (5).

Arbeille et al. (6) compared the accuracy of seven Doppler parameters for quantifying the degree of carotid stenosis in 133 patients. The reference methods were the grades of spectral disturbance and the index of spectral disturbance (STI) by continuous wave, which have been validated against endarterectomy specimens.

The parameters measured were the following:

- Maximum velocity (Vmax) inside the stenosis (pulse wave),
- Grade and STI at the outlet of the stenosis (pulse wave and continuous wave),
- Ratio of velocities between internal and common carotid arteries (pulse wave),
- Ratio of vessel cross section, and
- Residual lumen area (% color) inside the stenosis (color Doppler).

Arbeille et al. (6) found a high correlation between the grades of spectral disturbance or STI measured by pulse wave and continuous wave, whereas for intrastenotic velocity the increase in Vmax was not proportional to the degree of stenosis. Ratio of velocities between internal and common carotids showed large fluctuations for the same degree of stenosis. These two parameters could be used to detect only two groups of ICA stenosis, >75% or >90% in area. Finally, color Doppler routinely overestimated the degree of stenosis by 10% to 15% but correlated better with the reference method.

Muller et al. (7) investigated the accuracy of color-flow Doppler imaging, power Doppler imaging (PDI), and frequency shift (PSF) for assessment of carotid artery stenosis with angiography used as gold standard. They used the measurement techniques used in NASCET and the European Carotid Surgery Trial (ECST) and showed a high reproducibility of the color Doppler and power Doppler measurements of carotid artery stenosis, providing an accuracy equal to PSF.

ARTERIAL WALL IMAGING

Both increased intima-media thickness (IMT) and protruding carotid plaques appear to be ultrasound markers of general atherosclerosis, the latter being a potential precursor of cerebrovascular events. A previous study showed that increased IMT is a physiologic effect of aging and corresponds to diffuse intimal thickening and that IMT is distinct from pathologic plaque formation (8). Compared with histologic results, in vivo ultrasound measurements of IMT are systematically larger (9). Hunt et al. (10) showed that detected carotid artery lesions (plaques) and acoustic shadowing serve as markers of atherosclerosis and thus are predictive of ischemic stroke. In the GENIC study, Touboul et al. (11) concluded that an increased CCA IMT was associated with brain infarction of all types and that an increased IMT could be a selection criterion for patients at high risk for stroke. However, there are limited data about the reproducibility of ultrasound assessment of carotid plaques occurrence, thickness, and morphology. Joakimsen et al. (12) showed substantial agreement of plaques occurrence and morphology between and within sonographers, whereas measurements of plaque thickness are subject to considerable error. To prone a more homogeneous approach in describing carotid plaques, an international consensus conference proposes a five-step classification based (Table 10-1) on permutations of echo intensities and the distribution of echogenic zones within plaques, but its interobserver reproducibility still needs to be confirmed (13).

Anechoic echogenicity is standardized against blood. The consensus classifies the luminal surface into three classes: regular, irregular (0.4–2 mm depth), and ulcerated (>2 mm depth) (13). It has been suggested that many embolic events might coincide with recent intraplaque hemorrhage, which can be seen as echolucent areas with caps of echodense material. Almost all lesions with intraplaque hemorrhage contained microscopic hypoechoic components. This finding suggests that hypoechoic compo-

---

TABLE 10-1. *Five-step classification of carotid plaques*

Class I: *Uniformly anechoic plaques,* which are associated with a higher risk of causing embolic events than isoechoic or hyperechoic plaques

Class II: *Predominantly hypoechoic or anechoic plaques,* which contain hypoechoic signals within an area corresponding to ≥50% of the cross-sectional area

Class III: *Predominantly echoic or isoechoic plaques,* which exhibit hypoechoic zones occupying <50% of their total cross-sectional area; recent studies have not been able to link plaques of class II and III with an increased risk of stroke incidence

Class IV: *Uniformly isoechoic or hyperechoic plaques,* which are not associated with a higher risk of calcified stroke

Class V: *Unclassified calcified plaques* with zones of acoustic shadowing obscuring the deep aspect of the arterial wall as well as the vessel lumen; further studies are needed to confirm that these plaques (V) are not correlated with a higher risk of stroke

---

From de Bray JM, Baud JM, Dauzat M on behalf of the Consensus Conference Concerning the morphology and the risk of carotid plaques. *Cerebrovasc Dis* 1997;7:289–296.

nents are closely related to hemorrhage (14). A study conducted by Lammie et al. (15) suggests that lucent areas in the carotid plaques (corresponding to necrosis or hemorrhage) and the thickness of the fibrous cap can be determined reliably with ultrasound (7.5-MHz probe and color Doppler imaging). In their study based on 42 endarterectomy specimens, features corresponding to active atheromatous plaque were found to be similar for carotid and coronary arteries: thin fibrous cap, large necrotic core, ulceration, and inflammation. Lammie et al. (15) showed that the best agreement between ultrasound and pathologic categorization of atheromatous carotid plaques components was the fibrous cap (thick versus thin).

APPLICATIONS OF COLOR DUPLEX FLOW IMAGING AND POWER DOPPLER IMAGING

Power Doppler Imaging for Internal Carotid Artery Stenosis

In a study of 34 middle-grade stenoses, 32 high-grade stenoses, and 7 complete occlusions of the ICA diagnosed by digital subtraction angiography (DSA), Griewing et al. (16) showed that PDI visualized stenosis significantly more frequently and accurately than color duplex flow imaging (CDFI). CDFI tended to overestimate and underestimate both middle- and high-grade ICA stenosis, whereas PDI was superior to both CDFI and DSA with regard to differentiation of plaque surface morphology. One of the advantages of PDI compared with CDFI is that in PDI, noise can be assigned a homogeneous background, even when the gain is increased greatly over the level at which noise begins to obscure the CDFI image. Another advantage of PDI over CDFI is that PDI is essentially angle independent, which allows PDI to be relatively free of artifactual bias and able to display blood flow even when the mean Doppler frequency shift is zero, as is the case in high-grade carotid stenosis. Steinke et al. (17) performed the largest study devoted to PDI, consecutively investigating 128 ICA stenoses and 12 ICA occlusions by means of PDI, CDFI, and angiography. Reduction of the intrastenotic lumen was measured on longitudinal (diameter stenosis) and transverse (area stenosis) views of PDI and CDFI. PDI provided excellent or good visualization of plaque configuration and intrastenotic lumen of the 128 ICA stenoses more frequently (92%) than CDFI (79%), particularly in complicated high-grade stenosis. CDFI failed to detect the stenosis or provided poor displays of the vascular lumen surfaces significantly more frequently than PDI. Measurement of the diam-

eter stenosis was feasible in 97% of the ICA stenoses on PDI and in 93% on CDFI. Area stenosis could be reliably evaluated in more cases with PDI (94%) than with CDFI (88%), but the difference was not statistically significant (12). This study revealed the highest agreement between PDI and CDFI for area reduction in high-grade (80%–99%) ICA stenosis, supporting the view that measurements of lumen reduction on transverse views were probably the closest to the "true anatomic degree of stenosis." Steinke et al. (17) observed a moderate accordance between sonographic imaging and angiographic methods. Both ECST and CC methods frequently overestimated the stenoses, whereas the NASCET method led to significant underestimation compared to both PDI and CDFI. With regard to these findings, it can be postulated that modern sonographic methods such as PDI and CDFI used in combination because complementary, providing the best approximation of ICA stenosis degree because of their ability to directly visualize the intrastenotic residual lumen diameter and the distance between vessel wall at the same site. Angiographic methods suffer from the inability to delineate the outer vessel boundary, but sonographic techniques have limitations in consistently visualizing the residual vessel lumen, particularly with severe plaque calcification. This postulate for CDFI and PDI ideally should be correlated with anatomic specimens from carotid endarterectomy. Because PDI does not provide hemodynamic information about flow velocity and direction, we believe that PDI should be combined with CDFI.

Power Doppler Imaging for Vertebral Arteries

In a study of 49 consecutive patients with transient ischemic attacks (TIAs) or stroke depending on the posterior circulation, Ries et al. (18) showed that amplitude-modulated CDFI provided a significantly superior visualization of the intertransversal vertebral artery (VA_2), whereas display of the intracranial segment (VA_4) was significantly improved on CDFI (18).

Power Doppler Imaging for Intracranial Arteries

Postert et al. (19) found that the superiority of PDI was statistically significant for A_2, M_2, M_3, P_1, P_2, P_3, BA, and posterior communicating artery (PcoA) segments in 38 subjects without history or signs of cerebrovascular disease. P_3 segments and PcoA could be depicted by PDI exclusively. In contrast, no artery identified by transcranial color-coded duplex sonography (TCCD) was not visible by PDI. TCCD after contrast injection was superior to PDI for detection of the BA, PcoA, and P_3 segments but was inferior to PDI with respect to the selectivity in differentiating arteries with a close anatomic relationship. About one third of A_1 and P_1 segments could be detected exclusively by PDI. Results of the study by Postert et al. (19) suggest a superiority of PDI over conventional TCCD with regard to the depiction of central, as well as peripheral arterial segments of intracranial vasculature, but there are too few studies to definitively assess a superiority of PDI over TCCD. In contrast, Baumgartner et al. (20) concluded that until now, PDI has not provided important advantages but several unimportant limitations compared to TCCD. The main disadvantage of PDI is the missing information about flow direction because PDI is unable to demonstrate a collateral pathway through the anterior communicating artery (AcoA) for instance. For the same reasons as those for carotid duplex, we believe that PDI and CDFI are complementary and should be used together for cerebral arteries.

CONTRAST- OR ECHO-ENHANCED TRANSCRANIAL DUPLEX IMAGING: BENEFIT IN CLINICAL PRACTICE?

TCCD has been widely accepted for evaluation of cerebrovascular BFV associated with occlusive and stenotic disease of intracranial arteries with a sensitivity and specificity of 75% to 92%/50% to 79% and 92% to 99%/80% to 100% for M_1/MCA and VA/BA, respectively (21). However, the major limitation of TCCD is the thickness of the skull at the temporal window level, which renders clinical interpretation and diagnosis difficult or impossible, particularly when a temporal hyperostosis is present. A technically adequate transcranial study is believed to be unobtainable in 10% to 15%, mainly in patients older than 60 years and in elderly African-American women. Other obstacles to an adequately diagnostic Doppler study are the depth of the insonated vessel—the distal segment of the BA is impossible to insonate in approximately 30%—and vessels of slow or low flow volume. As for neuroimaging [computed tomography (CT), magnetic resonance imaging, DSA), a possible solution to inadequate Doppler signal is the use of an agent to enhance the intensity of the reflected ultrasound signal. Of such contrast agents, Levovist (SHU 508A) is the most detailed agent used in TCCD examinations at this time. Levovist is an intravenously administered galactose/palmitic acid–based echo enhancement agent that survives the cardiopulmonary circulation to provide signal enhancement of the entire blood pool, including the

intracranial circulation. To date, the largest study reported is the international European phase III clinical trial (22,23), which has confirmed previous results. This study was conducted in 1,255 patients, 86 of whom were undergoing TCD or TCCD for diagnosis of suspected cerebrovascular disease. In these 86 patients, initial unenhanced (baseline) TCD or TCCD findings were judged nondiagnostic in 97% of cases and were equivocal at best in the remaining 3%. After enhancement by Levovist, a firm diagnosis could be established with TCCD in approximately 87% of patients; examination was improved in an additional 12% of cases, although diagnosis was not specified. In this series, Levovist administration resulted in signal-to-noise ratios of 14 to 20 dB and a mean duration of enhancement examination time of more than 4 minutes (range 2–8 minutes). In this study, the final diagnosis after Levovist was normal in 62% and pathologic (microangiopathy, stenosis, occlusion) in 25%, whereas diagnosis was impossible in 2% and not finally specified in 12% (24). It seems that a Levovist concentration of 300 mg/mL provides optimal image enhancement and fewer side effects (color artifacts). In all of the studies, Levovist injections were well tolerated and safe. The most commonly reported side effects, which resolved quickly without medical intervention, were mild paresthesia, a general feeling of warmth, and pain at the injection site. To date, the literature has suggested that use of Levovist may increase signal to a sufficient degree and length of time safely in patients with inadequate or uninterpretable baseline TCCD examinations (22,23). Baumgartner et al. (25) reported that ultrasonic agents significantly increased the number of completely detected cerebral arteries to 69% to 81% on the side ipsilateral to the ultrasound transducer and 25% to 66% on the side contralateral to the ultrasound transducer. These authors showed that contrast TCCD provided conclusive examinations in two thirds of patients with ischemic cerebrovascular events and ultrasound refractory temporal windows. Moreover, precontrast TCCD identified no arterial Doppler signals in patients with inconclusive contrast TCCD (25). In contrast, precontrast identification of any basal cerebral artery predicted a conclusive contrast TCCD with an overall accuracy of 97% (25). Thus, the application of the previously mentioned criterion may prevent inappropriate use of a contrast agent, thus reducing costs. Levovist TCCD could increase the ability to diagnose cerebrovascular diseases. Further studies are needed to confirm this advantage and compare it to other noninvasive vascular diagnostic means, such as magnetic resonance angiography (MRA) and CT angiography in pathologic cases.

In a multicenter study, Kaps et al. (26) using TCCD showed the safety, good tolerance, and diagnostic potential of a new ultrasound contrast agent (SonoVue). They demonstrated that the administration of SonoVue to patients with ischemic cerebrovascular disease who undergo TCCD examination of cerebral vessels improves the visualization of intracranial arteries, providing dose-dependent contrast enhancement and a clinically useful duration of signal enhancement related to the dose. Droste et al. (27) demonstrated that in patients with a severe ICA stenosis characterized by poor precontrast depiction of the circle of Willis, echo contrast-enhanced TCCD is helpful in assessing the intracranial collateral pathways. Collateral flow via the AcoA and PcoA could be demonstrated in 25 and 32 echo contrast-enhanced TCCD, respectively, in comparison with only one demonstration of each collateral pathway in precontrast TCCD. In addition, flow velocity in the MCA could be measured in 45 cases after contrast compared with only 26 cases before contrast. Another study by Gahn et al. (28) showed the usefulness of contrast-enhanced TCCD in stroke-age patients with limited temporal acoustic windows, which is the case in 20% to 30% of patients in this age group. Gahn et al. (28) tested contrast-enhanced TCCD in 49 patients with ischemia in the MCA territory in whom precontrast TCCD revealed no detectable color-flow signals from the circle of Willis. The age of these 49 patients was 70.5 ± 10.6 years. Contrast-enhanced TCCD enabled full visualization of the circle of Willis bilaterally in 38 of 49 patients and unilaterally in another 5 patients. Moreover, contrast-enhanced TCCD revealed an MCA stenosis in 6 of 43 (on the symptomatic side in three) and a MCA occlusion in 3 of 43 (all on the symptomatic side). These MCA stenoses or occlusions were confirmed by CT angiography, MRA, or DSA in all of these nine cases. Gerriets et al. (29) also found stenoses or occlusions of basal cerebral arteries by contrast-enhanced TCCD in 28 (60%) of 47 patients whose basal arteries could not be assessed adequately. In the study by Goertler et al. (30), contrast-enhanced TCCD enabled diagnosis of intracranial vascular pathology in 20 affected hemispheres (from 23 consecutive patients with an anterior circulation stroke in whom contrast-enhanced TCCD was performed within 5 hours of stroke onset), whereas unenhanced TCCD and TCD were conclusive in 7 and 14 hemispheres, respectively. In this study, contrast-enhanced TCCD was superior in evaluating distal ICA (T-bifurcation) occlusion and differentiating major vessel occlusions from patent arteries with flow velocity diminution. Nabavi et al. (31) estimate that in approximately three fourths of 25 patients examined within 48 hours of the onset of stroke with insufficient native ultrasound investigations, contrast-enhanced TCCD enabled a reliable neurovascular diagnosis, which allowed cancellation of additive neurovascular imaging procedures in half of our cohort. In the series of Nabavi et al. (31), contrast-enhanced TCCD disclosed another three occlusions and four stenoses of the intracranial arteries compared with precontrast investigations.

HARMONIC CONTRAST IMAGING

Harmonic imaging (second harmonic TCCD) uses the following phenomenon. Gas bubbles from ultrasound contrast agents passing the capillary bed of the lungs are highly resonant at the frequency used for diagnostic ultrasound. When a gas bubble vibrates at near resonance, it produces harmonics or multiples of the transmitted frequency. Second harmonic Doppler systems work to transmit at one frequency (fundamental) and receive at twice that frequency (second harmonic). The advantage of this procedure is that the tissues primarily respond at the fundamental frequency and that the bubbles of the ultrasound contrast agents respond at the fundamental and the second harmonic frequencies. The ultrasound system removes the unwanted fundamental frequency (noise), leaving only the second harmonic frequency from the ultrasound contrast agent. Therefore, signal-to-noise and signal-to-tissue artifacts are reduced by second harmonic Doppler and parenchymal imaging (32). Use of this method of ultrasound is supposed to provide higher spatial resolution than conventional TCCD. For this reason, Seidel et al. (32) used this method to evaluate the vertebrobasilar system in transnuchal insonation in 13 healthy volunteers. Their clinical study evaluated three different methods for imaging the vertebrobasilar arteries: baseline TCCD, Levovist TCCD, and Levovist–second harmonic TCCD. The number of visible arterial segments of the vertebrobasilar system was increased using Levovist in the TCCD and second harmonic TCCD modes. There was no difference in the imaging of the major branches (VA$_4$ segment and BA) and only a minor increase in the number of detected cerebellar arteries when comparing Levovist TCCD and second harmonic TCCD, but a striking difference existed between these two modalities with regard to the spatial resolution of the branches of the cerebellar arteries, in favor of the second harmonic TCCD. The duration of blooming artifact was significantly reduced and the duration of diagnostically useful signal enhancement was significantly increased, whereas the maximal investigation depth was significantly reduced with second harmonic TCCD. For these authors, the best choice for the vertebrobasilar system is a fundamental frequency between 1 and 2 MHz because the resulting second harmonic frequency is between 2 and 4 MHz, which is a compromise between low spatial resolution (2 MHz) and decreasing maximal investigation depth (4 MHz). Even if there are few available data regarding the interest in second harmonic TCCD, the findings of Seidel et al. (32) are promising but whether this diagnosis is useful in patients with ischemia in the vertebrobasilar circulation, which is classically less conclusive than carotid system with baseline TCCD, will need to be confirmed. Wiesmann and Seidel (33) used harmonic gray-scale imaging with Optison, a perfluoro-propane-containing ultrasound contrast agent that shows strong echo enhancement in the brain parenchyma. By calculating color-coded perfusion maps, they visualized human brain tissue perfusion at the patient's bedside. Postert et al. (34) investigated two patients with acute cerebral infarction by second harmonic TCCD to prove that this technique detects focal abnormalities of cerebral echo-contrast enhancement. They could detect in both patients demarcated focal abnormalities of cerebral contrast enhancement, which were in accordance with the findings of follow-up CT scans. The patients with complete MCA infarction showed missing contrast enhancement in the entire hemisphere of the affected side during follow-up second harmonic imaging examinations. They concluded that this technique may identify focal abnormalities of echo-contrast enhancement and helps to determine size, localization, and prognosis of the ischemic region (34). Additional studies on harmonic imaging of the brain parenchyma using new ultrasound contrast agents containing perfluorobutane are still being evaluated in an animal model (35).

THREE-DIMENSIONAL TRANSCRANIAL POWER DOPPLER ULTRASOUND IMAGING

With second harmonic TCCD, 3D transcranial ultrasound imaging represents the most recent sonographic technique. The 3D system allows immediate inspection of vascular structures after reconstruction of registered, adjacent two-dimensional (2D) images. A data acquisition system for 3D ultrasound using a

TABLE 10-2. *Ipsilateral versus contralateral vessels successfully imaged*

	Two-dimensional imaging	Three-dimensional imaging
ACA	90%/60%	100%/90%
MCA	90%/30%	100%/80%
PCA	60%/10%	100%/100%
PcoA	60%/70% (29)	100%/100%

ACA, anterior cerebral artery, MCA, middle cerebral artery; PCA, posterior cerebral artery; PcoA, posterior communicating artery.

magnetic sensor for spatial localization now is available and eliminates the need for mechanical data acquisition, thus improving transducer mobility. This new 3D modality can be associated with power mode imaging combined with an echo-contrast agent. With an electromagnetic position sensor for 3D imaging, acquisition of the volume sweep dataset required 20 to 30 seconds, whereas routine study with 2D imaging required 15 to 20 minutes; reprojection requires less than 2 minutes (36,37). With 3D imaging, Lyden and Nelson (36) revealed more cerebral vessels more rapidly in normal volunteers. Frequently color blotches identified equivocal vessels or artifacts, which appeared as part of branching or looping vessels after reconstruction for 3D imaging. A_1 (ACA) segments and PcoA were identifiable by 3D imaging in all subjects. 3D-imaging was able to follow the MCA and ACA out of the trifurcation and the callosal-marginal branch, respectively, in many subjects. The top of the BA with bilateral P_1 (PCA) and the AcoA with proximal A_2 (ACA) were clearly identifiable in almost half of the subjects (36). When using power mode with Levovist injections to create 3D reconstruction, the ipsilateral versus contralateral (%/%) vessels that were imaged successfully are listed in Table 10-2.

Taking into account the very small number of subjects in this series (37) (most of them without history of stroke and without stenosis or occlusion of cerebral artery on angiography), the authors postulate that 3D imaging could allow an easier distinction between an asonic segment due to a loop of the vessel rather than a true occlusion. Future studies are needed to confirm this hypothesis, particularly in older patients with cerebral vessel patency.

MICROEMBOLIC SIGNALS

Microembolic signals (MES) currently is one of the most exciting field of neurosonology, but many questions remain concerning their depiction, incidence, nature, and prognostic value for increased risk for stroke. An obstacle to a better understanding of the MES phenomenon is the absence of an international agreement in the use and interpretation of criteria to identify MES. In 1998, a new international consensus on microembolus detection by TCD was published to provide guidelines for the use of embolus detection in clinical practice, as well as in scientific investigations (38). This consensus suggested recommendations based on several parameters: ultrasound device, transducer type and size, insonated artery, insonation depth, algorithms for signal intensity measurements, scale settings, detection of decibel threshold, axial extension of sample volume, fast Fourier transform (FFT) size, FFT length, FFT overlap, transmitted ultrasound frequency, high-pass filter settings, and recording time. For the crucial question of the distinction between artifacts and real circulating emboli, the consensus proposes the multigated Doppler technique, which traces the moving embolus in different depths of the same artery and takes the time delay of its appearance as the crucial criterion. Moreover, the multigated Doppler technique has been used in an attempt at automatic embolus detection. However, there was agreement in this consensus that no current system of automatic embolus detection has the required sensitivity and specificity for clinical use.

Microembolic Signals in Acute Stroke

Nineteen patients with MCA ischemic events (16 strokes and 3 TIAs) were investigated for MES within 24 hours after ischemia onset. Droste et al. (39) performed six 1-hour recordings on days 1, 2, 3, 4, 7, and 14 from the affected MCA. Eight of 19 patients showed MES (1–53) in at least one of these six recordings. Variability was high and there was no uniform tendency with respect to time since onset of symptoms or treatment. In this study, no MES was recorded in patients with lacunar stroke (39). Even more interesting, two patients with MES suffered recurrent TIAs in the follow-up period, whereas none of the patients without MES presented a recurrent ischemic event (37). In contrast, Serena et al. (40) found that early recurrent stroke occurred more frequently in patients with MES than in patients without MES, although the difference was not statistically significant. In the series of Serena et al. (40), no MES was detected in lacunar stroke. The multiple logistic regression analysis showed that MES increased the risk of dependency on discharge independent of age, stroke severity on admission, and presence of an arterial cardiac embolic source (40).

Carotid Diseases and Microembolic Signals

ICA stenosis is associated with an increased risk for stroke in the brain territory supplied by this artery, and this is believed to be predominantly embolic. Both asymptomatic and mainly symptomatic ICA stenoses are linked to an increased risk for ipsilateral cerebral ischemia. Sitzer et al. (41) examined the ipsilateral MCA in symptomatic severe (>70%) ICA stenoses and depicted embolic signals in 77% of cases at a mean of 14 per hour, whereas embolic signals were detected in 16% at a mean rate of 0.35 per hour among asymptomatic ICA stenoses. Sitzer et al. (42) reported a strong association between plaque ulceration, intraluminal thrombosis, and downstream MES, and the same authors noted that a rate of MES ≥2/hour had a positive predictive value of 0.88 for recent ischemic symptoms in patients with high-grade (≥70%) ICA stenosis (42). Furthermore, Sitzer et al. (42) observed that the number of MES significantly dropped after carotid endarterectomy. Ries et al. (43) also observed a tendency of MES to be associated with heterogeneous echogenicities and surface irregularities of ICA plaques and a significantly higher occurrence of MES in symptomatic rather than asymptomatic ICA stenosis (≥60%). However, Droste et al. (44) found that echolucency of the plaque was not related to an increased number of MES; their results showed that increasing degree of stenosis and presence of symptoms similarly affected macroembolic and microembolic risk. The results of their study indirectly support the possible relationship of microembolic events and macroembolic risk. Interestingly, MES occurred significantly less often during effective anticoagulation (41). A study by Tegeler et al. (45) suggested that territorial infarct on CT was the most frequent pattern seen in patients with MES recorded in CCAs, suggesting that proximal artery-to-artery embolism or cardioembolism are uncommon mechanisms for lacunar stroke. Babikian et al. (46) showed that MES were significantly more frequently depicted in symptomatic than asymptomatic vessels in patients with cerebrovascular diseases. Moreover, the frequency of MES was significantly higher in the groups of ICA occlusive or severe stenoses (≥70%) than in groups with ICA stenoses less than 70%, but there is no significant association between the degree of ICA stenosis and recurrent cerebral/retinal events. However, the difference between MES-positive and MES-negative arteries with regard to recurrent events was significant. Georgiadis et al. (47) found a prevalence of MES in 28% of patients with carotid disease. Their study provided evidence of a significant difference in MES prevalence and counts in the symptomatic MCA, as well as symptomatic patients (44). With serial TCD monitoring (within 72 hours of stroke onset, after an additional 24 hours, and after 7 days), Del Sette et al. (48) noted an overall prevalence of MES of 12%, and MES were recorded only in the symptomatic MCA, irrespective of the etiologic categories of stroke. Koennecke et al. (49) suggested an association between MES and cerebral ischemia in patients with acute carotid dissection. MES were depicted in the MCA ipsilateral to the ICA dissection in 3 of the 4 patients with cerebral ischemia and none of the patients with other presenting symptoms.

Carotid Endarterectomy, Coronary Artery Bypass Grafting, and Microembolic Signals

Among many presumed mechanisms of perioperative carotid endarterectomy stroke, the major recognized causes include embolism, hyperperfusion after release of the clamps, postoperative occlusive thrombosis, and hypoperfusion. Stroke is the more serious complication observed after coronary artery bypass grafting (CABG). Ultrasonographic studies of the carotid arteries have shown showers of embolic material that probably comes from atheromatous aorta and which is released during the manipulation of the aorta that is required by the CABG procedure (50). A study by Newman et al. (51) confirmed that cognitive decline complicates early recovery after CABG. TCD monitoring can provide hemodynamic and embolic information and could identify, in real time, these major causes of perioperative stroke so that preventive measures can be undertaken to avoid them. The studies of Spencer (52) and Levi et al. (53) confirmed that the intraoperative (52) and postoperative (53) occurrence of MES was strongly associated with cerebrovascular complications. Furthermore, Levi et al. (53) noted that the positive predictive value of counts greater than 50 MES/hour for cerebral ischemia postoperatively was 0.71, suggesting a strong association between rates greater than 50 MES/hour and focal ischemic signs and could help identify patients at higher risk for postoperative

embolic stroke. In the study by Spencer (52), embolism appears to be the main cause (54%) of cerebrovascular complications from carotid endarterectomy, whereas hyperperfusion (29%) and hypoperfusion (17%) were the second and third causes, respectively. In the study by Arnold et al. (54), TCD alone was sensitive enough to depict potential hemodynamic complications, which can be prevented by selective shunt insertion. The criteria for cross-clamp shunting were a decrease of ipsilateral MCA mean velocity greater than 70% (55,56), or stump pressure less than 40 mm Hg, 1 minute after clamping (56).

In the study by Finocchi et al. (56), patients with cerebral complications had a significantly longer clamping duration and the decrease of MCA mean velocity upon clamping was significantly greater, whereas stump pressure was not significantly different and MES were not associated with cerebrovascular complications. Embolism, which is increasingly considered the more common mechanism of brain ischemia (57), occurs during the dissection phase of surgery, upon shunt insertion and clamp release, and during the 12 hours immediately after surgery (58). Ackerstaff et al. (59) reported that intraoperative monitoring with TCD can identify patients at increased risk for perioperative stroke. They found that microemboli that occurred during dissection and wound closure was associated with stroke, whereas microemboli that occurred upon clamp release and during shunting were clinically irrelevant (59). They also reported that =90% decrease of MCA PSV at cross clamping and =100% of the pulsatile index of the Doppler at clamp release were associated with operative stroke (59). Further studies will distinguish patients with a higher risk for developing an embolic event from those who will develop hemodynamic intraoperative or postoperative stroke.

Vertebrobasilar Disease and Microembolic Signals

There are few data about stroke-related MES in the posterior cerebral circulation, although approximately 25% of brain infarcts involve the vertebrobasilar territory. To date, only Koennecke et al. (61) have described MES of the PCAs in 19.2% of patients with acute or recent vertebrobasilar ischemia. Potential cardiac sources were significantly associated with MES, whereas this study failed to prove a relationship between MES and vessel abnormalities. The prevalence of stenoses or occlusions of the VA (in particular proximal) and BA may have been underestimated because almost 50% of the patients did not undergo MRA or arteriography.

Prosthetic Cardiac Valves and Microembolic Signals

The higher occurrence of MES in patients with prosthetic cardiac valves suggested to most of the investigators that these signals could correspond to cavitation bubbles and could not represent solid material. Moreover, the overwhelming majority of these MES remain clinically asymptomatic, at least with regard to evident neurologic sequelae. A major step in favor of investigators who believe that circulating MES are mainly gaseous in patients with mechanical prosthetic cardiac valves has been accomplished by recent works. Droste et al. (62) compared the influence of 6 L of oxygen per minute inhalation on the MES occurrence recorded on MCA or PCA in patients with mechanical prosthetic heart valves (MPHV) or with ipsilateral extracranial carotid/vertebrobasilar artery disease or in control subjects. These authors observed a significant decrease of MES under oxygen in patients with MPHV but not in patients with large-artery embolic source; no MES were detected in control subjects (62). Georgiadis et al. (63) observed a significantly higher MES counts in children with MPHV compared to a corresponding group of adults. These two studies argue that the majority of clinically silent circulating microemboli in patients with MPHV are gaseous in nature. Oxygen inhibits the cavitation process of MPHV or speeds up redissolution of gas bubbles produced by cavitation. Oxygen inhalation cannot suppress presumed solid—nongaseous—microemboli originating from an arterial embolic source. The study by Georgiadis et al. (63) supports this hypothesis because the difference in MES counts between children and adults with MPHV has only two explanations: (a) the shorter distance between aortic valve and MCA because cavitation bubbles have a short lifespan and will dissolve with time and (b) the faster heart rate in children, which results in a greater number of valves closures per minute that probably generate a more important cavitation process, that is, formation of gaseous bubbles.

These works suggest that approximately 85% of the embolic signals are gaseous and only 15% correspond to solid material.

Technical Aspects of Microembolic Signal Detection

The problem of recognizing a so-called high-intensity transient signal (HITS) within the signal of the normal blood flow, and then to decide whether the HITS is an MES and not an artefact, is referred to as MES detection (Fig. 10-1). There are several signal processing techniques for isolating HITS within the background noise of normal blood flow, such as the classic FFT or the wavelet transform. A method by

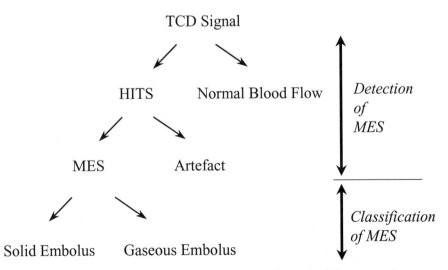

FIG. 10-1. Decision tree for microemboli signal detection and solid/gas separation.

which the signal can be "cleaned" from the background noise by means of the wavelet transform in order to retain only the part that may correspond to the MES is shown in Fig. 10-2. Whatever technique is used, it is easy to find a strong HITS and difficult to recognize a weak HITS (whose intensity is low). There is no clear-cut borderline, and not all experts agree whether a low-intensity signal perturbation is a potential MES or is just random noise.

Artifacts usually originate from some movement of the brain tissues (e.g., the patient is coughing), head, or probe. The great majority of artifacts are low-frequency signals and thus is easy to eliminate (64,65). However, to improve the differentiation between MES and artifacts, most machines use the dual-gate principle. The MCA is insonated at two different depths. An embolus is supposed to travel through the deeper region (proximal volume) first and then through the region closer to the skull (distal volume). This produces a time delay, as shown in Fig. 10-2. There is no time delay for artifacts. Another method is to place a "gate" inside the MCA and another

"gate" outside the MCA. An MES should produce a signal only in the internal gate.

For MES detection, the performance of an automatic system is measured against a panel of human experts. If this comparison is made with a large number of signals coming from a variety of patients, it appears that a good automatic system reaches both a sensitivity and a specificity on the order of 95%.

Automatic Differentiation Between Solid and Gaseous Emboli

Classification of MES into solid or gaseous emboli is a difficult task. Ideally, it should be performed on-line, as for MES detection. No expert is able to carry out such a task, except for saying that an intense MES is likely to be a bubble, whereas a weak MES is likely to be a clot. The differentiation between solid and gaseous emboli has important clinical implications; thus, an automatic system would be highly desirable. Such a system calculates on-line a set of parameters

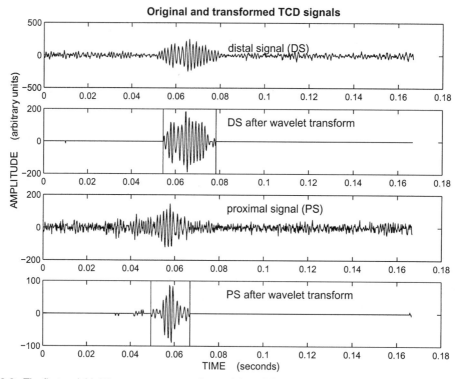

FIG. 10-2. The first and third time sequences are those of the original signals. The second and fourth sequences are those of the wavelet-transformed signals. The *vertical bars* indicate the likely start and end times of the two high-intensity transient signals (HITS). Note the time delay between the proximal and distal HITS. These two HITS come from a patient with carotid stenosis and correspond to a solid embolus.

from signals and then reaches a decision by combining these parameters. Obviously, one of the parameters measures the relative intensity of the MES, through the so-called mean embolus power ratio. Other parameters may include information on the frequency content of the signal, the shape of the signal envelope, and different statistical features.

To test such an automatic system, it is necessary to preselect the patients. Usually, patients with a carotid stenosis are chosen as providers of solid emboli. Patients with a patent foramen ovale (PFO) and no other embolic source provide gaseous emboli (see next section). The result of such a test, again with a large number of embolic signals coming from a variety of patients, shows that it is possible to build such an automatic system, but its sensitivity and its specificity do not exceed 85%. This is sufficient for research studies, where we are interested in deriving statistical trends, but not for routine clinical applications.

The automatic signal processing system attempts to extract in an optimal way the (hidden) information carried by the signals, but it cannot add information. It appears that improved signal acquisition is required to provide signals that contain more information with respect to separation of solid and gas. We recall that the current equipment is based on single radiofrequency (usually 2 MHz) and two gates. At least three avenues can be explored. First, we could keep a single radiofrequency, to be denoted by the letter f, and two gates, but instead of recovering echoes only around the basic frequency f, we also may recover harmonic frequencies, such as two or three times f. The rationale behind such an approach is that the gas/liquid interface of bubbles is more flexible than the solid/liquid interface of clots. As a result, the wall of the bubble is more likely to vibrate and produce harmonics (66,67). Second, we could use two different radiofrequencies, such as 2 and 2.5 MHz, as described by Russell and Brucher (68). It has been argued that solid microemboli reflect more ultrasound power at higher frequency, whereas the opposite is true for gaseous microemboli. Whether this effect is systematic remains hotly debated. Third, some evidence suggests that using more than two sample gates (up to around 30) may help in discriminating between solid and gaseous microemboli, as the profile of the embolus through a vessel ought to be different for clots or bubbles (69).

PATENT FORAMEN OVALE

The last few years have contributed to improvement of the diagnostic method, but some differences remain between centers depending on the contrast used (saline solution, gelatin, or Echovist), the timing of the Valsalva strain (before, during, or after contrast injection) and its duration, and whether the delay in detecting air microbubbles on MCA, ACA, or PCA is considered to reflect an interatrial right-to-left shunting rather than a pulmonary right-to-left shunting. Droste et al. (70) assessed the time window after injection of the contrast agent and the numbers of the detected microbubbles. Fifty-eight patients were investigated in this study by both transesophageal echocardiography (TEE) and bilateral TCD of the MCA. They found that TCD performed twice with Valsalva maneuver for 5 seconds injected after 5 seconds of the beginning of contrast Echovist injection is the most appropriate test comprised of the test without Valsalva strain. The highest sensitivity was achieved with a diagnostic time window of 40 seconds (70). In another study from this group, comparisons of two contrast agents (agitated saline and the galactose-based agent Echovist) and of simultaneous bilateral to unilateral recordings and the end of the distribution of the microbubbles were assessed in 54 patients (71). There was a symmetrical distribution of MES in the right and left MCAs. Both bilateral and repeated recordings increased the sensitivity of contrast TCD (71). With this method, contrast TCD detected the TEE-proven right-to-left shunts with a sensitivity of 95% and a specificity of 75% (71). Each type of procedure for detection of PFO by contrast TCD must be locally validated with contrast TEE. Contrast TCD and contrast TEE are highly sensitive and specific techniques for diagnosing PFO, but false-negative results exist for each procedure (72). One must bear in mind that these contrast TEE false-negative results probably are related to small PFOs for which the clinical impact probably is low. To date, the risk of stroke recurrence according to the presumed size of PFO is not well known (72).

In our experience, we assume that contrast TEE and contrast TCD are complementary rather than opposite for diagnosis of PFO for at least three reasons (72): (a) to avoid false-negative results that are possible in each method; (b) to evaluate more precisely the importance of the right-to-left shunting, which seems more reliable with contrast TCD for obtaining results from studies focusing on the stroke recurrence risk as a function of PFO size; and (c) contrast TEE is irreplaceable for investigating the anatomy of the interatrial septum, particularly for depicting an association with an interatrial septal aneurysm. Although right-to-left shunting has been reported to occur significantly more frequently in young patients with cryptogenic stroke, its relevance in a nonselected population of acute ischemic stroke is not well known. Serena et al. (73) investigated 208 patients with TIA or acute cerebral infarction and 100 healthy controls by means of bilateral TCD after intravenous application of agitated saline. The magnitude of right-to-left shunting was quantified by counting the number of MES in one MCA during Valsalva maneuver. They found large right-to-left shunts in 40 (19.7%) patients and in 21 (21%) control subjects (70). A large right-to-left shunt was present in 4.7% of atherothrombotic strokes, 10.5% of cardioembolic strokes, 15.4% of lacunar strokes, and 45.3% of cryptogenic strokes ($p < 0.001$). Although the overall frequency of right-to-left shunts was not significantly different between patients and control subjects, the detection of larger shunts by TCD was associated with a higher risk of stroke, particularly with cryptogenic strokes (70). In a prospective study about 143 patients, Serena et al. (74) determined with contrast TCD the importance of right-to-left shunt and its magnitude as a risk factor for stroke recurrence in patients with cryptogenic stroke (TOAST criteria). They showed that the detection of curtain (uncountable signals) or shower (>25 signals) patterns by contrast TCD was significantly associated with higher risk of recurrent stroke. A follow-up study of 581 patients (18–55 years old) was designed to assess the absolute and relative risks of recurrent cerebrovascular events in young patients with septal disorders who were receiving aspirin (75). The results showed that patients with PFO and atrial septal aneurysm who suffered from cryptogenic stroke had a higher risk of recurrent stroke while taking aspirin than patients without septal abnormality or with septal abnormality alone (75). This suggests that in young patients who had an isolated PFO and a single otherwise unexplained ischemic stroke, secondary prevention with aspirin is sufficient (75). In contrast with the results of the study by Serena et al., the degree of right-to-left interatrial shunting was not correlated to the stroke rate recurrence (75). The role of the importance of right-to-left in stroke patients with PFO is still controversial.

REFERENCES

1. de Bray JM, Glatt B. Quantification of atheromatous stenosis in the extracranial internal carotid artery. Cerebrovasc Dis 1995;5:414–426.
2. Carpenter JP, Lexa FJ, Davis JT. Determination of duplex Doppler ultrasound criteria appropriate to the North American symptomatic carotid endarterectomy trial. Stroke 1996;27:695–699.
3. Schwartz SW, Chambless LE, Baker WH, et al. Consistency of Doppler parameters in predicting arteriographically confirmed carotid stenosis. Stroke 1997;28: 343–347.
4. Alexandrov AV, Vital D, Brodie DS, et al. Grading carotid stenosis with ultrasound. An interlaboratory comparison. Stroke 1997;28:1208–1210.
5. Wilterdink JL, Feldmann E, Furie KL, et al. Transcranial Doppler ultrasound battery reliably identifies severe internal carotid artery stenosis. Stroke 1997;28: 133–136.
6. Arbeille P, Bouin-Pineau MH, Herault S. Accuracy of the main Doppler methods for evaluating the degree of carotid stenoses (continuous wave, pulsed wave, and color Doppler). Ultrasound Med Biol 1999;25:65–73.
7. Muller M, Ciccotti P, Reiche W, et al. Comparison of color-flow Doppler scanning, power Doppler scanning, and frequency shift for assessment of carotid artery stenosis. J Vasc Surg 2001;34:1090–1095.
8. Homma S, Hirose N, Ishida H, et al. Carotid plaque and intima-media thickness assessed by b-mode ultrasonography in subjects ranging from young adults to centenarians. Stroke 2001;32:830–835.
9. Schulte-Altedorneburg G, Droste DW, Felszeghy S, et al. Accuracy of in vivo carotid B-mode ultrasound compared with pathological analysis (intima-media thickening, lumen diameter, and cross-sectional area). Stroke 2001;32:1520–1524.
10. Hunt KJ, Evans GW, Folsom AR, et al. Acoustic shadowing on B-mode ultrasound of the carotid artery predicts ischemic stroke: the Atherosclerosis Risk in Communities (ARIC) study. Stroke 2001;32:1120–1126.
11. Touboul PJ, Elbaz A, Koller C, et al. Common carotid artery intima-media thickness and brain infarction: the Etude du Profil Genetique de l'Infarctus Cerebral (GENIC) case-control study. The GENIC Investigators. Circulation 2000;102:313–318.
12. Joakimsen O, Bønaa KH, Stensland-Bugge E. Reproducibility of ultrasound assessment of carotid plaque occurrence, thickness and morphology. The Tromsø Study. Stroke 1997;28:2201–2207.
13. de Bray JM, Baud JM, Dauzat M, on behalf of the Consensus Conference. Consensus concerning the morphology and the risk of carotid plaques. Cerebrovasc Dis 1997;7:289–296.
14. Kagawa R, Moritake K, Shima T, et al. Validity of B-mode ultrasonographic findings in patients undergoing carotid endarterectomy in comparison with angiographic and clinicopathologic features. Stroke 1996;27: 700–705.
15. Lammie GA, Wardlaw J, Allan P, et al. What pathological components indicate carotid atheroma activity and can these be identified reliably using ultrasound? Eur J Ultrasound 2000;11:77–86.
16. Griewing B, Morgenstern C, Driesner C, et al. Cerebrovascular disease assessed by color-flow and power Doppler ultrasonography: comparison with digital subtraction angiography in internal carotid artery stenosis. Stroke 1996;27:95–100.
17. Steinke W, Ries S, Artemis N, et al. Power Doppler imaging of carotid artery stenosis. Comparison with color Doppler flow imaging and angiography. Stroke 1997;28:1981–1987.
18. Ries S, Steinke W, Devuyst G, et al. Amplitude modulated and frequency modulated color duplex flow imag-

ing for the evaluation of normal and pathological verte-bral arteries. *Cerebrovasc Dis* 1997, 7[Suppl 4]:1–88.

19. Postert T, Meves S, Börnke C, et al. Power Doppler compared to color-coded duplex sonography in the assessment of the basal cerebral circulation. *J Neuroimaging* 1997;7:221–226.
20. Baumgartner RW, Mattle HP, Aaslid R, et al. Transcranial color-coded duplex sonography in arterial cerebrovascular disease. *Cerebrovasc Dis* 1997;7:57–63.
21. Dafer RM, Ramadan NM. Transcranial Doppler sonography and stroke. In: *Primer on cerebrovascular diseases.* Academic Press, 1997.
22. Levovist® Transcranial Study Group. Echo enhanced transcranial Doppler and duplex imaging with Levovist®: clinical results of phase III trials. *Angiology* 1996;47:S9–S18
23. Ries F. Clinical experience with echo-enhanced transcranial Doppler and duplex imaging. *J Neuroimaging* 1997;7[Suppl 1]:S15–S21.
24. Kenton AR, Martin PJ, Abbott RJ, et al. Comparison of transcranial color-coded sonography and magnetic resonance angiography in acute stroke. *Stroke* 1997;28:1601–1606.
25. Baumgartner RW, Arnold M, Gönner F, et al. Contrast-enhanced transcranial color-coded Duplex sonography in ischemic cerebrovascular disease. *Stroke* 1997;28:2473–2478.
26. Kaps M, Legemate DA, Ries F, et al. SonoVue in transcranial Doppler investigations of the cerebral arteries. *J Neuroimaging* 2001;11:261–267.
27. Droste DW, Jurgens R, Weber S, et al. Benefit of echocontrast-enhanced transcranial color-coded duplex ultrasound in the assessment of intracranial collateral pathways. *Stroke* 2000;31:920–923.
28. Gahn G, Gerber J, Hallmeyer S, et al. Contrast-enhanced transcranial color-coded duplex sonography in stroke patients with limited bone windows. *AJNR Am J Neuroradiol* 2000; 21:509–514.
29. Gerriets T, Seidel G, Fiss I, et al. Contrast-enhanced transcranial color-coded duplex sonography: efficiency and validity. *Neurology* 1999;52:1133–1137.
30. Goertler M, Kross R, Baeumer M, et al. Diagnostic impact and prognostic relevance of early contrast-enhanced transcranial color-coded duplex sonography in acute stroke. *Stroke* 1998;29:955–962.
31. Nabavi DG, Droste DW, Kemeny V, et al. Potential and limitations of echocontrast-enhanced ultrasonography in acute stroke patients: a pilot study. *Stroke* 1998;29:949–954.
32. Seidel G, Kaps M. Harmonic imaging of the verte-brobasilar system. *Stroke* 1997;28:1610–1613.
33. Wiesmann M, Seidel G. Ultrasound perfusion imaging of the human brain. *Stroke* 2000;31:2421–2425.
34. Postert T, Federlein J, Weber S, et al. Second harmonic imaging in acute middle cerebral artery infarction. Preliminary results. *Stroke* 1999;30:1702–1706.
35. Seidel G, Meyer K, Algermissen C, et al. Harmonic imaging of the brain parenchyma using a perfluorobutane-containing ultrasound contrast agent. *Ultrasound Med Biol* 2001;27:915–918.
36. Lyden PD, Nelson TR. Visualization of the cerebral circulation using three-dimensional transcranial power Doppler ultrasound imaging. *J Neuroimaging* 1997;7:35–39.
37. Delcker A, Turowski B. Diagnostic value of three-dimensional transcranial contrast duplex sonography. *J Neuroimaging* 1997;7:139–144.
38. International Consensus Group on Microembolus Detection. Consensus on microembolus detection by TCD. *Stroke* 1998;29:725–729.
39. Droste DW, Ritter M, Kemény V, et al. Microembolus detections at follow-up in 19 patients with acute stroke. *Cerebrovasc Dis* 2000;10:272–277.
40. Serena J, Segura T, Castellanos M, et al. Microembolic signal monitoring in hemispheric acute ischaemic stroke: a prospective study. *Cerebrovasc Dis* 2000;10:278–282.
41. Sitzer M, Muller W, Siebler W et al. Plaque ulceration and lumen thrombus are the main source of cerebral microemboli in high-grade internal carotid artery stenosis. *Stroke* 1995;26:1231–1233.
42. Sitzer M, Siebler M, Steinmetz H. Silent emboli and their relation to clinical symptoms in extracranial carotid artery disease. *Cerebrovasc Dis* 1995;5:121–123.
43. Ries S, Schminke U, Daffertshoffer M, et al. High intensity transient signals and carotid artery disease. *Cerebrovasc Dis* 1995;5:124–127.
44. Droste DW, Dittrich R, Kemény V, et al. Prevalence and frequency of microembolic signals in 105 patients with extracranial carotid artery occlusive disease. *J Neurol Neurosurg Psychiatry* 1999;67:525–528.
45. Tegeler CH, Knappertz VA, Nagaraja D, et al. Relationship of common carotid artery high intensity transient signals in patients with ischemic stroke to white matter versus territorial infarct pattern on brain CT scan. *Cerebrovasc Dis* 1995;5:128–132.
46. Babikian VL, Wijman CAC, Hyde C, et al. Cerebral microembolism and early recurrent cerebral or retinal ischemic events. *Stroke* 1997;28:1314–1318.
47. Georgiadis D, Lindner A, Manz M. Intracranial microembolic signals in 500 patients with potential cardiac or carotid embolic source and in normal controls. *Stroke* 1997;28:1203–1207.
48. Del Sette M, Angeli S, Stara I, et al. Microembolic signals with serial transcranial Doppler monitoring in acute focal ischemic deficit. A local phenomenon? *Stroke* 1997;28:1310–1313.
49. Koennecke HC, Trocio SS, Mast H, et al. Microemboli on transcranial Doppler in patients with spontaneous carotid artery dissection. *J Neuroimaging* 1997;7:217–220.
50. Selnes OA, McKhann GM. Coronary-artery bypass surgery and the brain [Editorial]. *N Engl J Med* 2001;344:451–452.
51. Newman MF, Kirchner JL, Phillips-Bute B, et al. Longitudinal assessment of neurocognitive function after coronary-artery bypass surgery. *N Engl J Med* 2001;344:395–402.
52. Spencer MP. Transcranial Doppler monitoring and causes of stroke from carotid endarterectomy. *Stroke* 1997;28:685–691.
53. Levi CR, O'Malley HM, Fell G, et al. Transcranial Doppler detected cerebral microembolism following carotid endarterectomy. High microembolic signal loads predict postoperative cerebral ischaemia. *Brain* 1997;120:621–629.
54. Arnold M, Sturzenegger M, Schäffer L, et al. Continuous intraoperative monitoring of middle cerebral artery blood

flow velocities and electroencephalography during carotid endarterectomy. A comparison of the two methods to detect cerebral ischemia. *Stroke* 1997;28:1345–1350.

55. Gossetti B, Martinelli O, Guerricchio R, et al. Transcranial Doppler in 178 patients before, during and after carotid endarterectomy. *J Neuroimaging* 1997;7:213–216.
56. Finocchi C, Gandolfo C, Carissimi T, et al. Role of transcranial Doppler and stump pressure during carotid endarterectomy. *Stroke* 1997;28:2448–2452.
57. Krul JM, van Gijn J, Ackerstaff RG, et al. Site and pathogenesis of infarcts associated with carotid endarterectomy. *Stroke* 1989;20:324–328.
58. Babikian VL, Cantelmo NL, Wijman CA. Cerebrovascular monitoring during carotid endarterectomy. In: Babikian VL, Wechsler LR, eds. *Transcranial Doppler ultrasonography.* Boston: Butterworth Heinemann, 1999:231–245.
59. Ackerstaff RGA, Moons KGM, van de Vlasakker CJW, et al. Association of intraoperative transcranial Doppler monitoring variables with stroke from carotid endarterectomy. *Stroke* 2000;31:1817–1823.
60. Babikian VL, Cantelmo NL. Cerebrovascular monitoring during carotid endarterectomy [Editorial]. *Stroke* 2000;31:1799–1801.
61. Koennecke HC, Mast H, Trocio SS, et al. Microemboli in patients with vertebrobasilar ischamia. Association with vertebrobasilar and cardiac lesions. *Stroke* 1997;28:593–596.
62. Droste DW, Hansberg T, Kemény V, et al. Oxygen inhalation can differentiate gaseous from nongaseous microemboli detected by transcranial Doppler ultrasound. *Stroke* 1997;28:2453–2456.
63. Georgiadis D, Preiss M, Lindner A. Doppler microembolic signals in children with prosthetic cardiac valves. *Stroke* 1997;28:1328–1329.
64. Markus H, Culliname M, Reid G. Improved automated detection of embolic signals using a novel frequency filtering approach. *Stroke* 1999;30:1610–1615.
65. Devuyst G, Darbellay GA, Vesin JM, et al. Automatic classification of HITS into artifacts or solid or gaseous emboli by a wavelet representation combined with dual-gate TCD. *Stroke* 2001;32:2803–2809.
66. Leighton TG. *The acoustic bubble.* London: Academic Press, 1994.
67. Palanchon P, Bouakaz A, van Blankenstein JH, et al. New technique for emboli detection and discrimination based on nonlinear characterization of gas bubbles. *Ultrasound Med Biol* 2001;27:801–808.
68. Russell D, Brucher R. Discrimination of cerebral microemboli. *Cerebrovasc Dis* 2001;11:4(abst).
69. Moehring M. Axial lengths of power m-mode microembolus tracks are proportional to sample volume size. *Cerebrovasc Dis* 2001;11:4(abst).
70. Droste DW, Silling K, Stypmann J, et al. Contrast transcranial Doppler ultrasound in the detection of right-to-left shunts. Time window and threshold in microbubble numbers. *Stroke* 2000;31:1640.
71. Droste DW, Reisener M, Kemény V, et al. Contrast transcranial Doppler ultrasound in the detection of right-to-left shunts. Reproducibility, comparison of 2 agents, and distribution of microemboli. *Stroke* 1999;30:1014–1018.
72. Devuyst G, Despland PA, Bogousslavsky J, et al. Complementarity of contrast transcranial Doppler and contrast transesophageal echocardiography for the detection of patent foramen ovale in stroke patients. *Eur Neurol* 1997;38:21–25.
73. Serena J, Segura T, Perez-Ayuso MJ, et al. The need to quantify right-to-left shunt in acute ischemic stroke. A case-control study. *Stroke* 1998;29:1322–1328.
74. Serena J, Silva Y, Castellanos M, et al. Risk of recurrent stroke associated with massive right-to-left shunt: a prospective study. *Stroke* 2002;45:370(abst).
75. Mas JL, Arquizan C, Lamy C, et al. Recurrent cerebrovascular events associated with patent foramen ovale, atrial septal aneurysm, or both. *N Engl J Med* 2001;345:1740—1746.

Ischemic Stroke: Advances in Neurology, Vol. 92. Edited by
H.J.M. Barnett, Julien Bogousslavsky, and Heather Meldrum.
Lippincott Williams & Wilkins, Philadelphia © 2003.

11

Amyloidosis of Cerebral Arteries

Harry V. Vinters and Emad S. Farag

*Department of Pathology and Laboratory Medicine, UCLA Medical Center,
Los Angeles, California, U.S.A.*

Cerebral amyloid (congophilic) angiopathy (CAA) describes a microvascular lesion of significance in the pathophysiology of stroke (especially cerebral hemorrhage) and Alzheimer's disease (AD). It is recognized in routine histologic specimens of brain tissue by examination of cerebral parenchymal and leptomeningeal microvasculature. CAA is suspected when the normal arteriolar media, which is composed of smooth muscle cells (SMC), is replaced by a hyaline eosinophilic material. In cases of severe CAA, amyloid can be seen "leaking" into the perivascular brain parenchyma (1,2). CAA also can involve brain capillaries, in which case the eosinophilic amyloid material often appears to "radiate" from the capillary lumen into surrounding neuropil. Confirmation of the presence of CAA can be done by either (a) staining a histologic section with classic "amyloid stains" and then viewing the section with appropriate optics, for example, Congo red stain with polarization or (b) demonstrating amyloid protein in vessel walls by immunohistochemistry, using a primary antibody directed against the suspected amyloid protein, most commonly Abeta (Aβ) protein, central nervous system (CNS) deposition of which is believed to be a key event in the pathogenesis of AD (3,4).

Although CAA is easy to recognize pathologically, it often cannot be confirmed clinically in a given patient unless it produces intracerebral hemorrhage (ICH). Criteria that can be used to predict the likelihood that a given individual harbors CAA have been promulgated (2).

CLINICOPATHOLOGIC SPECTRUM OF CEREBRAL AMYLOID ANGIOPATHY

CAA is a diagnosis that can be suspected clinically, but it is made definitively at necropsy. Increasingly, however, it also is seen in the course of brain biopsy or clot evacuation in the case of ICH. The diagnosis even may be made in the course of an intraoperative consultation (frozen section). Two brief clinical vignettes highlight ways in which CAA may present.

Case 1: An 87-year-old woman was hospitalized after family members noted that she had become confused and had difficulty moving her extremities on the right side. Past medical history included hypertension, coronary artery disease, ischemic cerebral infarct, and chronic renal insufficiency. Neurologic examination revealed right hemiparesis and a right homonymous hemianopia. Acute cerebral infarct was suspected. Neuroimaging was consistent with acute ischemia involving much of the left cerebral hemisphere and a smaller subcortical parietal region in the right cerebral hemisphere (Fig. 11-1). The presence of bilateral lesions with significant mass effect prompted further investigation, culminating in a right parietal biopsy that showed severe (Abeta-immunoreactive) CAA (Fig. 11-2). CAA was thought to be a contributing factor to the patient's extensive brain infarcts.

Case 2: A 78-year-old woman with a history of uncomplicated migraine experienced sudden onset of headache and left-sided weakness. She had no history of hypertension or cerebral infarct. In the emergency room, she gradually became obtunded and required intubation. Computed tomographic scan showed right temporal intraparenchymal hemorrhage (Fig. 11-3). Evacuation of the hematoma with anterior temporal lobectomy was performed. Severe CAA was seen in fragments of brain evacuated with the hematoma. The patient was weaned from mechanical ventilation and started on rehabilitation, although she remained significantly hemiparetic.

CAA (regardless of the biochemical composition of the amyloid subunit deposited in the vessel wall) has various clinical and neuroradiographic manifesta-

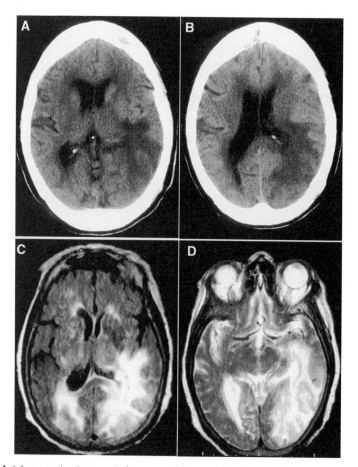

FIG. 11-1. A, B: Axial noncontrast computed tomographic scan showing a large irregular area of low density in the left posterior parietal and temporal lobes causing compression of the left lateral ventricle. Axial fluid-attenuated inversion recovery **(C)** and axial T2-weighted magnetic resonance imaging **(D)** scans show left temporo-occipital cortical and subcortical white matter hyperintensity with areas of periventricular hyperintensity, most severe in the right occipital region. The findings are consistent with acute ischemic infarct superimposed on chronic ischemic white matter disease.

tions, of which ICH is the most common (1,2,5–11). Other uncommon presentations of CAA include subarachnoid hemorrhage, leukoencephalopathy, angiitis/vasculitis, and recurrent intermittent neurologic symptoms resembling transient ischemic attacks, the latter possibly a result of small hemorrhages and/or microinfarcts within brain parenchyma (1,2,12–15). The possible role of CAA in cerebral ischemia has been controversial, but mounting evidence suggests such an association (16). Given the large and growing number of elderly individuals, many with mild-to-severe AD and almost all of whom by definition have some degree of CAA, ICH is relatively rare in these patients. However, in one series of more than 100 consecutive autopsies on AD patients, CAA-related cerebral hemorrhage had occurred in over 5% (17).

CAA may be the second most common cause of spontaneous ICH, accounting for as many as 10% of all cases (18).

CAA causes ICHs with highly distinctive features (6–10). Bleeds characteristically occur as "lobar" hemorrhages in the cortex and subcortical white matter, with frequent extension into the subarachnoid space. The distribution of hematomas reflects the topography of CAA, which is primarily a meningo-cortical microangiopathy (19). CAA can readily be detected in fragments of brain parenchyma adjacent to a surgically evacuated hematoma (20,21), provided the pathologist's index of suspicion is appropriately high and the patient's "profile" fits that of a patient likely to present with this type of stroke. Patients usually are in their 70s or 80s and may be demented

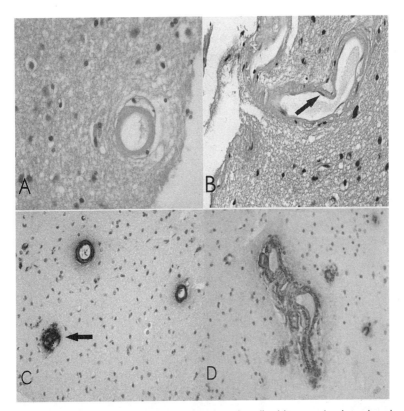

FIG. 11-2. Photomicrographs of biopsy sections from patient described in case 1, whose imaging studies are shown in Fig. 11-1. Hematoxylin and eosin-stained intraparenchymal **(A)** and leptomeningeal perforating **(B)** amyloid-laden arterioles show hyaline thickening of the tunica media with loss of smooth muscle cells and preserved endothelium *(arrow,* **B)**. Intraparenchymal vessels and a senile plaque *(arrow)* are immunoreactive with antibodies to amyloid Abeta 1-42 **(C)** and Abeta 1-40 **(D)**.

before the occurrence of hemorrhage. Hematomas may occur sequentially in various lobes of the cerebral hemispheres over months or years. Rarely, cerebellar hemorrhage occurs with CAA, but brainstem hemorrhage has never been documented (9). A review that undertook an analysis of all papers reporting CAA-related hemorrhage up to the late 1980s noted that approximately one third of affected patients also had clinical evidence of hypertension (10).

CAA occurs frequently in elderly individuals with or without hypertension. It usually appears to be "well tolerated," although the impact of CAA on surrounding CNS parenchyma, short of hemorrhage, is not completely understood (1,2,10). The majority of brains from patients with (AD- or age-related) CAA show no evidence of large or small bleeds. Cerebral hemorrhage is the defining feature of familial CAA syndromes (e.g., Dutch, Icelandic forms) in which vascular amyloidosis is generally more severe than in senescence or AD (2,22). Reports on cerebral

hematomas that occur in the presence of CAA stress the following: (a) spontaneous occurrence of the bleed, with or without associated hypertension (6,7,23); (b) traumatic aggravating factors in some cases (although the role of trauma in precipitating CAA-related bleeds has been questioned) (2,24); and (c) occasional formation of microaneurysms on arterioles involved by CAA (7,8,25,26). Amyloid gradually causes atrophy of the medial SMC layer of leptomeningeal and cortical arteries and veins. This gradual replacement of SMC leads to progressive changes in the vessel walls, impairing their function by reducing their flexibility and by limiting the ability of the vessel wall to respond to changes in blood flow and/or pressure (7,27).

Microaneurysms and fibrinoid necrosis affecting amyloid-laden arterioles appear to play a critical role in the genesis of lobar hemorrhage (7,8,25,27). In autopsy brain specimens with severe CAA and cerebral hemorrhages, serial sections have shown a clear

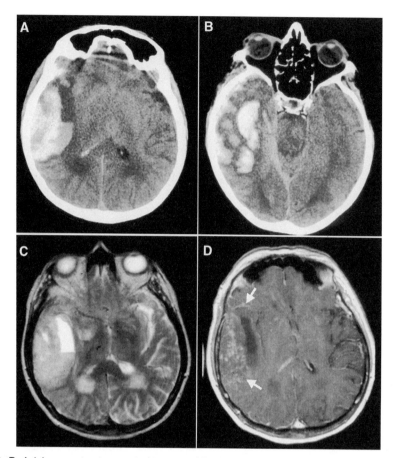

FIG. 11-3. A, B: Axial noncontrast computed tomographic scan showing a large intraparenchymal hemorrhage in the right temporal, parietal, and frontal opercular regions. Hemorrhage extends to the subarachnoid space. **C:** Axial T2-weighted magnetic resonance image showing the area of hemorrhage. **D:** Axial postcontrast T1-weighted image showing petechial enhancement in the region of the hemorrhage *(arrows).*

relationship between fibrinoid necrosis and the site of vascular rupture (8). The absence of blood leakage at sites of vessel wall fragmentation and presence of fibrin clots suggests that, in some cases, rupture of the wall might be sufficiently gradual to allow the clotting cascade to prevent a bleed. Microaneurysms, possibly a result of previous fibrinoid necrosis (with scarring and repair) of amyloid-laden arterioles, may play an important part in CAA-related hemorrhage, based upon studies of patients with Dutch familial CAA, i.e. hereditary cerebral hemorrhage with amyloidosis, Dutch type (HCHWA-D) (26). Additional factors that may increase the likelihood of hemorrhage include angiitis or simply the presence of foreign body giant cells around vascular amyloid (1,2,12). Systemic risk factors for CAA-related cerebral hemorrhage include administration of anticoagulants and thrombolytic agents (2).

CEREBRAL AMYLOID ANGIOPATHY-ASSOCIATED MICROANGIOPATHIES

Mandybur (27) first conceptualized cerebral amyloid angiopathy-associated microangiopathies (CAA-AMs) as vasculopathies that are, in poorly defined ways, associated with CAA (27). CAA-AMs may represent the immediate cause(s) of CAA-associated vascular rupture leading to hemorrhage. Morphologic features of CAA-AM include (a) glomerular formations, (b) microaneurysms, (c) obliterative intimal changes, (d) "double barreling," (e) chronic inflammatory infiltrates, (f) hyaline arteriolar degeneration (sometimes with formation of microaneurysms), (g) fibrinoid necrosis, and (h) rarely calcification of involved vessels. There is nothing in the clinical presentation of a given patient, with the possible exception of hemorrhage itself, to indicate who might have severe CAA-AM. The role of obliterative intimal change in causing microinfarcts is suspected but not proved. Vessel wall inflammation may aggravate a tendency to microaneurysm formation.

CAA-AMs occur with high frequency in a rare Dutch familial form of Abeta CAA, HCHWA-D (28). Examining CAA-AM (and its possible role in CAA-related stroke) is simplified by studying patients in whom CAA evolves with a somewhat predictable set of complications and time course. In autopsy brain tissue from patients with HCHWA-D, the severity and extent of HCHWA-D was evaluated to yield a CAA-AM "score" for each brain. This score was correlated (retrospectively) with clinical features of the patients, including the numbers of cerebrovascular lesions (hemorrhages/infarcts) they had experienced while alive, duration of illness, and presence or severity of hypertension and systemic atherosclerosis (26,28). An association was found between CAA-AM and the number of cerebrovascular lesions. Microaneurysmal dilation of CAA-affected arterioles appeared to be the most significant "predictor" of CAA-related stroke. A modest association was noted between atherosclerosis and the CAA-AM score, but hypertension did not show a significant association with CAA-AM in this unique patient group.

SPORADIC VERSUS ALZHEIMER'S DISEASE-RELATED CEREBRAL AMYLOID ANGIOPATHY

Considering the brains of patients with autopsy-confirmed AD, 83% show at least mild CAA and approximately 25% show moderate-to-severe CAA, affecting brain microvessels in one or more cortical regions (29). Brains with moderate-to-severe CAA also show a significantly higher frequency of ischemic or hemorrhagic lesions than do those with negligible CAA. A case control study using brain biopsy material has shown that CAA, but not amyloid plaque formation, is significantly more common in individuals with ischemic brain infarcts than in age-matched controls with nonvascular lesions, that is, CAA appears to be a significant risk factor for cerebral ischemic infarct (16). In a comparative study of AD- and age-matched controls, CAA was noted to be present in 86% of AD cases, more than twice as frequently as in controls (30). If one considers an unselected autopsy population of the elderly, estimates of CAA—both its frequency and severity—depend upon how carefully this lesion is sought. In one study, moderate-to-severe CAA showed a range from 2.3% (age group 65–74 years) to 8% (age range 75–84 years) to 12.1% (age 85 years or older). Consecutive autopsies on patients with AD from the same center showed 25.6% with moderate-to-severe CAA and over 5% with CAA-related ICH (17,31). CAA becomes more widespread and severe with advancing age, and it is significantly worse in those with AD than those without it (19,32).

A (clinically) poorly defined subset of patients who present with either dementia or cerebral hemorrhage (sometimes without dementia) shows CAA as the major defining manifestation of CNS Abeta deposition. Considering all patients with AD-type dementia, the extent and severity of CAA (in relation to parenchymal senile plaques and neurofibrillary tangles) is extremely variable. Widely divergent cellular and molecular mechanisms may lead to senile plaque and vascular amyloid deposition (33).

PATHOGENESIS OF CEREBRAL AMYLOID ANGIOPATHY

Our understanding of the complexity of brain amyloids has evolved together with an appreciation for the genetic and biochemical heterogeneity of systemic amyloids (34). Selected avenues leading to insights into CAA warrant brief consideration. Important questions in the etiology and manifestations of sporadic or AD-associated CAA include the following. (a) Why does fibrillar amyloid localize selectively to, or predominantly in, vessel walls in some AD patients? (b) What approaches can be used to investigate the evolution of CAA? (c) What, if any, injury to surrounding brain parenchyma results from severe CAA, in the absence of cerebral hemorrhage?

Familial Syndromes of Cerebral Amyloid Angiopathy

Two forms of familial syndromes of CAA (fCAA; i.e., CAA associated with Dutch and Icelandic hereditary cerebral hemorrhage) have been briefly considered. A previous review summarized molecular genetic features of several forms of fCAA, including recently discovered variants (35). Although several of these entities show CNS microvascular amyloid deposition, cerebral hemorrhage or ischemic lesions do not always result. The forms of fCAA that probably are of greatest relevance for understanding the neurobiology of sporadic/age- or AD-associated CAA are those seen with the three different mutations in the gene encoding the amyloid precursor protein (from which Abeta is cleaved): APP, and HCHWA-I/HCCAA.

The Dutch form of fCAA (HCHWA-D), first discovered in coastal Holland, results from a codon 693 mutation in the gene encoding APP, resulting in a Gln-for-Glu substitution at residue 22 of Abeta. The effect of this mutation on brain microvasculature is profound (2,28). Severe Abeta CAA and secondary microvascular degeneration occur, with cerebral hemorrhage in affected patients (26,28). A rare familial dementia (found in Belgium) associated with a codon 692 APP mutation appears to result from CAA (which may produce ICH), extensive parenchymal deposits of amyloid, and leukoencephalopathy (36). An Iowa kindred with familial dementia and an APP codon 694 mutation has been shown to have extensive CAA with marked similarities to HCHWA-D (37,38). HCHWA-I/HCCAA, caused by a mutation in the gene encoding a cysteine protease inhibitor, seems to result from a structurally unstable variant of the cystatin C protein. In this disease, amyloid deposition is almost purely vascular. Frequently fatal cerebral hemorrhages occur in young individuals, often in the third or fourth decade of life (2,5,39).

Why Vascular Deposition of Fibrillar Amyloid?

Several hypotheses have been put forth in an attempt to explain (Abeta) amyloid deposition in cerebral vessel walls. In situ hybridization studies confirm that many cellular components of cerebral arterial walls are capable of synthesizing APP (40). It is possible that Abeta simply accumulates in the arteriolar wall, with resultant injury to medial SMCs. The toxicity of various wild type and mutant forms of Abeta is demonstrable when human cerebral-derived SMCs or endothelial cells in culture are exposed to a variety of Abeta peptides (41,42). Another model of Abeta deposition within vessel walls proposes that this peptide accumulates in cerebral perivascular interstitial fluid drainage pathways. In AD, this may be the result of increased Abeta production, possibly by neurons; reduced solubility of Abeta peptides; or interference with Abeta drainage along periarterial interstitial fluid drainage pathways in the CNS and

adjacent meninges due to "aging factors" in cerebral arteries (43). Autopsy studies of human brain show that once Abeta deposition "seeds" some cerebral vessels, progression from asymptomatic to advanced (symptomatic) CAA results from progressive accumulation of amyloid in these vessels rather than "recruitment" of new arteries/arterioles (44). There is a complex relationship between apolipoprotein E (apoE) genotype and progression of CAA, including CAA-related brain hemorrhage. Whereas the apoE ε4 allele is associated with increased severity of Abeta CAA in AD, apoE ε2 allele appears to be a risk factor for CAA-related brain hemorrhage (2,45,46).

Does Cerebral Amyloid Angiopathy Damage the Central Nervous System?

Brain injury that results from a CAA-related bleed is obvious. What other deleterious effects, if any, does CAA produce in proximity to the microvascular lesion? In rare cases of AD with severe CAA, indirect immunohistochemical evidence of periarterial brain injury (including "neuritic" change) can be found (4). Whether this results from induction of proinflammatory molecules secreted by microglia/astrocytes, direct toxicity to neuronal processes, or simply relative ischemia to the surrounding brain remains to be determined. This is a question that may be fundamental to understanding the interface between vascular biology and neurodegenerative disease.

ACKNOWLEDGMENTS

Work in Dr. Vinters' laboratory was supported by NIH Grants P50AG16570 and P01AG12435. Dr. Farag was supported by PHS Training Grants T32-NS07356 and T32AG00093-21.

REFERENCES

1. Vinters HV, Wang ZZ, Secor DL. Brain parenchymal and microvascular amyloid in Alzheimer's disease. *Brain Pathol* 1996;6:179–195.
2. Verbeek MM, de Waal RMW, Vinters HV, eds. *Cerebral amyloid angiopathy in Alzheimer's disease and related disorders.* Dordrecht, The Netherlands: Kluwer Academic Publishers, 2000.
3. Selkoe DJ. Alzheimer's disease: a central role for amyloid. *J Neuropathol Exp Neurol* 1994;53:438–447.
4. Cummings JL, Vinters HV, Cole GM, et al. Alzheimer's disease. Etiologies, pathophysiology, cognitive reserve, and treatment opportunities. *Neurology* 1998;51[Suppl 1]:S2–S17.
5. Olafsson I, Thorsteinsson L, Jensson O. The molecular pathology of hereditary cystatin C amyloid angiopathy

causing brain hemorrhage. *Brain Pathol* 1996;6: 121–126.

6. Gilbert JJ, Vinters HV. Cerebral amyloid angiopathy: incidence and complications in the aging brain. I. Cerebral hemorrhage. *Stroke* 1983;14:915–923.

7. Okazaki H, Reagan TJ, Campbell RJ. Clinicopathologic studies of primary cerebral amyloid angiopathy. *Mayo Clin Proc* 1979;54:22–31.

8. Vonsattel JP, Myers RH, Hedley-Whyte ET, et al. Cerebral amyloid angiopathy without and with cerebral hemorrhages: a comparative histological study. *Ann Neurol* 1991;30:637–649.

9. Vinters HV. Cerebral amyloid angiopathy. In: Barnett HJM, Mohr JP, Stein BM, et al., eds. *Stroke: pathophysiology, diagnosis, and management,* 3rd ed. New York: Churchill Livingstone, 1998:945–962.

10. Vinters HV. Cerebral amyloid angiopathy. A critical review. *Stroke* 1987;18:311–324.

11. Coria F, Rubio I. Cerebral amyloid angiopathies. *Neuropathol Appl Neurobiol* 1996;22:216–227.

12. Fountain NB, Eberhard DA. Primary angiitis of the central nervous system associated with cerebral amyloid angiopathy: report of two cases and review of the literature. *Neurology* 1996;46:190–197.

13. Ohshima T, Endo T, Nukui H, et al. Cerebral amyloid angiopathy as a cause of subarachnoid hemorrhage. *Stroke* 1990;21:480–483.

14. Gray F, Dubas F, Roullet E, et al. Leukoencephalopathy in diffuse hemorrhagic cerebral amyloid angiopathy. *Ann Neurol* 1985;18:54–59.

15. Greenberg SM, Vonsattel JPG, Stakes JW, et al. The clinical spectrum of cerebral amyloid angiopathy: presentations without lobar hemorrhage. *Neurology* 1993; 43:2073–2079.

16. Cadavid D, Mena H, Koeller K, et al. Cerebral beta amyloid angiopathy is a risk factor for cerebral ischemic infarction. A case control study in human brain biopsies. *J Neuropathol Exp Neurol* 2000;59:768–773.

17. Greenberg SM. Cerebral amyloid angiopathy. Prospects for clinical diagnosis and treatment. *Neurology* 1998; 51:690–694.

18. Fisher M. *Clinical atlas of cerebrovascular disorders.* London: Mosby Wolfe, 1994.

19. Vinters HV, Gilbert JJ. Cerebral amyloid angiopathy: incidence and complications in the aging brain II. The distribution of amyloid vascular changes. *Stroke* 1983; 14:924–928.

20. Yong WH, Robert ME, Secor DL, et al. Cerebral hemorrhage with biopsy-proved amyloid angiopathy. *Arch Neurol* 1992;49:51–58.

21. Hinton DR, Dolan E, Sima AAF. The value of histopathological examination of surgically removed blood clot in determining the etiology of spontaneous intracerebral hemorrhage. *Stroke* 1984;15:517–520.

22. Luyendijk W, Bots GTAM, Vegter-van der Vlis M, et al. Hereditary cerebral haemorrhage caused by cortical amyloid angiopathy. *J Neurol Sci* 1988;85:267–280.

23. Cosgrove GR, Leblanc R, Meagher-Villemure K, et al. Cerebral amyloid angiopathy. *Neurology* 1985;35: 625–631.

24. Greene GM, Godersky JC, Biller J, et al. Surgical experience with cerebral amyloid angiopathy. *Stroke* 1990; 21:1545–1549.

25. Ferreiro JA, Ansbacher LE, Vinters HV. Stroke related

to cerebral amyloid angiopathy: the significance of systemic vascular disease. *J Neurol* 1989;236:267–272.

26. Natté R, Vinters HV, Maat-Schieman MLC, et al. Microvasculopathy is associated with the number of cerebrovascular lesions in hereditary cerebral hemorrhage with amyloidosis, Dutch type. *Stroke* 1998;29: 1588–1594.

27. Mandybur TI. Cerebral amyloid angiopathy: the vascular pathology and complications. *J Neuropathol Exp Neurol* 1986;45:79–90.

28. Vinters HV, Natté R, Maat-Schieman MLC, et al. Secondary microvascular degeneration in amyloid angiopathy of patients with hereditary cerebral hemorrhage with amyloidosis, Dutch type (HCHWA-D). *Acta Neuropathol* 1998;95:235–244.

29. Ellis RJ, Olichney JM, Thal LJ, et al. Cerebral amyloid angiopathy in the brains of patients with Alzheimer's disease: the CERAD experience, part XV. *Neurology* 1996;46:1592–1596.

30. Bergeron C, Ranalli PJ, Miceli PN. Amyloid angiopathy in Alzheimer's disease. *Can J Neurol Sci* 1987;14: 564–569.

31. Greenberg SM, Vonsattel J-PG. Diagnosis of cerebral amyloid angiopathy. Sensitivity and specificity of cortical biopsy. *Stroke* 1997;28:1418–1422.

32. Masuda J, Tanaka K, Ueda K, et al. Autopsy study of incidence and distribution of cerebral amyloid angiopathy in Hisayama, Japan. *Stroke* 1988;19:205–210.

33. Verbeek MM, Eikelenboom P, de Waal RMW. Differences between the pathogenesis of senile plaques and congophilic angiopathy in Alzheimer disease. *J Neuropathol Exp Neurol* 1997;56:751–761.

34. Glenner GG. Amyloid deposits and amyloidosis. The beta-fibrilloses. *N Engl J Med* 1980;302:1283–1292, 1333–1345.

35. Frangione B, Vidal R, Rostagno A, et al. Familial cerebral amyloid angiopathies and dementia. *Alzheimer Dis Assoc Disord* 2000;14[Suppl 1]:S25–S30.

36. Roks G, Van Harskamp F, De Koning I, et al. Presentation of amyloidosis in carriers of the codon 692 mutation in the amyloid precursor protein gene (APP692). *Brain* 2000;123:2130–2140.

37. Grabowski TJ, Cho HS, Vonsattel JPG, et al. Novel amyloid precursor protein mutation in an Iowa family with dementia and severe cerebral amyloid angiopathy. *Ann Neurol* 2001;49:697–705.

38. Vinters HV. Cerebral amyloid angiopathy: a microvascular link between parenchymal and vascular dementia? *Ann Neurol* 2001;49:691–693.

39. Wang ZZ, Jensson O, Thorsteinsson L, et al. Microvascular degeneration in hereditary cystatin C amyloid angiopathy of the brain. *APMIS* 1997;105:41–47.

40. Natté R, de Boer WI, Maat-Schieman MLC, et al. Amyloid beta precursor protein-mRNA is expressed throughout cerebral vessel walls. *Brain Res* 1999;828: 179–183.

41. Wang Z, Natté R, Berliner JA, et al. Toxicity of Dutch (E22Q) and Flemish (A21G) mutant amyloid beta proteins to human cerebral microvessel and aortic smooth muscle cells. *Stroke* 2000;31:534–538.

42. Eisenhauer PB, Johnson RJ, Wells JM, et al. Toxicity of various amyloid beta peptide species in cultured human blood-brain barrier endothelial cells: increased toxicity of Dutch-type mutant. *J Neurosci Res* 2000;60:804–810.

43. Weller RO, Massey A, Kuo Y-M, et al. Cerebral amyloid angiopathy: accumulation of Abeta in interstitial fluid drainage pathways in Alzheimer's disease. *Ann N Y Acad Sci* 2000;903:110–117.

44. Alonzo NC, Hyman BT, Rebeck GW, et al. Progression of cerebral amyloid angiopathy: accumulation of amyloid-beta 40 in affected vessels. *J Neuropathol Exp Neurol* 1998;57:353–359.

45. Olichney JM, Hansen LA, Hofstetter CR, et al. Association between severe cerebral amyloid angiopathy and cerebrovascular lesions in Alzheimer disease is not a spurious one attributable to Apolipoprotein E4. *Arch Neurol* 2000;57:869–874.

46. Nicoll JAR, Burnett C, Love S, et al. High frequency of apolipoprotein E epsilon 2 allele in hemorrhage due to cerebral amyloid angiopathy. *Ann Neurol* 1997;41:716–721.

Ischemic Stroke: Advances in Neurology, Vol. 92. Edited by
H.J.M. Barnett, Julien Bogousslavsky, and Heather Meldrum.
Lippincott Williams & Wilkins, Philadelphia © 2003.

12

Moyamoya Disease

*†Yasuhiro Yonekawa and †Nadia Kahn

*Department of Neurosurgery, University of Zürich and †Department of Neurosurgery, University
Hospital Zürich, Zürich, Switzerland*

INTRODUCTION

Moyamoya disease once was thought to be confined to Japan because of its initial discovery and reporting in 1955 and of the high prevalence of the disease in that country (1). We now know that this disease has a worldwide distribution, although its lower prevalence, especially in Europe and North America, now is known (2). The word *moyamoya* means "something hazy just like a puff of cigarette smoke drifting in the air" and expresses the angiographic abnormal vascular networks at the base of the brain (Fig. 12-1) (3). These abnormal vascular networks are considered to function as collateral circulation in the presence of stenotic or occlusive lesions at the terminal portions of the internal carotid arteries (ICAs).

Recent publications indicate that Japanese and Euro-American patients differ somewhat in the clinical expression of the disease (2,4,5).

EPIDEMIOLOGY AND ETIOLOGY

Moyamoya disease is most prevalent in Japan and Asian countries. There are believed to be around 4,000 persons with moyamoya disease in Japan, with 0.35 new patients per 100,000 population per year at the time of the Japanese nationwide survey of 1995. The male:female ratio is 1:1.8. Ten percent of cases

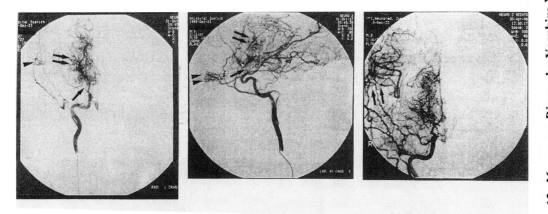

FIG. 12-1. Typical angiographic findings of moyamoya disease. **Left:** Anteroposterior (AP) view showing typical stenosis at the carotid fork *(arrow)* with typical abnormal vasculature (moyamoya) in the basal ganglia *(double arrows)*. A vault moyamoya *(arrowhead)* supplied by the middle meningeal artery is seen. **Middle:** Lateral view showing typical stenosis at the carotid fork *(arrow)*. Ethmoidal moyamoya *(double arrow head)* supplied by the ophthalmic artery is seen. **Right:** AP view of postoperative angiography showing a functional bypass with good arterial supply of the middle cerebral artery *(double arrows)* through the superficial temporal-middle cerebral artery bypass.

Chapter 12: *Moyamoya Disease* by Yasuhiro Yonekawa and Nadia Khan, pages 113–118
Dr. Nadia Khan's name is misspelled on page 113 and in the table of contents on page viii, and the list of contributors
on page xv. The correct spelling of Dr. Khan's name is as printed in this statement.

have familial incidence (6). The incidence and prevalence of the disease in Europe is believed to be around one tenth that in Japan (2).

The etiologic cause of moyamoya disease is unknown, but the possibility that it is a long-term result of an infection or of multifactorial inheritance, among other factors, has been presumed (7). Recent endeavor has been directed to identifying an etiologic gene for moyamoya disease carried on chromosomes 1 through 22. The markers D6S441 (chromosome 6), chromosome 3p24.2–p26 (chromosome 3), and 17q25 (chromosome 17) have been suggested to have possible linkage to familial moyamoya disease (2,8).

Basic fibroblastic growth factor (bFGF), a pluripotent peptide, and its receptor have been detected in increased amounts in the superficial temporal artery (endothelial cells, thickened intimal layer, and tunica media) (9) and in the diseased wall of the ICA of patients with moyamoya disease (10). As the cerebrospinal fluid concentration of bFGF reportedly is higher in moyamoya patients than in control patients with atherosclerosis or other diseases (11), its role in the etiology has been seriously discussed because some imbalance of various cytokines also is presumed to be related to the pathologic thickening of the intima of the cerebral vessels (12). Elevation of nitric oxide metabolites (13) and detection of some specific polypeptides in cerebrospinal fluid (14) have been reported to be specific for moyamoya disease. These possibilities should be followed carefully.

DIAGNOSTIC GUIDELINES

The disease presents itself at two age peaks: a higher incidence in children at age 5 years and a lower peak at age 30 to 40 years (2).

In children with peak age around 5 years, the disease generally presents either with frequent transient ischemic attacks (TIAs) manifesting as motor disturbances (70%–80%) due to cerebral ischemia or with epileptic seizures (20%–30%). The typical presentation in adults (especially women in their 30s) is headache associated with disturbance of consciousness due to intracranial bleeding. It is our impression and observation of other authors, however, that cerebral ischemia and not bleeding is the usual presentation in Europe and North America (2,4).

Once the diagnosis of moyamoya disease is suspected based on clinical findings, it can be confirmed by neuroradiologic studies on the basis of diagnostic guidelines (15). The most important finding is stenosis or occlusion of the terminal portion of the ICA (carotid fork) bilaterally, associated with abnormal vascular networks at the base of the brain. These can be demonstrated typically by angiography (Fig. 12-1) or by magnetic resonance imaging (MRI) (Fig. 12-2) and magnetic resonance angiography (MRA).

The following additional points may be important in making the diagnosis of moyamoya disease. The typical neuroradiologic findings may be present in association with other diseases, such as Down's syndrome and sickle cell anemia. This occurrence should be termed moyamoya syndrome and not moyamoya dis-

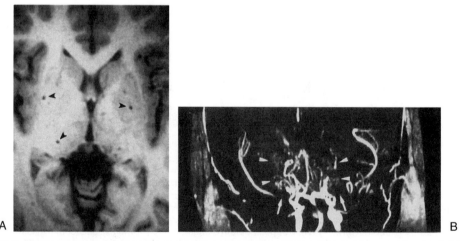

FIG. 12-2. Magnetic resonance imaging of a patient with moyamoya disease showing an extensive left hemispheric cortical infarct.

ease, which is a separate, idiopathic entity. Prevalence of moyamoya syndrome is not well known. It is our impression that moyamoya syndrome or related angiopathies are more frequent in Europe than in Japan (2). From the therapeutic, especially surgical, point of view, differentiation between the disease and the syndrome would not make sense (16). Treatment, namely revascularization procedure for cerebral ischemia, is the same and relies only on clinical presentation and specifically on the cerebral blood flow (CBF) findings.

Cases that have the typical neuroradiologic findings of moyamoya disease on only one side and normal vessels on the other side should be treated as probable cases or probable moyamoya disease. Up to 50% of such patients, especially children, will have bilateral findings on follow-up study within 1 to 2 years (17).

CLINICAL PRESENTATION, NATURAL HISTORY, AND PROGNOSIS

The disease generally presents with cerebral ischemia in children, manifesting itself as monoparesis or hemiparesis, sensory deficit, or dysphasia. These deficits characteristically are made worse by hyperventilation, such as while crying, blowing on hot food to cool it, or playing a harmonica or another wind instrument, and result from a reduction of CBF below adequate levels. Hyperventilation decreases P_aCO_2 and thereby CBF through an autoregulatory mechanism, bringing an already subnormal CBF even lower into the range where neurologic deficits occur. From 70% to 80% of children with moyamoya disease present with manifestations of cerebral ischemia, more usually as TIAs than as cerebral infarction (4:3 ratio). A rapid progression is rare and frequently seen in combination with febrile or infectious diseases. Mental retardation is present in more than half of the juvenile cases. The early onset of ischemic findings (before age 4 years) is associated with progressive mental retardation (18).

Involuntary movements may be observed, either in combination with ischemic phenomena or independently. These movements usually take a benign, self-limited course.

In adults, intracranial bleeding is the most frequent presenting event (in >60% of cases), manifesting as a disturbance of consciousness and/or hemiparesis. It occurs markedly more frequently in women. The bleeding is mostly intraventricular or intracerebral, and not subarachnoid. It is considered to originate from either abnormal vascular networks or aneurysms (discussed later). It is estimated that approximately one third of these patients go on to have further hemorrhages after a variable interval (days to years).

Again, this adult type of bleeding seems to occur less frequently in Euro-American patients compared with Japanese patients (2). A patient may have more than one manifestation, for example, first ischemia and then bleeding, or vice versa.

Mortality in the acute stage has been reported to be low, 2.4% in the infarction type and 16.4% in the hemorrhagic type (2).

The natural history of moyamoya disease is not yet definitively known. From 75% to 80% of cases are thought to have a benign course with regard to life expectancy with or without surgical treatment. These patients perform well independently, carrying out the activities of daily living. Nonetheless, adaptability to social or school life has been reported to be limited (19).

NEUROIMAGING AND CEREBRAL BLOOD FLOW STUDY

Computed Tomographic Scan

Forty percent of cases presenting with cerebral ischemia reportedly had abnormal findings on computed tomographic (CT) scan (20), such as low-density areas in the cerebral cortex or/and white matter (usually not in the basal ganglia) and cerebral atrophies, indicating chronic cerebral ischemia. Cases with hemorrhage show high-density areas corresponding to bleeding in the basal ganglia, thalamus, ventricle, subcortex, and cortex, in decreasing order of frequency.

Magnetic Resonance Imaging

In addition to the ischemic findings mentioned earlier, MRI may detect infarcts too small to be seen on CT scans without special techniques. These infarcts typically are corticosubcortical, located either unilaterally or bilaterally (Fig. 12-2). MRI and MRA are now effective tools in the diagnosis instead of cerebral angiography.

Cerebral Angiography

Angiography is the most common method of diagnosing the disease and is indispensable for planning the revascularization procedures. Care should be taken when performing the angiography because many major complications have occurred in the past. Technical expertise is required, as is adequate hydration of the patient, particularly those in the pediatric group.

Suzuki and Takaku (3) have classified the disease into six stages according to the angiographic findings. Progression from stage 1 to stage 6 has been observed in only a limited number of cases. Stage 4 is encountered most frequently. The posterior circulation usually is not affected.

Cerebral aneurysms are detected in about 10% of cases, either incidentally during angiography or because of hemorrhage, and they can be multiple (21–27).

Aneurysms associated with moyamoya disease occur in three locations: (a) in the circle of Willis (60%), mainly in the posterior circulation; (b) in the peripheral arteries (20%), such as the posterior choroidal artery, anterior choroidal artery, posterior cerebral artery, and Heubner's artery; and (c) in the abnormal moyamoya vascular networks (20%). Combination of arteriovenous malformation with moyamoya disease or syndrome is rare.

Cerebral Blood Flow Measurement

CBF can be measured in three dimensions with xenon-enhanced CT, single photon emission computed tomography, or positron emission tomography (PET). Moyamoya disease may be associated with a diffuse reduction of CBF, particularly in the frontal lobes. CBF in the basal ganglia is relatively well preserved. Reduction of CBF reserve capacity can be demonstrated by the acetazolamide (Diamox) loading technique (2,28). In the PET examination, the regional cerebral blood volume (rCBV) has been reported to be diffusely elevated; hence, the ratio rCBF/rCBV is diffusely reduced (29).

Electroencephalogram

Use of the electroencephalogram to detect a "rebuildup" phenomenon on hyperventilation once was considered an important test for moyamoya disease (30), but nowadays it confers no additional help in making the diagnosis.

TREATMENT

Because the etiology factor is unknown, there is no specific treatment. Acetylsalicylic acid (ASA, aspirin) or other antiplatelet drugs often are given because studies have revealed that platelet aggregation may have an influence on the progression of vascular stenosis. Empirical steroid therapy is given when there are frequent ischemic attacks or involuntary movements.

Surgical revascularization procedures are used to augment CBF, which is a goal no nonsurgical therapy can accomplish. The following revascularization procedures currently are in use (32–37):

1. Direct revascularization procedures
   A. Superficial temporal-middle cerebral artery bypass
   B. Extracranial-intracranial bypass to anterior or posterior cerebral artery (ACA, PCA)
2. Indirect revascularization procedures
   A. Encephalo-duro-arterio-synangiosis (EDAS), encephalo-myo-synangiosis (EMS), etc.
   B. Indirect revascularization with anastomosis: intracranial omental transplantation, muscle transplantation (latissimus dorsi, gracilis)

The cohort study performed by these research committees registered 884 patients with a long-term follow-up of 6.6 ± 5.6 years. The patients in the surgical group tended to perform better in their activities of daily living than those in the nonsurgical group (2). Effectiveness of revascularization procedures has been reported to improve IQ or preventing its deterioration, which correlated well with an increase of mean CBF (38).

In our opinion, a direct and multiple extracranial-intracranial bypass procedure is the first choice of revascularization procedures when feasible, whether the recipient vessel is the MCA, ACA, or PCA, depending upon findings of CBF study. Indirect revascularization, such as EDAS, is performed additionally or without any direct bypass procedure when the latter is not feasible.

When such revascularization procedures are performed, appropriate general perioperative management, including operation during a relatively stable clinical condition without frequent ischemic episodes, adequate hydration, normocapnia, and judicious selection of anesthetic agents, is of cardinal importance to prevent serious ischemic complications (39,40), which have been reported to occur at rates up to 10% or more.

CONCLUSION

Moyamoya disease is a rare disease of unknown etiology. Its predominant clinical manifestations are cerebral ischemia in children and intracranial bleeding in adults. These conditions are due to stenosis or occlusion of the ICA at its terminal portion bilaterally, with resulting formation of abnormal collateral vessels *(moyamoya)* that is most pronounced in the basal part of the brain. The disease is treated medically with ASA to prevent progression of the disease and surgically with revascularization procedures to augment CBF.

REFERENCES

1. Tekeuchi K, Shimizu K. Hypoplasia of the bilateral internal carotid arteries. *Brain Nerve (Tokyo)* 1957;9: 37–43.
2. Yonekawa Y, Taub E. Moyamoya disease: status 1998. *Neurologist* 1999;5:13–23.
3. Suzuki J, Takaku A. Cerebrovascular "moyamoya" disease: disease showing abnormal net-like vessels in base of the brain. *Arch Neurol* 1969;20:288–299.
4. Chiu D, Shedden P, Bratina P, et al. Clinical features of moyamoya disease in the United States. *Stroke* 1998;29: 1347–1351.
5. Han DH, Kwon OK, Byun BJ, et al. A co-operative study: clinical characteristic of 334 Korean patients with moyamoya disease treated at neurosurgical institutes (1976–1994). The Korean Society for Cerebrovascular Disease. *Acta Neurochir (Wien)* 2000;142: 1263–1273.
6. Wakai K, Tamakoshi A, Ikezaki K, et al. Epidemiological features of moyamoya disease in Japan: findings from a nation wide survey. *Clin Neurol Neurosurg* 1997;99[Suppl 2]:1–5.
7. Fukuyama Y, Sugawara N, Osawa M. A genetic study of idiopathic spontaneous multiple occlusion of the circle of Willis. In: Yonekawa Y, ed. *Annual report of the research committee on spontaneous occlusion of the circle of Willis (Moyamoya disease) 1990.* Japan: Ministry of Health and Welfare, 1991:139–144.
8. Inoue T, Ikezaki K, Sasazuki T, et al. Linkage analysis of Moyamoya disease on chromosome 6. *J Child Neurol* 2000;15:179–182.
9. Hoshimaru M, Takahashi JA, Kikuchi H, et al. Possible roles of basic fibroblast growth factor in the pathogenesis of moyamoya disease: an immunohistochemical study. *J Neurosurg* 1991;75:267–270.
10. Hosoda Y, Hirose S, Kameyama K. Histopathological and immunohistochemical study of growth factor in spontaneous occlusion of the circle of Willis. In: Fukui M, ed. *Annual report of the research committee on spontaneous occlusion of the circle of Willis (Moyamoya disease) 1993.* Japan: Ministry of Health and Welfare, 1994:25–28.
11. Yoshimoto T, Houkin K, Takahashi A, et al. Angiogenetic factors in moyamoya disease. *Stroke* 1996;27: 2160–2165.
12. Aoyagi M, Fukai N, Yamamoto M, et al. Early development of intimal thickening in superficial temporal arteries in patients with moyamoya disease. *Stroke* 1996;27: 1750–1754.
13. Noda A, Suzuki M, Takayasu K, et al. Elevation of nitric oxide metabolites in the cerebrospinal fluid of patients with moyamoya disease. *Acta Neurochir (Wien)* 2000; 142:1275–1280.
14. Hojo M, Houshimaru M, Miyamoto S, et al. A cerebrospinal fluid protein associated with moyamoya disease: report of three cases. *Neurosurgery* 1999; 45:170–174.
15. Fukui M, Members of the Research Committee on Spontaneous Occlusion of the Circle of Willis (Moyamoya Disease) of the Ministry of Health on Welfare, Japan. Guideline for the diagnosis and treatment of spontaneous occlusion of the circle of Willis (Moyamoya disease). Ministry of Health and Welfare, Japan. *Clin Neurol Neurosurg* 1997;99[Suppl 2]:238–240.
16. Peerless SJ. Risk factors of moyamoya disease in Canada and the USA. *Clin Neurol Neurosurg* 1997; 99[Suppl 2]:45–48.
17. Kawano T, Fukui M, Hashimoto N, et al. Follow-up study of patients with "unilateral" moyamoya disease. *Neurol Med Chir (Tokyo)* 1994;34:744–747.
18. Moritake H, Handa H, Yonekawa Y, et al. Follow-up study on the relationship between age at onset of illness and outcome in patients with moyamoya disease. *No Shinkei Geka* 1986;14:957–963.
19. Imaizumi T, Hayashi K, Saito K, et al. Long-term outcomes of pediatric moyamoya disease monitored to adulthood. *Pediatr Neurol* 1998;18:321–325.
20. Handa J, Nakano Y, Okuno T, et al. Computerized tomography in moyamoya syndrome. *Surg Neurol* 1977;7:315–319.
21. Kodama N, Suzuki J. Moyamoya disease associated with aneurysm. *J Neurosurg* 1978;48:565–569.
22. Furuse S, Matsumoto S, Tanaka Y, et al. Moyamoya disease associated with a false aneurysm. Case report and review of the literature. *No Shinkei Geka (Tokyo)* 1982; 10:1005–1012.
23. Kwak R, Ito S, Yamamoto N, Kadoya S. Significance of intracranial aneurysms associated with moyamoya disease. Part I. Differences between intracranial aneurysms associated with moyamoya disease and usual saccular aneurysms (part I). Review of the literature. *Neurol Med Chir (Tokyo)* 1984;24:97–103.
24. Kwak R, Emori T, Nakamura T, et al. Significance of intracranial aneurysms associated with moyamoya disease (part II.) Cause and site of hemorrhage. Review of the literature. *Neurol Med Chir (Tokyo)* 1984;24:104–109.
25. Waga S, Tochio H. Intracranial aneurysm associated with Moyamoya disease in childhood. *Surg Neurol* 1985;23:237–243.
26. Sadato A, Yonekawa Y, Morooka Y, et al. A case of moyamoya disease with repeated intraventricular hemorrhage due to ruptured pseudoaneurysm. *Neurol Surg (Tokyo)* 1988;17:755–758.
27. Kawaguchi S, Sakaki T, Morimoto T, et al. Characteristics of intracranial aneurysms associated with moyamoya disease. A review of 111 cases. *Acta Neurochir (Wien)* 1996;138:1287–1294.
28. Horowitz M, Yonas H, Albright AL. Evaluation of cerebral blood flow and hemodynamic reserve in symptomatic moyamoya disease using stable xenon-CT blood flow. *Surg Neurol* 1995;44:251–262.
29. Taki W, Yonekawa Y, Kobayashi A, et al. Cerebral circulation and oxygen metabolism in moyamoya disease of ischemic type in children. *Childs Nerv Syst* 1988;4: 259–262.
30. Yoshii N, Kudo T. Electroencephalographical study on occlusion of the Willis arterial ring. *Clin Neurol (Tokyo)* 1968;8:301–309.
31. Hosoda Y. A pathological study of so-called "spontaneous occlusion of the circle of Willis" (cerebrovascular moyamoya disease). *Folia Angiol* 1976;24:85.
32. Krayenbïhl H. The moyamoya syndrome and the neurosurgeon. *Surg Neurol* 1975;4:353–360.
33. Matsushima Y, Fukai N, Tanaka K, et al. A new surgical treatment of moyamoya disease in children: a preliminary report. *Surg Neurol* 1981;15:313–320.
34. Yonekawa Y, Yasargil MG. Brain vascularization by transplanted omentum: a possible treatment of cerebral ischemia. *Neurosurgery* 1977;1:256–259.

35. Karasawa J, Touho H, Ohnishi H, et al. Cerebral revascularization using omental transplantation for childhood moyamoya disease. *J Neurosurg* 1993;79:192–196.

36. Iwama T, Hashimoto N, Miyake H, et al. Direct revascularization to the cerebral artery territory in patients with moyamoya disease. Report of five cases. *Neurosurgery* 1998;42:1157–1161.

37. Mizoi K, Kayama T, Yoshimoto T, et al. Indirect revascularization for moyamoya disease: is there a beneficial effect for adult patients? *Surg Neurol* 1996;45:541–548.

38. Ishii R, Takeuchi S, Ibayashi K, et al. Intelligence in children with moyamoya disease: Evaluation after surgical treatments with special reference to changes in cerebral blood flow. *Stroke* 1984;15:873–877.

39. Iwama T, Hashimoto N, Yonekawa Y. The relevance of hemodynamic factors to perioperative ischemic complications in childhood moyamoya disease. Clinical studies. *Neurosurgery* 1996;38:1120–1126.

40. Sato K, Shirane R, Yoshimoto T. Perioperative factors related to the development of ischemic complications in patients with moyamoya disease. *Childs Nerv Syst* 1997;13:68–72.

Ischemic Stroke: Advances in Neurology, Vol. 92. Edited by
H.J.M. Barnett, Julien Bogousslavsky, and Heather Meldrum.
Lippincott Williams & Wilkins, Philadelphia © 2003.

13

Cervical Arterial Dissection

John W. Norris and *Vadim Beletsky

*Department of Neurology and *Stroke Research Unit, University of Toronto, Toronto, Ontario, Canada*

Excellent comprehensive reviews of cervical arterial dissection have been published (1–3). The brief review written in 1985 by Hart and Easton (4) remains one of the best synopses of the clinical and radiologic features of dissection.

Awareness of the frequency of stroke from cervical arterial dissection is a relatively recent phenomenon. Before 1987, no cases of carotid dissection had been reported in the population of Rochester, Minnesota (5). Based more upon inspiration than data (there were only 41 patients in the study), Bogousslavsky and Regli (6) suggested that arterial dissection probably was the most frequent cause of stroke in persons younger than 45 years, and subsequent large series and meta-analyses proved them right (7). In recent years since newer, safer forms of neuroimaging became available, it is clear that carotid and vertebral dissections are relatively frequent and seriously underestimated causes of stroke.

Cervical arterial dissection remains an infrequent cause of cerebral ischemic stroke. About 5% of all ischemic strokes occur in patients younger than 45 years, and because 20% of these are due to dissection, they account for only about 1% overall. Schievink (3) estimated the frequency of carotid dissections as 2.5 per 100,000 and vertebral dissection as 1 to 1.5 per 100,000.

ETIOLOGIC FACTORS

Although traditionally labeled as "spontaneous," careful history taking often will reveal sudden neck movement or trauma, with the typical neck or head pain, occurring at the time of dissection. In the study of dissection presently in progress by the Canadian Stroke Consortium, only 20 (12%) of 165 patients had no attributable trauma, and in 41 patients the given history was considered inadequate, as in one patient who collapsed doing "press-ups" and was designated as "spontaneous." Immediate neck pain or headache is a useful marker for the moment of dissection in up to 75% to 80% of cases (8), but often the trauma is so trivial, such as painting, golfing, skiing, basketball, and trampoline exercises (1) that it is overlooked by both patients and physicians (Fig. 13-1).

A variety of putative risk factors have been described, including migraine, oral contraceptives, hypertension, and smoking (2), but the evidence is conflicting. In the few case control studies available, the numbers are too small to be statistically convincing (9). This will remain a contentious issue until a properly controlled prospective study with sufficiently robust numbers of patients is performed.

Although it is postulated that concurrent infections make the arterial walls vulnerable to dissection (10), heavy coughing and sneezing produce typically violent flexion-extension movements severe enough to produce intimal tears. The effect of vertebral artery compression with or without intimal damage is underestimated, and brainstem infarctions have been described after otherwise uneventful anesthetic intubation (11). Dizziness due to vertebral arteries compression produced by forcible extension of the neck over the washbasin probably is responsible for the "beauty parlor syndrome" (12).

Dissection occurring after neck manipulation by chiropractors, physiotherapists, and physicians is well documented (2,13) and occurred in 17% (20/116) of patients in our current prospective series (Canadian Stroke Consortium data, 2002, unpublished data). However, its occurrence remains so rare that the exact incidence is difficult to document with any accuracy.

In a case control study, Rothwell et al. (14) compared hospitalization records of 582 patients with vertebrobasilar strokes to 2,328 matched controls without stroke and found that the stroke group were

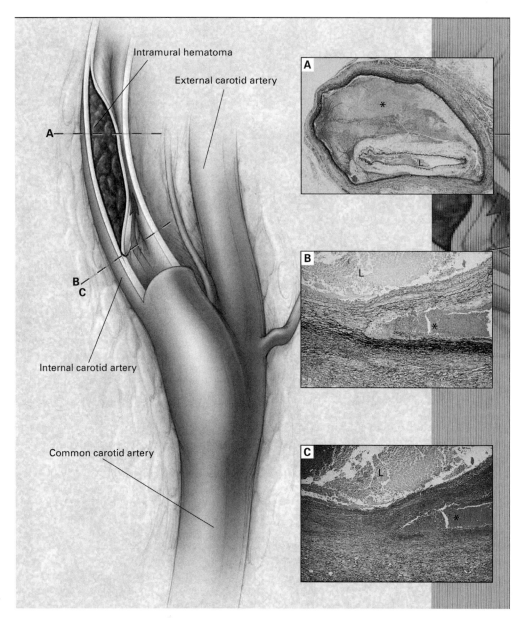

FIG. 13-1. Internal carotid artery dissection. **A:** Intramural hemorrhage (van Gieson stain). **B:** Fragmentation of elastic tissue (van Gieson stain). **C:** Cystic medial necrosis (Alcian blue). (From Schievink WI. Spontaneous dissection of the carotid and vertebral arteries. *N Engl J Med* 2001;12:898–906, with permission.)

five times more likely to have undergone neck manipulation in the previous week than the controls.

Canadian Heart and Stroke Foundation data for 2000 indicate an annual ischemic stroke-patient incidence of about 70,000, 5% of whom were younger than 45 years (mean age of our series). Because the incidence of cervical dissection in the Canadian Con-

sortium data is 13% (15), the estimated national stroke rate due to neck manipulation is 77 patients per year. However, because the gross reporting rate almost certainly is seriously underestimated (16), the true rate probably is considerably larger. Unfortunately, all these data must remain speculative until chiropractors and physicians collaborate to produce a reliable estimate based on consecutive cases in a prospective study.

HEREDITARY AND GENETIC INFLUENCES

The occasional familial occurrence of cervical arterial dissection (17,18) and the relatively frequent relationship with other hereditary disorders of connective tissues indicate an underlying genetic disorder affecting both the etiology and recurrence of dissection. Such disorders include Ehlers-Danlos and Marfan's syndromes, pseudoxanthoma elasticum, neurofibromatosis, polycystic kidneys, osteogenesis imperfecta, and cerebral aneurysms, as well as bicuspid aortic valve (3,18).

Fibromuscular dysplasia is seen in 15% of cases, and cystic medial fibrosis (3) indicates generalized selective vulnerability of the arterial wall not just localized to the neck but present in other arteries of the body. It also explains the simultaneous dissection of multiple neck arteries with minimal trauma. One patient in the Canadian Consortium series bent down to pick up a heavy weight and immediately experienced bilateral neck pain due to simultaneous bilateral carotid artery dissections.

PATHOLOGIC MECHANISMS

Although difficult to prove, it is generally believed that most dissections begin with an intimal tear that allows the force of blood in the arterial lumen to gain access and split the media, tracking upwards to reenter the lumen distally and create a double lumen or break through to the adventitia. This can cause pseudoaneurysm formation or subarachnoid hemorrhage, depending on the location of the arteries (Fig. 13-2).

Most series show a carotid preponderance, with carotid/vertebral ratios of 150:37 in the Mayo series (18,19) and 66:15 in the Swiss series (20), but in the current Canadian series this ratio is reversed, 58:107. Whether this represents a referral bias due to overenthusiastic reporting of traumatic stroke above others is uncertain, but there may be a carotid bias in the published series because angiographic confirmation is more likely in anterior rather than vertebral basilar strokes.

INTRACRANIAL VERSUS EXTRACRANIAL DISSECTIONS

Extracranial carotid arterial dissection is the most commonly reported. The extracranial carotid is embedded in soft tissues in the neck, but it is relatively tethered at the C2 area so that dissection occurs more distal to the bifurcation than atheromatous plaque. The vertebral artery is most vulnerable at the C1–2 junctions, where it winds around the atlas before penetrating the dura, so any stretching will easily tear the vessel. This explains the occurrence of high vertebral tears resulting from extreme rotation of the neck, as occur in motor vehicle accidents or neck manipulation.

If dissection tracks toward the intimal-medial area, the artery may occlude; if it tracks to the adventitial area, a pseudoaneurysm may form. Concomitant

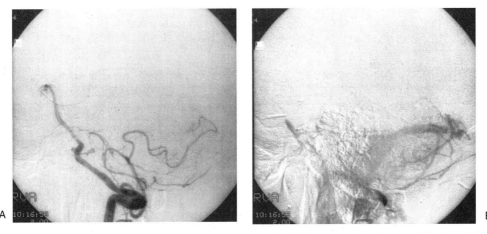

FIG. 13-2. Angiograms showing traumatic dissection of the right vertebral artery at C1 level **(A)** after a fall with hyperextension of the head. Contrast still is visible in pseudoaneurysm **(B)**, which remains a potential source of embolism.

hypertension may produce overexpansion of the artery at the bifurcation with each heartbeat, and it is recommended that patients accordingly be kept normotensive immediately after the dissection (18). Angiograms in the subacute stage show that the lesions are in a dynamic state. Occluded vessels often open within days, and aneurysms resolve or even expand in the first few weeks; therefore, follow-up angiograms in the first few months may detect newly formed aneurysms or an irregular luminal surface that could be a nidus for clot and therefore guide continuing anticoagulant therapy (21).

Intracranial dissections are much rarer, occurring in younger age groups, usually about 20 to 30 years, and carry a poorer prognosis (22). Vertebrobasilar dissections are more likely to cause cerebral ischemic damage because of their proximity to the brain or cause fatal subarachnoid hemorrhage. Intracranial carotid dissections with subintimal dissection lead to embolism and cerebral infarction and less frequently subarachnoid hemorrhage. In vertebral intracranial dissections, the blood tracks to the adventitia and is more likely to produce subarachnoid hemorrhage (23).

The structure of the cerebral arteries changes when the vessel penetrates the dura. The medial and adventitial layers become thinner and weaker intracranially, and they lack developed external elastic lamina. Gap defects have been described in the internal elastic lamina (23). Increased blood pressure from physical activity may stretch this honeycombed elastica, thus allowing tearing of the intima at bifurcations. Paradoxically, atherosclerosis of the aging artery may protect against this, thus possibly explaining the higher incidence of intracranial vertebral dissections in the young when they are involved in vigorous physical activity (24).

DIAGNOSTIC NEUROIMAGING

Intraarterial digital subtraction angiography (IA-DSA) obstinately remains the most accurate method of diagnosis, with various profiles including "rat's tail" of the carotid stump, "string of pearls," pseudoaneurysms, and intimal flaps the most characteristic of all the double lumen. Due to the invasive nature of IA-DSA, however, noninvasive techniques such as magnetic resonance angiography (MRA) usually are preferred (1,2).

Although there are advocates (16), the results of ultrasound imaging, in general, are disappointing because the carotid lesions are too high for good ultrasound resolution, especially the vertebral artery,

which is too small caliber for sufficient resolution. Ultrasound may be up to 79% sensitive, but it lacks specificity (25).

A combination of MRA and magnetic resonance imaging (MRI; with its characteristic crescentic defect on arterial cross section) are almost as good as IA-DSA and can safely detect 90% of angiographically demonstrated lesions (25,26). Stenoses and hematomas tend to resolve, whereas occlusions and vessel irregularity tend to persist. In our present series, the most common abnormality in 116 angiograms was irregularity of the lumen (44%), whereas "rat's tail" stenosis (28%) and occlusion (28%) occurred less frequently. We favor the suggestion of Auer et al. (25) that catheter angiography should be considered only if MRA/MRI imaging fails (Fig. 13-3).

Brain imaging, either computed tomography or MRI, commonly shows cerebellar or medullary infarcts in vertebral basilar lesions where the brunt of ischemia is more commonly found in areas supplied by the post-inferior cerebellar artery. The cortical location of many of these lesions lends credibility to the suggestion that most arise from the site of the tear and are embolic and not hemodynamic (27). Continuing microembolic activity documented with transcranial Doppler (28) may prove to be a useful guide to anticoagulant therapy in the future.

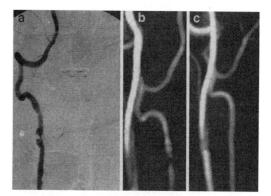

FIG. 13-3. Vertebral artery dissection. **A:** Intraarterial digital subtraction angiography of the vertebral artery. **B:** Baseline three-dimensional phase-contrast magnetic resonance angiography (MRA) showing mid vertebral artery irregularity. **C:** Follow-up MRA at 3 months showing normal vertebral artery. (Adapted from Rhodes RH, Phillips S, Booth FA, et al. Dissecting hematoma of intracranial internal carotid artery in an 8-year-old girl. *Can J Neurol Sci* 2001;28:357–364, with permission.)

CLINICAL FEATURES OF CERVICAL ARTERIAL DISSECTION

The clinical hallmark of cervical arterial dissection is head or neck pain that often is severe and present in 76% to 81% of patients (29,30) especially in vertebral dissections (8). In the Canadian Consortium study (in which symptoms are recorded prospectively and so should be more reliable), pain occurred in 83% of vertebral lesions and 61% of carotid lesions.

Pain is more commonly occipital in vertebral lesions and anterior in carotid lesions, but severe pain at the moment of dissection is seen in the face, ears, or eyes, always ipsilateral to the affected artery. In intracranial dissections, posterior headache is more common than neck pain. The pain usually disappears in days, but it may persist for months or even years (8). Sometimes pain overshadows minor neurologic symptoms masquerading as subarachnoid hemorrhage and prompts angiography, revealing dissections and not the anticipated cerebral aneurysm.

In vertebral dissection there are various cerebellar and brainstem symptoms, such as lateral medullary ischemia or even posterior fossa compression by large pseudoaneurysms. In carotid dissections, hemispheric transient ischemic attacks or strokes may have associated Horner's syndrome ipsilateral to the dissected artery, or sometimes isolated lower cranial nerve palsies. In some patients, only headache or Horner's syndrome is present, and many asymptomatic dissections probably go unrecognized.

The interval between dissection and symptoms usually is a few hours, but autopsy studies have shown that strokes may occur months later (31,32). In one case, stroke occurred 2 years after an attempted suicide by hanging (33). Presumably these cases represent embolism from pseudoaneurysms or permanent arterial wall irregularities.

MANAGEMENT

Medical Management

Immediate and sometimes prolonged courses of anticoagulation or antiplatelet therapy are recommended (1,2,16,34), but there is no evidence-based data to support any specific management strategy. As Saver and Easton (2) caustically comment, "Most patients do well either because of or despite of treatment."

Anticoagulants theoretically could worsen the dissection of the arterial wall, but because the major cause of stroke probably is embolism from the arterial tear rather than hemodynamic obstruction (13),

some form of antithrombotic therapy seems rational but is of unproven value. The low annual recurrence of stroke and the uncertainty as to whether this represents new dissection or fresh emboli are unknown. According to our calculations based on the Canadian Consortium data, a therapeutic trial would require about 1,000 patients in each arm (antiplatelet vs. anticoagulants); use of placebo may not be wise.

The duration of anticoagulant therapy remains speculative, but if MRI/MRA demonstrates no residual abnormality by 3 months, this would be a natural stopping point (2,35). Follow-up by ultrasound often is advocated (16,30,36), but even with improved technology, we believe that the specificity is too unreliable to form the basis of such critical decision-making.

The presence of unsuspected subarachnoid hemorrhage in patients with intracranial dissections adds an extra risk to anticoagulant therapy. Lumbar puncture should be considered before anticoagulant therapy is given, although MRI scanning probably is more practical under the circumstances.

The role of thrombolytic therapy remains anecdotal, and the hazards of giving tissue plasminogen activator (tPA) to patients with undiagnosed aortic dissection presenting with cervical artery dissection have been emphasized (37). A small study by a French group established the safety of intravenous thrombolysis in dissection, but in 9 of their 11 cases, the vessel remained occluded and there was no convincing evidence of a therapeutic effect (38). Use of the intraarterial route to deliver the thrombolytic directly to the embolus beyond the site of the dissection might prove a more effective method.

Surgical Management

The relatively benign prognosis counsels against any surgical intervention, and previously used procedures need strong justification. Pseudoaneurysms require excision if they bleed. Ligation of the vertebral or carotid artery, sometimes with cerebral bypass procedures, has been advocated. Stents sometimes are used empirically (3). Schievink (39) advises a conservative approach: because most dissections heal spontaneously, the natural outcome in most patients is good, and associated aneurysms rarely cause problems later so surgical correction is seldom needed.

CONCLUSION

Carotid and vertebral artery dissections, although relatively rare, probably are the most common causes of stroke in patients younger than 45 years and still are largely underdiagnosed despite the characteristic clinical picture.

MRI/MRA or computed tomographic angiography are the best imaging technologies for both initial diagnosis and follow-up. Use of IA-DSA should be reserved for cases where results of neurovascular imaging remain ambiguous. Duplex imaging is of limited value.

In general, the outcome is much better than in other forms of stroke. Until a therapeutic trial becomes feasible, the use of anticoagulants, antiplatelet agents, tPA, and invasive procedures remains a question of individual clinical judgment without benefit of evidence-based data.

REFERENCES

1. Leys D, Christian L, Marc G, et al. Cervical Artery Dissections. *Eur Neurol* 1997;37:3–12.
2. Saver JL, Easton JD. Dissection and trauma of cervicocerebral arteries. In: Barnett HJM, Mohr JP, Stein BM, et al., eds. *Stroke pathophysiology, diagnosis, and management,* 3rd ed. New York: Churchill Livingstone, 1998:769–786.
3. Schievink WI. Spontaneous dissection of the carotid and vertebral arteries. *N Engl J Med* 2001;12:898–906.
4. Hart RG, Easton JD. Dissection. *Stroke* 1985;16: 925–927.
5. Schievink WI, Mokri B Whisnant JP. Internal carotid artery dissection in a community. *Stroke* 1993;24: 1678–1680.
6. Bogousslavsky J, Regli F. Ischemic stroke in adults younger than 30 years of age. *Arch Neurol* 1987;44:479.
7. Martin PJ, Enevoldson TP, Humphrey PRD. Causes of ischemic stroke in the young. *Postgrad Med J* 1997;73: 8–16.
8. Silbert PL, Mokri B, Schievink WI. Headache and neck pain in spontaneous internal carotid and vertebral artery dissections. *Neurology* 1995;45:1517–1522.
9. D'Anglejan-Chatillon J, Ribeiro V, Mas JL, et al. Migraine: a risk factor for dissection of cervical arteries. *Headache*1989;29:560–561.
10. Constatinescu CS. Association of varicella-zoster virus with cervical artery dissection in 2 cases [Letter]. *Arch Neurol* 2000;57:427.
11. Gould DB, Cunningham K. Internal carotid artery dissection after remote surgery. *Stroke* 1994;25: 1276–1278.
12. Weintraub MI. Stroke after visit to the hairdresser [Letter]. *Lancet* 1997;350:1777–1778.
13. Norris JW, Beletsky V, Nadareishvili G. Sudden neck movement and cervical artery dissection. *CMAJ* 2000; 163:38–40.
14. Rothwell DM, Bondy SJ, Williams JI. Chiropractic manipulation and stroke. *Stroke* 2001;32:1054–1060.
15. Chan MTY, Nadareihvili ZG, Norris JW. Diagnostic strategies in young patients with ischemic stroke in Canada. *Can J Neurol Sci* 2000;27:120–124.
16. Stapf C, Elkind SV, Mohr JP. Carotid artery dissection. *Annu Rev Med* 2000;51:329–347.
17. Schievink WI, Mokri B, Piepgras DG, et al. Recurrent spontaneous arterial dissections. *Stroke* 1996;27: 622–624.
18. Schievink WI, Michels VV, Piepgras DG. Neurovascular manifestations of heritable connective tissue disorders. *Stroke* 1994;25:889–903.
19. Schievink WI, Mokri B, O'Fallon WM. Recurrent spontaneous cervical-artery dissection. *N Engl J Med* 1994; 330:393–397.
20. Bassetti C, Carruzzo A, Sturzenegger M, et al. Recurrence of cervical artery dissection. *Stroke* 1996;27: 1804–1807.
21. Nakagawa K, Touho H, Morisako T, et al. Long-term follow-up study of unruptured vertebral artery dissection: clinical outcomes and serial angiographic findings. *J Neurosurg* 2000;93:19–25.
22. Caplan LR, Baquis GD, Pessin MS, et al. Dissection of the intracranial vertebral artery. *Neurology* 1998;38: 868–877.
23. Deck JHN. Pathology of spontaneous dissection of intracranial arteries. *Can J Neurol Sci* 1987;14:88–91.
24. Rhodes RH, Phillips S, Booth FA, et al. Dissecting hematoma of intracranial internal carotid artery in an 8-year-old girl. *Can J Neurol Sci* 2001;28:357–364.
25. Auer A, Felber S, Schmidauer C, et al. Magnetic resonance angiographic and clinical features of extracranial vertebral artery dissection. *J Neurol Neurosurg Psychiatry* 1998;64:474–481.
26. Kasner SE, Hankins LL, Bratina P, et al. Magnetic resonance angiography demonstrates vascular healing of carotid and vertebral artery dissections. *Stroke* 1997;28: 1993–1997.
27. Lucas C, Moulin T, Deplanque D, et al. Stroke patterns of internal carotid artery dissection in 40 patients. *Stroke* 1998;29:2646–2648.
28. Droste DW, Junker K. Stogbauer F, et al. Clinically silent circulating microemboli in 20 patients with carotid or vertebral artery dissection. *Cerebrovasc Dis* 2001;12:181–185.
29. Mokri B, Houser OW, Sandok BA, et al. Spontaneous dissections of the vertebral arteries. *Neurology* 1988;38: 880–885.
30. de Bray JM, Penisson-Besnier I, Dubas F, et al. Extracranial and intracranial vertebrobasilar dissections: diagnosis and prognosis. *J. Neurol Neurosurg Psychiatry* 1997;63:46–51.
31. Auer RN, Kreek J, Butt JC. Delayed symptoms and death after minor head trauma with occult vertebral artery injury. *J Neurol Neurosurg Psychiatry* 1994;57: 500–502.
32. Viktrup L, Knudsen GM, Hansen SH. Delayed onset of fatal basilar thrombotic embolus after whiplash injury. *Stroke* 1995;26:2194–2196.
33. Noguchi K, Matsuoka Y, Hohada K, et al. A case of common carotid artery stenosis due to hanging. *Neurol Surg.* 1992;20:1185–1188.
34. Biousse V, D'Anglejan-Chatillon J, Touboul PJ, et al. Time course of symptoms in extracranial carotid artery dissections. *Stroke*1995;26:235–239.
35. Jacobs A, Lanfermann H, Neveling M, et al. MRI and MRA-guided therapy of carotid and vertebral artery dissection. *J Neuro Sci* 1997;147:27–34.
36. Bartels E, Flugel KA. Evaluation of extracranial vertebral artery dissection with duplex color-flow imaging. *Stroke* 1996;27:290–295.

37. Fleming KD, Brown RD. Acute cerebral infarction caused by aortic dissection: caution in the thrombolytic era. *Stroke* 1999;30:477–478.

38. Derex L, Nighoghossian N, Turjman F, et al. Intravenous tPA in acute ischemic stroke related to internal carotid artery dissection. *Neurology* 2000;54:2159–2161.

39. Schievink WI. The treatment of spontaneous carotid and vertebral artery dissections. *Cardiology* 2000;15:316–321.

Ischemic Stroke: Advances in Neurology, Vol. 92. Edited by
H.J.M. Barnett, Julien Bogousslavsky, and Heather Meldrum.
Lippincott Williams & Wilkins, Philadelphia © 2003.

14

Fibromuscular Dysplasia

*†Gian Luigi Lenzi and *Marco Calabresi

Department of Neurological Sciences, 1st University of Roma "La Sapienza" and
†Department of Neurology, Policlinico Umberto I, Rome, Italy

Fibromuscular dysplasia (FMD) is an uncommon segmental disease affecting small- to medium-sized arteries. Its etiology is uncertain. Histology of the arterial wall shows fibrous tissue proliferation; smooth muscle hyperplasia; and elastic fiber destruction, alternating with atrophy. There is frequent involvement of more than one artery in the same individual, particularly of the renal arteries (60%–75%), which causes hypertension, and of the cervicocranial arteries (25%–30%) and less frequent involvement of visceral (9%) and limb arteries (5%) (1).

EPIDEMIOLOGY

Depending on the population sampled and the diagnostic techniques, the incidence of cervicocranial FMD (ccFMD) varies. Contradictory figures have been reported.

A retrospective review of more than 33,000 consecutive carotid artery angiograms reported alterations consistent with ccFMD in 0.5% to 0.9% of cases (2). In contrast, histologic evidence of FMD affecting the extracranial portions of the internal carotid artery (ICA) was found in only 4 (0.02%) of 20,244 consecutive autopsies performed at the Mayo Clinic between 1968 and 1992. During the same 25-year period, FMD was observed in only six surgical specimens (3).

At least 80% of patients with renal artery or ICA FMD are women (4–6). The Caucasian population seems to be at a higher risk than the black population (2). ICA FMD has been described in children and adolescents (7), but the majority of FMD cases occur in adults in their 50s to 70s.

PATHOLOGY

Pathology of FMD is characterized by smooth muscle hyperplasia or thinning; elastic fiber destruc-

tion; fibrous tissue proliferation leading to arterial wall disorganization and atrophy, without inflammation; necrosis; lipid accumulation; and calcification.

Guidelines for FMD classification were proposed by Harrison and McCormack (8) in 1971. Three main varieties were identified according to the principal arterial wall layer involved: intimal fibroplasia, medial dysplasia, and adventitial (periarterial) fibroplasia. Medial dysplasia was divided further into medial fibroplasia, perimedial fibroplasia, and medial hyperplasia. A more simplified approach has been proposed (9), but the original histopathologic classification still is used with cervical artery involvement.

Patients with ccFMD may show a higher incidence of intracranial "berry" aneurysms (2), mainly located in the ICA and middle cerebral artery, with a distribution and histology similar to that of patients without FMD. Multiple aneurysms have been reported, as has de novo formation in one case (10).

A 21% to 51% frequency of intracranial aneurysms in ccFMD patients has been reported (2); however, a recent meta-analysis suggests this is an overestimate, with the true incidence closer to 7% (11).

ETIOLOGY

Despite a variety of theories, the etiology of FMD remains unknown. A genetic factor is present. In a study of 20 families, Rushton (12) found that the inheritance pattern in 60% of cases suggested an autosomal dominant trait with variable penetrance. A heterozygotic α_1-antitrypsin deficiency has been reported to be a risk factor (13,14).

The higher prevalence of disease among women implies that hormonal factors are important, particularly the influence of estrogen stimulation over smooth muscular cells (15).

Ischemia of the arterial wall, lesions of the vasa vasorum of the affected arteries, and viral infection have been proposed as etiologic factors.

It is unlikely that a simple unifying explanation would be sufficient because FMD may represent a nonspecific reaction to a noxa of the arterial wall.

CLINICAL FEATURES

Complaints reported by patients with ccFMD vary depending on the observing physician (5). The relationship between disease and symptoms is not always clear. Cervicocranial FMD has been reported as an asymptomatic disease in 8.1% to 15% of a total of 40 patients (5,16,17). The only postmortem series report describes 4 of 10 cases as asymptomatic (3).

Three mechanisms may produce symptoms in ccFMD: (a) direct or indirect effect on the arterial wall; (b) focal cerebral ischemia; and (c) global cerebral hypoperfusion (2).

Headache is common and its localization corresponds strikingly to the angiographically demonstrated lesion. The pain often is unilateral, usually described as a widespread throbbing or pressure (6).

Arterial dysplastic lesions could create a turbulence of blood flow, producing a cervical bruit, isolated or associated with other symptoms, in 69% to 100% of patients (4,17,18). The bruits are perceived by patients as a pulsatile tinnitus (4–6,19). It is uncertain if tinnitus is heard as a direct result of the dysplastic arterial wall lesion or of secondary vascular abnormalities.

Other findings are carotidynia (sometimes extending to the homolateral facial area) (6); Horner's syndrome (20,21); Collet-Sicard syndrome (22,23); giant carotid aneurysms (10,24–27); and carotid and vertebral arteriovenous fistulas (28,29), which in one case spontaneously obliterated (30).

Focal symptoms in FMD have been related to transient ischemic attacks (TIAs) or cerebral ischemia. In a review of literature, however, Healton (2) concluded that the association between FMD and stroke was thought in some studies to be fortuitous and common in others, with the method of patient selection heavily influencing the incidence of stroke, ranging from 0% to 28%. Well-documented cases of focal ischemic symptoms due to FMD are scanty (4–7,31) and often are reported as atypical FMD (32,33) or associated with dissection of the ICA (34–36) of the vertebral (37) or intracranial arteries (10). However, in most of these reports, the occurrence of ccFMD was not proven histologically; therefore, other causes of brain ischemia could not be excluded. In particular, many patients show involvement of renal arteries with hypertension, which is a well-recognized risk factor for cerebral ischemia. Cervicocranial FMD may represent a pathogenetic cofactor for focal brain damage because both head turning and neck trauma are known to have preceded cerebral infarction in ccFMD patients (34,38).

Cervicocranial FMD should be sought in cases of cerebral focal symptoms only when more common causes of disease have been excluded.

Syncope, seizures, dizziness, vertigo, and scintillating scotomata have been rarely reported and attributed to the global cerebral hypoperfusion produced by ccFMD (16,18); however, the mechanisms underlying these symptoms are unclear, and a causal relationship is unproved (2).

ANGIOGRAPHY AND OTHER DIAGNOSTIC TESTS

FMD has been associated with three main angiographic patterns. The first, more typical pattern is defined as a "string of beads," with artery segments of constriction alternating with normal or dilated segments. This form is present in more than 80% of cases, mostly of the medial dysplasia histologic type.

A smooth concentric tubular lesion is seen in about 10% of cases, associated with all the histologic types. This second pattern is associated with other clinical conditions, including Takayasu arteritis, arterial hypoplasia, and the arterial spasm induced by a catheter.

The third (uncommon) pattern, described as atypical FMD, consists of an eccentric outpouching *(diverticulum)* that may progress to a full aneurysmal formation. Differential diagnosis includes atherosclerotic aneurysm and posttraumatic pseudoaneurysm (Fig. 14-1).

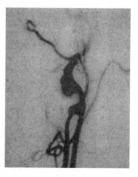

FIG. 14-1. Carotid angiography. Fibromuscular dysplasia of the internal carotid artery (ICA). Diffuse and irregular multiple dilations of the ICA up to the cranial base are seen.

A very rare angiographic finding is the noncircumferential weblike stenosis *(septum)*. Severe to complete occlusions have been reported (32,33).

Sonographic studies of ccFMD are few (39,40), but these lesions in most carotid cases and all vertebral cases are inaccessible.

Magnetic resonance angiography (MRA) has been used in few cases complicated with ICA dissection (37,41). Two-dimensional time-of-flight MRA is a useful noninvasive modality for evaluation of narrowing of the carotid artery bifurcation (42).

Cervicocranial FMD is characteristic in terms of location. Lesions are present in the ICA in 95% and are bilateral in 60% to 85% of cases. Vertebral artery FMD has been reported in 12% to 43% of affected patients, but a complete angiographic study has not always been performed. Most patients with vertebral lesions also are affected in the ICA.

Typically, the abnormalities involve the middle portion of the vessels, with the C2 level the most common location in both the ICA and vertebral artery. The origins of the arteries are uncommonly affected. This is helpful in differentiating these lesions from atherosclerosis (42). We have found only 16 patients with proximal ICA disease. It is not possible to exclude *a priori* the possibility of a fibromuscular dysplastic lesion on a topographic basis. There have been many reports of intraosseous or intracranial ICA FMD (10,43), either alone or as an extension of cervical abnormalities.

NATURAL HISTORY

Longitudinal studies of the evolution of ccFMD lesions are lacking, and only single case reports have described anatomic progression or resolution of ccFMD (2).

There have been two retrospective studies of neurologic outcome in patients with FMD. In the first study, 5 years of follow-up data with specific reference to cerebral ischemic events were collected in 79 of an initial cohort of 82 patients (5). The patients were divided into four groups according to the cause that led to the diagnosis: cerebral focal ischemia in 13; incidental discovery of FMD during investigation of an intracranial mass lesion in 29; FMD found in association with cerebral aneurysm in 10; and FMD found in association with other disorders in the remaining 27. Three of the 13 patients with focal neurologic symptoms were treated medically and four surgically; all were asymptomatic during follow-up. Of the 66 untreated patients, three had strokes during the observation period. In one of these cases, a 71-

year-old patient, the stroke that occurred 216 months after angiographic diagnosis was in the same vascular territory of the ccFMD.

In the second study, patients were followed-up for an average of 3.8 years; 9 patients were not treated, 7 received anticoagulation or antiplatelet therapy, and 1 had surgery (18). Two of the untreated patients (ages 60 and 79 years), who presented with concomitant cerebral atherosclerosis, had a stroke 18 and 30 months after diagnosis.

TREATMENT

There have been no controlled trials of therapy in ccFMD. Medical therapy is administration of antiplatelet and anticoagulant agents. Angioplasty is the most utilized surgical procedure, followed by endarterectomy, resection, arterial bypass, and other procedures. The medical and surgical groups both show a good outcome (no complication or mortality in the medical group, n = 51; 7.7% complications and 0.9% mortality in the surgery group, n = 222) as reported by Healton (2).

These positive results must take into account the favorable natural course of the disease. The recommendations for a conservative approach, made almost 20 years ago (44), still hold true. In asymptomatic patients, as well as those with stroke or TIA, antiplatelet therapy carries a lower risk than surgery (2).

Hemodynamically significant stenosis or recurrent symptoms despite medical therapy may suggest a surgical treatment, as well as the presence an atypical presentation such as a giant carotid bulb, with and without *septum*. In these cases, anticoagulant therapy should be tried initially, with close clinical and morphologic follow-up that may lead to surgery (32,33).

ACKNOWLEDGMENTS

The authors thank Professor Luigi Bozzao, Chair of Neuroradiology, for kindly providing the ccFMD image. Professor Vittorio Di Piero reviewed the draft and suggested important modifications.

REFERENCES

1. Begelman SM, Olin JW. Fibromuscular dysplasia. *Curr Opin Rheumatol* 2000;12:41–47.
2. Healton EB. Fibromuscular dysplasia. In: Barnett HJM, ed. *Stroke: pathophysiology, diagnosis and management.* New York: Churchill Livingstone, 1992:749–760.
3. Schievink WI, Bjornsson J. Fibromuscular dysplasia of the internal carotid artery: a clinicopathological study. *Clin Neuropathol* 1996;15:2–6.

4. So EL, Toole JF, Dalal P, et al. Cephalic fibromuscular dysplasia in 32 patients: clinical findings and radiologic features. *Arch Neurol* 1981;38:619–622.

5. Corrin LS, Sandok BA, Houser OW. Cerebral ischemic events in patients with carotid artery fibromuscular dysplasia. *Arch Neurol* 1981;38:616–618.

6. Mettinger KL, Ericson K. Fibromuscular dysplasia and the brain. I. Observations on angiographic, clinical and genetic characteristics. *Stroke* 1982;13:46–52.

7. Emparanza JI, Aldamiz-Echevarria L, Perez-Yarza E, et al. Ischemic stroke due to fibromuscular dysplasia. *Neuropediatrics* 1989;20:181–182.

8. Harrison EG, McCormack LJ. Pathologic classification of renal arterial disease in renovascular hypertension. *Mayo Clin Proc* 1971;46:161–167.

9. Mercier C, Pèllissier JF, Piquet P, et al. Fibromuscular disease of the renal artery: a new histopathologic classification. *Ann Vasc Surg* 1992;6:220–224.

10. Nakamura M, Rosahl SK, Vorkapic P, et al. De novo formation of an aneurysm in a case of unusual intracranial fibromuscular dysplasia. *Clin Neurol Neurosurg* 2000; 102:259–264.

11. Cloft HJ, Kallmes DF, Kallmes MH, et al. Prevalence of cerebral aneurysms in patients with fibromuscular dysplasia: a reassessment. *J Neurosurg* 1998;88:436–440.

12. Rushton AR. The genetics of fibromuscular dysplasia. *Arch Intern Med* 1980;140: 233–236.

13. Bofinger A, Hawley C, Fisher P, et al. Polymorphisms of the renin-angiotensin system in patients with multifocal renal arterial fibromuscular dysplasia. *J Hum Hypertens* 2001;15:185–190.

14. Schievink WI, Meyer FB, Parisi JE, et al. Fibromuscular dysplasia of the internal carotid artery associated with alpha1-antitrypsin deficiency. *Neurosurgery* 1998; 43:229–233.

15. Luscher TF, Lie JT, Stanson AW, et al. Arterial fibromuscular dysplasia. *Mayo Clin Proc* 1987;62:931–952.

16. Starr DS, Lawrie GM, Morris GC Jr. Fibromuscular disease of carotid arteries: long term results of graduated internal dilatation. *Stroke* 1981;12:196–199.

17. Effeney DJ, Ehrenfeld WK, Stoney RJ, et al. Why operate on carotid fibromuscular dysplasia? *Arch Surg* 1980;115:1261–1265.

18. Wells RP, Smith RR. Fibromuscular dysplasia of the internal carotid artery: a long term follow-up. *Neurosurgery* 1982;10:39–43.

19. Weissman JL, Hirsch BE. Imaging of tinnitus: a review. *Radiology* 2000;216:342–349.

20. Laing C, Thomas DJ, Mathias CJ, et al. Headache, hypertension and Horner's syndrome. *J R Soc Med* 2000;93:535–536.

21. Gelmers HJ. The pericarotid syndrome. A combination of hemicrania, Horner's syndrome, and internal carotid artery wall lesion. *Acta Neurochir (Wien)* 1981;57: 37–42.

22. Sturzenegger M, Huber P. Cranial nerve palsies in spontaneous carotid artery dissection. *J Neurol Neurosurg Psychiatry* 1993;56:1191–1199.

23. Havelius U, Hindfelt B, Brismar J, et al. Carotid fibromuscular dysplasia and paresis of lower cranial nerves (Collect-Sicard syndrome). Case report. *J Neurosurg* 1982;56:850–853.

24. Rhee RY, Gloviczki P, Cherry KJ Jr, et al. Two unusual variants of internal carotid artery aneurysms due to fibromuscular dysplasia. *Ann Vasc Surg* 1996;10: 481–485.

25. Faggioli GL, Freyrie A, Stella A, et al. Extracranial internal carotid artery aneurysms: results of a surgical series with long-term follow-up. *J Vasc Surg* 1996;23: 587–594; discussion 594–595.

26. Bour P, Taghavi I, Bracard S, et al. Aneurysms of the extracranial internal carotid artery due to fibromuscular dysplasia: results of surgical management. *Ann Vasc Surg* 1992;6:205–208.

27. Ouchi Y, Tagawa H, Yamakado M, et al. Clinical significance of cerebral aneurysm in renovascular hypertension due to fibromuscular dysplasia: two cases in siblings. *Angiology* 1989;40:581–588.

28. Kaufman HH. Spontaneous arteriovenous fistulas with fibromuscular dysplasia. *Neurosurgery* 1986;19:673.

29. Hieshima GB, Cahan LD, Mehringer CM, et al. Spontaneous arteriovenous fistulas of cerebral vessels in association with fibromuscular dysplasia. *Neurosurgery* 1986;18:454–458.

30. Canova A, Esposito S, Patricolo A, et al. Spontaneous obliteration of a carotid-cavernous fistula associated with fibromuscular dysplasia of the internal carotid artery. *J Neurosurg Sci* 1987;31:37–40.

31. Uncommon causes of stroke. *Lancet* 1989;1:26.

32. Kubis N, Von Langsdorff D, Petitjean C, et al. Thrombotic carotid megabulb: fibromuscular dysplasia, septae, and ischemic stroke. *Neurology* 1999;52:883–886.

33. Morgenlander JC, Goldstein LB. Recurrent transient ischemic attacks and stroke in association with an internal carotid artery web. *Stroke* 1991;22:94–98.

34. Duncan MA, Dowd N, Rawluk D, et al. Traumatic bilateral internal carotid artery dissection following airbag deployment in a patient with fibromuscular dysplasia. *Br J Anaesth* 2000;85:476–478.

35. Schievink WI, Bjornsson J, Piepgras DG. Coexistence of fibromuscular dysplasia and cystic medial necrosis in a patient with Marfan's syndrome and bilateral carotid artery dissections. *Stroke* 1994;25:2492–2496.

36. Amarenco P, Seux-Levieil ML, Cohen A, et al. Carotid artery dissection with renal infarcts. Two cases. *Stroke* 1994;25:2488–2491.

37. Provenzale JM, Morgenlander JC, Gress D. Spontaneous vertebral dissection: clinical, conventional angiographic, CT, and MR findings. *J Comput Assist Tomogr* 1996;20:185–193.

38. Eachempati SR, Sebastian MW, Reed RL 2nd. Posttraumatic bilateral carotid artery and right vertebral artery dissections in a patient with fibromuscular dysplasia: case report and review of the literature. *J Trauma* 1998; 44:406–409.

39. Schlagenhauff RE, Khatri A. Fibromuscular dysplasia of internal carotid arteries. With Doppler ultrasonic studies. *N Y State J Med* 1983;83:234–236.

40. Edell SL, Huang P. Sonographic demonstration of fibromuscular hyperplasia of the cervical internal carotid artery. *Stroke* 1981;12:518–520.

41. Klufas RA, Hsu L, Barnes PD, et al. Dissection of the carotid and vertebral arteries: imaging with MR angiography. *AJR Am J Roentgenol* 1995;164:673–677.

42. Heiserman JE, Drayer BP, Fram EK, et al. MR angiography of cervical fibromuscular dysplasia. *Am J Neuroradiol* 1992;13:1454–1457.

43. Belen D, Bolay H, Firat M, et al. Unusual appearance of intracranial fibromuscular dysplasia. A case report. *Angiology* 1996;47:627–632.

44. Sandok BA. Fibromuscular dysplasia of the internal carotid artery. *Neurol Clin* 1983;1:17–26.

Ischemic Stroke: Advances in Neurology, Vol. 92. Edited by
H.J.M. Barnett, Julien Bogousslavsky, and Heather Meldrum.
Lippincott Williams & Wilkins, Philadelphia © 2003.

15

Vertebrobasilar Disease

Louis R. Caplan

*Department of Neurology, Harvard Medical School and Cerebrovascular Service, Beth Israel
Deaconess Medical Center, Boston, Massachusetts, U.S.A.*

About one fifth of the blood supplying the brain courses through the vertebrobasilar circulation. Strokes within the vertebrobasilar arterial territory share the same etiologies as anterior circulation strokes with minor differences in frequencies. In this discussion, I rely heavily on data from the New England Medical Center Posterior Circulation Registry (NEMC-PCR), a collection of 407 prospectively entered, thoroughly investigated patients with posterior circulation strokes and transient ischemic attacks (TIAs) (1,2).

In the NEMC-PCR, we found that an anatomic classification scheme based on vascular supply territories was very useful (1,2). We categorized brain and vascular lesions as proximal, middle, and distal. *Proximal intracranial posterior circulation territory* includes regions supplied by the intracranial vertebral arteries (ICVAs): the medulla oblongata and the posterior inferior cerebellar artery (PICA)-supplied region of the cerebellum. *Middle intracranial posterior circulation territory* includes the portion of the brain supplied by the basilar artery (BA) up to its superior cerebellar artery (SCA) branches: the pons and the anterior inferior cerebellar artery (AICA)-supplied portions of the cerebellum. *Distal intracranial posterior circulation territory* includes all of the territory supplied by the rostral BA and its SCA, posterior cerebral artery (PCA), and the penetrating artery branches of these vessels: midbrain, thalamus, SCA-supplied cerebellum, and PCA territories. This distribution is shown diagrammatically in Fig. 15-1.

FREQUENCY OF VARIOUS ETIOLOGIES

Table 15-1 lists the frequencies of the various stroke mechanisms in the NEMC-PCR. As in the anterior circulation, embolism was the most frequent cause of brain ischemia. The source of embolism was

the heart, aorta, and proximal arteries. The most frequent arterial sources were the proximal extracranial vertebral artery (ECVA) and the ICVAs. In the NEMC-PCR, the aorta was not systematically evaluated so that this source was underestimated.

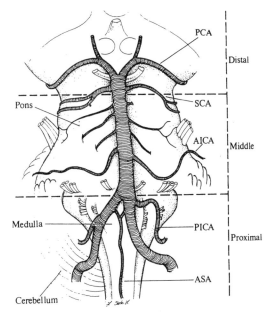

FIG. 15-1. Sketch of the base of the brain showing the intracranial vertebral and basilar arteries and their branches. The section is divided into proximal intracranial territory, middle intracranial territory, and distal intracranial territory. AICA, anterior inferior cerebellar artery; ASA, anterior spinal artery; PCA, posterior cerebral artery; PICA, posterior inferior cerebellar artery; SCA, superior cerebellar artery. (Drawn by Laurel Cook-Lowe. From Caplan LR. *Posterior circulation disease. Clinical findings, diagnosis, and management.* Boston: Blackwell Science, 1996, with permission.)

TABLE 15-1. *Frequency of diagnosis of stroke mechanisms in the New England Medical Center Posterior Circulatory Registry*

Stroke mechanism	Single most likely	Range of possible
Embolism	40%	40%–54%
Cardiac or aortic origin	24%	24%–33%
Intraarterial	14%	14%–18%
Cardiac and intraarterial sources	2%	2%–3%
Large artery disease	32%	32%–35%
Penetrating artery disease	14%	14%–17%
Migraine	3%	3%–4%
Dissection and other etiologies	10%	10%–14%

Large artery occlusive disease was the second most frequent etiology. At times, brain ischemia was due to stenotic plaques or thrombus blocking blood flow through penetrating and circumferential branches arising from the obstructed artery. These cases were classified as *large artery disease*. When infarction occurred distal to occlusive thrombi, for example, an occipital lobe infarct in a patient with recent occlusion of the ECVA, then the mechanism was classified as *intraarterial embolism.* Sometimes it is impossible to separate these two classifications. In some patients, there is both local and distant ischemia due to embolism from the local thrombus, for example, a patient with PICA territory cerebellar infarction related to an occlusion of the ipsilateral ICVA occluding the PICA orifice and occipital lobe infarction caused by an embolus from the ICVA to the PCA. Penetrating artery disease consisting of lipohyalinosis and atheromatous branch disease, migraine, dissections, fibromuscular dysplasia, drug abuse, and other rare arteriopathies accounted for the remainder of the cases.

Cardiac origin embolism (Section on *Heart and Brain*), arterial dissection (Chapter 13), and penetrating artery disease (Chapter 16) are discussed elsewhere in this text, so I will concentrate herein on large artery disease and intraarterial embolism within the posterior circulation.

DISTRIBUTION OF ATHEROMATOUS LARGE ARTERY LESIONS

Necropsy (3,4), angiographic, and ultrasound studies show that extracranial atheromatous plaques that cause luminal stenosis are most common within the proximal subclavian arteries and at the origins of the ECVAs in the neck. Plaques within the subclavian arteries often extend into the ECVAs at their origins. The first 1 to 2 cm of the ECVAs are frequent sites of atherosclerotic stenosis (3–5). Flat plaques often form a ladderlike arrangement opposite osteophytes and cervical discs, but these lesions in the second portion of the vertebral artery (VA) usually do not impinge significantly on the ECVA lumens. Plaques and stenosis occasionally occur within the proximal innominate arteries.

The most common regions of predilection for fibrous plaques, stenosis, and occlusion within the intracranial posterior circulation arteries are within the ICVAs, especially within the distal ICVAs near or at the ICVA-BA junction and the proximal ICVAs just after dural penetration (1–4,6-8). ICVA disease often is bilateral (6,7). Plaques are commonly found along the BA but are most likely to cause stenosis in the proximal portion of the BA and in its most distal segment near the BA bifurcation into the PCAs (9–11). Plaques also occur often in the mid-BA near the origins of the long circumferential cerebellar arteries (AICAs and SCAs). The proximal portions of the PCAs are another site for plaque deposition.

There are important racial and gender differences in the distribution of atherosclerotic lesions (12–14). White men have more severe disease of the extracranial arteries, in the subclavian and proximal ECVAs. They have a high frequency of coronary artery atherosclerosis, peripheral vascular occlusive disease in the limbs, and hypercholesterolemia. White men also often have involvement of the ICVAs and the BA, in addition to lesions in the extracranial arteries. In contrast, blacks and individuals of Chinese, Japanese, and Thai ancestry tend to have more intracranial atherosclerosis, especially affecting the PCAs, the origins of the long cerebellar arteries (PICAs, AICAs, and SCAs), and the distal BA. The ICVAs also show plaques in these groups, but the subclavian arteries and the ECVAs usually are relatively spared. Although they often have hypertension, black, Chinese, Japanese, and Thai individuals have a lower incidence of coronary, peripheral vascular, and main renal artery atherosclerotic stenosis and occlusion, more diabetes, and less hypercholesterolemia than white men. Premenopausal women tend to have a pattern of distribution of atherosclerosis similar to that found in black people, and those of Chinese, Japanese, and Thai ancestry. Postmenopausal white women have a distribution of atherosclerosis similar to that of white men.

CLINICAL FINDINGS IN PATIENTS WITH VARIOUS POSTERIOR CIRCULATION OCCLUSIVE LESIONS

Table 15-2 lists the most frequent sites of atherostenosis in the NEMC-PCR.

Subclavian and Innominate Artery Occlusive Disease

Among 407 patients with posterior circulation TIAs and ischemic strokes in the NEMC-PCR, only two had symptoms (TIAs) attributable to significant subclavian or innominate artery disease (1).

Now, most often, subclavian artery disease is detected when patients with coronary or peripheral vascular occlusive disease involving the lower extremities are referred to ultrasound laboratories for noninvasive testing. Most patients with subclavian artery disease are asymptomatic. In patients with symptoms, most complaints are related to arm ischemia. Coolness, weakness, and pain upon use of the arm are common but usually not severe. In a large series of patients with subclavian steal detected by ultrasound, one third of patients reported pain, numbness, or fatigue in the arm, but only 15 (4.8%) of 324 had objective physical signs of brachial ischemia or embolism (15). Neurologic symptoms are uncommon

unless there is accompanying carotid artery disease. Among 155 patients, 116 (74%) who had a unilateral subclavian steal shown by ultrasonography had no neurologic symptoms (15).

When VA flow is compromised (either decreased antegrade flow or retrograde flow), patients may report dizzy spells. Dizziness is by far the most common neurologic symptom of the subclavian steal syndrome and usually has a spinning or vertiginous character. Diplopia, decreased vision, oscillopsia, and staggering all occur, but less frequently, often accompanying dizziness. The attacks are brief and occasionally are brought on by exercising the ischemic arm. In most patients, exercise of the ischemic limb does not provoke neurologic symptoms or signs. Although some patients with subclavian steal may have frequent vestibulocerebellar ischemic attacks, development of a posterior circulation stroke is rare.

Atherosclerosis of the proximal subclavian artery usually is accompanied by occlusive disease in other large arteries, typically the coronary, lower extremity, and other extracranial arteries. Baseball pitchers and cricket bowlers are at risk for developing innominate and subclavian artery disease, which is related to their arm mechanics during throwing. A cervical rib or chronic use of an arm crutch can lead to stenosis or aneurysmal dilation of the subclavian artery. Clot can form in the diseased vessel and periodically embolize to individual finger arteries, causing findings that can be confused with unilateral Raynaud's syndrome. When the lesion affects the innominate artery, signs and symptoms of anterior circulation ischemia can occur related to embolism into the right internal carotid artery territory. Occasional patients who had recurrent arm and brain ischemia caused by embolization of floating thrombi within the innomi-

TABLE 15-2. *Frequency of arterial lesions (>50% stenosis or occlusion) on vascular imaging in the New England Medical Center Posterior Circulation Registry*

Artery	Total lesions	Only lesions
Innominate	2	0
Subclavian	5	1
ECVA	131 (29 bilateral)	52 (15 bilateral)
ICVA	132 (37 bilateral)	40 (12 bilateral)
BA	108	46
PICA	14	5
AICA	2	0
SCA	10	3
PCA	38 (4 bilateral)	14

AICA, anterior inferior cerebellar artery; BA, basilar artery; ECVA, extracranial vertebral artery; ICVA, intracranial artery; PCA, posterior cerebral artery; PICA, posterior inferior cerebellar artery; SCA, superior cerebellar artery.

nate artery have been reported (16,17). Innominate artery disease is less common than subclavian artery disease (18,19).

Most patients with innominate artery disease are cigarette smokers. In a series of patients with innominate artery disease, women were affected more often than men, in contrast to a series of patients with carotid, subclavian, and peripheral vascular occlusive disease, in which there is a male preponderance. Although right subclavian steal is much less frequent than left, it is more serious and more important to treat. Two early cases reported by Symonds (20) describe right subclavian artery occlusion with spread of clot into the innominate and carotid arterial systems. A more recent case report described the events in a professional baseball pitcher (21). The pitcher noted his throwing arm suddenly went dead. Angiography showed occlusion of the right subclavian artery just proximal to the medial edge of the first rib. Five days later, while exercising, he suddenly developed a left hemiplegia and confusion (21). Angiography showed that clot had propagated proximally to block the innominate artery and had embolized into ICA branches intracranially (21). A combination of ipsilateral arm and eye ischemia accompanied by anterior and/or posterior circulation ischemia is diagnostic of innominate artery disease.

Occlusive Disease of the Proximal Extracranial Vertebral Artery

The most frequently reported symptom during TIAs due to ECVA origin disease is dizziness. The attacks are indistinguishable from those described by patients with subclavian steal, except that TIAs in patients with ECVA disease are not precipitated by effort or arm exertion. Although dizziness is the most common symptom, it is seldom the only neurologic symptom. Usually, in at least some attacks, dizziness is accompanied by other more definite signs of hindbrain ischemia. Diplopia, oscillopsia, weakness of both legs, hemiparesis, or numbness often is mentioned if the patient is closely questioned. Repeated attacks of unaccompanied dizziness are rarely attributable to VA disease. In most patients with TIAs related to ECVA occlusive disease, the attacks stop spontaneously after days or weeks. Two important anatomic facts explain why ECVA-origin lesions seldom cause chronic hemodynamically significant low flow to the vertebrobasilar system. (a) The VAs are paired vessels that unite to form a single BA. Only rarely is there complete atresia of one VA, although

asymmetries are frequent. (b) The VA gives off numerous muscular and other branches as it ascends in the neck. In contrast, there are no nuchal branches of the ICA. In the VA system, there is much more potential for development of adequate collateral circulation. Even when there is bilateral occlusion of the VAs at their origins, patients usually do not develop posterior circulation infarcts. ECVA-origin disease is thus much more benign than ICA origin disease from a hemodynamic standpoint (1,2,22,23). Thrombi can develop, engrafted upon ulcerative plaques or stenotic lesions, and embolize into the intracranial posterior circulation arteries (1,2,23–27).

Embolization of white platelet fibrin and red erythrocyte fibrin thrombi from atherostenotic occlusive lesions is the most important presentation of VA origin disease (1,2,23–27). A similar situation is well known in the anterior circulation. A patient is admitted with a small middle cerebral artery (MCA) territory infarct, and ultrasound or angiography shows an occlusion at the ICA origin. The recently formed occlusive thrombus has fragmented and embolized distally. Among 407 patients in the NEMC-PCR, 80 had severe stenosis or occlusion of the proximal VA. In 45 (56%) of these 80 patients, embolization from the ECVA lesion was the most likely cause of brain ischemia (23). Only 13 (16%) of 80 were considered to have hemodynamic-related TIAs, and 12 of these 13 had severe bilateral VA occlusive disease. The only patient with unilateral ECVA disease had bilateral ICA occlusions. Intraarterial embolism to the intracranial posterior circulation arteries occurs much more often than is presently recognized.

Most often emboli arising from ECVA disease go to the ipsilateral ICVA and/or the distal BA and its branches. The most frequent sites of infarction are in the proximal and distal posterior circulation territories, especially PICA- and SCA-supplied cerebellum, and the PCA territories of the cerebellar hemispheres. Occasionally, a "top of the basilar" syndrome occurs (1,28,29).

Intracranial Vertebral Artery Disease

ICVA disease presents in several different ways. (a) Ischemia within the proximal intracranial territory supplied by a stenotic or occluded ICVA. The findings conform to common syndromes: lateral medullary syndrome, medial medullary syndrome, hemimedullary syndrome in which both the medial and lateral medulla on one side are ischemic, and

PICA territory cerebellar infarction. (b) Intraarterial embolism arising from the ICVA, most often to the distal BA and its branches (SCA and PCA). Sometimes the symptoms include local ischemia in the medulla and PICA cerebellum accompanied by distal territory infarcts. (c) Frequent TIAs in patients with severe flow-limiting ICVA disease. These attacks often are positional and may include elements of both proximal and distal intracranial territory symptoms.

Local Proximal Intracranial Territory Ischemia and Infarction

Lateral Medullary Infarction

The most common vascular lesion is occlusion of the proximal or middle portion of the ICVA. Penetrating branches to the lateral medulla arise from the middle and distal two thirds of the ICVAs and penetrate through the lateral medullary fossa to reach and supply the lateral medullary tegmentum. The medial branches of the PICAs supply only a small portion of the dorsal medullary tegmentum (1). ICVA occlusive lesions decrease flow in lateral medullary tegmental penetrators. Less often, lateral medullary infarction is caused by occlusion of small medullary branches or the medial PICA branch. Important symptoms and signs of lateral medullary infarction are recalled best by visualizing the lateral medullary nuclei and tracts.

Nucleus and descending spinal tract of nerve V. Symptoms include sharp jabs or stabs of pain in the ipsilateral eye and face and facial numbness. Examination usually shows decreased pinprick and temperature on the ipsilateral face and a reduced corneal reflex.

Vestibular nuclei and their connections. Dizziness, frank vertigo, or instability of the environment results from dysfunction of the vestibular system and may invoke vomiting. Examination usually shows nystagmus with coarse rotatory eye movements when looking to the ipsilateral side and small-amplitude faster nystagmus when looking contralaterally. Sometimes the eyes forcibly deviate to the side of the lesion, so-called lateral pulsion (1).

Spinothalamic tract. Lesions of this structure usually produce decreased pinprick and temperature in the contralateral limbs and body. This sensory loss is seldom spontaneously recognized or reported by patients and usually is noticed only after detection on examination. Sometimes the pain and temperature loss extend to the contralateral face because of involvement of the crossed quintothalamic tract, which appends itself medially to the spinothalamic tract. Rarely the loss of pain and temperature sensation is totally contralateral and involves the face, arm, trunk, and leg.

Restiform body (inferior cerebellar peduncle). Symptoms include veering or leaning toward the side of the lesion and clumsiness of the ipsilateral limbs. Examination shows hypotonia and exaggerated rebound of the ipsilateral arm. When standing or sitting, patients often lean or tilt to the side of the lesion.

Autonomic nervous system nuclei and tracts. The descending sympathetic system traverses the lateral medulla in the lateral reticular formation. Dysfunction causes an ipsilateral Horner's syndrome. The dorsal motor nucleus of the vagus sometimes is affected, leading to tachycardia and a labile increased blood pressure.

Nucleus ambiguus. When the infarct extends medially and ventrally, it often affects this nucleus, causing hoarseness and dysphagia. The pharynx and palate are weak on the side of the lesion, often leading to retention of food within the piriform recess of the pharynx. A crowlike cough results from an attempt to extricate food from this area. At times, there is ipsilateral facial weakness, related to ischemia of the caudal part of the seventh nerve nucleus just rostral to the nucleus ambiguus or involvement of corticobulbar fibers going toward the seventh nerve nucleus.

Abnormal respiratory control. Initiation and control of respiration are known to involve the lateral pontine and medullary tegmentum. Poliomyelitis and bilateral medullary infarcts are well known to cause decreased respiratory drive. Hypoventilation or apnea probably is related to involvement of the nucleus of the solitary tract, the nucleus ambiguus, the nucleus retroambiguus, and the nuclei parvocellularis and gigantocellularis (1).

Medial and Hemimedullary Infarction

In medial medullary infarction, branches from the anterior spinal artery branch of the ICVA are affected, causing damage to structures in the medial medulla including the pyramidal tract, medial lemniscus, and hypoglossal nerve nucleus and nerve. The syndrome of the medial medulla consists of three main findings: contralateral hemiparesis, slight contralateral paresthesias and minor loss of posterior column sensory modalities, and ipsilateral tongue paresis.

Ischemia in the medial medulla has been reported much less often than lateral medullary ischemia. Ischemia in the medial medullary base often has accompanied lateral medullary ischemia. These hemimedullary infarcts are caused by occlusions of the ipsilateral ICVA. In some patients, ischemia involves the medial medulla bilaterally; in these cases, the vascular lesion has been either multiple embolic obstructions of anterior spinal artery branches or presumed occlusion of a dominant anterior spinal artery branch of one ICVA (1). Unilateral medial medullary infarction can result from atheromatous branch disease or the vascular pathology within penetrating anterior spinal artery branches that underlies lacunar infarction, in which case the infarct usually is limited to one medullary pyramid.

The most consistent feature of medial medullary ischemia is a contralateral hemiparesis. Usually, the hemiparesis is complete and flaccid at onset. Later, increased tone and spasticity develop. Sometimes the face is involved. Facial involvement is explained by caudal looping of supranuclear corticobulbar fibers that synapse at the facial nucleus. These fibers descend into the medulla before turning craniad to go to the nucleus of nerve VII in the lower pons. The next most frequent sign of involvement of medial medullary structures relates to ischemia to the medial lemniscus located just dorsal and medial to the medullary pyramid. Some patients report paresthesias or less often dysesthesias in the contralateral lower limb and trunk. Less often sensory symptoms occur in the arm and hand. In many patients with sensory symptoms, there are no objective signs of touch, vibration, or position sense loss. Ipsilateral tongue paralysis is the least common but most topographically localizing sign of medial medullary infarction. Tongue weakness probably is most often related to involvement of the intraparenchymal twelfth nerve fibers as they pass ventrally to exit at the medullary base rather than to infarction of the hypoglossal nucleus in the tegmentum.

Posterior Inferior Cerebellar Artery Territory Cerebellar Infarcts

The infarct can involve either the medial (mPICA) or lateral (lPICA) branches or the entire PICA-supplied territory of the cerebellum. The vermis and a small portion of the dorsal medulla are supplied by mPICA. Ischemia in this territory produces primarily vestibulocerebellar symptoms of vertigo and gait ataxia. The syndrome mimics an attack of Ménière's disease. In lPICA, infarcts veering or leaning to the side of the infarct upon standing and walking and ipsilateral arm hypotonia are the major signs.

Frequent Transient Ischemic Attacks in Patients with Severe Bilateral Intracranial Vertebral Artery Occlusive Disease

Bilateral ICVA disease is common. Twenty-one percent of patients in the NEMC-PCR had severe ICVA occlusive disease and 10% had bilateral severe ICVA occlusive disease. Both ICVAs could be stenotic or occluded. Unilateral occlusive disease could be accompanied by a hypoplastic contralateral ICVA or an ICVA that ended in the PICA. Early symptoms often are referable to the cerebellum and lateral medulla. Because of a low-flow system, the symptoms often are positionally sensitive, worsening with sitting or standing or when blood pressure falls either spontaneously or after treatment. TIAs usually are multiple and stereotyped. Symptoms and signs may progress gradually in some patients. Cerebellar and pyramidal signs and symptoms predominate. At times, ischemia of the PCA territories leads to abnormalities of vision, memory, and behavior. Bilateral ICVA occlusive lesions are most common in hypertensive and diabetic patients.

Basilar Artery Occlusive Disease

Occlusion of the BA often causes an extensive pontine infarct that involves most often the paramedian base and tegmentum. Blockage of the mid-BA at the orifice of the AICAs often is accompanied by infarction in the anterior inferior cerebellum on one or both sides. At times, the distribution of infarction conforms to the supply of a penetrating branch in which case a BA plaque obstructs that branch. Occlusion or severe stenosis of the distal portion of the BA can cause midbrain and thalamic infarction, as well as ischemia in the territories of the SCA and the PCAs. More often, the "top of the basilar" syndrome is caused by embolism from the heart, aorta, or VAs.

Occlusion of the Proximal or Middle Portion of the Basilar Artery

The infarct usually affects the midline and paramedian structures in the basis pontis (1,10,30). Collateral circulation is generally through the circumferential arteries that course around the lateral portions of the brainstem and supplies the lateral base, tegmentum, and cerebellum. The tegmentum of the pons has a rich collateral blood supply but depends primarily on the SCAs that originate from the rostral BA just before it bifurcates. The cerebellar hemispheres are mostly nourished by the PICA, which originates before the BA, and the SCA, which is preserved when the basilar artery clot does not extend to the distal BA. BA occlusion most often causes ischemia in the pontine base bilaterally, sometimes extending into the medial tegmentum on one or both sides (10,30). Predominant signs are motor and oculomotor. The spinothalamic tracts and cerebellum often are spared so that sensory and cerebellar abnormalities are not common, in contradistinction to the findings in patients with ICVA disease.

Descending corticospinal and corticobulbar tracts and bulbar motor nuclei. Weakness usually is bilateral but may be asymmetric. Stiffness, hyperreflexia, and extensor plantar reflexes are found upon examination of the weak limbs. Some patients present with a hemiparesis but have, on examination, some weakness and reflex abnormalities in the limbs contralateral to the hemiparesis. Hemiparesis was more common than quadriparesis in patients with BA occlusion studied in the NEMC-PCR (1). Paralysis of the face, palate, pharynx, neck, or tongue on one or both sides is common, as are symptoms of dysarthria, dysphonia, hoarseness, and dysphagia. The pontine lesion can involve cranial nerve fifth and seventh motor nuclei. The ischemia often interrupts corticofugal-descending fibers destined for the ninth to twelfth nerve nuclei located within the medullary tegmentum below the level of the infarct. Exaggerated jaw and facial reflexes, increased gag reflex, and emotional incontinence with excessive laughing or crying accompany the bulbar weakness. In some cases, the limb and bulbar paralysis is so severe that the patient is "locked in" and cannot communicate either verbally or by gesture.

Oculomotor nuclei and their connection. The sixth nerve nuclei, medial longitudinal fasciculi, and pontine lateral gaze centers all are located in the paramedian pontine tegmentum. Lesions of the sixth nerve or nucleus cause paralysis of abduction of the eye. A medial longitudinal fasciculi lesion causes an internuclear ophthalmoplegia characterized by loss of adduction of the ipsilateral eye, on gaze directed to the opposite side, and nystagmus of the contralateral abducting eye. The internuclear ophthalmoplegia can be bilateral. Lesions of the paramedian pontine tegmentum may affect the paramedian pontine reticular formation, the so-called pontine lateral gaze center, which mediates gaze to the same side. A lesion of this region causes an ipsilateral conjugate gaze paresis. A unilateral lesion can affect both the paramedian

pontine reticular formation and the medial longitudinal fasciculi on the same side. The resulting syndrome was called the "one- and one-half syndrome" by Fisher because only one half of gaze (scoring 1 for gaze to each side) is preserved (1,31). The vestibular nuclei and their connections are commonly affected, causing vertical and horizontal nystagmus. Ptosis, small pupils, and ocular skewing are found often.

Reticular activating system. If the lesion interrupts function of the medial pontine tegmentum bilaterally, coma may develop. Reduced consciousness is a poor prognostic sign, but care must be taken in differentiating reduced alertness from the locked-in state.

Infarction in the Distribution of a Penetrating Branch or Anterior Inferior Cerebellar Artery

Plaques within the BA may block or extend into the orifices of BA branches that penetrate into the pons from the BA (32–34). The resulting infarcts usually are restricted to the territory of the individual branches. Hemiplegia affecting the contralateral arm and leg (and often the face) and ataxic hemiparesis with or without dysarthria are the predominant syndromes.

Infarction involving the AICA territory causes a syndrome identical to that found in patients with lateral medullary infarction, except that cranial nerves VII and VIII are involved (35,36). The internal auditory artery is most often a branch of AICA so that ischemia to the vestibule, cochlea, and eighth nerve can accompany pontine infarction. Ipsilateral facial palsy and deafness can occur. When AICA territory infarction is caused by a thrombus within the BA, there often are accompanying motor or reflex signs (35,36).

Distal Brainstem, Superior Cerebellar Artery, and Posterior Cerebral Artery Territory Infarction: "Top of the Basilar" Syndromes (28,29)

Occlusion of the distal BA most often is due to embolism from the heart, aorta, or vertebral arteries. Emboli small enough to pass through the VAs usually will not lodge in the proximal BA, a vessel larger than each ICVA, but will reach the distal BA or its branches. The distal BA supplies the midbrain and diencephalon through small arteries that pierce the posterior perforated substance. Signs of dysfunction in this region are related to the paramedian structures in the midbrain tegmentum and posterior thalamus near the posterior commissure.

Pupillary abnormalities. The lesion may interrupt the afferent reflex arc by interfering with fibers going toward the Edinger-Westphal nucleus. The third nerve nucleus sometimes is involved, as well as the rostral descending sympathetic system. The pupils usually are abnormal and can be small, mid position, or dilated, depending on the location and extent of the lesion. Decreased pupillary reactivity and eccentricity of the pupil are found.

Eye movement abnormalities. Vertical gaze abnormalities are common. The paralysis may affect upward gaze, downward gaze, or both. The eyes may be skewed and may be deviated at rest, most often downward and inward. Hyperconvergence, retractory nystagmus, and pseudo sixth nerve paresis are other oculomotor abnormalities.

Altered alertness. Hypersomnolence or frank coma can result from ischemia affecting the bilateral rostral portion of the reticular activating system in the regions adjacent to the cerebral aqueduct and paramedian thalamus.. After the acute phase, the patient may remain relatively inert and apathetic.

Dysmemory. Memory loss can accompany thalamic infarction. Patients may be unable to make new memories and may have no recall of events just preceding their stroke. There may be other behavioral abnormalities, including agitation, hallucinations, and abnormalities that mimic lesions of the frontal lobe.

Cerebellar infarcts in territory supplied by the SCAs usually causes limb dysmetria and dysarthria (1,37,38). Gait ataxia and vertigo are less common than in PICA cerebellar infarcts.

Posterior Cerebral Artery Occlusive Disease

The great majority of PCA territory infarcts are embolic, with the source arising from the heart, aorta, or proximal posterior circulation arteries (1,39,40). Occasionally PCA stenosis with superimposed occlusion can cause PCA territory ischemia and infarction, in which case the clinical picture usually is TIAs that include hemianopic visual symptoms with or without paresthesiae (41).

The most common finding in patients with PCA territory infarction is a *hemianopia* (1, 39–43). Hemianopia is caused by infarction of the striate visual cortex on the banks of the calcarine fissure or interruption of the geniculocalcarine tract as it nears the visual cortex. If only the lower bank of the calcarine fissure is involved (lingual gyrus), a superior quadrant field defect results. An inferior quadrantanopia results if the lesion affects the cuneus on the upper bank of the calcarine fissure. When infarcts are restricted to the striate cortex and do not extend into adjacent parietal cortex, patients are fully aware of the visual defect. Patients usually recognize that they must focus extra attention to the hemianopic field. In patients with occipital lobe infarcts, physicians can reliably map out the visual fields by confrontation. At times, the central or medial part of the field is spared, so-called macular sparing. Optokinetic nystagmus is normal. Although some patients can detect motion or the presence of objects in their hemianopic field, they cannot identify the nature, location, or color of that object. When the full PCA territory is involved, visual neglect often accompanies hemianopia.

In patients with PCA territory infarcts, lateral thalamic ischemia is the major reason for *somatosensory symptoms and signs* (1,44,45). The lateral thalamus is the site of the major somatosensory relay nuclei, the ventroposteromedial and ventroposterolateral nuclei. Ischemia to these nuclei or to the white matter tracts carrying fibers from the thalamus to somatosensory cortex (postcentral gyrus and the sensory II region in the parietal operculum) produces changes in sensation, usually without paralysis. Patients describe paresthesias or numbness in the face, limbs, and trunk. On examination, their touch, pinprick, and position senses are reduced. The combination of hemisensory loss with hemianopia without paralysis is virtually diagnostic of infarction in the PCA territory. The occlusive lesion is within the PCA before the thalamogeniculate branches to the lateral thalamus. Rarely, occlusion of the proximal portion of the PCA can cause a hemiplegia (1,46,47). Penetrating branches from the proximal PCA penetrate into the midbrain to supply the cerebral peduncle. Proximal PCA occlusions cause hemiplegia due to midbrain peduncular infarction, accompanied by a hemisensory loss due to lateral thalamic infarction and hemianopia due to occipital lobe infarction.

When the left PCA territory is infarcted, there may be several other findings (1,42,43).

Alexia without agraphia. Infarction of the left occipital lobe and splenium of the corpus callosum is associated with loss of reading ability while writing and spelling abilities are preserved (1,43,48,49). In some patients, the disorder extends to objects, as well as written words, in which case the disorder is called associative visual agnosia (1,43,49). These patients with left PCA infarction have difficulty naming and describing the nature and use of objects presented visually. They can trace with their fingers and copy objects, which shows that visual perception is preserved. They can name objects if the objects are presented in their hand, explored by touch, or verbally described.

Anomic or transcortical sensory aphasia. Some patients with left PCA territory infarction have difficulty naming; others can repeat but not understand spoken language (50).

Gerstmann's syndrome. PCA territory infarction can undercut the angular gyrus, leading to findings usually lumped together as Gerstmann's syndrome (1). These findings include difficulty telling right from left; difficulty naming digits on their own or on others' hands; constructional dyspraxia; agraphia; and difficulty in calculating. In any single patient, all features may appear together, or one or more may occur in isolation.

Altered memory. A defect in acquisition of new memories is common when both medial temporal lobes are damaged, but it also occurs when lesions are limited to the left temporal lobe (1,49,51). The memory deficit in unilateral lesions is not permanent but has lasted up to 6 months. Patients cannot recall what has happened recently; when given new information, they cannot recall it moments later. They often repeat statements and questions spoken only minutes before.

Infarcts of the right PCA territory often are accompanied by *prosopagnosia,* which is difficulty in recognizing familiar faces (1,52). Disorientation to place and an inability to recall routes or to read or revisualize the location of places on maps are common findings in patients with right PCA territory infarcts (53). Patients with right occipitotemporal infarcts may have difficulty revisualizing what a given object or person should look like. Dreams may be devoid of visual imagery. Visual neglect is much more common after lesions of the right than of the left PCA territory.

When the PCA territory is infarcted bilaterally, the most common findings are cortical blindness, amnesia, and agitated delirium (1,54–56). Most often, bilateral PCA territory infarction is due to embolism, with blockage of the distal basilar bifurcation. Cortically blind patients cannot see or identify objects in either visual field but have preserved pupillary light reflexes Amnesia due to bilateral medial temporal lobe infarction may be permanent and closely resembles Korsakoff's syndrome. Infarction of the hippocampus, fusiform, and lingual gyri, usually bilaterally, leads to an agitated hyperactive state that can be confused with delirium tremens (1,55,56).When infarction is limited to the lower banks of the cal-

carine fissures bilaterally, the major findings are prosopagnosia and defective color vision (1,52,57, 58).

REFERENCES

1. Caplan LR. *Posterior circulation disease. Clinical findings, diagnosis, and management.* Boston: Blackwell Science, 1996.
2. Caplan LR. Posterior circulation ischemia: then, now, and tomorrow. The Thomas Willis lecture—2000. *Stroke* 2000;31:2011–2023.
3. Fisher CM, Gore I, Okabe N, et al. Atherosclerosis of the carotid and vertebral arteries—extracranial and intracranial. *J Neuropathol Exp Neurol* 1965;24:455–476.
4. Moosy J. Morphology, sites, and epidemiology of cerebral atherosclerosis. *Res Publ Assoc Res Nerv Ment Dis* 1966;51:1–22.
5. Hutchinson E, Yates P. The cervical portion of the vertebral artery, a clinico-pathological study. *Brain* 1956; 79:319–331.
6. Muller-Kuppers, Graf KJ, Pessin MS, et al. Intracranial vertebral artery disease in the New England Medical Center Posterior Circulation Registry. *Eur Neurol* 1997; 37:146–156.
7. Shin H-K, Yoo K-M, Chang HM, et al. Bilateral intracranial vertebral artery disease in the New England Medical Center Posterior Circulation Registry. *Arch Neurol* 1999;56:1353–1358
8. Fisher CM, Karnes W, Kubik C. Lateral medullary infarction: the pattern of vascular occlusion. *J Neuropathol Exp Neurol* 1961;20:323–379.
9. Cornhill J, Akins D, Hutson M, et al. Localization of atherosclerotic lesions in the human basilar artery. *Atherosclerosis* 1980;35:77–86.
10. Kubik CS, Adams RD. Occlusion of the basilar artery: a clinical and pathological study. *Brain* 1946;69:73–121.
11. Pessin MS, Gorelick PB, Kwan E, et al. Basilar artery stenosis—middle and distal segments. *Neurology* 1987; 37:1742–1746.
12. Caplan LR, Gorelick PB, Hier DB. Race, sex, and occlusive cerebrovascular disease: a review. *Stroke* 1986;17:648–655.
13. Gorelick PB, Caplan LR, Hier DB, et al. Racial differences in the distribution of posterior circulation occlusive disease, *Stroke* 1985;16:785–790.
14. Wityk R, Lehman D, Klag M, et al. Race and sex differences in the distribution of cerebral atherosclerosis *Stroke* 1996;27:1974–1980.
15. Hennerici M, Klemm C, Rautenberg W. The subclavian steal phenomenon: a common vascular disorder with rare neurologic deficits. *Neurology* 1988;38:669–673.
16. Martin R, Bogousslavsky J, Miklossy J, et al. Floating thrombus in the innominate artery as a cause of cerebral infarction in young adults. *Cerebrovasc Dis* 1992;2:177–181.
17. Ferriere M, Negre G, Bellecoste JF, et al. Thrombus flottant sous-clavier responsible d'un syndrome encephalo-digital, deux observations. *La Presse Med* 1984;13:27–29.

18. Brewster DC, Moncure AC, Darling C, et al. Innominate artery lesions: problems encountered and lessons learned. *J Vasc Surg* 1985;2:99–112.

19. Hennerici M, Aulich A, Sandemann W, et al. Incidence of asymptomatic extracranial occlusive disease. *Stroke* 1981;12:750–758.

20. Symonds C. Two cases of thrombosis of subclavian artery with contralateral hemiplegia of sudden onset, probably embolic. *Brain* 1927;50:259–260.

21. Fields WS, LeMak NA, Ben-Menachem Y. Thoracic outlet syndrome: review and reference to a stroke in a major league pitcher. *AJNR Am J Neuroradiol* 1986;7:73–78.

22. Fisher CM. Occlusion of the vertebral arteries. *Arch Neurol* 1970;22:13–19.

23. Wityk RJ, Chang H-M, Rosengart A, et al. Proximal extracranial vertebral artery disease in the New England Medical Center Posterior Circulation Registry. *Arch Neurol* 1998;55:470–478.

24. Pelouze GA. Plaque ulcerie de l'ostium de l'artere vertebrale. *Rev Neurol* 1989;145:478–481.

25. George B, Laurian C. Vertebrobasilar ischemia with thrombosis of the vertebral artery: report of two cases with embolism. *J Neurol Neurosurg Psychiatry* 1982;45:91–93.

26. Caplan LR, Tettenborn B. Embolism in the posterior circulation. In: Bergner R, Caplan LR, eds. *Vertebrobasilar arterial disease.* St. Louis: Quality Medical Publishers, 1991:50–63.

27. Caplan LR, Amarenco P, Rosengart A, et al. Embolism from vertebral artery origin occlusive disease. *Neurology* 1992;42:1505–1512.

28. Caplan LR. Top of the basilar syndrome: selected clinical aspects. *Neurology* 1980;30:72–79.

29. Mehler MF. The rostral basilar artery syndrome: diagnosis, etiology, prognosis. *Neurology* 1989;39:9–16.

30. LaBauge R, Pages C, Marty-Double JM, et al. Occlusion du tronc basilaire. *Rev Neurol* 1981;137:545–571.

31. Fisher CM. Some neuro-ophthalmological observations. *J Neurol Neurosurg Psychiatry* 1967;30:383–392.

32. Fisher CM, Caplan LR. Basilar artery branch occlusion: a cause of pontine infarction. *Neurology* 1971;21:900–905.

33. Fisher CM. Bilateral occlusion of basilar artery branches. *J Neurol Neurosurg Psychiatry* 1977;40:1182–1189.

34. Caplan LR. Intracranial branch atheromatous disease: a neglected, understudied and underused concept. *Neurology* 1989;39:1246–1250.

35. Amarenco P, Hauw JJ. Cerebellar infarction in the territory of the anterior inferior cerebellar artery: a clinicopathological study of 20 cases. *Brain* 1990;118:139–155.

36. Amarenco P, Rosengart A, DeWitt LD, et al. Anterior inferior cerebellar artery territory infarcts. Mechanisms and clinical features. *Arch Neurol* 1993;50:154–161.

37. Amarenco P, Hauw JJ. Cerebellar infarction in the territory of the superior cerebellar artery: a clinicopathologic study of 33 cases. *Neurology* 1990;40:1383–1390.

38. Amarenco P. Cerebellar stroke syndromes. In: Bogousslavsky J, Caplan LR, eds. *Stroke syndromes,* 2nd ed.

Cambridge: Cambridge University Press, 2001:540–546.

39. Pessin MS, Lathi E, Cohen M, et al. Clinical features and mechanism of occipital infarction. *Ann Neurol* 1987;21:290–299.

40. Yamamoto Y, Georgiadis AL, Chang HM, et al. Posterior cerebral artery territory infarcts in the New England Medical Center (NEMC) Posterior Circulation Registry. *Arch Neurol* 1999;56:824–832.

41. Pessin MS, Kwan E, DeWitt LD, et al. Posterior cerebral artery stenosis. *Ann Neurol* 1987;21:85–89.

42. Chaves C, Caplan LR. Posterior cerebral artery. In: Bogousslavsky J, Caplan LR, eds. *Stroke syndromes,* 2nd ed. Cambridge: Cambridge University Press, 2001:479–489.

43. Barton JS, Caplan LR, Cerebral visual dysfunction. In: Bogousslavsky J, Caplan LR, eds. *Stroke syndromes,* 2nd ed. Cambridge: Cambridge University Press, 2001:87–110.

44. Georgiadis AL, Yamamoto Y, Kwan ES, et al. The anatomy of sensory findings in patients with posterior cerebral artery (PCA) territory infarction. *Arch Neurol* 1999;56:835–838.

45. Caplan LR, DeWitt LD, Pessin MS, et al. Lateral thalamic infarcts. *Arch Neurol* 1988;45:959–964.

46. Benson DF, Tomlinson EB. Hemiplegic syndrome of the posterior cerebral artery. *Stroke* 1971;2:559–564.

47. Hommel M, Besson G, Pollak P, et al. Hemiplegia in posterior cerebral artery occlusion. *Neurology* 1990;40:1496–1499.

48. Geschwind N, Fusillo M. Color naming defect in association with alexia. *Arch Neurol* 1966;15:137–146.

49. Caplan LR, Hedley-White T. Cuing and memory dysfunction in alexia without agraphia. *Brain* 1974;97:251–262.

50. Kertesz A, Sleppard A, MacKenzie R. Localization in transcortical sensory aphasia. *Arch Neurol* 1982;39:475–479.

51. Ott B, Saver JL. Unilateral amnestic stroke. Six new cases and a review of the literature. *Stroke* 1993;24:1033–1042.

52. Damasio A, Damasio H, Van Housen G. Prosopagnosia: anatomic basis and behavioral mechanisms. *Neurology* 1982;32:331–341.

53. Fisher CM. Disorientation to place. *Arch Neurol* 1982;39:33–36.

54. Symonds C, McKenzie I. Bilateral loss of vision from cerebral infarction. *Brain* 1957;80:415–455.

55. Medina J, Rubino F, Ross E. Agitated delirium caused by infarctions of the hippocampal formation and fusiform and lingual gyri: a case report. *Neurology* 1974;24:1181–1183.

56. Horenstein S, Chamberlain W, Conomy J. Infarction of the fusiform and calcarine regions: agitated delirium and hemianopsia. *Trans Am Neurol Assoc* 1962;92:357–367.

57. Meadows J. Disturbed perception of colors associated with localized cerebral lesions. *Brain* 1974;97:615–632.

58. Damasio A, Yamada T, Damasio H, et al. Central achromatopsia: behavioral, anatomic, and physiologic aspects. *Neurology* 1980;30:1064–1071.

Ischemic Stroke: Advances in Neurology, Vol. 92. Edited by
H.J.M. Barnett, Julien Bogousslavsky, and Heather Meldrum.
Lippincott Williams & Wilkins, Philadelphia © 2003.

16

Small-Vessel Disease with Lacunes

Domenico Inzitari and Maria Lamassa

*Department of Neurological and Psychiatric Sciences, University of Florence and Department of
Neurology, Careggi University Hospital, Florence, Italy*

The term *lacune* appeared in the French literature in the mid-to-late nineteenth century (1). It was applied in 1901 by Marie (2) and in 1902 Ferrand (3) to two cases of capsular and pontine infarction, respectively, with specific symptoms.

Fisher (4) established the term *lacunar syndrome* in the 1960s. Users of this term accept the hypothesis that, among patients with cerebral infarction of diverse cause, there exist a few distinct clinical syndromes that are associated with small infarcts or lacunes seated in selective deep areas of the brain, including deep white matter, basal ganglia, internal capsule, thalamus, and brainstem. The infarcts were supposed to result from occlusion of one of the perforating arteries supplying each of these areas. Five main lacunar syndromes were described: pure motor stroke, pure sensory stroke, ataxic hemiparesis, dysarthria–clumsy hand, and sensory motor stroke, all of which remain up-to-date with the most frequent syndromes (5–9).

VASCULAR PATHOLOGY

After Fisher's work, the cause of occlusion was attributed to distinct vascular lesions specifically affecting small-caliber arteries: lipohyalinosis, microatheroma, fibrinoid necrosis, and Charcot-Bouchard aneurysms (4,10–12).

Lipohyalinosis is the term used by Fisher to describe degenerative changes with replacement of muscle and elastic laminae by collagen and hyaline material. At the arteriole level, these changes confer rigidity with loss of the autoregulatory capacity.

Microatheroma consists of subintimal accumulation of foam cells and other atheromatous changes. Microatheroma may involve both the orifice and the initial segment of a penetrating artery having a diameter from 300 to 700 μm, with possible hemodynamic

effect. Some authors consider microatheroma to be the most common angiopathy underlying the development of lacunar infarct (13,14). The lumen becomes either narrowed or occluded by this microplaque. Microdissection, hemorrhage within the plaque, and superimposed thrombi made of platelets, as well as fibrin, may contribute to obstruction (12). *Fibrinoid necrosis,* which may occur in arterioles of patients who have extremely high blood pressure, is characterized by finely granular or homogeneous brightly eosinophilic deposits in the connective tissue of small blood vessels. These deposits likely result from a combination of necrotic smooth muscle cells and extravasated plasma proteins.

Lipohyalinosis, fibrinoid necrosis, and microatheroma may be associated with areas of focal dilation called *Charcot-Bouchard aneurysms.* Thrombosis into Charcot-Bouchard aneurysms or emboli from these areas may be another cause of vessel occlusion. Whether Charcot-Bouchard aneurysms represent true aneurysms or result from a dissection into the wall of a microatheroma is controversial (10–12). Using modern histopathologic techniques, Challa et al. (15) concluded that microaneurysms are uncommon and that the abnormalities called microaneurysms frequently are coils, twists, and overlapping loops of the affected intraparenchymal vessels.

There is indirect evidence supporting the embolic (from large arteries or from the heart) origin of occlusion of small vessels in selected cases (16–20). Reduced perfusion in the territory of large precerebral vessels may interact with an already narrowed lumen of small vessel, increasing the hemodynamic effect. These mechanisms, together with the fact that large- and small-vessel diseases share common vascular risk factors, may explain the lacunar stroke presentation in patients with carotid artery stenosis. In the North American Symptomatic Carotid Endarterectomy Trial (NASCET) (21), patients who presented with lacunar stroke had a lower degree of stenosis, and intervention with carotid endarterectomy showed less benefit in these patients than in patients with other types of events, suggesting that this combination more likely is coincidental than causal.

EPIDEMIOLOGY AND RISK FACTORS

Before the computed tomography (CT) scan era, diagnosis of lacunar infarct lacked accuracy because lacunar syndromes due to nonischemic causes are not rare (22). Small hemorrhages and nonvascular lesions may cause lacunar syndromes. This notwithstanding, in many studies frequency data continue to be based only on the clinical definition.

Using the same clinical criteria (discussed later), the Oxfordshire Community Stroke Project (OCSP) in England (23) and the Studio Epidemiologico Prevalenza Incidenza Vasculopatia Acuta Cerebrale (SEPIVAC) in Italy (24), both community-based stroke registries, found the proportion of lacunar infarcts from total ischemic strokes to be 24.4% and 28.9%, respectively. A similar figure (26.7%) was reported from the European BIOMED Study of Stroke Care, a large multicenter hospital-based registry (25). Compared with the other stroke types, no selective effect by age, gender, and race was noted in the different studies (19,22,26,27).

Whether the other conventional risk factors play a specific role in lacunar infarct is controversial. Considering the type of vascular pathology, hypertension has been regarded the principal determinant (28–30). However, most often, no selective effect was noted when patients with lacunar stroke were compared with those with nonlacunar stroke types (atherothrombotic or cardioembolic) in either hospital- or population-based stroke patient series (27,31). The importance of hypertension as a specific determinant of lacunar stroke was demonstrated definitively by comparison of patients with lacunar stroke and age-matched nonstroke controls (32).

Diabetes is reported as a definite risk factor for lacunar infarct in some but not all studies (28,33,34). In NASCET, a history of diabetes and abnormal blood glucose values were associated with lacunar stroke independent of other risk factors (21). In the same study, hyperlipidemia was found to be an independent determinant of lacunar stroke. Moreover, abnormal low-density lipoprotein cholesterol values and diabetes showed a synergistic effect when the two factors were combined (Inzitari et al., unpublished

data). These observations suggest that the effect of lipid factors in relation to lacunar stroke probably is undervalued. Data are accumulating on the role of genetic polymorphisms, such as that of angiotensin-converting enzyme (35), that have a selective relationship with lacunar infarct. Finally, recent observations in the hospital setting suggest that risk factor profile and outcome differ, depending on whether multiple asymptomatic lacunar lesions are seen on imaging at the initial presentation of a lacunar stroke or only a single (symptomatic) lesion is evidenced. Hypertension was found to be more closely linked to the presence of multiple lacunar infarcts on CT scan, suggesting lipohyalinosis (arteriolosclerosis) as the most probable underlying vascular pathology in these patients and microatheroma in patients with a single lesion (36,37).

CLINICAL DEFINITION

Currently, in vivo diagnosis of lacunar infarct is based on the description of the clinical syndrome, which eventually is corroborated by the typical findings on brain imaging studies, CT, or magnetic resonance (MR).

Clinically, lacunar stroke can be identified based on patterns of symptoms/signs related to the dysfunction/lesion of the areas supplied by the small perforating arteries, after excluding the presence of symptoms/signs resulting from a cortical or more extensive subcortical lesion.

The OCSP (23) has proposed and validated (against the CT scan appearance of lacunar lesions) a clinical definition of lacunar infarct that has been adopted by many population- or hospital-based studies. To be defined as a lacunar cerebral infarct patient, the patient must present with one of the classic syndromes after the presence of symptoms/signs characterizing other brain syndromes with involvement of the cortical areas are excluded. This definition also requires that only patients presenting with facio-brachial and brachiocrural involvement be included in the lacunar cerebral infarct category; those with more restricted (i.e., only face, arm, or leg) deficits are not included (23). However, in NASCET (21), more than 10% of patients whose CT scan showed a congruent lacunar lesion had only one segment of the hemibody affected. Several clinicoradiologic studies reported a variety of syndromes in which symptoms and signs were combined differently, were expressed partially, or were atypical with respect to the classic syndromes (38). Table 16-1 lists the most common syndromes, the possible variants of neurologic pre-

TABLE 16-1. *Main lacunar syndromes with variants an possible lesion sites.*

Lacunar syndromes	Clinical features	Lesion site
Pure sensory stroke	Transient or persistent numbness, mild sensory loss over the one entire side of the body	Thalamus
	Objective sensory deficit may be absent	Corona radiata (parietal, also extending to centro semiovale)
	No associated hemiparesis	Pons
Pure motor stroke	Motor deficit/weakness	Internal capsule
	Proportional (face + arm + leg)	Pons
	Not proportional:	Mesencephalon
	• Face + arm type (more frequent in supratentorial lacunes)	Corona radiata
	• Arm + leg type (more frequent in lower pontine lacunes)	
	• Facial paresis (upper motor type) with or without dysarthria	
	• Faciolingual paresis	
	• Faciopalatal paresis	
	Transient numbness of the affected limbs may be associated at the onset of the motor deficit	
Sensory motor stroke	Numbness, mild sensory loss over the one entire side of the body + motor deficit/weakness (face + arm + leg)	Thalamocapsular
Ataxic hemiparesis	Ipsilateral motor deficit/weakness associated with cerebellar-like dysfunction	Internal capsule
	Transient paresthesia or other sensory symptoms may be presented at onset	Thalamus
	Sensory disturbances may be persistent, affecting various modalities, particularly, position sense	Corona radiata
	Special types	Pons
	Hemispheral	
	• Relative or complete facial sparing	
	• No dysarthria	
	• No nystagmus or sensory disturbances	
	Brainstem	
	• Face + arm involvement	
	• Dysarthria and dysphagia present	
	• Nystagmus, vertigo, or dyplopia event if transient	
	• Lack of sensory disturbances	
Dysarthria–clumsy hand	Facial weakness	Pons
	Severe dysarthria	Genu internal capsule
	Slight weakness and clumsiness of the hand (writing impaired most when dominant side affected)	Deep capsular region
	Some degree of weakness of arm or even leg, at least in the early phase	Junction internal capsule + corona radiata

From Fisher CM. Lacunar stroke and infarcts: a review. *Neurology* 1982;32:871–876.

sentation within each syndrome, and the possible sites of lesion.

In addition to the classic syndromes, several other syndromes have been described in relation to lacunar infarcts, mostly in terms of their location in the inferior striatum, subthalamic area, or brainstem (39). These syndromes are less specific because they may depend merely on the site and the restricted area of infarct and may not necessarily reflect the involvement of single perforating vessels. Unilateral movement disorders, including hemichorea, hemiballis-

mus, focal dystonia, and asterixis, are the syndromes that most consistently have been related to "sensu strictiori" lacunar infarcts. Lesions usually are located in inferior striatum, corpus of Luys, or other basal ganglia. Isolated eye movement disorders may result from upper brainstem lacunar lesions interrupting intraaxial oculomotor nerves tracts, especially the third and sixth cranial nerves. Midbrain syndromes occasionally may be due to lacunar infarcts. Conjugate gaze disorders, including internuclear ophthalmoplegia, vertical gaze palsy, and other oculomotor

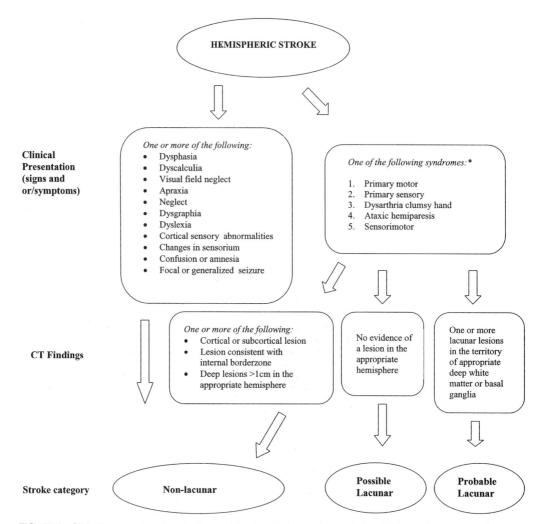

FIG. 16-1. Clinical and radiologic criteria used to classify hemispheric stroke. *The syndromes were based on signs or symptoms in one or more areas involving the face, arm, or leg. A lacunar lesion was identified as round or oval in shape, measuring ≤1 cm, located in a territory supplied by deep or superficial small perforating arteries, not in the cortical territories, and without characteristics of internal border zone infarcts. (From Inzitari D, Eliasziw M, Sharpe BL, et al. Risk factors and outcome of patients with carotid artery stenosis presenting with lacunar stroke. *Neurology* 2000;54:660–666, with permission.)

disorders, isolated or in combination with long tracts disorders, rarely occur as a consequence of brainstem lacunar infarcts. Cognitive deterioration, parkinsonism, and pseudobulbar palsy likely represent the effect of multiple bilateral lacunar infarcts in the subcortical deep regions of the brain (lacunar state), where they alter function by interrupting subcortical connections among cortical areas involved in cognition (subcortical vascular dementia) (40), motor tracts, or basal ganglia of both sides.

IMAGING DEFINITION

On neuroimaging, lacunar infarct commonly appears as an area of reduced attenuation on CT scan, hypointensity on T1-weighted magnetic resonance imaging (MRI) sequence, or hyperintensity on T2-weighted sequence. This area usually is round or oval in shape and is seated alternatively in the corona radiata, internal capsule, basal ganglia, or upper brainstem. The margins of old lesions usually are sharp;

those of recent lesions may be less defined because of the so-called *foggy* effect. Different maximum diameters have been used in different studies (<2, <1.5, or <1 cm) to define lacunar lesions. The size used most frequently in the literature is <1.5 cm. Lesions with a diameter <1 cm probably are more consistent with occlusion of a single perforating artery. There is a time profile for the appearance of this lesion after the clinical event. This differs when comparing CT and MRI, given the different sensitivities of the two techniques. Using CT imaging, the lowest prevalence of positive images occurs in the first week after the event. From reported data, early CT positivity for lesions congruent with a clinically defined lacunar infarct ranges from 12% (41) to 50% of patients (42). In the first few days, MRI is reported to show a recent lacunar infarct in up to 94% of patients (42). MRI sensitivity increases with use of contrast enhancement (43). Although MR is more sensitive, it may be less specific, for example, in identifying a lesion congruent with the recent clinical event from among several older symptomatic or asymptomatic lesions. Compared with conventional MRI, diffusion-weighted magnetic resonance imaging (DW-MRI) seems to be more sensitive in detecting early small infarcts and differentiating acute from nonacute lesions. In one study, DW-MRI performed after 3 days was 95% sensitive and 94% specific for revealing an acute lacunar infarct (44).

COMBINED DEFINITION

In practice, diagnosis of lacunar stroke can be achieved with the greatest precision by combining the clinical and the imaging definitions. The algorithm proposed by the NASCET Study Group for definition of lacunar stroke patients is shown in Fig. 16-1. This definition has proved to be reproducible based on sufficiently detailed and reliable clinical and CT information (21).

REFERENCES

1. Poirier J, Derouesné C. Le concept de lacune cérébrale de 1838 à nous jour. *Rev Neurol (Paris)* 1985;141:3–17.
2. Marie P. Des foyers lacunaire de desintegration et de differents autres etats cavitaires du cerveau. *Rev Med* 1901;21:281–298.
3. Ferrand J. *Essai sur l'hémiplégie des viellards. Les lacunes de désintégration cérébrale.* Thesis, Rousset, Paris, 1902.
4. Fisher CM. Lacunes: small deep cerebral infarcts. *Neurology* 1965;15:774–784.
5. Fisher CM, Curry HB. Pure motor hemiplegia of vascular origin. *Arch Neurol* 1965;13:30–44.
6. Fisher CM. Pure sensory stroke involving face, arm and leg. *Neurology* 1965;15:76–80.
7. Fisher CM, Cole M. Homolateral ataxia and crural paresis: a vascular syndrome. *J Neurol Neurosurg Psychiatry* 1965;28:48–55.
8. Fisher CM. A lacunar stroke. The dysarthria-clumsy hand syndrome. *Neurology* 1967;17:614–617.
9. Mohr JP, Kase CS, Meckler RJ, et al. Sensorimotor stroke due to thalamocapsular ischaemia. *Arch Neurol* 1977;34:734–741.
10. Mohr JP. Lacunes. *Stroke* 1982;13:3–11.
11. Bamford JM, Warlow CP. Evolution and testing of the lacunar hypothesis. *Stroke* 1988;19:1074–1082.
12. Ho KL, Garcia JH. Neuropathology of the small blood vessels in selected diseases of the cerebral white matter. In: Pantoni L, Inzitari D, Wallin A, eds. *The matter of white matter. Clinical and pathophysiological aspects of white matter disease related to cognitive decline and vascular dementia.* Utrecht, The Netherlands, Academic Pharmaceutical Productions, 2000: 247–273.
13. Fisher CM. Lacunar strokes and infarcts: a review. *Neurology* 1982;32:871–876.
14. Caplan LR. Intracranial branch atheromatous disease: a neglected, understudied, and underused concept. *Neurology* 1989;39:1246–1250.
15. Challa VR, Moody DM, Bell MA. The Charcot-Bouchard aneurysm controversy: impact of a new histologic technique. *J Neuropathol Exp Neurol* 1992;51: 263–271.
16. Santamaria J, Graus F, Rubio F, et al. Cerebral infarction of the basal ganglia due to embolism from the heart. *Stroke* 1983;14:91100–914.
17. Gorsselink EL, Peeters HP, Lodder J. Causes of small deep infarcts detected by CT. *Clin Neurol Neurosurg* 1984;86:271–273.
18. Kappelle LJ, Koudstaal PJ, van Gijn J, et al. Carotid angiography in patients with lacunar infarction. A prospective study. *Stroke* 1988;19:1093–1096.
19. Ghika J, Bogousslavsky J, Regli F. Infarcts in the territory of the deep perforators from the carotid system. *Neurology* 1989;39:507–512.
20. Jung DK, Devuyst G, Maeder P, et al. Atrial fibrillation with small subcortical infarcts. *J Neurol Neurosurg Psychiatry* 2001;70:344–349.
21. Inzitari D, Eliasziw M, Sharpe BL, et al. Risk factors and outcome of patients with carotid artery stenosis presenting with lacunar stroke. *Neurology* 2000;54: 660–666.
22. Anzalone N, Landi G. Nonischaemic causes of lacunar syndromes: prevalence and clinical findings. *J Neurol Neurosurg Psychiatry* 1989;52:1188–1190.
23. Bamford J, Sandercock P, Dennis M, et al. Classification and natural history of clinically identifiable subtypes of cerebral infarction. *Lancet* 1991;337: 1521–1536.
24. Ricci S, Celani MG, Guercini G, et al. First-year results of a community-based study of stroke incidence in Umbria, Italy. *Stroke* 1989;20:853–857.
25. Di Carlo A, Lamassa M, Pracucci G, et al. Stroke in the very old: clinical presentation and determinants of 3-month functional outcome: a European perspective. European BIOMED Study of Stroke Care Group. *Stroke* 1999;30:2313–2319.
26. Bamford J, Sandercock P, Jones L, et al. The natural his-

tory of lacunar infarction: the Oxfordshire Community Stroke Project. *Stroke* 1987;18:545–551.

27. Hajat C, Dundas R, Stewart JA, et al. Cerebrovascular risk factors and stroke subtypes: differences between ethnic groups. *Stroke* 2001;32:37–42.

28. Gandolfo C, Caponnetto C, Del Sette M, et al. Risk factors in lacunar syndromes: a case-control study. *Acta Neurol Scand* 1987:7:22–26.

29. Tegeler CH, Shi F, Morgan T. Carotid stenosis in lacunar stroke. *Stroke* 1991;22:1124–1128.

30. Boiten J, Lodder J. Lacunar infarcts. Pathogenesis and validity of the clinical syndromes. *Stroke* 1991;22:1374–1378.

31. Lodder J, Bamford JM, Sandercock PA, et al. Are hypertension or cardiac embolism likely causes of lacunar infarction? *Stroke* 1990;21:375–381.

32. Boiten J, Luijckx GJ, Kessels F, et al. Risk factors for lacunes. *Neurology* 1996;47:1109–1110.

33. Loeb C, Gandolfo C, Mancardi GL, et al. The lacunar syndromes: a review with personal contribution. In Lechner H, Meyer JS, Ott E, eds. *Cerebrovascular disease: research and clinical management,* vol. 1. Amsterdam: Elsevier, 1986:107–156.

34. Moulin T, Tatu L, Vuillier F, et al. Role of a stroke data bank in evaluating cerebral infarction subtypes: patterns and outcome of 1,776 consecutive patients from the Besancon stroke registry. *Cerebrovasc Dis* 2000;10:261–271.

35. Markus HS, Barley J, Lunt R, et al. Angiotensin-converting enzyme gene deletion polymorphism. A new risk factor for lacunar stroke but not carotid atheroma. *Stroke* 1995;26:1329–1333.

36. Spolveri S, Baruffi MC, Cappelletti C, et al. Vascular risk factors linked to multiple lacunar infarcts. *Cerebrovasc Dis* 1998;8:152–157.

37. Boiten J, Lodder J, Kessels F. Two clinically distinct lacunar infarct entities? A hypothesis. *Stroke* 1993;24:652–656.

38. Orgogozo JM, Bogousslavsky J. *Vascular disease, part II, Vinken and Bruyn's handbook of clinical neurology.* 1989:235–269.

39. Besson G, Hommel M. Lacunar syndromes. In: Pullicino PM, Caplan LR, Hommel M, eds. *Cerebral small artery disease. Advances in neurology, vol. 62.* New York: Raven Press, 1993:141–160.

40. Erkinjuntti T, Inzitari D, Pantoni L, et al. Research criteria for subcortical vascular dementia in clinical trials. *J Neural Transm Suppl* 2000;59:23–30.

41. Toni D, Iweins F, von Kummer R, et al. Identification of lacunar infarcts before thrombolysis in the ECASS I study. *Neurology* 2000;54:684–688.

42. Stapf C, Hofmeister C, Hartmann A, et al. Predictive value of clinical lacunar syndromes for lacunar infarcts on magnetic resonance brain imaging. *Acta Neurol Scand* 2000;101:13–18.

43. Miyashita K, Naritomi H, Sawada T, et al. Identification of recent lacunar lesions in cases of multiple small infarctions by magnetic resonance imaging. *Stroke* 1988;19:834–839.

44. Lai PH, Li JY, Chang CY, et al. Sensitivity of diffusion-weighted magnetic resonance imaging in the diagnosis of acute lacunar infarcts. *J Formos Med Assoc* 2001;100:370–376.

Ischemic Stroke: Advances in Neurology, Vol. 92. Edited by
H.J.M. Barnett, Julien Bogousslavsky, and Heather Meldrum.
Lippincott Williams & Wilkins, Philadelphia © 2003.

17

CADASIL

Cerebral Autosomal Dominant Arteriopathy with Subcortical Infarcts and Leukoencephalopathy

*Hugues Chabriat and *†Marie Germaine Bousser

*Department of Neurology, Hôpital Lariboisière and,
†Department of Neurology, Faculte de Medicine, Paris, France

CADASIL is the acronym for *cerebral autosomal dominant arteriopathy with subcortical infarcts and leukoencephalopathy.* It is an inherited arterial disease of mid-adulthood caused by mutations of the *Notch3* gene on chromosome 19 (1,2). The presumed key mechanism of cerebral lesions in CADASIL is "chronic ischemia" secondary to severe ultrastructural alterations within the wall of the small arteries of the brain (3,4). Secondary inflammatory processes within the tissue, alterations of exchanges through the arteriolar wall, and wallerian degeneration are other important associated factors (5–7). The genetic testing to confirm the diagnosis of the disease has been available since 1996 (8). The disease was first reported in European families, but now it has been diagnosed in American, African, and Asiatic pedigrees, indicating that the condition is present worldwide and suggesting its frequency may be much higher than currently thought. This is supported by the recent identification of the first sporadic case pointing to the occurrence of de novo mutations of the *Notch3* gene causing the disease (9). No treatment currently has been evaluated for this condition.

CLINICAL PRESENTATION

The mean age at onset of symptoms is 45 years. The duration of the disease varies between 10 and 40 years. Mean age at death is about 65 years, but it varies from 30 to 80 years in the affected pedigrees (10–12).

Stroke is the most frequent clinical manifestation of the disease. About 85% of symptomatic patients suffer transient ischemic attacks (TIA) or completed strokes (12,13). Most frequently, the events occur in the absence of vascular risk factors. The ischemic events occur at a mean age of 49 years, with a large range from 27 to 65 years. All temporal profiles of ischemic manifestations are observed: TIA, reversible ischemic neurologic deficits, and completed strokes. The ischemic deficits are of the subcortical type. Two thirds of occurrences are classic lacunar syndromes: pure motor stroke, ataxic hemiparesis, pure sensory stroke, and sensory motor stroke. Some episodes of focal deficits occur in association with headache. During the course of the disease, the total number of TIAs varies from one to tens. In most cases, the maximal number of completed strokes is fewer than five during life. In the largest series of affected families (12,13), 40% of affected members with ischemic manifestations had TIAs, 70% had completed strokes, and 10% had both.

Dementia is the other main clinical manifestation of CADASIL. It is reported in one third of symptomatic patients. Dementia is observed at a mean age of 60 years and in 90% of patients before death (11,12). Eighty percent of CADASIL patients older than 65 years are demented. The exact onset of cognitive impairment in CADASIL is difficult to ascertain; however, Taillia et al. (14) showed that nondemented symptomatic patients, the younger of whom was aged 35 years, had altered performances using tasks very sensitive to frontal dysfunction. In 90% of cases, cognitive impairment occurs in steps and is associated with recurrent stroke events. In 10% of cases, neuropsychologic decline is isolated and mimics the course of Alzheimer's disease (12,13). Cognitive deficit is of the subcortical type, with predominating frontal symptoms and memory impairment. Dementia often is associated with pyramidal signs, pseudobulbar palsy, gait difficulties, and/or urinary incontinence.

From 20% to 30% of affected subjects suffer attacks of migraine with aura. This symptom is present in 40% of CADASIL families, but its frequency varies from 0% to 85% of patients within affected pedigrees. When present, migraine with aura is the earliest clinical manifestation of the disease, with a mean age at onset of 30 years. As usually observed in migraine with aura, the most frequent neurologic symptoms associated with headache are visual and/or sensitive. The frequency of attacks with basilar, hemiplegic, or prolonged aura, according to IHS diagnosis criteria, is noticeably high. In some families, migraine with aura appears as the main and sole symptom of the disease (12,13,15,16).

Nearly 20% of CADASIL patients present with severe mood disturbances. The frequency of such manifestations is widely variable between families. Most patients have severe depression of the melancholic type, sometimes alternating with typical manic episodes. The diagnosis of bipolar mood disorder was considered in some subjects until the magnetic resonance imaging (MRI) examination was performed (17). The exact cause of mood disturbances in CADASIL remains undetermined. The location of ischemic lesions in basal ganglia or in frontal white matter may play a key role in their occurrence (18).

NEUROIMAGING

MRI is always abnormal in symptomatic subjects. Signal abnormalities can be detected during a presymptomatic period of variable duration. MRI signal abnormalities are observed as early as 20 years of age. After age 35 years, all subjects with the affected gene have an abnormal MRI (2).

MRI shows on T1-weighted images punctiform or nodular hyposignals in basal ganglia and white matter. T2-weighted images show hypersignals in the same regions associated with widespread areas of increased signal in the white matter (Fig. 17-1) (19). T2 hypersignals may be observed in the absence of T1 lesions in one third of affected subjects (20). The severity of MRI lesions dramatically increases with age. The frequency of signal abnormalities in the external capsule (two thirds of cases) and particularly within the anterior part of the temporal lobes are noteworthy and might be helpful for differential diagnosis (21). Brainstem lesions are observed mainly in the pons. The mesencephalon and medulla usually are spared. Cortical or cerebellar lesions are exceptional.

Ultrasound studies and echocardiography usually are normal. Cerebral angiography is normal, showing a narrowing of small arteries only in rare cases. Angiography with contrast agents should be avoided when the diagnosis of CADASIL is suspected

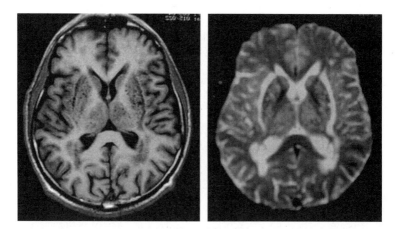

FIG. 17-1. T1- and T2-weighted magnetic resonance imaging of a symptomatic CADASIL patient showing typical hyperintensities on T2-weighted images predominating within the deep and periventricular white matter associated with hyposignals in the same areas on T1-weighted images. Note the increased signal within the external capsules on T2-weighted images and the presence of punctiform hyposignals within the lentiform nuclei on T1-weighted images.

because confusion or coma have been reported as secondary effects in several affected subjects (22).

Cerebrospinal fluid examination usually is normal, but oligoclonal bands with pleocytosis have been reported. A monoclonal immunoglobulin was detected in two cases of our first family but not in other affected pedigrees (23).

PATHOLOGIC EXAMINATION

Macroscopic examination of the brain shows a diffuse myelin pallor and rarefaction of the hemispheric white matter sparing the U fibers (Fig. 17-2). Lesions predominate in the periventricular areas and centrum semiovale (3). They are associated with lacunar infarcts located in the white matter and basal ganglia. In the brainstem, the lesions are more marked in the pons and are similar to the pontine rarefaction of myelin of ischemic origin described by Pullicino et al. (3,7).

Microscopic investigations show that the wall of cerebral and leptomeningeal arterioles is thickened

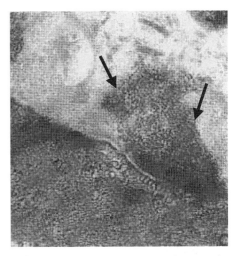

FIG. 17-3. Granular material within the vessel wall (*arrows*) observed with electron microscopy after skin biopsy. (Courtesy of Pr. M.M. Ruchoux, Service de Neuropathologie, CHRU Lille.)

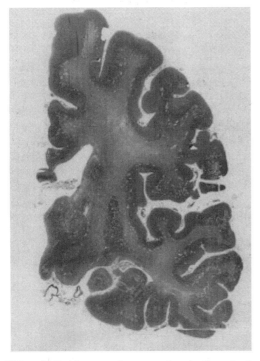

FIG. 17-2. Macroscopic aspect of the brain (hemateine eosin staining) in a CADASIL patient showing small deep infarcts associated with demyelination sparing the U fibers. (Courtesy of Pr. M.M. Ruchoux, Service de Neuropathologie, CHRU Lille.)

and their lumen is significantly reduced. Such abnormalities also can be detected by leptomeningeal biopsy (24). The media is thickened. It contains abnormal smooth muscle cells, often degenerated, with multiple nuclei and an eosinophilic nonamyloid material. Sometimes smooth muscle cells are not detectable and are replaced by collagen fibers. The endothelium usually is spared. On electron microscopy, the eosinophilic material appears dense, granular, and osmiophilic. Staining for amyloid substance and elastin is negative (3). Ruchoux et al. (4,25) made the crucial observation that the vascular abnormalities observed in the brain also were detectable in other organs. The granular material surrounding the smooth muscle cells as seen with electron microscopy also is present in the media of arteries located in the spleen, liver, kidneys, muscle, and skin. The presence of this material in the skin, muscle, and nerve vessels allowed confirmation of the *intra vitam* diagnosis of CADASIL in several patients (Fig. 17-3) (11,25,26). Joutel et al. (27) proposed use of immunostaining with anti-Notch3 antibodies after skin biopsy, which seems to be much easier and more sensitive for diagnosis.

GENETICS

The defective gene in CADASIL is the *Notch3* gene located on chromosome 19. This gene encodes a large transmembrane receptor (1,28). Its exact role in the occurrence of the disease remains undetermined. Numerous missense mutations of *Notch3* gene have been detected in CADASIL patients. They are located in the epidermal growth factor-like (EGF-like) repeats in the extracellular domain of the protein. They invariably lead to an odd number of cysteine residues. Most of the causative mutations are clustered within two exons (3 and 4), which allowed proposal of a genetic test able to routinely detect 70% of mutations causing the disease (8). For the other mutations, in the absence of an already known target (known mutation within the family), genetic testing is hampered by the numerous exons requiring analysis. In such cases, skin biopsy with immunostaining of the Notch3 protein is particularly useful (27).

REFERENCES

1. Joutel A, Corpechot C, Ducros A, et al. Notch3 mutations in CADASIL, a hereditary adult-onset condition causing stroke and dementia. *Nature* 1996;383: 707–710.
2. Tournier-Lasserve E, Joutel A, Melki J, et al. Cerebral autosomal dominant arteriopathy with subcortical infarcts and leukoencephalopathy maps to chromosome 19q12. *Nat Genet* 1993;3:256–259.
3. Baudrimont M, Dubas F, Joutel A, et al. Autosomal dominant leukoencephalopathy and subcortical ischemic strokes: a clinicopathological study. *Stroke* 1993;24:122–125.
4. Ruchoux MM, Guerrouaou D, Vandenhaute B, et al. Systemic vascular smooth muscle cell impairment in cerebral autosomal dominant arteriopathy with subcortical infarcts and leukoencephalopathy. *Acta Neuropathol* 1995;89:500–512.
5. Molko N, Pappata S, Mangin JF, et al. Diffusion tensor imaging study of subcortical gray matter in CADASIL. *Stroke* 2001;32:2049–2054.
6. Rocca MA, Filippi M, Herzog J, et al. A magnetic resonance imaging study of the cervical cord of patients with CADASIL. *Neurology* 2001;56:1392–1394.
7. Ruchoux MM, Maurage CA. CADASIL: cerebral autosomal dominant arteriopathy with subcortical infarcts and leukoencephalopathy. *J Neuropathol Exp Neurol* 1997;56:947–964.
8. Joutel A, Vahedi K, Corpechot C, et al. Strong clustering and stereotyped nature of Notch3 mutations in CADASIL patients. *Lancet* 1997;350:1511–1515.
9. Joutel A, Dodick DD, Parisi JE, et al. De novo mutation in the Notch3 gene causing CADASIL. *Ann Neurol* 2000;47:388–391.
10. Chabriat H, Joutel A, Vahedi K, et al. CADASIL (cerebral autosomal dominant arteriopathy with subcortical infarcts and leukoencephalopathy). *J Mal Vasc* 1996;21: 277–282.
11. Chabriat H, Joutel A, Vahedi K, et al. CADASIL. Cerebral autosomal dominant arteriopathy with subcortical

12. Chabriat H, Vahedi K, Iba-Zizen MT, et al. Clinical spectrum of CADASIL: a study of 7 families. Cerebral autosomal dominant arteriopathy with subcortical infarcts and leukoencephalopathy. *Lancet* 1995;346: 934–939.
13. Dichgans M, Mayer M, Uttner I, et al. The phenotypic spectrum of CADASIL: clinical findings in 102 cases. *Ann Neurol* 1998;44:731–739.
14. Taillia H, Chabriat H, Kurtz A, et al. Cognitive alterations in non-demented CADASIL patients. *Cerebrovasc Dis* 1998;8:97–101.
15. Desmond DW, Moroney JT, Lynch T, et al. The natural history of CADASIL: a pooled analysis of previously published cases. *Stroke* 1999;30:1230–1233.
16. Verin M, Rolland Y, Landgraf F, et al. New phenotype of the cerebral autosomal dominant arteriopathy mapped to chromosome 19: migraine as the prominent clinical feature. *J Neurol Neurosurg Psychiatry* 1995; 59:579–585.
17. Kumar SK, Mahr G. CADASIL presenting as bipolar disorder [Letter]. *Psychosomatics* 1997;38:397–398.
18. Aylward ED, Roberts-Willie JV, Barta PE, et al. Basal ganglia volume and white matter hyperintensities in patients with bipolar disorder. *Am J Psychiatry* 1994;5: 687–693.
19. Skehan SJ, Hutchinson M, MacErlaine DP. Cerebral autosomal dominant arteriopathy with subcortical infarcts and leukoencephalopathy: MR findings. *Am J Neuroradiol* 1995;16:2115–2119.
20. Chabriat H, Levy C, Taillia H, et al. Patterns of MRI lesions in CADASIL. *Neurology* 1998;51:452–457.
21. Auer DP, Putz B, Gossl C, et al. Differential lesion patterns in CADASIL and sporadic subcortical arteriosclerotic encephalopathy: MR imaging study with statistical parametric group comparison. *Radiology* 2001;218: 443–451.
22. Dichgans M, Petersen D. Angiographic complications in CADASIL [Letter]. *Lancet* 1997;349:776–777.
23. Tournier-Lasserve E, Iba-Zizen MT, Romero N, et al. Autosomal dominant syndrome with stroke-like episodes and leukoencephalopathy. *Stroke* 1991;22: 1297–1302.
24. Lammie GA, Rakshi J, Rossor MN, et al. Cerebral autosomal dominant arteriopathy with subcortical infarcts and leukoencephalopathy (CADASIL)—confirmation by cerebral biopsy in 2 cases. *Clin Neuropathol* 1995; 14:201–206.
25. Ruchoux MM, Chabriat H, Bousser MG, et al. Presence of ultrastructural arterial lesions in muscle and skin vessels of patients with CADASIL. *Stroke* 1994;25: 2291–2292.
26. Goebel HH, Meyermann R, Rosin R, et al. Characteristic morphologic manifestation of CADASIL, cerebral autosomal-dominant arteriopathy with subcortical infarcts and leukoencephalopathy, in skeletal muscle and skin. *Muscle Nerve* 1997;20:625–627.
27. Joutel A, Favrole P, Labauge P, et al. Skin biopsy immunostaining with a Notch3 antibody for CADASIL diagnosis. *Lancet* 2001;15:2049–2051.
28. Joutel A, Tournier-Lasserve E. Notch signalling pathway and human diseases. *Semin Cell Dev Biol* 1998;9: 619–625.

Ischemic Stroke: Advances in Neurology, Vol. 92. Edited by
H.J.M. Barnett, Julien Bogousslavsky, and Heather Meldrum.
Lippincott Williams & Wilkins, Philadelphia © 2003.

18

Biochemistry of Ischemic Stroke

Philip A. Barber, Andrew M. Demchuk, *Lorenz Hirt, and Alastair M. Buchan

*Department of Clinical Neurosciences, University of Calgary and Foothills Medical Centre,
Calgary, Alberta, Canada; *Department of Neurology, Centre Hospitalier Universitaire Vaudois,
Lausanne, Switzerland*

Acute cerebral ischemia begins with the mechanical occlusion of cerebral blood vessels, usually by embolus and occasionally by thrombus (1). During moderate to severe cerebral ischemia, cerebral blood flow (CBF) is reduced, and autoregulation is impaired. At blood flow levels around 20 mL/100 g/min, the oxygen extraction fraction becomes maximal, the cerebral metabolic rate for oxygen begins to fall (2), normal neuronal function of the cerebral cortex is affected, and cortical electroencephalographic activity ceases (3). This degree of ischemia represents a threshold for loss of neuronal electrical function. At levels below 10 mL/100 g/min, cell membranes and function are severely affected (4). At this threshold, lack of oxygen inhibits the mitochondrial metabolism and activates the inefficient anaerobic metabolism of glucose, causing a local rise in lactate production and so a fall in pH, leading to intra- and extracellular acidosis. The energy-dependent functions of cell membranes to maintain ion homeostasis become progressively impaired. Potassium ions leak out of cells into the extracellular space, Na^+ and water enter cells (cytotoxic edema), and Ca^{2+} enters the cell, where it impairs mitochondrial function and compromises intracellular membranes to control subsequent ion fluxes, leading to further cytotoxicity. This degree of ischemia represents a threshold for loss of cellular ion homeostasis.

These two concepts of critical thresholds of electrical and membrane failure define the upper and lower flow limits of the ischemic penumbra. This is defined as fundamentally reversible (5) and is perhaps pragmatically characterized by a response to pharmacologic agents (6). However, recent studies of functional and metabolic disturbances suggest a more complex pattern of thresholds. During the initial few hours of vascular occlusion, different brain functions break down at widely varying CBF levels. At declining flow rates in both global and focal models of ischemia, protein synthesis is first inhibited in neurons, followed by anaerobic glycolysis, the release of neurotransmitters, impaired energy metabolism, and finally membrane depolarization (7).

The extent of the brain injury is ultimately dependent on critical thresholds of reduced CBF, the duration of the ischemic insult, the tissue temperature, the blood glucose level, and other physiologic variables. Some neurons are thought to be more vulnerable to hypoxia and decreased CBF than other neurons, such as the CA1 cells in the hippocampus, termed "selective vulnerability." Mechanisms that give rise to ischemic cell death occur via three major mediators: unregulated increases of Ca^{2+} concentration intracellularly, tissue acidosis, and nitric oxide (NO) and free radical production. Ischemic brain injury is modulated by inflammatory processes, by the induction of immediate early genes, and later by apoptotic mechanisms (Fig. 18-1).

CALCIUM ION HOMEOSTASIS

Extracellular Ca^{2+} concentrations are several thousand times greater than intracellular concentrations, and the mechanisms that control this gradient are energy dependent. Calcium enters the cell predominantly through two types of channels: voltage controlled and receptor operated (8). There are several agonists that increase permeability to Ca^{2+} when bound to specific receptors, namely, excitatory amino acids (glutamate, nucleotides, and cyclic nucleotides) (9,10). The export of Ca^{2+} from neurons into the extracellular environment occurs via processes that

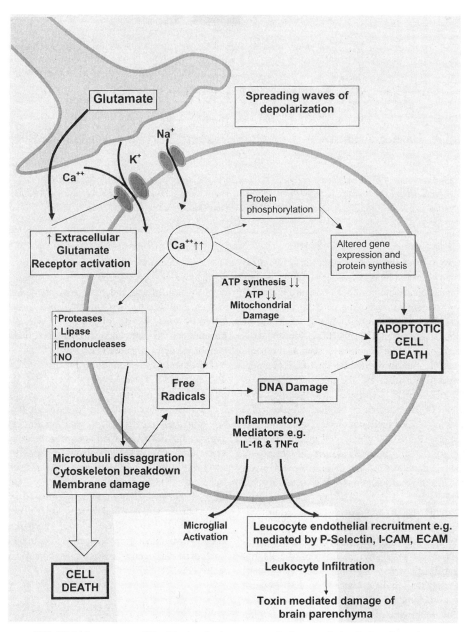

FIG. 18-1. A summary of the biochemical processes that occur during ischemic stroke.

are linked directly or indirectly to the utilization of energy (11,12). In the former category is the adenosine triphosphate (ATP)-dependent calcium pump and in the second is the Na^+/Ca^{2+} exchanger that utilizes energy stored in the sodium electrochemical gradient. The exchanger can operate in either direction so that when the Na^+ gradient falls, it can import, rather than export, Ca^{2+}. Substantial amounts of Ca^{2+} are stored within intracellular organelles, mainly the

mitochondria and endoplasmic reticulum. Release of Ca^{2+} from mitochondria requires energy, which is either Na^+ dependent or independent. The accumulation of Ca^{2+} in the endoplasmic reticulum requires energy and is mediated by an ATP-consuming pump (Fig. 18-2).

Calcium enters cells by ionotropic-operated calcium channels, which are gated predominately by glutamate receptors of the N-methyl-D-aspartate

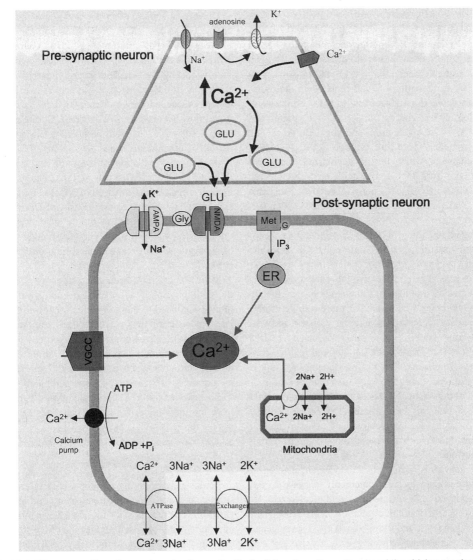

FIG. 18-2. Diagram outlines the routes of entry and exit of calcium from the cytosol and the driving mechanisms maintaining calcium homeostasis. Calcium entering the cell under nonischemic conditions is either bound by calcium-bound proteins or sequestered by the endoplasmic reticulum (ER). Entry of calcium into the mitochondria activates a number of enzymes for pyruvate, isocitrate, etc. During ischemia, excessive release of the neurotransmitter glutamate activates α-amino-3-hydroxy-5-methyl-4-isoxazole-4-propionic acid (AMPA), *N*-methyl-D-aspartate (NMDA), and metabotropic (Met) glutamate receptors. Activation of AMPA receptors causes membrane depolarization and opens voltage-sensitive calcium channels (VSCQs). Activation of NMDA receptors opens a receptor-gated calcium channel. Activation of metabotropic receptors stimulates, via a second messenger inositol 1,4,5-trisphosphate (IP_3), the release of calcium. Calcium extrusion from the cell normally occurs through a calcium-activated adenosine triphosphatase (ATPase) and through 3 Na^+/Ca^{2+} exchangers.

(NMDA) type and by voltage-sensitive calcium channels. When glutamate is released from presynaptic endings, it activates two types of ionotropic glutamate receptors, the non-NMDA type being selectively activated by α-amino-3-hydroxy-5-methyl-4-isoxazole-4-propionic acid (AMPA). The AMPA receptor gates a channel that is permeable to monovalent cations (Na^+, K^+, H^+), whereas the NMDA-gated channel is also permeable to Ca^{2+}. This channel is blocked by Mg^{2+}, which is released when the cell membrane depolarizes following AMPA receptor activation. Depolarization also allows Ca^{2+} to enter via voltage-sensitive calcium channels (13).

The decline in CBF and the accompanying loss of oxygen supply result in impaired energy metabolism and measurable decreases in ATP and phosphocreatine. The combination of ATP breakdown and compensatory anaerobic glycolysis leads to cellular acidification. With energy depletion, the membrane potential is lost, and neurons and glia depolarize (14). This triggers Ca^{2+} influx through voltage-sensitive Ca^{2+} channels, which further depolarizes the membrane, and excitatory amino acids are released into the extracellular space. Energy-dependent processes such as glutamate reuptake are impaired, which further increases extracellular glutamate, resulting in prolonged activation of membrane glutamate receptors and Ca^{2+} influx (15). Sodium and Cl^- enter the neuron via channels for monovalent ions (11). Water follows passively, and the ensuing edema can affect the perfusion of regions surrounding the focally injured brain, as well as having more remote effects that produce increased intracranial pressure and vascular compression.

The consequences of the unregulated rise in intracellular cytoplasmic Ca^{2+} during ischemia are linked with glutamate excitotoxicity to a number of biochemical processes that result in further detrimental injury to ischemic brain tissue (15). Some of these events continue irrespective of reoxygenation, whereas others are provoked or triggered during reperfusion.

The activation of lipolysis produces an increase in free fatty acids, which are potentially neurotoxic, and the oxidation of arachidonic acid (catalyzed by cyclooxygenase and lipoxygenase) yields prostaglandins, leukotrienes, and thromboxane A_2. These agents, together with platelet-activating factor, can damage cellular membranes and act additionally as chemoattractants (15). This activation also produces oxygen free radicals. These reactions can produce sustained damage to the cell membranes and receptors, further accelerating the toxic effects of glutamate by impaired uptake.

Many of the enzymatic processes involved in the phosphorylation of proteins are Ca^{2+} mediated. An alteration in protein kinase and phosphatase activity during ischemia provokes changes in ion membrane and receptor activity, as well as affecting gene transcription and translation. The effect of these processes may perhaps explain the long-term effects of ischemia on membrane function and integrity, facilitating free radical peroxidation, as well as unmasking processes leading to programmed cell death (apoptosis).

During ischemia, other Ca^{2+}-mediated reactions are accelerated, such as proteolysis and the assembly/reassembly of microtubules (12). Cytoskeletal proteins are degraded when Ca^{2+} level rises intracellularly. Several Ca^{2+}-dependent enzymes trigger reactions that produce reactive oxygen species. These events proceed during ischemia if there is residual blood flow but are greatly accelerated during reperfusion. Some of the reactions involved result in the oxidation of arachidonic acid (by cyclooxygenase and lipoxygenase), oxidation of xanthine and hypoxanthine to $O_2\cdot$ and H_2O_2 (via xanthine oxidase), and those leading to the formation of $NO\cdot$ (by nitric oxide synthase). However, the vast majority of reactive oxygen species are produced by the mitochondrial respiratory chain, and as the mitochondria contains superoxide dismutase, the result is the formation of $O_2\cdot$ and H_2O_2.

Mitochondria have been increasingly implicated in the pathophysiology of ischemic brain injury. Free radical-mediated disruption of the inner mitochondrial membrane and the oxidation of proteins that mediate electron transport impair their function. The mitochondrial membrane becomes leaky, and eventually mitochondria become overloaded with Ca^{2+}, resulting in impaired ATP production and ultimately energy and membrane failure (15). Cytochrome c is released from the mitochondria and has been suggested as a trigger for apoptosis (16).

ACIDOSIS

Acidosis arises during ischemia, contributes to tissue damage, and may mitigate recovery during reoxygenation. The mechanisms include edema formation, inhibition of H^+ extrusion, inhibition of lactate oxidation, and impairment of mitochondrial respiration (11,12). Cellular acidosis may promote intracellular edema formation by inducing Na^+ and Cl^- accumulation in the cell via coupled Na^+/H^+ and Cl^-/HCO_3^- exchange; acidosis activates Na^+/H^+ exchange; and H^+ leaks back into the cell via the Cl^-/HCO_3^- antiporter, causing accumulation of Na^+ and Cl^- in the cell, with water entering the cell by osmosis. In addition, extracellular acidosis may compete with Na^+ at the external site of the Na^+/H^+ antiporter, thereby retarding or preventing H^+ movement from the cells. Finally, acidosis may block the lactate oxidase form of the lactate dehydrogenase complex, retarding both oxidation of lactate accumulated during ischemia and oxidative phosphorylation in isolated mitochondria, impairing ATP production. It has also been hypothesized that acidosis enhances the production of free radicals and triggers deoxyribonucleic acid (DNA) fragmentation.

FREE RADICAL FORMATION

Free radicals are produced in small quantities in cells during aerobic metabolism. Mitochondria are the major producer of free radicals in biological systems. Superoxide (O_2·) is formed during the operation of complexes I and II of the mitochondrial electron transport chain. However, it is extremely toxic, causing damage to DNA, proteins, lipids, and components of the extracellular matrix. Polyunsaturated fats and sulfur-containing amino acids that are found in high concentration within the brain are particularly vulnerable. Free radical scavengers such as tocopherol and vitamin C and enzymes that metabolize free radicals (superoxide dismutase and catalase) maintain the balance physiologically.

During severe ischemia, insufficient O_2 is available to accept electrons passed along the mitochondrial electron transport chain. Free radicals are also generated during ischemia by the release of iron from ferritin stores within ischemic neurons (17). As the cerebrospinal fluid has a low concentration of ferritin-binding proteins, much of the iron released from damaged brain cells remains unbound and is therefore available to catalyze the generation of radical hydroxyl (OH·), leading to iron-induced lipid peroxidation. This process is further compounded by the fact that the central nervous system is relatively depleted of superoxide dismutase, which scavenges OH· and controls the release of iron from intracellular stores.

The commonest free radicals produced during cerebral ischemia are O_2· and OH·, and these, like other free radicals, react with and exacerbate damage of proteins, DNA, and lipids, particularly the fatty acid component of the cell membrane, causing changes in the permeability and integrity of the cell membranes (lipid peroxidation).

It has been shown, using salicylate trapping of OH·, that brain undergoing ischemia/reperfusion produces oxygen free radicals during the reperfusion phase after ischemia (18). Activated leukocytes produce oxygen free radicals, which, during ischemia, become localized on the brain microvessels through the action of P-selectin, exposing the microvascular endothelium to high levels of oxygen free radicals, causing oxidative damage to specific local sites. This contributes to the breakdown of the blood–brain barrier and brain edema.

INFLAMMATION

Astrocytes, microglia, leukocytes, and endothelial cells are activated by ischemia and begin to produce cytokines (19). In addition, there is evidence for peripherally derived cytokines by phagocytes, T-lymphocytes, natural killer cells, and polymorphonuclear leukocytes, which can exacerbate central nervous system inflammation and gliosis. In support of this, peripheral irradiation or treatment with colchicine attenuates inflammation, wound healing, and gliosis (20).

The early accumulation of neutrophils in ischemic brain has been confirmed histologically (21–25), by biochemical studies (26,27), and in radiolabeled leukocyte studies (28,29). Brain ischemia is associated with expression of a number of inflammatory mediators [interleukin (IL) 1 and tumor necrosis factor-α (TNF-α)] and chemokines [IL-8 for neutrophils, macrocyte chemoattractant protein-1 for monocytes, β-chemokine regulated upon activation, normal T-cell expressed and secreted (RANTES), leukotriene B4, and interferon-inducible protein (IP) 10], and up-regulation of adhesion molecules [intercellular adhesion molecule-1 (ICAM-1), selectins] maintains leukocyte recruitment to the vascular endothelium (30). Cytokines such as TNF-α and IL-1β are responsible for the accumulation of inflammatory cells in the injured brain and may affect the survival of damaged neurons. During ischemia, cytokines attract leukocytes and stimulate the production of adhesion receptors on leukocytes and endothelial cells (Fig. 18-3). Leukocytes promote infarction through their toxic byproducts and phagocytic action and by the immune reaction. This inflammatory reaction not only contributes to lipid membrane peroxidation but also exacerbates the degree of tissue injury caused by the rheologic effects of "sticky" leukocytes in the blood, which interfere with microvascular perfusion. Injury is also mediated through the product of leukocyte neurotoxic products (31,32). Increased expression of TNF-α ribonucleic acid (RNA) occurs rapidly after middle cerebral artery occlusion in rats at 1 to 3 h (33,34). The fact that TNF-α messenger RNA expression precedes neutrophil migration into the brain parenchyma suggests that it is involved in this response.

Like TNF-α, IL-1β has many proinflammatory properties, and receptors for this cytokine have been demonstrated in the central nervous system (35,36). It is produced in microglia, astrocytes, neurons, and endothelium. It has been demonstrated in focal transient cerebral ischemia in the rat (37,38), and the exacerbation of stroke injury has been demonstrated following the administration of exogenous IL-1β

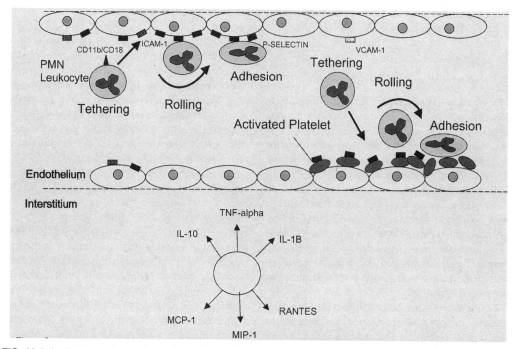

FIG. 18-3. Leukocyte rolling is dependent on the selectin family of adhesion molecules. P-Selectin expression is induced within minutes on endothelium. Firm adhesion is mediated by the integrins including B2-integrin (CD I I/CD 18) and BI-integrin. However, the α4-integrin [vascular cell adhesion molecule-I (VCAM-I) ligand] can also mediate leukocyte rolling, especially in delayed inflammatory processes. Leukocyte recruitment can also occur when platelets adhere to endothelium (**right**), express P-selectin, and function as a bridge to tether and adhere leukocytes. Once adherent, the leukocytes can cause endothelial dysfunction, transvascular protein leakage, and edema, leading to brain injury. These changes in leukocyte behavior are mediated by increased brain inflammatory cytokines (tumor necrosis factor-α, interleukins-1β and -8, etc.), chemokine expression, as well as adhesion molecules as described above in the ischemic brain.

(39). IL-1 receptor antagonist is a naturally occurring inhibitor of IL-1 activity, whereas exogenous administration of IL-1 antagonists attenuates infarct size (40,41).

Cytokines induce the expression of the adhesion receptors such as ICAM-1, vascular cell adhesion molecule-1, P-selectin, and endothelial cell adhesion molecule-1. Adhesion receptors interact with complementary surface receptors on neutrophils [CD11/CD18, MAC-1 (chemoattractant activation-dependent molecule), LFA-1 (leukocyte function-associated antigen one)]. The neutrophils in turn adhere to the endothelium, cross the vascular wall, and enter the brain parenchyma. Macrophages and monocytes follow neutrophils and migrate into ischemic brain. Modification of this postischemic inflammation has been shown in some studies to alleviate ischemic brain injury. Antiinflammatory approaches may be of benefit by improvement in postischemic blood flow (36).

Production of toxic mediators by activated inflammatory cells and injured neurons has important consequences. Infiltrating neutrophils produce inducible nitric oxide synthase (NOS), an enzyme that produces toxic amounts of NO. The pathogenic importance of NO is reflected by the observation that pharmacologic inhibitors of inducible NOS reduce ischemia. The inflammatory process might also be linked to apoptosis because antibodies against adhesion molecules attenuate postischemic inflammation and reduce apoptotic cell death in ischemic brain (42).

Focal ischemia is a very powerful stimulus to elicit genomic responses in the brain in the form of multiple early gene expression. In addition to the genes expressed for TNF-α and IL-1β, many other inflammatory genes are expressed during focal ischemia. Depending on the severity of the ischemia and the intrinsic nature of the neuronal populations, it is thought that a stress response and changes in gene expression are elicited by ischemia, which may be vital to cell survival and repair. Following focal ischemia, immediate early genes are the first to be regulated, as shown by the identification of c-fos, c-jun, and zinc finger genes, but the expression is only transient (43,44). A second phase consists of the heat shock proteins. The third phase comprises increased cytokine gene expression as previously described for TNF-α and IL-1β but also includes IL-6 (45) and IL-1 receptor antagonist (46). Chemokines such as IL-8 (47) and IP-10 (48) are also elevated and probably play an important role in neutrophil and mononuclear cell infiltration. After middle cerebral artery occlusion in rats, both ICAM-1 (49) and endothelial–leukocyte adhesion molecule-1 (50) messenger RNA were expressed in the first 1 to 3 h. After stroke in primates, both P-selectin and ICAM-1 have been shown to be up-regulated on the postcapillary microvessels in the ischemic penumbra (51). In addition, growth factors such as nerve growth factor, brain-derived nerve growth factor (BDNF), and tumor suppressor gene p53 (52) are also increased. This third phase is considered to be very important in the infiltration of neutrophils into ischemic brain.

A fourth phase of new gene expression involves the transcription of proteolytic enzymes (metalloproteinases), which are implicated in the remodeling of the extracellular matrix (53,54), and their endogenous proteinase inhibitor, tissue inhibitor matrix metalloproteinase (55). The expression of the enzymes is associated with a breakdown of the blood–brain barrier and an infiltration of inflammatory cells that may cause secondary injury. The fifth phase involves the transcription of mediators such as transforming growth factor-β (48) and osteopontin (56), which appear to be important in tissue remodeling and as barriers to protect the residual brain tissue.

Although TNF-α appears to precipitate leukocyte endothelium recruitment and infiltration into injured brain, it does not appear to be directly toxic to neurons (57), and some investigators have even suggested that it has a protective effect on the neurons. Studies using TNF receptor knock-out mice (p55 and p750) in cerebral ischemia suggested increased sensitivity to brain ischemia, highlighting the potential beneficial effects of TNF (58,59). This has also been supported by the observations that repeated exogenous administration of both TNF and IL-1 displays a capacity of inducing ischemic tolerance (60,61). Although these studies contradict much of the data that show that TNF and IL-1 augmentation is injurious and that blocking these cytokines is neuroprotective, these cytokines are clearly also involved in the later repair and remodeling of damaged brain. Antiinflammatory interventions that limit the degree of

damage have been shown to interfere with nervous regeneration and recovery (62).

Much interest has focused on the involvement of nuclear factor-κB (NFκB) during ischemia. NFκB is a well-characterized ubiquitous and inducible transcription factor that plays an important role in inflammation and also in apoptosis and the cell cycle (63). In nonstimulated neuronal cells, inhibitor-κB (IκB), which masks the nuclear transport signal, binds this dimer. Upon activation, inhibitor-κB (IκB) is degraded by the proteasome complex, revealing the nuclear localization signal, and NFκB translocates to the nucleus, where it activates the transcription of target genes such as cell adhesion molecules, inducible NOS (see above), cyclooxygenase-2, p53, Mn superoxide dismutase, and Bcl-2. *In vivo*, NFκB is strongly induced in animal models of focal cerebral ischemia (64,65). Different experiments suggest that NFκB can promote either cell death or survival, depending on the paradigm. Mice lacking the NFκB subunit p50 have significantly smaller lesions after focal cerebral ischemia. Inhibition of NFκB by a proteasome inhibitor (CVT-634) also reduces ischemia-induced damage (67). Both these experiments support the idea that overall NFκB is detrimental for neuronal survival. On the contrary, the capacity of NFκB to promote expression of antiapoptotic genes such as Bcl-2 and Mn superoxide dismutase suggests that NFκB can also promote cell survival (68). Along these lines, overexpression of NFκB *in vitro* renders neurons more resistant to glucose deprivation and to glutamate excitotoxicity (69). NFκB also promotes expression of nuclear apoptosis inhibitor protein (NAIP; see below), which renders neurons more resistant to ischemia *in vivo* (70,71). NFκB activates inducible NOS and cyclooxygenase-2 and plays a major role in later stages of inflammatory ischemic brain injury (72).

In conclusion, certain strategies may be required to intervene early in brain inflammation to reduce injury and neurodegeneration; other interventions may be needed to facilitate repair and recovery of regenerating processes after central nervous system injury (73,74). On the same lines, the timing of specific interventions may be critical to the development of significant neuroprotective antiinflammatory therapy.

APOPTOSIS

Cell death following cerebral ischemia has been described as either necrotic or apoptotic by histologic criteria. This rather arbitrary and sometimes misleading classification is more appropriately defined by a continuum of biochemical processes, which has apoptosis and necrosis at opposite poles. Ischemic cell death within the brain is an active process that requires energy, involves new gene expression, and is caspase mediated (apoptotic proteolytic pathways; Fig. 18-4) (12,75). The process of apoptosis refers to "programmed" cell death. Apoptosis occurs in the nervous system during development, as well as during a number of pathophysiologic processes such as neurodegeneration and ischemia. It is mediated by DNA cleavage and by other autolytic processes causing nuclear shrinkage, chromatin clumping, cytoplasmic blebbing, and `ultimate cell death. During ischemia, brain cells that are exposed to excessive glutamate receptor activation, Ca^{2+} overload, oxygen radicals, or mitochondria and DNA damage can die by necrosis or apoptosis. This may depend on the nature of the stimulus, the type of cell, and the stage it has reached in its development. Necrosis is the predominant mechanism that follows acute permanent focal vascular occlusion or global ischemia, whereas in milder injury, death may resemble apoptosis. The pathway of apoptosis is initiated by early involvement of mitochondria, which, in turn, leads to the triggering the genes for proteolytic processes, such as the

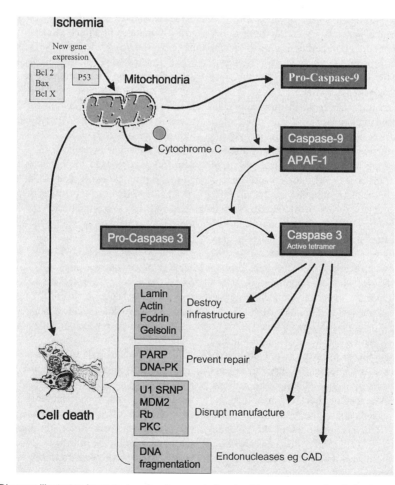

FIG. 18-4. Diagram illustrates important molecular events involved in programmed cell death. Following stroke, there is an early response in gene expression such as in the Bcl-2 family and p53. There then is a release of proapoptogenic molecules such as cytochrome *c* and apoptosis-inducing factor (AIF) from the mitochondria, which may result in increased leakiness of the mitochondrial permeability transition (MPT) pore. There is subsequent activation of the caspase cascade with formation of active tetramers of caspases (caspase-3). Such active effector caspases, in turn, cause the proteolytic demolition of key structural and functional systems of the cell, including shredding of the genome into ordered deoxyribonucleic acid (DNA) fragments. These lethal events culminate in the cell's morphology in the nucleus and atrophy of the dendritic tree.

caspases, as well as genes that suppress or augment cell death. Three major classes of genes control apoptosis. These include (a) those that prevent cell death, like bcl-2 and bcl-xL; (b) those that promote cell death, like bax and bcl-xs; and (c) those that promote the engulfment and destruction of cells. Drugs that block caspases (76) or enhance the action of bcl-2 (77) protect against ischemic injury. Of the 12 that have been identified, caspases-1 and -3 seem to have a pivotal role in ischemia-mediated apoptosis.

During ischemia, a sharp increase in the permeability of the mitochondria inner membrane occurs, termed the mitochondrial permeability transition (MPT). This has been known to occur in necrosis but has also been observed in apoptosis (78,79). The MPT leads to membrane depolarization, uncoupling of oxidative phosphorylation, release of intramitochondrial ions, and swelling, which, when severe, ruptures the outer membrane, releasing macromolecules into the cytoplasm. If membrane depolarization is incomplete, cellular recovery is possible. This release of apoptogenic substances activates a cascade of proteolytic caspase activity (80), leading to destruction of key structural and functional proteins, causing ultimate cell death. The Bcl-2 family of proteins are intimately involved in this mitochondrial release of killer molecules (81). If this programmed path is blocked, then ATP depletion due to energy failure will force the cell to necrosis.

During an ischemic insult, the mitochondria are extremely sensitive to ischemia. The ensuing acidosis, ATP depletion, depolarization, and Ca^{2+} overload are processes that ultimately damage the mitochondria. An MPT in mitochondria has been observed by 1 h (82). The inducibility of MPT depends on the cell type and brain region; for instance, hippocampus is more sensitive to ischemia than cortex, which is more sensitive than cerebellum. This also correlates with the susceptibility of these areas to ischemic damage (83).

The consequential release of mitochondrial components has been observed to result in the redistribution of cytochrome c in focal ischemia (84). A similar appearance of cytochrome c in the cytoplasm of ischemically vulnerable hippocampal CA necrosis was observed following global ischemia in the gerbil by a combination of cell fractionation and Western blotting methods (85). Another mitochondrial component, caspase-9, has also been identified to be involved in the proteolytic cascade (86).

Apoptotic cell death requires the expression of new genes. Genes related to the Bcl-2 family and those related to P53 have been identified to be important in the active cell death. Bcl-2 is an integral membrane protein, found predominantly in the mitochondrial outer membrane, which is targeted by translocation of Bax following a cell death signal. Bax may lead to the formation of pores through which killer molecules such as cytochrome c may escape. In nonneuronal cells, pathways leading to caspase activation are well characterized (87): BID is a 22-kDa cytosolic, proapoptotic Bcl-2 family member and plays a role in linking cell death receptor activation to downstream events (88,89). Death receptor activation (Fas/TNF family) activates caspase-8, which cleaves BID. Truncated BID is targeted to the outer mitochondrial membrane and induces conformational changes of Bak and Bax, leading to cytochrome c release (90–92). BID is expressed in the brain and plays a role in cerebral ischemia. Transcription factors such as P53 lie within a network of interrelated genes associated with cell death and can lead to up-regulation of target genes such as Bax and those involved in generating reactive oxygen species (93).

Transgenic and knock-out mice have been used to define the role of the Bcl-2 family members in ischemic cell death. Overexpression of antiapoptotic Bcl-2 reduced focal brain infarct by 42% at 7 days after middle cerebral artery occlusion (94). After focal cerebral ischemia, BID is cleaved by caspase-8, before cytochrome c release and caspase-3 activation. Cytochrome c release is reduced and infarct volumes are smaller in BID knock-out mice (95).

In focal ischemia, a disturbance in the ratio of Bax/Bcl-2 levels has been seen in rat cortex at 6 h at the border of the lesion (96) or overall at 24 h (97) and at 3 to 12 h in mice (98), which is consistent with the findings of increased Bcl-2 expression in surviving neurons at 24 h (99). Bcl-2 levels are also increased (without change in levels of Bax) after focal cerebral ischemia in mice lacking neuronal NOS. These mice are more resistant to focal cerebral ischemia, with smaller infarcts and fewer terminal deoxyribosyltransferase-mediated fluorescein-dUTP nick end labeling (TUNEL)-positive neurons than wild-type controls (100).

In global ischemia, hippocampal Bax levels were increased by 60% by 6 h and remained so for 72 h. Bax appeared to favor apoptosis by binding the antiapoptotic species Bcl-x (101), and other studies have shown an imbalance of proapoptotic Bax concomitant with a decrease in the antiapoptotic Bcl-2 and Bcl-x proteins (102). The outcome of the opposing actions of the genes will depend on the duration of the ischemia, location of the lesion, energy supply, and other modulating factors.

P53 has been reported to be elevated following focal cerebral ischemia (103), and both p53 messenger RNA and protein have shown to be elevated at the periphery of the infarct (104,105). In the absence of p53 gene, there was reduced infarct volume (106). In global ischemia, increased p53 has also been reported in both CA1 and CA3 at 24 h but only in CA1 by 48 h (107). The importance of this is not clear, especially as increased p53 levels have been identified in the ischemia-resistant CA3 neurons (108), which appears independent of the duration and severity of the ischemia.

Caspases are a family of cysteine proteases involved in regulating cytokine maturation and apoptosis (109), of which 14 have been identified and divided into three groups. Caspases can be classified according to their amino acid sequence homology into caspase-1, -3, and -9 subfamilies. The caspase-1 subfamily includes 1, 4, 5, and 11. As the predominant defect of caspase-1 knock-out mice is the inability to process pro-IL-1B, the major function of caspase-1 is believed to be regulating cytokine maturation (110). On the other hand, caspase-1 is responsible for the activation of executioner caspases, directly involved in apoptosis progression (111). Further evidence that caspase-1 activation could play a pivotal role in the ischemic neurodegeneration comes from caspase-1–/– mice and mice expressing a dominant negative mutant caspase-1 gene. Both of these genetically modified mouse strains are more resistant to ischemic insult than wild-type mice (112). The effects of caspase inhibition on cerebral ischemia induced neurodegeneration are seen by using the non-selective inhibitors z-VAD.fmk and z-DVED.fmk. Both inhibitors induced a significant neuroprotection in mouse models of transient cerebral ischemia (113–115), and z-VAD.fmk was neuroprotective also in transient and permanent models in the rat (116,117).

The caspase-3 subfamily is a group II member and includes caspase-3, -6, -7, -8, and -10, with long prodomains. Caspase-3 has been shown to be a major execution caspase that acts downstream in the apoptosis pathway and is involved in cleaving important substrates such as inhibitor of caspase-activated DNase (ICAD), which activates the apoptotic DNA ladder form activity (caspase-activated DNase) (117,118). Mice null for caspase-3 display neuronal expansion, usually resulting in death by the second week of life. Two known pathways that can activate procaspase-3 are through proteolytic cleavage by caspase-8 and -9. Activated caspase-8 can be detected in neurons after spinal cord ischemia (119). Peptide-based caspase inhibitors prevent neuronal loss. During transient focal ischemia, levels of NAIP become elevated. Therefore, increased NAIP levels may confer protection. This is supported by two treatments that elevate NAIP and that reduce ischemic damage: systemic administration of the bacterial K252a and intracerebral injection of an adenovirus vector capable of overexpressing NAIP *in vivo*.

Trophic factors are well known for their antiapoptotic role during development. They are also important in cerebral ischemia. Basic fibroblast growth factor protects neurons *in vitro* against various noxious stimuli (120). In focal cerebral ischemia, exogenous basic fibroblast growth factor up-regulates Bcl-2 in the penumbra (121) and protects synergistically with caspase inhibitors by reducing caspase-3 activation (122–127). Exogenous administration of BDNF and neurotrophin (NT) 4 reduces ischemic damage in different animal models of cerebral ischemia (123–126). Endogenous BDNF and NT-4 also exert a protective effect, as mice lacking either one allele of BDNF or both alleles of NT-4 are more vulnerable to focal cerebral ischemia (127). Surprisingly, conditional knock-out mice lacking NT-3 expression in the central nervous system develop smaller lesions than wild-type littermates (128). *In vitro*, NT-3 enhances oxygen/glucose deprivation-induced neuronal death, and this enhancement is blocked by the oxygen free radical chelator Trolox (Hoffman La Roche, Basel, Switzerland), suggesting that NT-3 potentiates oxygen radical-mediated neuronal death (128).

CONCLUSION

In conclusion, this review has outlined a complex cascade of biochemical and associated electrophysiologic mechanisms involved in ischemic brain injury. Several experiments of neuronal ischemic injury have produced evidence suggesting that neuronal death may be mediated by the effects of excitatory neurotransmitters such as glutamate, which promote Ca^{2+} entry into the cells, the release of oxygen free radicals, and the accumulation of lactic acid during a switch to anaerobic metabolism. In addition to these processes, there are a number of microcirculatory processes that precede or occur during these processes and may exacerbate injury. Polymorphonuclear leukocytes play several roles in the maturation of focal ischemia, especially during reperfusion. They contribute to the local hemostatic changes in the microcirculation and edema formation and increase postcapillary venule endothelial permeability, free radical generation, and ultimately infarct maturation. At the same time, the type of cell death encountered *in vivo* in several neuropathologic conditions and *in vitro* in neuronal cultures exposed to glutamate may depend on the intensity of the exposure and may involve temporally distinct phases. Necrotic cell death, for instance, may simply reflect the failure of neurons to carry out programmed cell death (as seen with apoptosis) used to dispose efficiently of aged or damaged cells simply because of severe energy failure. The maintenance of mitochondrial function may therefore be the limiting factor in determining the degree and progression of neuronal injury caused by excitotoxins.

REFERENCES

1. Raichle M. The pathophysiology of brain ischemia. *Ann Neurol* 1983;13:2–10.
2. Wise RJ, Rhodes CG, Gibbs JM, et al. Disturbance of oxidative metabolism of glucose in recent human cerebral infarcts. *Ann Neurol* 1983;14:627–637.
3. Heiss WD, Hayakawa T, Waltz AG . Cortical neuronal function during ischemia. Effects of occlusion of one middle cerebral artery on single-unit activity in cats. *Arch Neurol* 1976;33:813–820.
4. Hakim AM. The cerebral ischemic penumbra. *Can J Neurol Sci* 1987;14:557–559.
5. Astrup J, Siesjø BK, Symon L. Thresholds in cerebral ischemia—the ischemic penumbra. *Stroke* 1981;12:723–725.
6. Memezawa H, Smith M-L, Siesjø BK. Penumbral tissues salvaged by reperfusion following middle cerebral artery occlusion in rats. *Stroke* 1992;23:552–559.
7. Hossmann K-A. Disturbances of cerebral protein synthesis and ischemic cell death. In: Kogure K, Hossmann KA, Siesjø BK, eds. *Progress in brain research, vol 96: neurobiology of ischemic brain damage*, New York: Dana Press;1993:161–181.
8. Miller RJ. Multiple calcium channels and neuronal function. *Science* 1987;235:46–53.
9. Siesjø BK. Pathophysiology and treatment of focal cerebral ischemia. Part I: pathophysiology. *J Neurosurg* 1992;77:169–184.
10. Siesjö BK . Pathophysiology and treatment of focal cerebral ischemia. Part II: pathophysiology. *J Neurosurg* 1992;77:351–354.
11. Tyson RL, Sutherland GR, Peeling J. ^{23}Na nuclear magnetic resonance spectral changes during and after forebrain ischemia in hypoglycemic, normoglycemic, and hyperglycemic rats. *Stroke* 1996;27:957–964.
12. Baudry M, Bundman MC, Smith EK, et al. Micromolar calcium stimulates proteolysis and glutamate binding in rat brain synaptic membranes. *Science* 1981;212:937–938.
13. Siesjö BK, Kristian T, Katsura K. Overview of bioenergetic failure and metabolic cascades in brain ischemia In: Ginsberg MD, Bogousslavsky J, eds. *Cerebrovascular disease. Volume 1: Pathophysiology, diagnosis and management*. Malden, MA: Blackwell Science, 1998:3–13.
14. Katsura K, Kristian T, Smith ML, et al. Acidosis induced by hypercapnia exaggerates ischemic brain damage. *J Cereb Blood Flow Metab* 1994;14:243–250.
15. Budd SL. Mechanisms of neuronal damage in brain hypoxia/ischemia: focus on the role of mitochondrial

16. calcium accumulation. *Pharmacol Ther* 1998;80:203–229.
16. Dirnagl U, Iadecola C, Moskowitz MA. Pathobiology of ischaemic stroke: an integrated view. *Trends Neurosci* 1999;22:391–397.
17. Davalos A, Fernandez-Real JM, Rilart M. Iron related damage in acute ischemic stroke. *Stroke* 1994;24:1543–1546.
18. Cao W, Carney JM, Duchan A, et al. Oxygen free radical involvement in ischemia and reperfusion injury to brain. *Neurosci Lett* 1998;88:233–238.
19. Rothwell NJ. Cytokines and acute neurodegeneration. *Mol Psychiatry* 1997;2:120–121.
20. Guillian D, Chen J, Ingman JE, et al. The role of mononuclear phagocytes in wound healing after traumatic injury to adult mammalian brain. *J Neurosci* 1989;9:4410–4429.
21. Hallenbeck JM, Dutka AJ, Tanishima T, et al. Polymorphonuclear leukocyte accumulation in brain regions with low blood flow during the early postischemic period. *Stroke* 1986;17:246–253.
22. Chen H, Chopp M, Bodzin G. Neutropenia reduces the volume of cerebral infarct after transient middle cerebral artery occlusion in the rat. *Neurosci Res Commun* 1992;11:93–99.
23. Dereski MO, Chopp M, Knight RA, et al. Focal cerebral ischemia in the rat: temporal profile of neutrophil responses. *Neurosci Res Commun* 1992;11:179–186.
24. Clark RK, Lee EV, Fish CJ, et al. Development of tissue damage, inflammation and resolution following stroke: an immunohistochemical and quantitative planimetric study. *Brain Res Bull* 1993;35:623–639.
25. Ritter L, Coull B, Davisgomen G, et al. Leukocytes accumulate in the cerebral microcirculation during the first hour of reperfusion following stroke. *FASEB J* 1998;12:188.
26. Barone FC, Hillegass ZM, Rzimas MN, et al. Polymorphonuclear leukocyte infiltration into cerebral focal ischemic tissue: myeloperoxidase activity and histologic verification. *J Neurosci Res* 1991;29:336–345.
27. Barone FC, Hillegass ZM, Rzimas MN, et al. Time related changes in myeloperoxidase activity and leukotriene B4 receptor binding reflect leukocyte influx in cerebral focal stroke. *Mol Chem Neuropathol* 1995;24:13–30.
28. Pozzilli C, Lenzi GL, Argentino C, et al. Imaging of leukocyte infiltration in lumen cerebral infarcts. *Stroke* 1985;16:251–255.
29. Dukta AJ, Kochanek PM, Hallenbeck JM. Influence of granulocytopenia on canine cerebral ischemia induced by embolism. *Stroke* 1989;20:390–395.
30. Feuerstein GZ, Wang XK, Barone FC. Inflammatory mediators of ischemic injury: cytokine gene regulation in stroke. In: Ginsberg MD, Bogousslowsky J, eds. *Cerebrovascular disease: pathophysiology, diagnosis and management.* New York: Blackwell Science,1998:507–531.
31. Kochanek PM, Hallenback JM. Polymorphonuclear leukocytes and monocytes/macrophages in the pathogenesis of cerebral ischemia and stroke. *Stroke* 1992;23:1367–1379.
32. Del Zoppo GJ, Schmid-Schonbein GW, Mori E, et al. Polymorphonuclear leukocytes occlude capillaries following middle cerebral artery occlusion and reperfusion in baboons. *Stroke* 1991;22:1276–1283.

33. Liu T, Clark RK, McDonnell PC, et al. Tumor necrosis factor-α expression in ischemic neurons. *Stroke* 1994; 25:1481–1488.

34. Wang XK, Yue T-L, Barone FC, et al. Concomitant cortical expression of TNFα and IL-1β mRNA following transient focal ischemia. *Mol Chem Neuropathol* 1994;23:103–114.

35. Rothwell NJ. Functions and mechanisms of interleukin-1 in the brain. *Trends Pharmacol Sci* 1991;12: 430–435.

36. Dinarello CA. Biology of interleukin-1. *FASEB J* 1996;2:108–115.

37. Minami M, Kyraishi Y, Yabunchi K, et al. Induction of interleukin-1β mRNA in rat brain after transient forebrain ischemia. *J Neurochem* 1992;58:390–392.

38. Yababuchi K, Minami M, Katsumata S, et al. An in situ hybridisation study on interleukin-1β mRNA induced by transient forebrain ischemia in the rat brain. *Mol Brain Res* 1994;26:135–142.

39. Loddick SA, Rothwell NJ. Neuroprotective effects of human recombinant interleukin-1 receptor. *J Cereb Blood Flow Metab* 1996;16:932–940.

40. Betz AL, Yang G-Y, Davidson BL. Attenuation of stroke size in rats using an adenoviral vector to induce overexpression of interleukin-1 receptor antagonist in brain. *J Cereb Blood Flow Metab* 1995;15:547–551.

41. Relton JK, Martin D, Thompson RC, et al. Peripheral administration of interleukin-1 receptor antagonist inhibits brain damage after focal cerebral ischemia in the rat. *Exp Neurol* 1996;138:206–213.

42. Iadecola C, Zhang F, Casey R, et al. Delayed reduction of ischemic brain injury and neurological deficits in mice lacking the inducible nitric oxide synthase gene. *J Neurosci* 1997;17:9157–9164.

43. Hsu CY, An G, Liu JS, et al. Expression of immediate early gene and growth factor mRNAs in a focal cerebral ischemia model in the rat. *Stroke* 1993;24:178.

44. Wang XK, Yue TL, Young PR, et al. Expression of interleukin-6, c-fos, and zif268 mRNA in rat ischemic cortex. *J Cereb Blood Flow Metab* 1995;15: 166–171.

45. Wang XK, Yue TL, Barone FC, et al. Macrocyte chemoattractant protein-1 (MCP-1) mRNA expression in rat ischemic cortex. *Stroke* 1995;26:661–666.

46. Wang XK, Barone FC, Aiyar NV, et al. Increased interleukin-1 receptor and interleukin-1 receptor antagonist gene expression after focal stroke. *Stroke* 1997;28: 155–162.

47. Liu T, Young PR, McDonnell PC, et al. Cytokine-induced neutrophil chemoattractant mRNA expressed in cerebral ischemia. *Neurosci Lett* 1993;164: 125–128.

48. Wang XK, Ellison JA, Siren AL, et al. Prolonged expression of interferon inducible protein 10 in ischemic cortex after permanent occlusion of the middle cerebral artery in the rat. *J Neurochem* 1995;71: 1194–1204.

49. Wang XK, Siren AL, Yue TL, et al. Up-regulation of adhesion molecule-1 (ICAM-1) on brain microvascular endothelial cells in rat ischemic cortex. *Mol Brain Res* 1994;26:61–68.

50. Wang XK, Yue TL, Barone FC, et al. Demonstration of increased endothelial—leukocyte adhesion molecule 1 mRNA expression in rat ischemic cortex. *Stroke* 1995; 26:1665–1669.

51. Okada Y, Copeland BR, Mori E, et al. P-Selectin and intercellular adhesion molecule-1 expression after focal brain ischemia and reperfusion. *Stroke* 1994; 25: 202–211.

52. Li Y, Chopp M, Zhang ZG, et al. P53-immunoreactive protein and P53 mRNA expression after transient middle cerebral artery occlusion in rats. *Stroke* 1994;25: 849–856.

53. Rosenberg GA, Navratil M, Barone F, et al. Proteolytic cascade enzymes increase in focal cerebral ischemia in rat. *J Cereb Blood Flow Metab* 1996;16:360–366.

54. Romanic AM, White RF, Arleth AJ, et al. Matrix metalloproteinase expression increases following cerebral ischemia: inhibition of MMP-9 reduces infarct size. *Stroke* 1998;29:1020–1030.

55. Wang XK, Barone FC, White RF, et al. Subtractive cloning identifies tissue inhibitor matrix metalloproteinase-1 (TIMP-1) increased gene expression in focal stroke. *Stroke* 1998;29:516–520.

56. Ellison JA, Vellier JJ, Spera PA, et al. Osteopontin and its integrin receptor avb3 are up-regulated during formation of the glial scar following focal stroke. *Stroke* 1998;29:1698–1707.

57. Garcia JE, Nonner D, Ross D, et al. Neurotoxic components in normal serum. *Exp Neurol* 1992;118: 309–316.

58. Bruce AJ, Boling W, Kindy MS, et al. Altered neuronal and microglial responses to excitotoxic and ischemic brain in mice lacking TNF receptors. *Nat Med* 1996;2: 788– 794.

59. Rothwell NJ, Luheshi GN. Brain TNF: damage limitation or damaged reputation? *Nat Med* 1996;2: 746–747.

60. Ouktsuki T, Reutzler CA, Tasaki K, et al. Induction of tolerance to ischemia by preconditioned interleukin-1a in gerbil hippocampal neurons. *J Cereb Blood Flow Metab* 1996;16:1137–1142.

61. Nawashiro H, Tasaki K, Ruetzlav CA, et al. TNF-alpha pretreatment induces protective effects against focal cerebral ischemia in mice. *J Cereb Blood Flow Metab* 1997;17:483–490.

62. Hirschberg DL, Yoles E, Belkin M, et al. Inflammation after axonal injury has conflicting consequences for recovery of function: rescue of spared axons is impaired but regeneration is supported. *J Neuroimmunol* 1994;50:9–16.

63. Baeuerle PA, Baltimore D. NF-kappa B: ten years after. *Cell* 1996;87:13–20.

64. Carroll JE, Hess DC, Howard EF, et al. Is nuclear factor-kappaB a good treatment target in brain ischemia/reperfusion injury? *NeuroReport* 2000;11: R1–R4.

65. Salminen A, Liu PK, Hsu CY. Alteration of transcription factor binding activities in the ischemic rat brain. *Biochem Biophys Res Commun* 1995;212:939–944.

66. Schneider A, Martin-Villalba A, Weih F, et al. NF-kappaB is activated and promotes cell death in focal cerebral ischemia. *Nat Med* 1999;5:554–559.

67. Buchan AM, Li H, Blackburn B. Neuroprotection achieved with a novel proteasome inhibitor which blocks NF-kappa B activation. *NeuroReport* 2000;11: 427–430.

68. Mattson MP, Goodman Y, Luo H, et al. Activation of NF-kappaB protects hippocampal neurons against oxidative stress-induced apoptosis: evidence for induc-

tion of manganese superoxide dismutase and suppression of peroxynitrite production and protein tyrosine nitration. *J Neurosci Res* 1997;49:681–697.

69. Yu Z, Zhou D, Bruce-Keller AJ, et al. Lack of the p50 subunit of nuclear factor-kappaB increases the vulnerability of hippocampal neurons to excitotoxic injury. *J Neurosci* 1999;19:8856–8865.

70. Xu DG, Crocker SJ, Doucet JP, et al. Elevation of neuronal expression of NAIP reduces ischemic damage in the rat hippocampus. *Nat Med* 1997;3:997–1004.

71. Stehlik C, de Martin R, Binder BR, et al. Cytokine induced expression of porcine inhibitor of apoptosis protein (iap) family member is regulated by NF-kappa B. *Biochem Biophys Res Commun* 1998;243:827–832.

72. Iadecola C, Alexander M. Cerebral ischemia and inflammation. *Curr Opin Neurol* 2001;14:89–94.

73. Dopp J, de Vellis J. Strategies or therapeutic manipulation of cytokines and their receptors in inflammatory neurodegenerative diseases. *Ment Retard Dev Disabil Res Rev*1998;4:200–211.

74. Lazarov-Spiegler O, Rapalino O, Agranov G, et al. Restricted inflammatory reaction in CNS: a key impediment to axonal regeneration? *Mol Med Today* 1998;4:337–342.

75. Lee JL, Zipfel GJ, Choi DW. The changing landscape of ischaemic brain injury mechanisms. *Nature* 1999; 399[Suppl]:A7–A14.

76. Li H, Zhu H, Xu CJ, et al. Cleavage of BID by caspase 8 mediates the mitochondrial damage in the Fas pathway of apoptosis. *Cell* 1998;94:491–501.

77. Adams JM, Cory S. The Bcl-2 protein family: arbiters of cell survival. *Science* 1998;281:1322–1326.

78. Lemasters JJ, Qian T, Elmore SP, et al. Confocal microscopy of the mitochondrial permeability transition in necrotic cell killing, apoptosis and autophagy. *Biofactors* 1998;8:283–285.

79. Murphy AN, Fiskum G, Beal MF. Mitochondria in neurodegeneration: bioenergetic function in cell life and death. *J Cereb Blood Flow Metab* 1999;19: 231–245.

80. Eldadah BA, Faden AI . Caspase pathways, neuronal apoptosis and CNS injury. *J Neurotrauma* 2000;17: 811–829.

81. Graham SH, Chen J, Clark RSB. Bcl-2 family gene products in cerebral ischemia and traumatic brain injury. *J Neurotrauma* 2000;17:831–841.

82. Ouyang YB, Kuroda S, Kristian T, et al. Release of mitochondrial aspartate aminotransferase (mast) following transient focal cerebral ischemia suggests the opening of a mitochondrial permeability transition pore. *Neurosci Res Commun* 1997;20:167–173.

83. Friberg H, Connern C, Halestrap AP, et al. Differences in the activation of the mitochondrial permeability transition among brain regions in the rat correlate with selective vulnerability. *J Neurochem* 1999;72:2488–2497.

84. Fujimura M, Morita-Fujimura Y, Kawase M, et al. Manganese superoxide dismutase mediates the early release of mitochondrial cytochrome C and subsequent DNA fragmentation after permanent focal cerebral ischemia in mice. *J Neurosci* 1999;19:3414–3422.

85. Antonawich FJ. Translocation of cytochrome C following transient global ischemia in the gerbil. *Neurosci Lett* 1999;274:123–126.

86. Krajewski S, Krajewska M, Ellerby LM, et al. Release of caspase-9 from mitochondria during neuronal apoptosis and cerebral ischemia. *Proc Natl Acad Sci USA* 1999;96:5752–5757.

87. Strasser A, O'Connor L, Dixit VM. Apoptosis signaling [Review]. *Annu Rev Biochem* 2000;69:217–245.

88. Wang K, Yin XM, Chao DT, et al. BID: a novel BH3 domain-only death agonist. *Genes Dev* 1996;10: 2859–2869.

89. Nagata S. Biddable death. *Nat Cell Biol* 1999;1: E143–E145.

90. Li H, Colbourne F, Sun P, et al. Caspase inhibitors reduce neuronal injury after focal but not global cerebral ischemia in rats. *Stroke* 2000;31:176–182.

91. Zha J, Weiler S, Oh KJ, et al. Posttranslational *N*-myristoylation of BID as a molecular switch for targeting mitochondria and apoptosis. *Science* 2000;290: 1761–1765.

92. Wei MC, Lindsten T, Mootha VK, et al. tBID, a membrane-targeted death ligand, oligomerizes BAK to release cytochrome c. *Genes Dev* 2000;14: 2060–2071.

93. Sionov RV, Haupt Y. The cellular response to p53: the decision between life and death. *Oncogene* 1999;18: 6145–6157.

94. Martinou JC, Dubois-Dauphin M, Staple JK, et al. Overexpression of BCL-2 in transgenic mice protects neurons from naturally occurring cell death and experimental ischemia. *Neuron* 1994;13:1017–1030.

95. Plesnila N, Zinkel S, Le DA, et al. BID mediates neuronal cell death after oxygen/glucose deprivation and focal cerebral ischemia. *Proc Natl Acad Sci USA* 2001; 98:15318–15323.

96. Gillardon F, Lenz C, Waschke KF, et al. Altered expression of Bcl-2, Bcl-X, and c-Fos colocalizes with DNA fragmentation and ischemic cell damage following middle cerebral artery occlusion in rats. *Mol Brain Res* 1996;40:254–260.

97. Dubal DB, Shughrue PJ, Wilson ME, et al. Estradiol modulates bcl-2 in cerebral ischemia: a potential role for estrogen receptors. *J Neurosci* 1999;19:494–498.

98. Matsushita K, Matsuyama T, Kitagawa K, et al. Alterations of Bcl-2 family proteins precede cytoskeletal proteolysis in the penumbra, but not in infarct centres following focal cerebral ischemia in mice. *Neuroscience* 1998;83:439–448.

99. Chen J, Graham SH, Chan PH, et al. Bcl-2 is expressed in neurons that survive focal ischemia in the rat. *Neuroreport* 1995;6(2):394–398.

100. Elibol B, Söylemezoglu F, Ünal I, et al. Nitric oxide is involved in ischemia-induced apoptosis in brain: a study in neuronal nitric oxide synthase null mice. *Neuroscience* 2001;105:79–86.

101. Antonawich FJ, Krajewski S, Reed JC. Bcl-xL Bax interaction after transient global ischemia. *J Cereb Blood Flow Metab* 1998;18:882–886.

102. Krajewski S, Mai JK, Krajewska M. Up-regulation of Bax protein levels in neurons following cerebral ischemia. *J Neurosci* 1995;15:6364–6376.

103. Chopp M, Li Y, Zhang ZG, et al. P53 expression in brain after middle cerebral artery occlusion in the rat. *Biochem Biophys Res Commun* 1992;182:1201–1207.

104. Li Y, Chopp M, Zhang ZG, et al. P53 immunoreactive protein and P53 mRNA expression after transient middle cerebral artery occlusion in rats. *Stroke* 1994;25: 849–856.

105. Park SW, Kim YB, Hwang SN, et al. The effects of *N*-methyl-*N*-nitrosourea and azoxymethane on focal

cerebral infarction and the expression of p53, p21 proteins. *Brain Res* 2000;855:298–306.

106. Crumrine RC, Thomas AL, Morgan PF. Attenuation of p53 expression protects against focal ischemic damage in transgenic mice. *J Cereb Blood Flow Metab* 1994; 14:887–891.

107. McGrahan L, Hakim AM, Robertson GS. Hippocampal Myc and P53 expression following transient global ischemia. *Mol Brain Res* 1998;56:133–145.

108. Tomasevic G, Kamme F, Stubberod P, et al. The tumour suppressor p53 and its response gene p21WAF/Cip1 are not markers of neuronal death following transient global cerebral ischemia. *Neuroscience* 1999;90:781–792.

109. Cryns V, Yuan J. Proteases to die for. *Genes Dev* 1998; 12:1551–1570.

110. Kuida K, Loppke JA, Ku G, et al. Altered cytokine export and apoptosis in mice deficient in interlekin 1b converting enzyme. *Science* 1995;217:2000–2002.

111. Denner L. Caspases in apoptic death. *Exp Opin Invest Drugs* 1999;8:37–50.

112. Hara H, Fink K, Endres M, et al. Attenuation of transient focal cerebral ischemia injury in transgenic mice expressing a mutant ICE inhibitory protein. *J Cereb Blood Flow Metab* 1997;17:370–375.

113. Hara H, Friedlander RM, Gagliardini V, et al. Inhibition of interleukin 1? Converting enzyme family proteases reduce ischemic and excitotoxic neuronal damage. *Proc Natl Acad Sci USA* 1997;94:2007–2012.

114. Endres M, Namura S, Shimizu-Sasamota M, et al. Attenuation of delayed neuronal death after mild focal ischemia in mice by inhibition of the caspase family. *J Cereb Blood Flow Metab* 1998;18:238–247.

115. Ma J, Endres M, Moskowitz MA. Synergistic effects of caspase inhibitors and MK-801 in brain injury after transient focal cerebral ischemia in mice. *Br J Pharmacol* 1998;124:756–762.

116. Loddick SA, MacKenzie A, Rothwell NJ. An ICE inhibitor z-VAD-dbc attenuates ischaemic brain damage in the rat. *Neuroreport* 1996;7:1465–1468.

117. Enari M, Sakahira H, Yokoyama H, et al. A caspase activated DNase that degrades DNA during apoptosis, and its inhibitor ICAD. *Nature* 1998;391:43–50.

118. Sakahira H, Enari M, Nagata S. Cleavage of CAD inhibitor in CAD activation and DNA degradation during apoptosis. *Nature* 1998;391:96–99.

119. Matsushita K, Wu Y, Qiu J, et al. Fas receptor and neuronal cell death after spinal cord ischemia. *J Neurosci* 2000;20:6879–6887.

120. Mattson MP, Lovell MA, Furukawa K, et al. Neurotrophic factors attenuate glutamate-induced accumulation of peroxides, elevation of intracellular Ca^{2+} concentration, and neurotoxicity and increase antioxidant enzyme activities in hippocampal neurons. *J Neurochem* 1995;65:1740–1751.

121. Ay I, Sugimori H, Finklestein SP. Intravenous basic fibroblast growth factor (bFGF) decreases DNA fragmentation and prevents down-regulation of Bcl-2 expression in the ischemic brain following middle cerebral artery occlusion in rats. *Brain Res Mol Brain Res* 2001;87:71–80.

122. Ma J, Qiu J, Hirt L, et al. Synergistic protective effect of caspase inhibitors and bFGF against brain injury induced by transient focal ischaemia. *Br J Pharmacol* 2001;133:345–350.

123. Beck T, Lindholm D, Castren E, et al. Brain-derived neurotrophic factor protects against ischemic cell damage in rat hippocampus. *J Cereb Blood Flow Metab* 1994;14:689–692.

124. Tsukahara T, Yonekawa Y, Tanaka K, et al. The role of brain-derived neurotrophic factor in transient forebrain ischemia in the rat brain. *Neurosurgery* 1994;34: 323–331.

125. Chan PH. Reactive oxygen radicals in signaling and damage in the ischemic brain. *J Cereb Blood Flow Metab* 2001;21:2–14.

126. Schabitz WR, Schwab S, Spranger M, et al. Intraventricular brain-derived neurotrophic factor reduces infarct size after focal cerebral ischemia in rats. *J Cereb Blood Flow Metab* 1997;17:500–506.

127. Endres M, Fan G, Hirt L, et al. Ischemic brain damage in mice after selectively modifying BDNF or NT4 gene expression. *J Cereb Blood Flow Metab* 2000;20: 139–144.

128. Bates B, Hirt L, Thomas S, et al. Neurotrophin-3 promotes cell death induced by cerebral ischemia, oxygen-glucose deprivation, and oxidative stress: possible involvement of oxygen free radicals. *Neurobiol Dis* 2002;9:24–37.

Ischemic Stroke: Advances in Neurology, Vol. 92. Edited by
H.J.M. Barnett, Julien Bogousslavsky, and Heather Meldrum.
Lippincott Williams & Wilkins, Philadelphia © 2003.

19

Fifty Years at Framingham: Contributions to Stroke Epidemiology

Philip A. Wolf

Department of Neurology, Boston University School of Medicine, Boston, Massachusetts, U.S.A.

BACKGROUND

The Framingham Study, begun in 1948, is the longest-running prospective epidemiologic study of chronic disease in a free-living population. The Framingham Study has played an important role in defining the epidemiology of cardiovascular diseases including stroke. This chapter attempts to highlight and summarize the contributions to our understanding of cerebrovascular disease made by the Framingham Study investigators utilizing this unique general population sample.

After World War II, it was apparent that cardiovascular diseases and cancer were the major diseases affecting the U.S. population, with cardiovascular diseases approximately twice as common as cancer. By 1950, the toll of atherosclerotic disease had become apparent, with one man in three developing cardiovascular disease by age 60; one in every six coronary attacks presented as sudden death. In fact, sudden death was the initial symptom of the disease, and half of all coronary deaths were sudden, occurring outside the hospital. Clearly, a preventive approach was needed.

THE FRAMINGHAM STUDY

Dr. Gilcin F. Meadors, a young U.S. Public Health Service officer, began enrolling volunteers for a cardiovascular disease study in Framingham, MA, in 1948. The National Heart Institute was established in 1949, and the nascent Framingham Study was placed under the institute's jurisdiction. A career Public Health Service officer, Dr. Cassius J. Van Slyke, the first National Health Institute director, decided the study population needed to be more representative of the town rather than comprised solely of volunteers.

Based on rough estimates of disease incidence, a study sample of 5,000 adult men and women, 30 to 60 years of age, were recruited for an anticipated 20-year study. It was expected that sufficient numbers of cases would develop in this group to permit the study of both coronary heart disease and hypertension. Van Slyke appointed another career Public Health Service officer, Dr. Thomas R. Dawber, as director of the study, a post he held for 16 years (1).

The town of Framingham was selected because it was a small, self-contained community of approximately 28,000 individuals, 20 miles west of Boston. Community leaders, including the members of the medical community, welcomed the opportunity to participate in this effort. Framingham, incorporated in 1700, has an illustrious history, with 5,000 residents, one-third of the population, serving as part of a "TB Demonstration Program" from 1916 to 1923 (2).

CONDUCT OF THE STUDY

The initial examination of the 5,209 men and women began in 1950 and took 2 years to complete. Thereafter, subjects returned for 26 biennial exams, with 85% of the surviving cohort members attending each exam. Exam 27 began in 2002. In 1971, 5,124 children (and their spouses) of the original Framingham cohort were recruited as a second generation to facilitate the study of familial occurrence of risk factors for and incidence of atherosclerotic disease. Offspring exam 7 was completed in 2001 (3). Beginning in 2002, approximately 3,500 children of this offspring cohort, the third generation (Gen3), were recruited to facilitate genetic and family studies of disease and risk factors, representing the largest number of Framingham Study families for whom data, deoxyribonucleic acid (DNA), and immortalized cell lines are available.

In 1971, the Framingham Study, which had been an "off campus" intramural program of the National Heart, Lung, and Blood Institute, was transferred to a different administrative structure, and it has been supported by the institute, which works collaboratively through a contract with Boston University School of Medicine. Dr. Dawber, who had recently retired from the U.S. Public Health Service and had joined Boston University School of Medicine as chair of the Section of Preventive Medicine, served as the first principal investigator of the Framingham contract. He was succeeded in 1978 by William B. Kannel, M.D., M.P.H. (following his retirement from the U.S. Public Health Service and his tour as the second Framingham Study director), and in 1988 by the author.

STROKE IN THE FRAMINGHAM HEART STUDY

The earliest reports from Framingham focused on coronary heart disease, but hypertension, stroke, congestive heart failure, and peripheral vascular disease were also under study. In 1961, the initial definitive report, titled "Factors of Risk in the Development of Coronary Heart Disease—Six-Year Follow-Up Experience: The Framingham Study," was published (4). Notable were both the title and the contents. This appears to be the first time the term "risk factor" was used, and it was the first report based on prospective epidemiologic study of coronary heart disease in a defined general population sample. The report definitively linked prior hypertension, an enlarged heart (left ventricular hypertrophy on the electrocardiogram), and elevated serum cholesterol level to coronary disease incidence. The first publications on stroke followed in 1965. It is apparent, even from these earliest publications, that the founders of the Framingham Study appreciated the clinical aspects of stroke and eschewed the practice of epidemiologists of the day to study "cerebrovascular accidents" as a single homogeneous nosologic entity. In 1967, the author, upon completion of his training in clinical neurology at Massachusetts General Hospital and profoundly influenced by C. Miller Fisher, M.D., was recruited to provide clinical neurologic expertise for the study of stroke. From the beginning, there was a deliberate effort to distinguish stroke from other neurologic events and to separate infarction from hemorrhage. This effort was facilitated by in-hospital evaluation of all Framingham Study subjects at Framingham Union Hospital, the only hospital in

town, soon after admission. At the time, there were few useful diagnostic tests available: radiographs of the skull, lumbar puncture, electroencephalographs, and, less commonly, cerebral angiography via direct arterial puncture. Differential diagnosis was, and continues to be, greatly facilitated by a detailed clinical history from subject and family and neurologic assessment of the subject shortly after admission for stroke.

As the technology evolved, computed tomography (CT) scans of the head were routine by the mid-1970s and magnetic resonance imaging (MRI) studies approximately 10 years later. With use of noninvasive cardiac and neurovascular testing and brain imaging, it was frequently possible to distinguish between the varieties of ischemic stroke: lacunar infarction, large-artery atherothrombotic disease, embolic stroke, and infarction of undetermined cause. However, separating hemorrhage from aneurysm (subarachnoid hemorrhage) from intracerebral hemorrhage, deep or lobar, was facilitated by the advent of CT scans of the brain, which were available for virtually all hospitalized subjects and for 85% of stroke cases overall. Systematic neurologic examination by a stroke neurologist, functional assessment by a rehabilitation nurse, cognitive assessment by a neuropsychologist, MRI of the brain, and MR angiography of the intracranial and cervical arteries (in addition to an admission CT scan of the head and conventional medical evaluation) have been performed since 1981 under grant support from the National Institute of Neurological and Communication Disorders and Stroke.

In the initial articles, it was clear that the majority of stroke events, 63%, were "thrombotic brain infarction." This frequency is quite similar to data available from later Framingham tabulations (and other populations) showing that approximately two-thirds of stroke events are secondary to atherothrombotic disease. The authors, recognizing that differing pathologies underlying stroke might have differing risk factors, focused on the epidemiology of thrombotic stroke, comparing it with the epidemiology of myocardial infarction.

Apart from death certificate records, data on the incidence of stroke in men and women at different ages were sparse. Information on the frequency of specific stroke subtypes was not available, and the relative frequencies of hemorrhages versus nonhemorrhages were unknown. Stroke case series, particularly surgery or autopsy series, formed the bases of knowledge of the frequency and distribution of stroke.

Epidemiology has been defined as the study of the distribution and determinants of disease prevalence in humans (5). Therefore, determining the incidence of specific stroke subtypes permitted a more complete assessment of the distribution of cerebrovascular disease and its determinants (risk factors). The initial publications in 1965 were based on a total of 90 cases of stroke of all types arising over 12 years of follow-up of the 5,106 persons previously free of coronary heart disease or stroke (6–8). Incidence of brain infarction (n = 57) by age and sex, in contrast to myocardial infarction, showed only a modest male predominance. Brain infarction was, however, related to many of the same risk factors predisposing to myocardial infarction (n = 157), but the marked male predominance seen for myocardial infarction was not present. Hypertension and cardiac impairments (electrocardiographic evidence of left ventricular hypertrophy, intraventricular block, and persistent ST- and T-wave abnormalities or heart enlargement on radiography) were significantly related to incidence of brain infarction. While exerting a similar impact on brain infarction, these measures were not statistically significant risk factors for thrombotic stroke. Upon comparison of data recorded on the death certificates with available clinical information for Framingham Study subjects, it was apparent that death certificates were neither sensitive nor specific for the stroke diagnostic rubrics, particularly for non-fatal infarcts and in the elderly (9).

The initial detailed assessment of a key stroke risk factor in Framingham was published in 1970, "Epidemiologic Assessment of the Role of Blood Pressure in Stroke" (10). This report, based on 14 years of follow-up of the original Framingham cohort, focused on 135 stroke events, 86 of which fulfilled criteria for the diagnosis of "atherothrombotic brain infarction" (ABI), a term coined by William B. Kannel to designate nonembolic and nonhemorrhagic stroke. At the time, definite hypertension was defined as a blood pressure of 160/95 mm Hg or higher, normotension was present at pressures below 140/90 mm Hg, with the remainder considered borderline.

The abstract of the *Journal of the American Medical Association* article outlines the key findings:

Prospectively, hypertension proved the most common and potent precursor of ABI's. Its contribution was direct and could not be attributed to factors related both to stroke and hypertension. Asymptomatic, causal [*sic*] "hypertension" was associated with a risk of ABI about four times that of normotensives. The probability of occurrence of an ABI was predicted no better with both blood pressure mea-

surements or the mean arterial pressure than with systolic alone. Since there was no diminishing impact of systolic pressure with advancing age, the concept that systolic elevations are, even in the aged, innocuous is premature. Comparing normotensives and hypertensives in each sex, women did not tolerate hypertension better than men.

Thus, casual systolic elevation of blood pressure, even in persons of advanced age, was the key risk factor for ABI. Further, it was not solely hypertension but blood pressure level that influenced risk of stroke. Further, there was no evidence of a safe or critical level of blood pressure, and the impact of the various components of the blood pressure did not diminish with advancing age. That intermediate levels of blood pressure, systolic and diastolic, carried intermediate risk for stroke was also underappreciated. It was well known that intracerebral hemorrhage was related to hypertension; the Framingham report showed the association with cerebral infarction was no less certain. Definite hypertension was a more potent risk factor for brain infarction than for coronary heart disease or intermittent claudication (peripheral arterial disease) but less than for the development of congestive heart failure. Twenty-five years later, when the article was designated as a Landmark Article by the editor, Nils Lassen (a reviewer of the original paper) noted that a number of key insights derived from the data in 1970 had been borne out from trial data: in particular, the prediction that reduction in blood pressure would reduce stroke incidence (11,12). Prior speculation by influential members of the neurologic and medical communities that reducing elevated blood pressure in the elderly would precipitate stroke, an idea amazingly persistent even into the 1990s, has been discredited (13,14). Further studies of these points relating elevations of blood pressure to stroke risk and the augmentation of the blood pressure risk by associated risk factors are now widely accepted (15–17). Amplification of the blood pressure–stroke relationship included an examination of the role of isolated systolic hypertension as a risk factor for stroke in the elderly (18,19). Recently, it was shown that even high normal blood pressure levels of 130 to 139 mm Hg systolic increased cardiovascular mortality (20) and stroke incidence (unpublished data). That elevated level of blood pressure, prior to the index or current pressure at age 50, 60, or 70 years, provides additional information on heightened risk was not unexpected but could now be shown because repeated blood pressures were available from the wealth of biennial exam data in Framingham (Table 19-1) (21).

TABLE 19-1. *Regression of ischemic stroke incidence on current and antecedent blood pressure measurements, by blood pressure component[a]*

Blood pressure measurement	Women			Men		
	Systolic blood pressure	Diastolic blood pressure	Pulse pressure	Systolic blood pressure	Diastolic blood pressure	Pulse pressure
Baseline age of 60 yr						
	71 ischemic strokes in 2,197 subjects			71 ischemic strokes in 1,564 subjects		
Current: age 60 yr	2.03 (1.69–2.44)	1.85 (1.56–2.21)	1.78 (1.48–2.15)	1.39 (1.12–1.72)	1.42 (1.15–1.74)	1.23 (0.98–1.53)
Recent past: mean age 50–59 yr[b]	1.68 (1.25–2.25)	1.78 (1.33–2.38)	1.80 (1.34–2.42)	1.92 (1.39–2.66)	1.73 (1.28–2.38)	1.82 (1.14–2.58)
Remote past: mean age 40–49 yr[b]	1.48 (1.07–2.07)	1.57 (1.13–2.17)	1.60 (1.08–2.38)	1.54 (0.96–2.45)	1.30 (0.86–1.91)	1.50 (0.88–2.56)
Baseline age of 70 yr						
	130 ischemic strokes in 1,875 subjects			101 ischemic strokes in 1,174 subjects		
Current: age 70 yr	1.61 (1.44–1.94)	1.49 (1.27–1.75)	1.53 (1.31–1.18)	1.53 (1.28–1.83)	1.08 (0.89–1.31)	1.86 (1.39–1.99)
Recent past: mean age 60–69 yr[b]	1.66 (1.28–2.14)	1.44 (1.11–1.88)	1.72 (1.31–2.27)	1.30 (0.97–1.75)	1.14 (0.84–1.54)	1.37 (0.99–1.90)
Remote past: mean age 50–59 yr[b]	1.41 (1.17–1.69)	1.47 (1.23–1.75)	1.52 (1.20–1.93)	1.45 (1.14–1.86)	1.42 (1.13–1.80)	1.51 (1.10–2.08)
Baseline age of 80 yr						
	81 ischemic strokes in 791 subjects			37 ischemic strokes in 412 subjects		
Current: age 80 yr	1.40 (1.13–1.73)	1.14 (0.91–1.43)	1.37 (1.10–1.69)	1.25 (0.92–1.71)	0.99 (0.71–1.38)	1.30 (0.95–1.77)
Recent past: mean age 70–79 yr[b]	1.19 (0.84–1.70)	1.21 (0.86–1.70)	1.12 (0.75–1.67)	1.25 (0.78–2.04)	1.32 (0.79–2.21)	1.12 (0.67–1.87)
Remote past: mean age 60–69 yr[b]	1.05 (0.19–1.42)	1.14 (0.86–1.51)	1.01 (0.69–1.49)	1.25 (0.81–1.93)	1.20 (0.80–1.79)	1.26 (0.74–2.16)

[a]Data are given as relative risk (95% confidence interval). All relative risks are presented per SD change in blood pressure component at baseline age and are adjusted for diabetes mellitus and smoking status.

[b]Relative risks for antecedent blood pressure measurements are also adjusted for current (baseline) blood pressure measurements.

In these analyses, the relative risks of stroke per standard deviation increment in current blood pressure are shown. The relative risks of stroke for the antecedent blood pressure measurements, after adjustment for current blood pressure, are also presented. Higher levels of pressure at the time of risk prediction were associated with increases in the 10-year risk of stroke by up to 103%, depending on the age at the time of risk assessment and the blood pressure component used (systolic, diastolic, or pulse pressure) to predict risk (Table 19-1). The effect of current blood pressure was strongest at the age of 60 years and weakest at the age of 80 years, and the relative risks were more marked for systolic and pulse pressures than for diastolic pressure at the age of 80 years (21).

IMPAIRED CARDIAC FUNCTION AND RISK OF STROKE

Although coronary attacks were frequently unexpected and occurred in previously well middle-aged men, stroke often developed on a backdrop of hypertension, diabetes, and cardiac disease, overt or occult. Data from Framingham established atrial fibrillation (AF) as an independent risk factor for stroke with particular importance in the elderly, confirming the link between this most common sustained arrhythmia and cerebral infarction (22). Estimates of the increased stroke risk from AF in Framingham were utilized in planning the clinical trials of AF using warfarin for stroke prevention.

Although overall 14.7% of strokes occurred in the presence of AF, this cardiac rhythm disturbance exerted increasing impact on stroke risk with increasing age: from 6.7% at ages 50 to 59 years to 36.2% at ages 80 to 89 years (23). In confirmation of the clinical experience, AF-associated strokes were moderately severe, severely disabling, or fatal, and overall mortality was doubled in the presence of AF (24–26).

In men, there was a tripling and in women a doubling of the age-specific prevalence of AF in Framingham between 1968 and 1988, suggesting we can anticipate a continuing rise in the importance of this arrhythmia in stroke occurrence (27). The increase in AF prevalence likely reflects improved survival of persons with coronary heart disease and congestive heart failure. Of interest, risk factors for AF are largely the factors that predispose to these atherosclerotic vascular outcomes (28). Attention to these risk factors—control of elevated blood pressure, cessation of cigarette smoking, prevention of diabetes, prevention of congestive heart failure and myocardial infarc-

tion—should serve to prevent both this arrhythmia as well as ischemic strokes, embolic and nonembolic. Findings on echocardiography found to be associated with AF and to further increase stroke risk include mitral annular calcification and left atrial enlargement. Both of these cardiac conditions frequently are associated with increased left ventricular mass and congestive heart failure (28–32).

COMPLETING THE CLINICAL PICTURE OF STROKE

Over the years, studies in Framingham have provided information on the "natural history" of stroke, including incidence of stroke by age and sex, disability following stroke, survival and recurrence following stroke, transient ischemic attack and risk of stroke, temporal patterns of stroke onset, and secular trends in stroke incidence and severity (33–39). These data, derived from a general population sample, include the milder and nonhospitalized stroke cases and permit examination of changes over time. In contrast to case series comprising hospitalized patients from stroke centers or those fatal strokes coming to autopsy, Framingham data include all stroke cases. Further, as subjects were queried systematically every 2 years concerning neurologic symptoms, transient and brief episodes were often reported. Such reports were then followed by evaluation by the stroke neurologists associated with the Framingham Study. Subjects did not have to seek medical care for these symptoms to be counted, as is usually the case in medical care-based registries. These population-based observations, backed up with stroke expertise, have provided a more complete picture of the disease than that derived from other case selection methods. It has permitted the sorting out, for example, of transient visual obscurations in the elderly of a benign and probably migrainous etiology from episodes of monocular or visual field defects attributable to arterial embolism with more serious outcomes (40).

As spouses were often recruited in the initial cohort in 1948 and their offspring in 1971, it has been possible to demonstrate an increased propensity to stroke in family members of subjects with stroke. DNA has been extracted on approximately half the original cohort and more than 4,000 of the offspring and immortalized cell lines are available on more than 4,000 of these subjects. A 390-marker 10-cM genome scan has been performed on approximately 1,775 members of the 334 largest families. As noted above, approximately 3,500 members of the third Framingham generation are being recruited in 2002 to enhance further genetic studies of health and disease including stroke.

OTHER RISK FACTORS FOR STROKE

Reports from Framingham have often been the first to document, in a prospective epidemiologic study, the impact of traits on risk of stroke. Cigarette smoking, low levels of habitual physical activity, elevated hematocrit (within the normal range), glucose intolerance and diabetes, and fibrinogen level were found to independently increase stroke incidence significantly. In 1971, the initial Framingham stroke-risk handbook was published, based on 16 years of follow-up. A

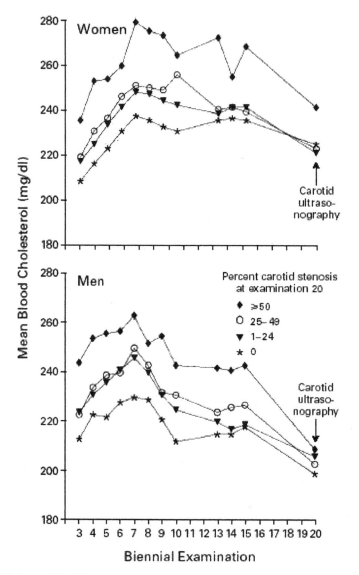

FIG. 19-1. Mean cholesterol levels in men and women at 12 biennial examinations spanning 34 years, according to the severity of carotid stenosis as determined by B-mode ultrasonography at the 20th biennial examination (1988). Subjects were categorized according to the degree of carotid stenosis, and mean levels of cholesterol are shown for the corresponding biennial examination. To convert values for cholesterol to millimoles per liter, multiply by 0.02586. From Wilson WF, Hoeg JM, D'Agostino RB, et al. Cumulative effects of high cholesterol levels, high blood pressure, and cigarette smoking on carotid stenosis. *N Engl J Med* 1997;337:516–522.

comprehensive, gender-specific Cox proportional hazards regression model was published, based on 36 years of follow-up (15,41). These models provide a simple formula for estimating the probabilities of stroke for specified levels of risk factors and variable lengths of follow-up. These equations permit the quantitative assessment of stroke probability, which is particularly useful for those individuals with borderline levels of multiple risk factors. It has proved to be a useful tool for physicians and patients and for estimating the impact of a particular therapeutic intervention or multiple risk factor modifications.

Because plasma and serum have been frozen and saved from several examinations during the last years, it has been possible to assay these specimens for more recently identified chemistries or risk markers. Hence, it was possible to measure homocysteine on exams 16 and 20 and plasma vitamins on exam 20 in the original cohort and relate these levels to the subsequent development of stroke and extracranial carotid artery atherosclerosis (42,43). Noninvasive testing using B-mode ultrasonography of the extracranial carotid artery was first performed on exam 20 in 1989 in the original cohort and on exam 5 in the offspring (it was repeated in the offspring on exam 6). These measures put into perspective the relative frequency of carotid artery stenosis in the general population. Carotid stenosis of greater than or equal to 50% was present in only 9% of men and 7% of women; more than half were in the under 70% range. Risk factors for carotid atherosclerosis were quite similar to those for stroke generally with the exception of elevated total serum cholesterol level, which was significantly related to carotid stenosis but not to stroke generally. The association between many risk factors and cardiovascular disease diminishes with advancing age, and the original cohort was quite elderly (66 to 93 years old) at the time of the carotid scans. For example, the total serum cholesterol levels at the time of the B-mode carotid scans were not significantly different in men with carotid stenosis ranging from 0 to 50% or higher (Fig. 19-1). However, with use of time-integrated measurements covering the previous 34 years (17 prior biennial exams), it is apparent that the higher degrees of carotid stenosis occur in persons with previously elevated cholesterol levels (44). The availability of decades of risk factor levels facilitates any number of these longitudinal analyses and promises to be of considerable use in defining phenotypes for future genetic studies. More recently, it has been possible to measure C-reactive protein levels and to relate these levels to risk of stroke in men and women (45).

SUMMARY

The author is obviously indebted to the many Framingham investigators and researchers over 35 years who have contributed to this remarkable enterprise. The reader is referred to the Framingham Study website (*http://www.nhlbi.nih.gov/about/framingham/index.hm*) for a more complete listing of publications and other background materials.

ACKNOWLEDGMENT

The Framingham Heart Study of the National Heart, Lung, and Blood Institute is supported by National Institutes of Health/National Heart, Lung, Blood Institute contract no. N01-HC-25195 and National Institutes of Health/National Institute of Neurological and Communication Disorders and Stroke grant no. 5R01 NS17950-21.

REFERENCES

1. Dawber TR. *The Framingham Study. The epidemiology of atherosclerotic disease.* Cambridge, MA: Commonwealth Fund /Harvard University Press, 1980.
2. Herring SW. *Framingham. An American town.* Framingham, MA Framingham Historical Society/Framingham Tercentennial Commission, 2000.
3. Feinleib M, Kannel WB, Garrison RJ, et al. The Framingham Offspring Study. Design and preliminary data. *Prev Med* 1975;4:518–525.
4. Kannel WB, Dawber TR, Kagan A, et al. Factors of risk in the development of coronary heart disease—six-year follow-up experience: the Framingham Study. *Ann Intern Med* 1961;55:33–50.
5. MacMahon B, Pugh TF, Ipsen J. *Epidemiologic methods.* Boston Little, Brown, 1960.
6. Dawber TR, Kannel WB, McNamara PM, et al. An epidemiologic study of apoplexy ("strokes"). Observations in 5,209 adults in the Framingham Study on association of various factors in the development of apoplexy. *Trans Am Neurol Assoc* 1965;90:237–240.
7. Kannel WB, Dawber TR, McNamara PM. Vascular disease of the brain—epidemiologic aspects: the Framingham Study. *Am J Public Health* 1965;55:1355–1366.
8. Dawber TR, Kannel WB. The Framingham Study; an epidemiological approach to coronary heart disease. *Circulation* 1966;34:553–555.
9. Corwin LE, Wolf PA, Kannel WB, et al. Accuracy of death certification of stroke: the Framingham Study. *Stroke* 1982;13:818–821.
10. Kannel WB, Wolf PA, Verter JI, et al. Epidemiologic assessment of the role of blood pressure in stroke; the Framingham Study. *JAMA* 1970;214:301–310.
11. Lassen NA. Epidemiologic assessment of the role of blood pressure in stroke. *JAMA* 1996;276:1279–1280.
12. Collins R, Peto R, MacMahon S, et al. Blood pressure, stroke, and coronary heart disease. Part 2, short-term reductions in blood pressure: overview of randomised drug trials in their epidemiological context. *Lancet* 1990;335:827–838.

13. Denny-Brown D. The treatment of recurrent cerebrovascular symptoms and the question of "vasopasm." *Med Clin North Am* 1951;35:1457–1474.

14. Evans JG, Williams TF, eds. *Oxford textbook of geriatric medicine.* New York: Oxford Medical Publications, 1992.

15. Wolf PA, D'Agostino RB, Belanger AJ, et al. Probability of stroke: a risk profile from the Framingham Study. *Stroke* 1991;22:312–318.

16. JNC-VI. The sixth report of the Joint National Committee on Prevention, Detection, Evaluation, and Treatment of High Blood Pressure. *Arch Intern Med* 1991;157: 2413–2446.

17. Executive Summary of the Third Report of the National Cholesterol Education Program (NCEP) Expert Panel on Detection, Evaluation, and Treatment of High Blood Cholesterol in Adults (Adult Treatment Panel III). *JAMA* 2001;285:2486–2497.

18. Kannel WB, Wolf PA, McGee DL, et al. Systolic blood pressure, arterial rigidity, and risk of stroke. The Framingham Study. *JAMA* 1981;245:1225–1229.

19. Wilking SV, Belanger A, Kannel WB, et al. Determinants of isolated systolic hypertension. *JAMA* 1988; 260:3451–3455.

20. Vasan RS, Larson MG, Leip EP, et al. Impact of high-normal blood pressure on the risk of cardiovascular disease. *N Engl J Med* 2001;345:1291–1297.

21. Seshadri S, Wolf PA, Beiser A, et al. Elevated midlife blood pressure increases stroke risk in elderly persons: the Framingham Study. *Arch Intern Med* 2001;161: 2343–2350.

22. Wolf PA, Dawber TR, Thomas HE Jr, et al. Epidemiologic assessment of chronic atrial fibrillation and risk of stroke: the Framingham Study. *Neurology* 1978;28: 973–977.

23. Wolf PA, Abbott RD, Kannel WB. Atrial fibrillation: a major contributor to stroke in the elderly. The Framingham Study. *Arch Intern Med* 1987;147:1561–1564.

24. Lin HJ, Wolf PA, Benjamin EJ, et al. Newly diagnosed atrial fibrillation and acute stroke. The Framingham Study. *Stroke* 1995;26:1527–1530.

25. Lin HJ, Wolf PA, Kelly-Hayes M, et al. Stroke severity in atrial fibrillation. The Framingham Study. *Stroke* 1996;27:1760–1764.

26. Benjamin EJ, Wolf PA, D'Agostino RB, et al. Impact of atrial fibrillation on the risk of death: the Framingham Heart Study. *Circulation* 1998;98:946–952.

27. Wolf PA, Benjamin EJ, Belanger AJ, et al. Secular trends in the prevalence of atrial fibrillation; the Framingham Study. *Am Heart J* 1996;131:790–795.

28. Benjamin EJ, Levy D, Vaziri SM, et al. Independent risk factors for atrial fibrillation in a population- based cohort. The Framingham Heart Study. *JAMA* 1994;271: 840–844.

29. Benjamin EJ, Plehn JF, D'Agostino RB, et al. Mitral annular calcification and the risk of stroke in an elderly cohort. *N Engl J Med* 1992;327:374–379.

30. Benjamin EJ, D'Agostino RB, Belanger AJ, et al. Left atrial size and the risk of stroke and death. The Framingham Heart Study. *Circulation* 1995;92:835–841.

31. Bikkina M, Levy D, Evans JC, et al. Left ventricular mass and risk of stroke in an elderly cohort. *JAMA* 1994;272:33–36.

32. Vaziri SM, Larson MG, Benjamin EJ, et al. Echocardiographic predictors of nonrheumatic atrial fibrillation. The Framingham Heart Study. *Circulation* 1994;89:724–730.

33. Gresham GE, Phillips TF, Wolf PA, et al. Epidemiologic profile of long-term stroke disability: the Framingham Study. *Arch Phys Med Rehabil* 1979;60:487–491.

34. Gresham GE, Fitzpatrick TE, Wolf PA, et al. Residual disability in survivors of stroke—the Framingham Study. *N Engl J Med* 1975;293:954–956.

35. Gresham GE, Kelly-Hayes M, Wolf PA, et al. Survival and functional status 20 or more years after first stroke: the Framingham Study. *Stroke* 1998;29:793–797.

36. Kelly-Hayes M, Wolf PA, Kannel WB, et al. Factors influencing survival and need for institutionalization following stroke: the Framingham Study. *Arch Phys Med Rehabil* 1988;69:415–418.

37. Kelly-Hayes M, Wolf PA, Kase CS, et al. Time course of functional recovery after stroke: the Framingham Study. *J Neurol Rehab* 1989;38:4:504–509.

38. Wolf PA, D'Agostino RB, O'Neal MA, et al. Secular trends in stroke incidence and mortality. The Framingham Study. *Stroke* 1992;23:1551–1555.

39. Sacco RL, Wolf PA, Kannel WB, et al. Survival and recurrence following stroke. The Framingham Study. *Stroke* 1982;13:290–295.

40. Wijman CA, Wolf PA, Kase CS, et al. Migrainous visual accompaniments are not rare in late life: the Framingham Study. *Stroke* 1998;29:1539–1543.

41. D'Agostino RB, Wolf PA, Belanger AJ, et al. Stroke risk profile: adjustment for antihypertensive medication, the Framingham Study. *Stroke* 1994;25:40–43.

42. Bostom AG, Rosenberg IH, Silbershatz H, et al. Non-fasting plasma total homocysteine levels and stroke incidence in elderly persons: the Framingham Study. *Ann Intern Med* 1999;131:352–355.

43. Selhub J, Jacques PF, Bostom AG, et al. Association between plasma homocysteine concentrations and extracranial carotid-artery stenosis. *N Engl J Med* 1995; 332:286–291.

44. Wilson PW, Hoeg JM, D'Agostino RB, et al. Cumulative effects of high cholesterol levels, high blood pressure, and cigarette smoking on carotid stenosis. *N Engl J Med* 1997;337:516–522.

45. Rost NS, Wolf PA, Kase CS, et al. Plasma concentration of C-reactive protein and risk of ischemic stroke and transient ischemic attack, the Framingham Study. *Stroke* 2001;32:2575–2579.

Ischemic Stroke: Advances in Neurology, Vol. 92. Edited by
H.J.M. Barnett, Julien Bogousslavsky, and Heather Meldrum.
Lippincott Williams & Wilkins, Philadelphia © 2003.

20

Nutritional and Metabolic Aspects of Stroke Prevention

J. David Spence

*Department of Clinical Neurological Sciences, University of Western Ontario;
Stroke Prevention and Atherosclerosis Research Centre, Robarts Research Institute,
London, Ontario, Canada*

THE IMPORTANCE OF DIET: VASTLY UNDERESTIMATED

With the advent of effective drug therapy for hyperlipidemia, an important misconception has become rather prevalent among both the public and physicians. Because these drugs are much more effective than is diet in reducing fasting lipid levels and because it is difficult to persuade patients to change the dietary patterns of a lifetime, many physicians believe that diet is unimportant. Nothing could be further from the truth. The problem lies in a faulty assumption that fasting lipid levels are all-important.

Several studies show that postprandial lipemia is more predictive of atherosclerotic risk than is fasting lipemia (1,2). However, the assessment of postprandial lipemia is complicated by the problem of knowing what to measure. The lipid/lipoprotein complexes that are routinely measured in the fasting state [total cholesterol, triglycerides, and high-density lipoprotein (HDL)] are essentially manufactured by the liver, mostly overnight. What goes into the bloodstream after a high-fat meal is a complex toxic soup of oxidized fats, trans fatty acids, and free radicals.

A healthy diet is not only low in harmful substances such as cholesterol and fat, it is high in beneficial substances. A Cretan Mediterranean diet high in fruits, vegetables, α-linolenic acid, lycopene, olive oil, antioxidants including vitamin E, vitamin C, bioflavonoids and phenolic substances in red wine (3), phytoestrogens, and probably other beneficial substances that are as yet unrecognized was shown in the Lyon Diet Heart Study to reduce myocardial infarction and death by 60% in 4 years compared with a diet similar to a Step I NCEP (National Cholesterol Education Program) diet (4). This effect was twice that of simvastatin in the Scandinavian Simvastatin Survival Study (5), which showed a 40% reduction of cardiac events in 6 years. A Step II diet involves reduction of saturated fats to 7% of total calories and total fat to 20% of total calories, an increase in complex carbohydrates, and a reduction of cholesterol intake to below 200 mg/day. This diet, though usually recommended after discharge from coronary care units, is probably not even close to what we should be recommending.

The Mediterranean diet was low in cholesterol and animal fats but achieved the same proportion of calories from fat (20%). Patients on the Mediterranean diet used olive oil and substituted canola margarine for butter. Importantly, there was no difference in fasting lipids between the two dietary groups at the end of the study and no difference in alcohol intake. Some experts have wondered if the observed effect of the diet was possible because there was no difference in fasting lipid levels; but what the study is telling us is that postprandial fat is much more important than fasting cholesterol levels.

Several studies have shown that diets high in fruits and vegetables are associated with reduced stroke rates; this has recently been reviewed (6–8).

The result of the Lyon Diet Heart Study is so important that it is quite surprising how little attention it has received; most dietitians in coronary care units are still prescribing a Step I NCEP diet, even though it was proven in that study to be much less efficacious than the Cretan Mediterranean diet.

Because control of hypertension is so critical to stroke prevention, it is particularly important to recognize the importance of dietary reduction of blood pressure. A diet low in meat, fish, and poultry, high in fruits and vegetables, and containing two daily low-fat servings of low-fat, high-calcium dairy products reduced systolic pressure by 11 mm Hg and diastolic by 5 mm Hg in a group of hypertensive patients (9). The follow-up study showed that sodium restriction further reduced blood pressure (10). The importance of lifestyle modification in control of hypertension has recently been reviewed (11).

For patients with vascular disease, target low-density lipoprotein (LDL) level is less than 2.6 mmol/L; β-hydroxymethylglutaryl coenzyme-A reductase inhibitors are recommended for patients with normal triglycerides and HDL, whereas fibrates or niacin may be more effective (or may need to be added to statin) for patients with high triglycerides and low HDL. In addition to medication for fasting lipids, it is important to understand that diet is much more important than we think; the reason is postprandial fats.

EFFECT OF DIETARY FAT ON ENDOTHELIAL FUNCTION

A single high-fat meal has been shown to impair endothelial function for several hours (12), and this effect can be reduced by pretreatment with vitamins C and E (13). A Mediterranean diet has been shown to improve endothelial function in hyperlipidemic men (14). This diet has a higher content of antioxidants and significantly lower indexes of plasma lipid peroxidation (15). Vogel et al. (16) studied the effect of components of the Mediterranean diet on endothelial function and found that the beneficial components appeared to be antioxidant-rich foods including vegetables, fruits, balsamic vinegar, and omega-3-rich fish and canola oil.

Dietary Cholesterol *Is* Important

Dietary cholesterol intake *is* important. Ginsberg et al. (17) showed a dose–response relationship between increases in plasma cholesterol and fasting dietary cholesterol in a study using eggs. Even though egg consumption increases fasting LDL by only about 10% (18), it increases oxidized LDL levels by 34% (19). An analysis from the Health Professionals Study and the Nurses' Study showed a doubling of coronary risk among diabetic individuals who consumed 1 egg/day versus fewer than 1/week (20). Egg yolks, therefore, are not an appropriate food for patients with vascular disease.

It is no longer good enough to prescribe a Step II NCEP diet for high-risk vascular patients. A diet approximating the Cretan Mediterranean diet is much more effective. It should include no egg yolks; the restriction to 4 oz every other day of the flesh of any animal (fish preferred); use of nonhydrogenated canola; margarine or olive oil instead of butter; avoidance of deep-fried foods and hydrogenated vegetable oils; a high intake of fruits, grains, vegetables, low-fat dairy products; and a low intake of salt (no added salt, salty foods avoided).

VITAMINS AND ANTIOXIDANTS

Because of lack of space, readers who want more detail on vitamins and antioxidants are referred elsewhere (21,22).

Vitamin B_{12} deficiency is relevant to stroke because it causes elevated homocysteine levels. This problem is much more common than is appreciated because there are a number of steps involved in absorption and handling. Dietary deficiency is most common in vegetarians. Gastric acid is required to strip B_{12} from food, whereas crystalline supplements can be absorbed without gastric acid. Achlorhydria can result from gastrectomy, atrophic gastritis, or proton pump inhibitors such as omeprazole (23–25).

Intrinsic factor from the gastric parietal cells is required for absorption and can be eliminated by antibodies. Pancreatic third factor and normal function of the last 2 ft of the ileum are also required, so that pancreatitis and Crohn's disease can result in deficiency. Finally, transport proteins including transcobalamin II are required to bring B_{12} from the ileal mucosa to the circulation and the liver, as well as for endocytosis. Some patients have antibodies to transcobalamin II; others have hereditary deficiency (26). Surveys using methylmalonic acid levels for diagnosis indicate that at least 15% of the elderly are deficient in B_{12}; the usual reason is atrophic gastritis (27,28). Only 3% of the elderly have pernicious anemia due to deficiency of intrinsic factor.

Evidence that antioxidant therapy including vitamin E improves endothelial function has recently been reviewed (29). Of particular interest, given the discussion above regarding the importance of postprandial lipemia, are studies showing that vitamins C and E reduce the impairment of endothelial function caused by a fatty meal (12,13).

The Cambridge Heart Antioxidant Study showed a significant 77% reduction of nonfatal myocardial infarction (30). A subsequent analysis related mortality significantly to noncompliance with vitamin E after the Cambridge trial (31).

A diet contains natural constituents in natural proportions, and it is likely that pharmacologic regimens may not achieve optimal proportions and combinations of antioxidants and other beneficial substances. We are only beginning to learn about the beneficial substances in foods. Antioxidant bioflavonoids are found in high concentrations in citrus juices, tea, red wine, seaweed, and other dietary sources. They tend to be highly flavored and strongly colored (e.g., lycopene is responsible for the red color of tomatoes and watermelon).

The intake of antioxidant flavonols such as quercetin has been linked to coronary mortality in a number of studies. In the Zutphen Elderly Study, the relative risk of a coronary event among men in the highest tertile of flavonoid intake was 0.47 (95% confidence interval 0.27–0.82) (32–34).

Grapefruit contains very high concentrations (approximately 125 mg in a 250-mL glass) of naringin, a bioflavonoid that is related to hesperitin in orange juice and genistein in soy protein. Grapefruit juice markedly reduces oxidation of a number of drugs by cytochrome P4503A4 in the gut wall, thus markedly increasing their bioavailability (35–37).

In addition to its effects on drug metabolism, naringin, like hesperitin and genistein, has effects on lipid metabolism and also phytoestrogen anticancer effects in animal models (38). Herbs also have antioxidant effects (39), as do polyphenols in cocoa (40) and tea (41). The putative benefits of garlic are unconvincing but merit further study (42).

HOMOCYSTEINE AND STROKE

Homocysteine, as measured in plasma, consists of several chemical species: homocysteine, homocystine, and mixed cysteine–homocysteine disulfide (43).

The original cause of high homocysteine levels in plasma, with homocystinuria, was discovered in 1962 (44,45): It was a deficiency of cystathionine β-synthase, which is very rare; only 1% or less of the population are heterozygous. Perhaps for that reason, homocystinuria was, for a long time, regarded as a rare problem.

McCully (46) suggested in 1969 that more moderate levels of hyperhomocysteinemia might be associated with atherosclerosis. Subsequently, Boers et al. (47) reported in 1985 that homocysteine levels above 14 μmol/L were present in about 30% of patients with premature peripheral and cerebrovascular disease but not coronary artery disease; this was (probably incorrectly) attributed to heterozygosity for cystathionine synthase deficiency. In 1991, Clarke et al. (48) confirmed that about 30% of patients with premature atherosclerosis had plasma homocysteine levels above 14 μmol/L. The relationship between plasma homocysteine levels and stroke has recently been reviewed (49).

How Does Homocysteine Contribute to Vascular Disease?

There are many mechanisms by which homocysteine may contribute to cerebral vascular disease; these include increased production of hydrogen peroxide, oxidative stress, and endothelial dysfunction with increased oxidation of LDL and changes in lipoprotein (α) and hypercoagulability (21). Hypercoagulability links homocysteine to cerebral infarctions due to venous thrombosis (50). Homocysteine inhibits thrombomodulin expression on the surface of endothelial cells and inactivates both thrombomodulin and protein C irreversibly (51). Probably via hypercoagulability, hyperhomocystinemia was associated with a threefold increase in the risk of stroke in patients with atrial fibrillation in a major trial (unpublished data).

Recently, homocysteine has been shown to be associated with the inflammatory mediators intercellular adhesion molecule-1 and vascular cell adhesion molecule (52) and with endoplasmic reticulum stress resulting in increased accumulation of lipids in hepatic cells and in macrophages and monocytes. One mechanism for the effects of homocysteine on endothelial function has been endoplasmic reticulum stress. Hyndman et al. (54) recently showed that 5-methyltetrahydrofolate attenuates superoxide production, thereby increasing nitric oxide production and improving endothelial function (54).

Treatment of Hyperhomocystinemia with Vitamins

Hyperhomocystinemia is very common because there are at least five enzymes and six nutritional factors that represent substrates or cofactors for those enzymes that are involved in homocysteine metabolism (Fig. 20-1). For most patients, a combination of folate, B_6, and B_{12} is effective in reducing levels. Patients with renal failure have very high levels, associated with very high risk, and respond only partially to vitamin therapy (55). Some patients require betaine (trimethylglycine), as well as the triple-vitamin therapy. We are currently exploring a new approach to treatment using dimercaptosuccinic acid.

Treatment of homocysteine with vitamins has recently been reviewed (56). Vitamin therapy not only

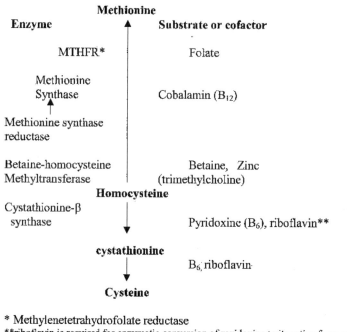

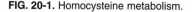

* Methylenetetrahydrofolate reductase
**riboflavin is required for enzymatic conversion of pyridoxine to its active form, pyridoxal 5'phosphate

FIG. 20-1. Homocysteine metabolism.

reduces plasma homocysteine levels, it additionally restores endothelial dysfunction (21). Vitamin therapy also reduces plasma levels of fibrinogen and lipoprotein (a) in patients with renal failure and very high levels of homocysteine (57).

The first evidence of an effect of vitamin therapy on progression of atherosclerosis in humans was reported by our group. We found in patients whose carotid plaque was progressing, despite therapy for traditional risk factors, that vitamin therapy for homocysteine (folate, B_6, and B_{12}) not only halted progression but, on average, achieved regression of plaque (58,59). Recently, Schnyder et al. (60) showed that treatment with folate, B_6, and B_{12} reduced restenosis and clinical events after coronary angioplasty.

WHAT IS THE LEVEL TO TREAT AND HOW LOW SHOULD TARGET LEVELS BE?

It appears likely, given the apparent response of carotid plaque to vitamin therapy as described above and given the epidemiologic evidence, that in the future we may consider treating patients with vascu-

lar disease to a low target level of plasma homocysteine, such as below 9 μmol/L, rather than selecting patients for treatment on the basis of very high levels. This approach would be analogous to approaches now taken to treatment of LDL–cholesterol in patients with vascular disease (61).

At least two secondary stroke prevention trials are under way. The first was the Vitamin Intervention in Stroke Prevention Trial, a randomized, controlled trial of high-dose versus low-dose folate, B_6, and cobalamin for secondary prevention of nondisabling stroke. VITAmins TO Prevent Stroke (VITATOPS), an Australian stroke prevention study, and approximately 10 coronary prevention trials are also being conducted. Results from the Vitamin Intervention in Stroke Prevention Trial should be known in early 2004.

SUMMARY

Epidemiologic evidence, animal studies, angiographic and ultrasound studies in humans, and a limited number of clinical trials suggest that vitamins C and E may be protective and that folate, B_6, and B_{12}, by lowering homocysteine levels, may reduce stroke.

However, these hypotheses require testing before widespread use of supplementary vitamins can be generally recommended (62). Clinical trials under way will test those hypotheses. In the meantime, it should be understood that the role of diet is much more important than is widely recognized. A diet low in saturated fat and cholesterol, low in sodium, high in potassium and calcium, and containing a lot of fruits and vegetables reduces blood pressure as much as an antihypertensive drug and in coronary patients is twice as effective as statin drugs in reducing death and myocardial infarction. Such a diet can therefore be confidently recommended as a source not only of natural proportions of vitamins and antioxidants but also for benefits that we are only beginning to define.

REFERENCES

1. Kirchmair R, Ebenbichler CF, Patsch JR. Post-prandial lipaemia. *Baillieres Clin Endocrinol Metab* 1995;9:705–719.
2. Ebenbichler CF, Kirchmair R, Egger C, et al. Postprandial state and atherosclerosis. *Curr Opin Lipidol* 1995;6:286–290.
3. de Lorgeril M, Salen P. Wine, ethanol, platelets, and Mediterranean diet. *Lancet* 1999;353:1067.
4. de Lorgeril M, Salen P, Martin JL, et al. Mediterranean diet, traditional risk factors, and the rate of cardiovascular complications after myocardial infarction: final report of the Lyon Diet Heart Study. *Circulation* 1999;99:779–785.
5. Scandinavian Simvastatin Survival Study Group. Randomized trial of cholesterol lowering in 4444 patients with coronary heart disease: the Scandinavian Simvastatin Survival Study (4S). *Lancet* 1994;344:1383–1389.
6. Gillman MW, Cupples LA, Gagnon D, et al. Protective effect of fruits and vegetables on development of stroke in men. *JAMA* 1995;273:1113–1117.
7. Joshipura KJ, Ascherio A, Manson JE, et al. Fruit and vegetable intake in relation to risk of ischemic stroke. *JAMA* 1999;282:1233–1239.
8. Renaud SC. Diet and stroke. *J Nutr Health Aging* 2001;5:167–172.
9. Appel LJ, Moore TJ, Obarzanek E, et al. A clinical trial of the effects of dietary patterns on blood pressure. *N Engl J Med* 1997;336:1117–1124.
10. Sacks FM, Svetkey LP, Vollmer WM, et al. Effects on blood pressure of reduced dietary sodium and the Dietary Approaches to Stop Hypertension (DASH) diet. DASH–Sodium Collaborative Research Group. *N Engl J Med* 2001;344:3–10.
11. Campbell NRC, Burgess E, Taylor G, et al. Lifestyle changes to prevent and control hypertension: do they work? *Can Med Assoc J* 1999;160:1341–1343.
12. Vogel RA, Corretti MC, Plotnick GD. Effect of a single high-fat meal on endothelial function in healthy subjects. *Am J Cardiol* 1997;79:350–354.
13. Plotnick GD, Corretti MC, Vogel RA. Effect of antioxidant vitamins on the transient impairment of endothe-lium-dependent brachial artery vasoactivity following a single high-fat meal. *JAMA* 1997;278:1682–1686.
14. Fuentes F, Lopez-Miranda J, Sanchez E, et al. Mediterranean and low-fat diets improve endothelial function in hypercholesterolemic men. *Ann Intern Med* 2001;134:1115–1119.
15. Mancini M, Parfitt VJ, Rubba P. Antioxidants in the Mediterranean diet. *Can J Cardiol* 1995;11[Suppl G]:105G–109G.
16. Vogel RA, Corretti MC, Plotnick GD. The postprandial effect of components of the Mediterranean diet on endothelial function. *J Am Coll Cardiol* 2000;36:1455–1460.
17. Ginsberg HN, Karmally W, Siddiqui M, et al. A dose–response study of the effects of dietary cholesterol on fasting and postprandial lipid and lipoprotein metabolism in healthy young men. *Arterioscler Thromb* 1994;14:576–586.
18. Schnohr P, Thomsen OO, Riis HP, et al. Egg consumption and high-density-lipoprotein cholesterol. *J Intern Med* 1994;235:249–251.
19. Levy Y, Maor I, Presser D, et al. Consumption of eggs with meals increases the susceptibility of human plasma and low-density lipoprotein to lipid peroxidation. *Ann Nutr Metab* 1996;40:243–251.
20. Hu FB, Stampfer MJ, Rimm EB, et al. A prospective study of egg consumption and risk of cardiovascular disease in men and women. *JAMA* 1999;281:1387–1394.
21. Spence JD. Vitamins and antioxidants. In: Bogous-slavsky J, ed. *Drug therapy for stroke prevention.* London: Taylor & Francis, 2001:231–252.
22. Brody T. *Nutritional chemistry.* 2nd ed. San Diego: Academic Press, 1999.
23. Koop H. Review article: metabolic consequences of long-term inhibition of acid secretion by omeprazole. *Aliment Pharmacol Ther* 1992;6:406.
24. Saltzman J, Kemp JA, Golner BB, et al. Effect of hypochlorhydria due to omeprazole treatment or atrophic gastritis on protein-bound vitamin B_{12} absorption. *J Am Coll Nutr* 1994;13:584–591.
25. Marcuard SP, Albernaz L, Khazanie PG. Omeprazole therapy causes malabsorption of cyanocobalamin (vitamin B_{12}). *Ann Intern Med* 1994;120:211–215.
26. Thomas PK, Hoffbrand AV. Hereditary transcobalamin II deficiency: a 22 year follow up [Letter]. *J Neurol Neurosurg Psychiatry* 1997;62:197.
27. Carmel R. Prevalence of undiagnosed pernicious anemia in the elderly. *Arch Intern Med* 1996;156:1097–1100.
28. Carmel R. Cobalamin, the stomach and aging. *Am J Clin Nutr* 1997;66:750–759.
29. Aminkabakhsh A, Mancini GBJ. Chronic antioxidant use and changes in endothelial function: a review of clinical investigations. *Can J Cardiol* 1999;15:895–903.
30. Stephens NG, Parsons A, Schofield PM, et al. Randomised controlled trial of vitamin E in patients with coronary disease: Cambridge Heart Antioxidant Study (CHAOS). *Lancet* 1996;347:781–786.
31. Mitchinson MJ, Stephens NG, Parsons A, et al. Mortality in the CHAOS trial. *Lancet* 1999;353:381–382.
32. Hertog MG, Feskens EJM, Kromhout D. Antioxidant

flavonols and coronary heart disease risk. *Lancet* 1997; 349:699.

33. Hertog MG, Sweetnam PM, Fehily AM, et al. Antioxidant flavonols and ischemic heart disease in a Welsh population of men: the Caerphilly Study. *Am J Clin Nutr* 1997;65:1489–1494.

34. Keli SO, Hertog MG, Feskens EJ, et al. Dietary flavonoids, antioxidant vitamins, and incidence of stroke: the Zutphen Study. *Arch Intern Med* 1996;156: 637–642.

35. Dresser GK, Spence JD, Bailey DG. Pharmacokinetic–pharmacodynamic consequences and clinical relevance of cytochrome P450 3A4 inhibition. *Clin Pharmacokinet* 2000;38:41–57.

36. Bailey DG, Malcolm J, Arnold O, et al. Grapefruit juice–drug interactions. *Br J Clin Pharmacol* 1998;46: 101–110.

37. Bailey DG, Spence JD, Munoz C, et al. Interaction of citrus juices with felodipine and nifedipine. *Lancet* 1991;337:268–269.

38. Borradaile NM, Carroll KK, Kurowska EM. Regulation of HepG2 cell apolipoprotein B metabolism by the citrus flavanones hesperetin and naringenin. *Lipids* 1999; 34:591–598.

39. Lionis C, Faresjö Å, Skoula M, et al. Antioxidant effects of herbs in Crete. *Lancet* 1998;352:1987–1988.

40. Kondo K, Hirano R, Matsumoto A, et al. Inhibition of LDL oxidation by cocoa. *Lancet* 1996;348:1514.

41. Luo M, Kannar K, Wahiqvist ML, et al. Inhibition of LDL oxidation by green tea extract. *Lancet* 1997;349: 360–361.

42. Beaglehole R. Garlic for flavour, not cardioprotection. *Lancet* 1996;348:1186–1187.

43. Mudd SH, Finkelstein JD, Refsum H, et al. Homocysteine and its disulfide derivatives: a suggested consensus terminology. *Arterioscler Thromb Vasc Biol* 2000; 20:1706.

44. Carson NAJ, Neill DW. Metabolic abnormalities detected in a survey of mentally backward individuals in Northern Ireland. *Arch Dis Child* 1962;37:505–513.

45. Gerritsen T, Vaughn JG, Waisman HA. The identification of homocystine in the urine. *Biochem Biophys Res Commun* 1962;9:493–496.

46. McCully KS. Vascular pathology of homocysteinemia: implications for the pathogenesis of atherosclerosis. *Am J Pathol* 1969;56:111–128.

47. Boers GHJ, Trijbels FJM, Fowler B, et al. Heterozygosity for homocystinuria in premature peripheral and cerebral occlusive arterial disease. *N Engl J Med* 1985;313: 709–714.

48. Clarke R, Daly L, Robinson K, et al. Hyperhomocysteinemia: an independent risk factor for vascular disease. *N Engl J Med* 1991;324:1149–1155.

49. Spence JD, Toole JF. Homocysteine and cerebral vascular disease. In: Carmel R, Jacobsen DW, eds. *Homocys-*

teine in health and disease. Cambridge: Cambridge University Press, 2001:384–392.

50. Franken DG, Vreugdenhil A, Boers GHJ, et al. Familial cerebrovascular accidents due to concomitant hyperhomocysteinemia and protein C deficiency type 1. *Stroke* 1993;24:1599–1600.

51. Lentz SR, Sadler JE. Inhibition of thrombomodulin surface expression and protein C activation by the thrombogenic agent, homocysteine. *J Clin Invest* 1991;88: 1906–1916.

52. Title LM, Cummings PM, Giddens K, et al. Effect of folic acid and antioxidant vitamins on endothelial dysfuction in patients with coronary artery disease. *J Am Coll Cardiol* 2000;36(3):758–765.

53. Werstuck GH, Lentz SR, Dayal S, et al. Homocysteine-induced endoplasmic reticulum stress causes dysregulation of the cholesterol and triglyceride biosynthetic pathways. *J Clin Invest* 2001;107(10):1263–1273.

54. Hyndman ME, Verma S, Rosenfield RJ, et al. Interaction of 5-methyltetrahydrofolate and tetrahydrobiopterin on endothelial function. *Am J Physiol Heart Circ Physiol* 2002;282(6):H2167–H2172.

55. Spence JD, Cordy P, Kortas C, et al. Effect of usual doses of folate supplementation on elevated plasma homocyst(e)ine in hemodialysis patients: no difference between 1 mg and 5 mg daily. *Am J Nephrol* 1998;19: 405–410.

56. Scott JM. Modification of hyperhomocysteinemia. In: Carmel R, Jacobsen DW, eds. *Homocysteine in health and disease.* Cambridge: Cambridge University Press, 2001:467–476.

57. Klinke K, Dziewanowski K, Staniewicz A, et al. [Effect of vitamin therapy on homocyst(e)ine, fibrinogen and Lp(a) in dialysis patients.] *Czynniki Ryzyka [Suppl]* 1998;4:28(abst).

58. Hackam DG, Peterson JC, Spence JD. What level of plasma homocyst(e)ine should be treated? Effects of vitamin therapy on progression of carotid atherosclerosis in patients with homocyst(e)ine levels above and below 14 mmol/L. *Am J Hypertens* 2000;13: 105–110.

59. Peterson JC, Spence JD. Vitamins and progression of atherosclerosis in patients with hyper-homocyst(e)inemia. *Lancet* 1998;351:263.

60. Schnyder G, Roffi M, Pin R, et al. Decreased rate of coronary restenosis after lowering of plasma homocysteine levels. *N Engl J Med* 2001;345:1593–1600.

61. Spence JD. Patients with atherosclerotic vascular disease: how low should plasma homocyst(e)ine levels go? *Am J Cardiovasc Drugs* 2001;1:85–89.

62. Tribble DD. Antioxidant consumption and risk of coronary heart disease: emphasis on vitamin C, vitamin E, and β-carotene. A statement for health care professionals from the American Heart Association. *Circulation* 1999;99:595.

Ischemic Stroke: Advances in Neurology, Vol. 92. Edited by
H.J.M. Barnett, Julien Bogousslavsky, and Heather Meldrum.
Lippincott Williams & Wilkins, Philadelphia © 2003.

21

Risk Factor Management to Prevent Stroke

Graeme J. Hankey

*Department of Medicine, The University of Western Australia; Stroke Unit, Royal Perth Hospital,
Perth, Australia*

The Framingham and other cohort studies (Chapter 19) show that up to two-thirds of all cases of first-ever ischemic stroke can be attributed to a few major causal risk factors: high blood pressure (BP), cigarette smoking, diabetes mellitus, atrial fibrillation, ischemic heart disease, and carotid artery stenosis (1). Other possible causal risk factors, which remain to be confirmed, include elevated C-reactive protein level and a high plasma total homocysteine concentration (2). Risk factors for recurrent stroke may differ qualitatively and quantitatively from those for first-ever stroke, but few data are available from large, prospective, community-based studies (3).

The appropriate management of the major causal risk factors for first-ever and recurrent stroke is one of the three main strategies of primary and secondary stroke prevention, respectively. The others are antithrombotic therapy and revascularization of symptomatic arteries.

This chapter will review the effectiveness of modifying major causal risk factors on the incidence of stroke among the general population (primary stroke prevention) and among patients with a previous stroke (secondary stroke prevention). The effectiveness of risk factor modification in reducing stroke incidence will be derived from a systematic review of all randomized, controlled trials of risk factor modification or, when not available, from single randomized, controlled trials or a systematic review of prospective observational cohort studies of adjusted associations between a risk factor and stroke.

PRIMARY PREVENTION OF STROKE AMONG THE GENERAL POPULATION

Lowering of Blood Pressure

Data from randomized, placebo-controlled trials in over 47,000 individuals with hypertension indicate that allocation to antihypertensive drug therapy (chiefly diuretics and β-blockers) for about 3 years reduces diastolic BP by 5 to 6 mm Hg and systolic BP by 10 to 12 mm Hg and the 3-year rate of stroke by 38% (SD 5%) from 3.2% (control) to 2.0% (antihypertensive therapy) (4,5). This is an annual absolute risk reduction (ARR) of 1.2% over 3 years, or 0.4%/year. Therefore, treating 1,000 hypertensive patients prevents about four strokes (0.4%) each year. The number of patients needed to treat (NNT) to prevent one stroke each year is 250. Of course, the magnitude of the ARR depends on the baseline risk of the hypertensive population, which is determined by many factors such as age, severity of hypertension [the relative hazard rate associated with a 10-mm Hg higher systolic BP is 1.22 (p = 0.02) for stroke (4)], and prevalence of other vascular risk factors in the population. Greater absolute benefits are seen in men than women, in people over age 70, and in those with prior cardiovascular events or wider pulse pressure. On average, every 1,000 person-years of treatment in older adults prevents about five strokes [95% confidence interval (CI): 2–8], three coronary events (95% CI: 1–4), and four cardiovascular deaths (95% CI: 1–8). Drug treatment in middle-aged adults prevents about one stroke (95% CI: 0–2) for every 1,000 person-years of treatment and does not significantly affect coronary events or mortality.

Lifestyle Strategies to Lower Blood Pressure

Physical Activity

Aerobic exercise reduces BP by about 4.7 mm Hg systolic (95% CI: 4.4–5.0 mm Hg) and 3.1 mm Hg diastolic (95% CI: 3.0–3.3 mm Hg), as well as body weight (6).

Weight Reduction

Modest weight reduction of 3% to 9% body weight, which is achievable in motivated middle-aged and older adults, may lead to modest reductions in BP of about 3 mm Hg systolic and 3 mm Hg diastolic in obese people with hypertension (7,8). However, many adults find it difficult to maintain weight loss.

Eating More Fruits and Vegetables

A high-fruit and -vegetable diet modestly reduces BP by about 2.8 mm Hg systolic (97.5% CI: 0.9–4.7 mm Hg) and 1.1 mm Hg diastolic (97.5% CI: 2.4-mm Hg decrease to 0.3-mm Hg increase; $p = 0.07$), and a combined low-fat and high-fruit and -vegetable diet reduces BP by about 5.5 mm Hg systolic (97.5% CI: 3.7–4.4 mm Hg) and 3.0 mm Hg diastolic (97.5% CI: 1.6-mm Hg decrease to 4.3-mm Hg increase; $p = 0.07$) (9).

Salt Restriction

Salt restriction may lead to modest reductions in BP, with more benefit in people older than 45 than in younger people (10). A mean reduction in sodium intake of 118 mmol (6.7 g)/day for 28 days leads to reductions of 3.9 mm Hg (95% CI: 3.0–4.8 mm Hg) in systolic BP and 1.9 mm Hg (95% CI: 1.3–22.5 mm Hg) in diastolic BP (11,12).

Potassium Supplementation

Potassium supplementation of about 60 to 100 mmol of potassium chloride daily (2,000 mg, which is roughly the amount contained in five bananas) is feasible for most adults and reduces BP a little, by about 4.4 mm Hg systolic (95% CI: 2.2–6.6 mm Hg) and 2.5 mm Hg diastolic (95% CI: 0.1–4.9 mm Hg) (13). It is not harmful in people without kidney failure and in people not taking drugs that increase serum potassium. Gastrointestinal adverse effects such as belching, flatulence, diarrhea, or abdominal discomfort occur in about 2% to 10% of people.

Fish Oil Supplementation

Fish oil supplementation in large doses of 3 g/day modestly lowers BP by about 4.5 mm Hg systolic (95% CI: 1.2–7.8 mm Hg) and 2.5 mm Hg diastolic (95% CI: 0.6–4.4 mm Hg) (14). There is inconclusive evidence regarding the effects of calcium supplementation, magnesium supplementation, and alcohol reduction on BP.

Reduced Alcohol Consumption

The association between alcohol consumption and BP is generally linear, although there does appear to be a threshold effect at about two to three standard drinks a day, below which (i.e., up to two drinks a day) any adverse effect on BP is either very small or nonexistent (15).

Pharmacologic Strategies to Lower Blood Pressure

Conventional antihypertensives (low-dose diuretics or low-dose β-blockers) and newer antihypertensives (calcium channel antagonists) are similarly effective in preventing stroke (16). In other words, it appears to be the size (intensity) of the reduction in BP, rather than the type of antihypertensive drug, which is important in preventing hard clinical outcome events (Table 21-1) (17). Furthermore, the costs of the conventional antihypertensives are substantially lower than those of the newer antihypertensives (18,19). However, two recent studies have suggested a major additional benefit of angiotensin-converting enzyme inhibitors (20) and angiotensin II receptor blockade (21) over and above the antihypertensive benefit.

Major Adverse Effects of Different Classes of Antihypertensive Agents

Despite some adverse effects, reduction of BP reduces stroke incidence and does not produce significant adverse effects of major clinical importance (22).

Target Diastolic Blood Pressure

One randomized, controlled trial (18,790 people, mean age 62 years, diastolic BPs between 100 and 115 mm Hg) aimed to evaluate the effects on cardiovascular risk of target diastolic BPs of 90, 85, and 80 mm Hg (23). However, the mean achieved diastolic BPs were 85, 83, and 81 mm Hg, and there were no significant differences in the three groups.

Lowering of Cholesterol

Observational studies do not support any association between increasing plasma cholesterol level and all types of stroke combined (24,25). This may be explained to some extent by a positive association between increasing cholesterol and ischemic stroke due to large-artery atherothrombosis being diluted by a weaker association with ischemic stroke due to intracranial small-vessel disease and a possible negative association with hemorrhagic stroke (25).

Clinical trials (n = 16) have shown that lowering plasma concentrations of cholesterol by means of β-

TABLE 21-1. *Effects of different blood pressure-lowering drugs from most recent updated systematic review of randomized trials*

	% (95% confidence interval).	
	Stroke: relative risk reduction	Major cardiovascular events[a]
Comparisons with placebo		
Diuretics or β-blockers	38 (28–48)	21 (13–28)
ACE inhibitors 30 (15–43)	21 (14–27)	
Calcium antagonist-based therapy	39 (15–36)	28 (13–41)
Direct head-to-head comparisons		
ACE inhibitor vs. diuretic/β-blocker	−5 (−19 to +8)	0 (−8–7)
Calcium antagonist vs. diuretic/β-blocker	13 (2–23) (just favors calcium antagonist)	−2 (−10 to +5)
ACE inhibitor vs. calcium antagonist	−2 (−21 to +15)	8 (−1 to +17)
More-intensive vs. less-intensive blood pressure-lowering strategies	20 (2–35) (favors more intensive)	15 (4–24)

ACE, angiotensin-converting enzyme.
[a]Major cardiovascular events: stroke, myocardial infarction, heart failure, or death from any cardiovascular cause.
From Blood Pressure Lowering Treatment Trialists' Collaboration. Effects of ACE inhibitors, calcium antagonists, and other blood pressure-lowering drugs: results of prospectively designed overviews of randomised trials. *Lancet* 2000;355:1955–1964, with permission.

hydroxymethylglutaryl coenzyme-A reductase inhibitors ("statins") in about 39,000 patients at low risk of stroke reduces the odds of stroke by about 25% (95% CI: 14%–41%) and the absolute risk of stroke by about 0.17% (i.e., 1.7 strokes/1,000 patient-years of treatment) (26–28). However, a significant reduction in the risk of stroke was apparent only among the patients with a history of coronary heart disease (29). The three primary prevention placebo-controlled trials of "statins" in a total of 7,361 individuals with hypercholesterolemia showed that after a mean follow-up of 3 to 4.9 years, those assigned "statins" manifested a 22% to 28% reduction in serum low-density lipoprotein–cholesterol levels and an overall nonsignificant 11% (95% CI: −31%–40%) reduction in stroke (control: 0.3%/year; "statin": 0.27%/year) (30–32). This is an ARR of about 0.03%/year. The NNT is 3,333.

Control of Diabetes Mellitus

Tight glycemic control significantly reduces the incidence of retinopathy, nephropathy, and neuropathy in patients with type 1 (33,34) and type 2 (33,35–37) diabetes mellitus. It is the tightness of the glycemic control, rather than the method of achieving it [e.g., diet alone, a sulfonylurea, metformin (if obese), or insulin], that is important in reducing the risk of microvascular complications (36,37). The

effect of glycemic control on macrovascular disease (e.g., stroke) is less certain (36,37).

Cessation of Cigarette Smoking

There is little doubt that cigarette smoking is a risk factor for stroke (38,39). However, there has been only one randomized, controlled trial of an intervention to stop smoking, and stroke was not studied as an outcome (40). Among 1,445 men aged 40 to 59 years who were randomized to receive advice and encouragement to stop smoking or not, a greater proportion of the men who were given advice to stop smoking gave up cigarettes (i.e., there was a 53% mean absolute reduction in men continuing to smoke after advice compared with control) (40). However, the trial found no evidence that men given advice to stop smoking had a significantly lower mortality from coronary heart disease (relative risk reduction 18%, 95% CI: −18%–43%) (40). The wide CIs mean that there could have been anything from a 43% decrease to an 18% increase in rates of coronary heart disease death in men given advice to quit, regardless of whether they actually gave up smoking.

Observational studies indicate that the risk of stroke falls when people stop smoking, but the risk can take many years to approximate that of nonsmokers, particularly in those with a history of heavy smoking. The risk of stroke is decreased in ex-smokers compared with smokers (relative risk of stroke, smokers versus ex-smokers 1.2, 95% CI not available) but remains raised for 5 to 10 years after cessation compared with those who had never smoked (relative risk of stroke ex-smokers versus never smokers 1.5, 95% CI not available) (41). A study of 7,735 middle-aged British men found that 5 years after smoking cessation, the risk of stroke in previously light smokers (under 20 cigarettes/day) was identical to that of lifelong nonsmokers, but the risk in previously heavy smokers (more than 21 cigarettes/day) was still raised compared with that of lifelong nonsmokers (relative risk of stroke, previously heavy smokers versus never smokers 2.2, 95% CI: 1.1–4.3) (42). Another study of 117,001 middle-aged female nurses also found a fall in risk on stopping smoking and no difference between previously light and previously heavy smokers (relative risk in all former smokers 2–4 years after stopping smoking 1.17, 95% CI: 0.49–2.23) (43).

SECONDARY PREVENTION OF STROKE AMONG PATIENTS WITH PREVIOUS STROKE

Lowering of Blood Pressure

Published data from 10 randomized, controlled trials suggest that lowering the BP of transient ischemic attack (TIA)/stroke patients by 5 to 6 mm Hg diastolic and 10 to 12 mm Hg systolic for 2 to 3 years, or 9/4 mm Hg for 4 years, reduces their relative risk of stroke by about 28% (95% CI: 15%–39%) (44,45). These results are consistent, irrespective of the pathologic type of stroke (ischemic or hemorrhagic), the patient's baseline BP level, the time since the previous stroke (as long as it was between about 2 weeks and 5 years since the stroke), and the patient's ethnic background (45). Furthermore, a preliminary report from another trial in China, in which 5,665 people with a prior stroke or TIA were randomized to receive either a diuretic (indapamide) or placebo, a reduction of about 2 mm Hg in diastolic BP over 2 years was associated with a reduction in stroke incidence of 29% (95% CI: 12%–42%) (46).

If the average annual risk of recurrent stroke among patients with prior stroke or TIA is about 7.0% (47), the above data suggest that antihypertensive therapy reduces this risk to 5.0%/year, which is a relative risk reduction of 28% and ARR of 2.0%. Treating 1,000 patients for 1 year would prevent about 20 strokes each year. The NNT is therefore about 50. However, the longer patients are treated with antihypertensive therapy, the greater is the relative and absolute risk reduction for recurrent stroke.

The implication of these data is that patients with a history of TIA or stroke of any type, with no con-

traindication to BP lowering, should, with lifestyle changes and antihypertensive medication, slowly but intensively lower BP over several months to less than 130/80 mm Hg (or the lowest BP level above 130/80 mm Hg that the patient can tolerate) and thereby reduce the risk of subsequent serious vascular events by at least one-quarter (45). However, it must be emphasized that the results of the above clinical trials cannot necessarily be extrapolated to the very elderly or to patients with severe bilateral carotid occlusive disease who may not tolerate aggressive BP lowering.

Inhibition of the Angiotensin-Converting Enzyme

The results of the Heart Outcomes Prevention Evaluation (HOPE) Trial (20) suggest that the addition of ramipril 10 mg/day to best medical therapy (e.g., vascular risk factor control, antiplatelet therapy, carotid revascularization) has an additional favorable effect in reducing the rate of recurrent stroke, myocardial infarction, or death from vascular causes by about one-quarter. The reduction in vascular events is larger than might be expected from just lowering the BP and suggests that angiotensin-converting enzyme inhibition may have an additional protective effect on the vasculature over and above that associated with lowering BP. This remains controversial, however.

Lowering of Cholesterol

Until recently, there was uncertainty about whether lowering serum cholesterol levels in patients with previous stroke would reduce the risk of recurrent stroke and other serious vascular events, without compromising the risk of hemorrhagic stroke. However, the interim results of the British Heart Foundation/Medical Research Council Heart Protection Study (BHF/MRC-HPS) indicate that simvastatin effectively prevents stroke and other serious vascular events among patients with previous stroke (48).

A total of 20,536 patients, aged 40 to 80 years, with a history of previous coronary heart disease, stroke, peripheral arterial disease, diabetes mellitus, or treated hypertension, who had a serum total cholesterol level of more than 3.5 mmol/L (more than 135 mg/dL), were randomized to receive 40 mg of simvastatin, antioxidants (vitamin C 250 mg, vitamin E 600 mg, and β-carotene 20 mg), both, or neither. About 3,000 patients had a past history of ischemic stroke or TIA, of whom 1,820 had a history of stroke and no history of coronary heart disease. The patients were followed up for about 5 years.

Among the 10,269 patients allocated to simvastatin treatment, the average serum cholesterol level over the 5 years was 0.96 ± 0.02 mmol/L (37 ± 0.8 mg/dL) lower than among the 10,267 patients allocated to no simvastatin.

Allocation to simvastatin therapy was associated with a reduction in subsequent stroke, myocardial infarction, or vascular death from 25.4% (no simvastatin) to 19.9% (simvastatin) over 5 years, which is an odds reduction of 24% (SE 2.6%, $2p < 0.00001$) and ARR of 5.5%. This means that among 1,000 patients allocated to simvastatin, there were 55 ± 5.8 fewer serious vascular events over 5 years.

Allocation to simvastatin therapy was also associated with a reduction in subsequent stroke from 6.0% (no simvastatin) to 4.4% (simvastatin) over 5 years, which is an odds reduction of 27% (SE 5.3%, $2p < 0.00001$). In addition to a statistically significant reduction in ischemic stroke, there was a nonsignificant trend toward a modest reduction in hemorrhagic stroke, but the number of outcome events was very small and the results imprecise.

The effect of simvastatin on major outcome events was consistent, irrespective of the patient's age, gender, qualifying disease, or baseline serum cholesterol concentration.

Among the patients with previous stroke, allocation to simvastatin therapy was associated with a reduction in subsequent stroke, myocardial infarction, or vascular death from 215 events (no simvastatin) to 182 events (simvastatin) over at least 5 years, which is an odds reduction of about 20% (95% CI: 3%–35%). This means that among 1,000 patients with previous stroke who were allocated to simvastatin, there were about 70 fewer serious vascular events over 5 years.

The risks of hepatic dysfunction (alanine transaminase more than 3 times the upper limit of normal: 0.8% simvastatin, 0.6% placebo) and myopathy (creatine kinase more than 10 times the upper limit of normal: 0.09% simvastatin, 0.05% placebo) were very low.

The results of the Stroke Prevention by Aggressive Reduction in Cholesterol Levels (SPARCL) Trial, which is comparing the effect of atorvastatin with placebo in 4,200 patients with minor stroke or TIA, on the rate of total stroke are awaited (*www.neuro.wustl.edu/stroke/trials*; recruitment completed in 2001).

Control of Diabetes Mellitus

There have been no randomized, controlled trials, but observational studies suggest that tight glycemic control reduces the risk of macrovascular as well as microvascular disease (33–37).

Stopping Smoking

There have been no randomized, controlled trials, but observational studies suggest that stopping smoking decreases the risk of stroke by at least 1.5 times and up to 3 times in people under the age of 55 years (39).

Estrogen Replacement Therapy

Two recent clinical trials of estrogen replacement therapy suggest that estrogen does not reduce mortality or recurrent stroke in postmenopausal women with previous recent ischemic stroke or TIA (49) or coronary heart disease (50). The ongoing Women's Health Initiative, a randomized trial, should help clarify the role of estrogen in the primary prevention of stroke and other vascular diseases (if any—given the small increase in risk of breast and uterine cancer and venous thromboembolism associated with estrogen replacement therapy).

Vitamin Therapy

It remains uncertain whether lowering plasma total homocysteine concentrations by means of multivitamin therapy (folic acid, vitamin B_{12}, and vitamin B_6) is effective in preventing recurrent stroke and other serious vascular events among patients with previous stroke and TIA. It is hoped that this issue will be resolved by the results of the ongoing Vitamins in Stroke Prevention (VISP) Trial (Bowman Gray School of Medicine, Winston-Salem, North Carolina U.S.A.) (51) and the VITAmins TO Prevent Stroke (VITATOPS) Study (Royal Perth Hospital, University of Western Australia, Perth, Western Australia) (52).

REFERENCES

1. Whisnant JP. Modeling of risk factors for ischemic stroke: the Willis lecture. *Stroke* 1997;28:1839–1843.
2. Hankey GJ, Eikelboom J. Homocysteine and vascular disease. *Lancet* 1999;354:407–413.
3. Hankey GJ, Jamrozik K, Broadhurst RJ, et al. Long-term risk of first recurrent stroke in the Perth Community Stroke Study. *Stroke* 1998;29:2491–2500.
4. Staessen JA, Gasowski J, Wang JG, et al. Risks of untreated and treated isolated systolic hypertension in the elderly: meta-analysis of outcome trials. *Lancet* 2000;355:865–872.
5. O'Brien AA, Rajkumar C, Bulpitt CJ. Blood pressure lowering for the primary and secondary prevention of

stroke: treatment of hypertension reduces the risk of stroke. *J Cardiovasc Risk* 1999;6:203–205.

6. Ebrahim S, Davey Smith G. Lowering blood pressure: a systematic review of sustained non-pharmacological interventions. *J Public Health Med* 1998;20:441–448.

7. Stevens VJ, Obarzanek E, Cook NR, et al. Long-term weight loss and changes in blood pressure: results of the trials of hypertension prevention, phase II. *Ann Intern Med* 2001;134:1–11.

8. Metz JA, Stern JS, Kris-Etherton P, et al. A randomized trial of improved weight loss with a prepared meal plan in overweight and obese patients. *Arch Intern Med* 2000;160:2150–2158.

9. Appel LJ, Moore TJ, Obarzanek E, et al. A clinical trial of the effects of dietary patterns on blood pressure. *N Engl J Med* 1997;336:1117–1124.

10. Sacks FM, Svetkey LP, Vollmer WM, et al. Effects on blood pressure of reduced dietary sodium and the Dietary Approaches to Stop Hypertension (DASH) diet. *N Engl J Med* 2001;344:3–10.

11. Graudal NA, Galloe AM, Garred P. Effects of sodium restriction on blood pressure, renin, aldosterone, catecholamines, cholesterols, and triglyceride. *JAMA* 1998;279:1383–1391.

12. Whelton PK, Appel LJ, Espelland MA, et al. Sodium reduction and weight loss in the treatment of hypertension in older persons: a randomized controlled trial of non pharmacologic interventions in the elderly (TONE). *JAMA* 1998;279:839–846.

13. Whelton PK, He J, Cutler JA, et al. Effects of oral potassium on blood pressure: meta-analysis of randomized controlled clinical trials. *JAMA* 1997;277:1624–1632.

14. Morris MC, Sacks F, Rosner B. Does fish oil lower blood pressure? A meta-analysis of controlled clinical trials. *Circulation* 1993;88:523–533.

15. Goldberg IJ, Mosca L, Piano MR, et al. Wine and your heart. *Stroke* 2001;103:591–594.

16. Blood Pressure Lowering Treatment Trialists' Collaboration. Effects of ACE inhibitors, calcium antagonists, and other blood-pressure-lowering drugs: results of prospectively designed overviews of randomised trials. *Lancet* 2000;355:1955–1964.

17. He J, Whelton PK. Selection of initial antihypertensive drug therapy. *Lancet* 2000;356:1942–1943.

18. Arnolda L. Containing the costs of managing hypertension. *Med J Aust* 2001;174:556–557.

19. Nelson MR, McNeil JJ, Peeters A, et al. PBS.RPBS cost implications of trends and guideline recommendations in the pharmacological management of hypertension in Australia 1994–1998. *Med J Aust* 2001;174:565–568.

20. Heart Outcomes Prevention Evaluation (HOPE) Study investigators. Effects of an angiotensin converting-enzyme inhibitor, ramipril, on cardiovascular events in high-risk patients. *N Engl J Med* 2000;342:145–153.

21. Dahlöf B, Devereux RB, Kjeldsen SE, et al. Cardiovascular morbidity and mortality in the Losartan Intervention for Endpoint Reduction in Hypertension Study (LIFE): a randomised trial against atenolol. *Lancet* 2002;359:995–1003.

22. Gueyffier F, Froment A, Gouton M. New meta-analysis of treatment trials of hypertension: improving the estimate of therapeutic benefit. *J Hum Hypertens* 1996;10:1–8.

23. Hansson L, Zanchetti AZ, Carruthers SG, et al. Effects of intensive blood pressure lowering and low-dose aspirin in patients with hypertension: principal results of the Hypertension Optimal Treatment (HOT) Trial. *Lancet* 1998;351:1755–1762.

24. Prospective Studies Collaboration. Cholesterol, diastolic blood pressure, and stroke: 13,000 strokes in 450,000 people in 45 prospective cohorts. *Lancet* 1995;346:1647–1653.

25. Eastern Stroke and Coronary Heart Disease Collaborative Research Group. Blood pressure, cholesterol and stroke in Eastern Asia. *Lancet* 1998;352:1801–1807.

26. Byington RP, Davis PR, Plehn J, et al. Reduction in stroke events with pravastatin: the Prospective Pravastatin Pooling (PPP) Project. *Circulation* 2001;103:387–392.

27. Di Mascio R, Marchioli R, Tognoni G. Cholesterol reduction and stroke occurrence: an overview of randomised clinical trials. *Cerebrovasc Dis* 2000;10:85–92.

28. Sandercock P. Statins for stroke prevention? *Lancet* 2001;357:1548–1549.

29. Crouse JR III, Byington RP, Furberg CD. HMG-CoA reductase inhibitor therapy and stroke risk reduction: an analysis of clinical trials data. *Atherosclerosis* 1998;138:11–24.

30. Furberg CD, Adams HP, Applegate WB, et al. Effect of lovastatin on early carotid atherosclerosis and cardiovascular events. *Circulation* 1994;90:1679–1687.

31. Mercuri M, Bond MG, Sirtori CR, et al. Pravastatin reduces carotid intima-media thickness progression in an asymptomatic hypercholesterolaemic Mediterranean population: the Carotid Atherosclerosis Italian Ultrasound Study. *Am J Med* 1996;101:627–634.

32. Shepherd J, Cobbe SM, Ford I, et al., for the West of Scotland Coronary Prevention Study Group. Prevention of coronary heart disease with pravastatin in men with hypercholesterolaemia. *N Engl J Med* 1995;333:1301–1307.

33. Palumbo PJ. Glycemic control, mealtime glucose excursions, and diabetic complications in type 2 diabetes mellitus. *Mayo Clin Proc* 2001;76:609–618.

34. Diabetes Control and Complications Trial Research Group. The effect of intensive treatment of diabetes on the development and progression of long-term complications in insulin-dependent diabetes mellitus. *N Engl J Med* 1993;329:977–986.

35. Ohkubo Y, Kishikawa H, Araki E, et al. Intensive insulin therapy prevents the progression of diabetic microvascular complications in Japanese patients with non-insulin-dependent diabetes mellitus: a randomised prospective 6 years study. *Diabetes Res Clin Pract* 1995;28:103–117.

36. U.K. Prospective Diabetes Study (UKPDS) Group. Intensive blood-glucose control with sulphonylureas or insulin compared with conventional treatment and risk of complications in patients with type 2 diabetes. *Lancet* 1998;352:837–853.

37. U.K. Prospective Diabetes Study (UKPDS) Group. Intensive blood-glucose control with metformin on complications in overweight patients with type 2 diabetes (UKPDS 34). *Lancet* 1998;352:854–865. Correction in *Lancet* 1998;352:1557.

38. Shinton R, Beevers G. Meta-analysis of relation between cigarette smoking and stroke. *Br Med J* 1989;298:789–794.

39. Hankey GJ. Smoking and risk of stroke. *J Cardiovasc Risk* 1999;6:207–211.

40. Rose G, Hamilton PJ, Colwell L, et al. A randomised controlled trial of anti-smoking advice: 10-year results. *J Epidemiol Community Health* 1982;36:102–108.

41. U.S. Department of Health and Human Services. *The health benefits of smoking cessation: a report of the Surgeon General.* DHHS publication (CDC) 90-8416. Rockville, MD: U.S. Department of Health and Human Services, Public Health Service, Centers for Disease Control, 1990.

42. Wannamethee SG, Shaper AG, Ebrahim S. History of parental death from stroke or heart trouble and the risk of stroke in middle-aged men. *Stroke* 1996;27:1492–1498.

43. Kawachi I, Colditz GA, Stampfer MJ, et al. Smoking cessation in relation to total mortality rates in women: a prospective cohort study. *Ann Intern Med* 1993;119: 992–1000.

44. INDANA (Individual Data Analysis of Antihypertensive Intervention Trials) Project Collaborators. Effect of antihypertensive treatment in patients having already suffered a stroke: gathering the evidence. *Stroke* 1997;28:2557–2562.

45. PROGRESS Collaborative Group. Randomised trial of a perindopril-based blood-pressure-lowering regimen among 6105 individuals with previous stroke or transient ischaemic attack. *Lancet* 2001;358:1033–11041.

46. PATS Collaborating Group. Post-stroke antihypertensive treatment study: a preliminary result. *Chin Med J* 1995;108:710–717.

47. Hankey GJ, Jamrozik K, Broadhurst RJ, et al. Long-term risk of recurrent stroke in the Perth Community Stroke Study. *Stroke* 1998;29:2491–2500.

48. British Heart Foundation/Medical Research Council Heart Protection Study (BHF/MRC-HPS) Group. Randomised trial of antioxidant vitamins and simvastatin in patients at high risk of vascular events. Presented at the American Heart Association Annual Scientific Meeting, Anaheim, CA, U.S.A., November 2001.

49. Viscoli CM, Brass LM, Kernan WN, et al. A clinical trial of estrogen-replacement therapy after ischemic stroke. *N Engl J Med* 2001;345:1243–1249.

50. Simon JA, Hsia J, Cauley JA, et al. Postmenopausal hormone therapy and risk of stroke: the Heart and Estrogen–Progestin Replacement Study (HERS). *Circulation* 2001;103:638–642.

51. Spence JD, Howard VJ, Chambless LE, et al., for the VISP investigators. Vitamin Intervention for Stroke Prevention (VISP) Trial: rationale and design. *Neuroepidemiology* 2001;20:16–25.

52. VITATOPS Trial Study Group. The VITATOPS (VITAmins TO Prevent Stroke) Trial: rationale and design of an international, large, simple, randomised trial of homocysteine-lowering multivitamin therapy in patients with recent transient ischaemic attack or stroke. *Cerebrovasc Dis* 2002;13:120–126.

Ischemic Stroke: Advances in Neurology, Vol. 92. Edited by
H.J.M. Barnett, Julien Bogousslavsky, and Heather Meldrum.
Lippincott Williams & Wilkins, Philadelphia © 2003.

22

An Overview of Nonseptic Cardioembolic Stroke

*Anthony J. Furlan and Stephen D. Samples

*Section of Stroke and Neurological Intensive Care, Department of Neurology,
Cleveland Clinic Foundation, Cleveland, Ohio, U.S.A.

There is a very close relationship between the heart and stroke. Although the relative risk varies (e.g., hypertension is a relatively stronger risk factor for stroke and hyperlipidemia for coronary disease), atherosclerotic-related stroke and cardiac disease share the same risk factors. Indeed, the most frequent long-term cause of death in atherosclerotic stroke populations is myocardial infarction (1).

Acute stroke may cause a variety of cardiac dysrhythmias and even subendocardial myonecrosis. A more frequent occurrence, however, is cardiogenic stroke. Embolism from the heart accounts for approximately 15% to 20% of all ischemic strokes (2,3). The prevalence of cardioembolic stroke is higher in patients under 45 years old and may be as high as 23% to 36% (4). The higher percentage of cardioembolic stroke in younger patients reflects the lower prevalence of atherosclerotic disease in the young.

CLINICAL FEATURES

Small cardiac emboli may be associated with transient symptoms, minor clinical infarcts, or clinically silent infarcts detectable only by neuroimaging (5). However, cardioembolic strokes tend to be large and disabling. Abrupt cerebral arterial occlusion by a large cardiac embolism does not allow for the development of collateral blood flow. The onset typically occurs in an awake, active patient. The neurologic deficit from cardioembolic stroke typically is maximal at or near onset; stuttering evolution can reflect clot fragmentation and distal embolization but is more suggestive of atherothrombosis or lacunar infarction. Spontaneous recanalization occurs within 72 h in 75% of patients; delayed reperfusion of

infarcted tissue results in a high rate of hemorrhagic transformation that is usually clinically silent (6). Spontaneous recanalization within 6 h of stroke onset occurs in less than 20% of patients but may be associated with abrupt neurologic improvement—the so-called "spectacular shrinking deficit" (7).

Another clinical hallmark of cardiac embolism is cerebral ischemic events in multiple vascular territories. The cerebral circulation receives 10% to 15% of cardiac output, with the anterior (carotid) circulation accounting for about 90%. The most common sites of cardioembolic occlusion are the main trunk and branches of the middle cerebral artery (MCA); the anterior cerebral artery accounts for about 7% of cardiac emboli (8). The posterior (vertebral basilar) circulation receives about 10% of cerebral emboli, which typically lodge at the top of the basilar artery or in the posterior cerebral artery territory (9). Concomitant clinical symptoms suggestive of cardiac embolism include isolated fluent (Wernicke) aphasia (MCA), isolated homonymous hemianopsia (posterior cerebral artery), or top-of-the-basilar syndromes.

DIAGNOSTIC EVALUATION

A retrospective analysis of 184 consecutive patients with focal cerebral ischemia admitted to an intensive care stroke unit illustrates the value of a thorough cardiac evaluation (10). There were 68 patients with a transient ischemic attack and 116 with a stroke. History and physical exam found cardiac disease in 18.4%. An electrocardiogram (ECG) detected another 14.1%: 3 with atrial fibrillation and 23 with silent myocardial infarctions, predominantly in diabetic individuals. Two-dimensional echocardiography was performed in two-thirds of patients and detected a potential cardiac source of emboli in another 11.9%: Eleven patients had dyskinetic segments, six had left ventricular thrombi, one had endocarditis, and one had global left ventricular dysfunction. All patients were monitored with continuous ECG for 48 h. Four additional cases of atrial fibrillation were detected. Approximately 25% of the 184 patients underwent more prolonged ECG monitoring. Two more cases of atrial fibrillation were detected in addition to a case of sick sinus syndrome. Hence, an unsuspected cardiac source of embolism was detected as the potential source of stroke in an additional 15.2% of patients, nearly as frequently as those suspected based on a cardiac history or cardiac signs.

Echocardiography

Echocardiography is indicated in young patients with unexplained cerebrovascular symptoms and all patients with symptoms or signs of heart disease. However, in the elderly patient without evidence of heart disease, routine echocardiography is of limited utility and is not cost-effective. Transthoracic echocardiography (TTE) gives valuable information about left ventricular size and function and valvular abnormalities such as unsuspected mitral valve prolapse or rheumatic valvular disease. The sensitivity of TTE for a left ventricular thrombus (larger than 4 mm) is 86% to 95% with a specificity of 86% to 95%. TTE cannot adequately visualize the left atrium and atrial appendage, which are the main areas involved in nonvalvular atrial fibrillation (NVAF). The sensitivity of TTE for left atrial thrombi is only 39% to 63% and the specificity is under 50%. A technically inadequate study can occur with obese patients and those with underlying pulmonary disease. Adding intravenous bubble contrast material is useful for detecting the presence of intraatrial shunting, but accuracy is highly dependent on the adequacy of the study (11,12). Transcranial Doppler can be combined with bubble contrast echocardiography to better document the cerebral embolic potential of patent foramen ovale (PFO) and other potential cardiac sources of embolism.

Employing a small probe lowered into the esophagus, transesophageal echocardiography (TEE) offers images of the left atrium and atrial septum and appendage unobscured by chest wall or lung that are superior to those of TTE. TEE is also the preferred method for assessing the aortic arch, an underestimated source of atheroembolism in older patients.

TEE detects potential occult sources of embolism such as aortic arch atheromatous plaques and PFO in up to 30% of selected populations (13–15). TEE is particularly adept at diagnosing small intraatrial communications such as PFO, atrial septal defects, and atrial septal aneurysms, which many series suggest are the most frequent occult potential cardiac sources of embolism. Whereas the sensitivity and specificity of TEE for left ventricular thrombi are similar to those of TTE, TEE is superior for left atrial thrombi (100% and 99%, respectively). Also, the sensitivity of TEE for PFO is 85% (100% specificity). Unfortunately, 0.6% of patients cannot tolerate the procedure, and there is a 0.18% morbidity (from pulmonary or cardiac bleeding) and 0.0098% mortality (esophageal tear).

Electrocardiographic Monitoring

Prolonged cardiac monitoring (Holter) may reveal a variety of dysrhythmias such as paroxysmal atrial fibrillation, which can cause stroke. Stroke may itself precipitate a dysrhythmia, and sometimes it is unclear if an arrhythmia is a result, rather than a cause, of the stroke (16). Prolonged monitoring should be reserved for patients with syncope or palpitations at onset and for those patients with unexplained stroke, especially younger patients or those with other cardiac symptoms or signs.

The algorithm for a cardiac workup for patients with an acute stroke differs from one geographic region to another or even one hospital to another (17). The American Heart Association (AHA) recommends an echocardiogram for patients with an embolic stroke and clinical evidence of heart disease. An echocardiogram is also appropriate for patients younger than 45 years (18). The AHA recognizes that echocardiography is frequently done in patients older than 45 with a suspicion of cardiogenic stroke without clinical evidence of cardiac disease but, owing to a divergence of opinion, does not recommend it.

Neuroradiologic Imaging

Computed Tomography and Magnetic Resonance Imaging

Several findings on computed tomography (CT) have been characteristically associated with embolic strokes: (a) the presence of a cortical infarct, particularly in the middle or posterior cerebral artery territories; (b) the demonstration of multiple acute infarcts in different territories; (c) a hyperdense MCA; and (d) hemorrhagic infarction (19,20). None of these "rules," however, is inviolable. For example, deep infarcts may be caused by cardiac embolism to a lenticulostriate perforating artery and atherothrombotic infarcts may involve the MCA (especially in non-Caucasians) and be hemorrhagic.

The rate of hemorrhagic transformation on CT is between 2% and 4 % within 6 h of stroke onset (21). Scans 2 to 4 days after infarct show a rate of transformation of between 10% and 20%. Another study using serial scans found a rate of 6.2% between 1 and 4 days, 27.5% at 10 days, and 40.6% at 1 month (6). As mentioned, most of the CT hemorrhages are clinically silent.

Recent advancements allow for more accurate examinations with CT. CT angiography allows evaluation of large intracranial vessels for embolic clots (22). CT angiography should prove more sensitive than the dense MCA sign for clot recognition. CT perfusion studies more readily identify areas of infarction and can provide quantitative assessment of cerebral blood flow. Also, ischemic regions in multiple territories should be more easily viewed.

MRI (magnetic resonance imaging) with magnetic resonance angiography (MRA) and diffusion-weighted and perfusion-weighted MRI have many of the same advantages as advanced CT (23). Early detection of hemorrhage can now be reliably achieved using gradient echo MR techniques. Diffusion-weighted MRI may identify multiple unsuspected acute infarcts suggesting a cardiac source of embolism. Whereas the sensitivity and specificity of diffusion- and perfusion-weighted MRI may be slightly greater than those of perfusion CT, CT is more readily available and takes significantly less time.

Whichever technique is used, the approach to imaging acute stroke is rapidly changing to provide the clinician with a more informative "stroke-o-gram."

Cerebral Angiography

The lack of atherosclerotic stenosis underlying an occlusion and the presence of branch occlusions or delayed perfusion of distal arterial branches in the absence of a more proximal arterial source of embolism on angiography are highly suggestive of a cardioembolic source. In the era of transcranial Doppler, MR angiography, and CT angiography, angiography is utilized less frequently except in cases of potential intraarterial thrombolysis (24). However, cerebral angiography can precisely localize the site of

arterial occlusion in patients with acute stroke and may suggest a cardiac source of embolism (25).

COMMON CARDIAC SOURCES OF EMBOLISM

The most frequent cardiac sources of embolic stroke are NVAF, acute myocardial infarction, ventricular aneurysm, rheumatic heart disease, and prosthetic cardiac valves. Certain common cardiac conditions, especially PFO and mitral valve prolapse, have also been linked with stroke in patients under the age of 45. It is important to emphasize that a cardioembolic mechanism cannot always be inferred by the presence of a potential cardioembolic source. In older patients, an estimated 30% of patients with a cardioembolic source (e.g., atrial fibrillation) have concomitant cerebrovascular atherosclerosis. In younger patients, the stroke mechanism (e.g., paradoxic embolism) may be difficult to prove and is often inferred by a process of elimination.

Atrial Fibrillation

Atrial fibrillation in the setting of rheumatic mitral valve disease has long been recognized to greatly increase the risk of stroke and systemic embolism. Chronic NVAF in the absence of rheumatic heart disease was subsequently found to increase stroke risk fivefold after adjustment for other risk variables (26). NVAF is now recognized as the most frequent cause of cardioembolic stroke. The prevalence of NVAF increases with advancing age from 6.7% for ages 50 to 59 to 36.2% for ages 80 to 89 (27,28). More than one-third of ischemic strokes occurring in the elderly are in the setting of atrial fibrillation, and one-third of patients with atrial fibrillation will experience a clinical stroke sometime during their lifetime. Clinically silent cerebral infarcts are also present on CT in more than one-third of patients (5). Risk factors for stroke in the setting of NVAF include left atrial hypertrophy, hypertension, heart failure, and a history of prior stroke (29–31).

Myocardial Infarction: Acute and Long-Term Risk

Prior to the advent of thrombolysis, stroke complicated 0.8% to 5.5% of acute myocardial infarctions (32–34). Strokes after acute myocardial infarction were almost uniformly ischemic and generally thought to be embolic. An embolic mechanism is supported by pathologic studies demonstrating left ventricular mural thrombi in 38% to 67% of cases, typically in the apex in the setting of anteroapical infarctions (35–37). TTE evidence of mural thrombi or severe wall motion abnormalities identifies patients at increased risk for embolic stroke, although embolization may occur even in the absence of detectable thrombus on echocardiography (38,39). Stroke distribution reflects cerebral blood flow patterns, with the majority affecting the anterior circulation, particularly the MCA. Although 90% of the cerebral embolic events occur within the first 2 weeks after acute myocardial infarction, stroke risk continues for 4 to 6 months with a minority of patients at lifelong risk. Risk factors for stroke include older age, prior history of stroke, paroxysmal atrial fibrillation, anterior or apical location, impaired left ventricular function, and severity of myocardial infarction as measured by levels of cardiac enzymes, congestive heart failure, or advanced Killip class (40–44).

Valvular Heart Disease

Rheumatic mitral stenosis increases stroke risk 6-fold, which increases to 18-fold when associated with atrial fibrillation. Embolism occurs with all degrees of rheumatic mitral stenosis but is less frequent with pure mitral regurgitation (45–47). The risk of prosthetic valve thromboembolism is higher for valves in the mitral position than in the aortic position, higher for caged ball valves than tilting disc or bileaflet bioprosthetic valves, and higher for multiple than single prosthetic valves. Additional risk factors for thromboembolism include prior thromboembolism, atrial fibrillation, coronary heart disease, an enlarged left atrium, or left atrial thrombus (48–50).

Impaired Myocardial Function

Clinical evidence of impaired cardiac function including coronary artery disease and congestive heart failure further doubles the stroke risk. In heterogeneous groups of patients with cerebrovascular disease, 86% have angiographic evidence of coronary artery disease that is severe in 40% as determined by stress radionuclide ventriculography or cardiac catheterization (51,52). The neurologic presentation does not predict the severity of coronary artery disease. There is a 2.0%/year risk of stroke in patients with low ejection fraction. The risk of stroke increases with decreasing ejection fraction because of the increased formation of fresh thrombus in the left ventricle. Chronic left ventricular dysfunction or an akinetic wall segment after acute myocardial infarction carries a lower risk of embolic stroke because

any underlying thrombus is often organized and sessile (53,54).

Patent Foramen Ovale and Atrial Septal Aneurysm

Common in the general population, the prevalence of PFO is much higher in young patients with stroke of unknown cause than in matched control subjects (1,55). Several series have reported a 50% frequency of PFO in patients under age 45 with stroke of unknown cause. In older stroke populations, the prevalence is about 20%. TEE is the most sensitive technique for identifying a PFO. TTE may miss a small PFO especially if bubble contrast material is not used. Transcranial Doppler can be combined with TTE or TEE to document the right-to-left embolic potential of a PFO after the injection of agitated saline (56,57). PFO size (greater than 2 mm), associated atrial septal aneurysm, "smoke" in the left atrium, and deep vein thrombosis are associated with an increased risk of stroke from PFO (58,59). However, deep vein thrombosis is usually not documented in young patients with cryptogenic stoke and a PFO (which may partly reflect the insensitivity of leg venous ultrasound). About 60% of patients with atrial septal aneurysm also have a PFO, although only a small minority of patients with PFO have an atrial septal aneurysm. It is not clear if stroke in patients with both PFO and atrial septal aneurysm is due to paradoxic embolism, local thrombus formation, or some combination (60,61).

Mitral Valve Prolapse

Analogous to PFO, the prevalence of mitral valve prolapse is much higher in young patients with stroke of unknown cause compared with matched controls (62). In addition to stroke, mitral valve prolapse has been linked to other neurologic disorders including migraine and seizures. A unifying mechanism may be platelet dysfunction, which has been documented in patients with mitral valve prolapse (63). The tell-tale "click" of mitral valve prolapse is easily missed, and echocardiography is required for firm diagnosis.

TREATMENT AND PREVENTION OF CARDIAC EMBOLISM

Heparin

Anticoagulation with heparin has traditionally been advocated to prevent early recurrence in patients with acute cardioembolic stroke (64). Contraindications include patients with hemorrhage on CT (microhemorrhages on MR with negative CT have not been routinely used to exclude anticoagulation), patients with large infarcts (e.g., National Institutes of Health Stroke Scale score higher than 18), and septic infarcts. Recently, two large randomized trials [International Stroke Trial (IST) and Trial of ORG 10172 in Acute Stroke Treatment (TOAST)] failed to show any benefit of anticoagulation with either heparin (subcutaneous) or a low-molecular-weight heparinoid (65, 66). It is perhaps not surprising that heparin was of little value in improving neurologic disability in these trials as both entered patients up to 24 h after stroke onset. Even within 6 h of stroke onset, heparin and antithrombotic therapy is best viewed as adjunctive therapy in the era of thrombolysis. The more surprising finding in both IST and TOAST, of relevance to cardiac embolism, was the very low rate of early recurrent embolism even in patients with atrial fibrillation. Even though the rate was low, both heparin and aspirin reduced the rate of early recurrent stroke in these trials. However, any benefit of heparin was lost because of an excess risk of hemorrhage. Given the low recurrence rate and the risk of hemorrhage, the routine use of immediate heparin in patients with nonhemorrhagic cardioembolic stroke cannot be recommended. However, heparin may still be justified in certain subgroups at especially high risk of recurrent embolism, for example, patients with multiple cardiac risk factors, soft intracardiac thrombus, or multiple clinical events. Hence, the role of heparin in acute ischemic stroke remains controversial (67,68).

Atrial Fibrillation

The 1980s produced a series of randomized clinical trials addressing primary prevention of stroke and systemic embolism with chronic anticoagulant or antiplatelet therapy in patients with NVAF (69). Combined data of four trials included 3,135 patients followed from 15 to 27 months. Treatment consisted of placebo, aspirin at dosages of 75 or 325 mg/day, and warfarin with a prothrombin time ranging from 1.2 to 1.9 times the control value and standardized by an international normalization ratio (INR). The primary endpoints were the thromboembolic complications of cerebral infarction and systemic embolism and treatment complications of intracranial hemorrhage, major hemorrhage (bleeding requiring hospitalization, transfusion, or surgery), and minor bleeding. Exclusion criteria typically included significant bleeding history including intracranial hemorrhage, predisposition to trauma, inability for adequate follow-up, uncontrolled hypertension, alcohol abuse, or a requirement for anticoagulant therapy.

In the Copenhagen AFASAK (Atrial Fibrillation, Aspirin, Anticoagulation) Trial (70), 60% of the cerebral infarcts occurred during subtherapeutic anticoagulation and one-third of the patients dropped out because of the inconvenience of monthly monitoring. The Boston Area Anticoagulation Trial for Atrial Fibrillation (BAATAF) randomized patients to anticoagulation or usual care in an unblinded fashion (71). The discretionary use of aspirin was carefully monitored, and 8 of 13 endpoints in the control group occurred in patients taking at least 325 mg/day of aspirin.

The Stroke Prevention in Atrial Fibrillation (SPAF) studies finally established anticoagulation as the prevention treatment of choice in patients with atrial fibrillation. SPAF I (72) consisted of Group I patients randomized to receive placebo, aspirin 325 mg/day, or warfarin and Group II patients who were ineligible for warfarin but received aspirin or placebo. The study was prematurely interrupted when active treatment (aspirin or warfarin) was found to be significantly superior to placebo for Group I patients. Insufficient endpoints occurred at the time of interruption to assess the relative value of aspirin versus warfarin. SPAF II (73) compared warfarin (prothrombin time 1.3 to 1.8 times control value) to aspirin 325 mg/day for 1,100 patients younger than 75 years and 385 patients older than 75. SPAF III (74) addressed low-intensity, fixed-dose warfarin plus aspirin 325 mg/day versus adjusted-dose warfarin. SPAF III was stopped prematurely when an interim analysis demonstrated that warfarin at an INR of 2.0 to 3.0 was clearly superior to low-dose warfarin plus aspirin.

Aggregate data from these trials show that chronic anticoagulation reduced relative stroke risk by 63% in patients with NVAF, from 5.8%/year to 2.6%/year. Relative risk reduction increases to an impressive 83% when target anticoagulation is achieved. Complications of anticoagulant treatment included intracerebral hemorrhage at a rate of 0.3%/year. Major hemorrhage occurred in 1.5%/year regardless of treatment, but minor bleeding was three times more frequent in anticoagulated patients. These studies clearly document the efficacy and safety of chronic adjusted-dose anticoagulation at an INR range of 2.0 to 3.0 in a heterogeneous population of eligible patients with NVAF.

Acute Myocardial Infarction

Three large randomized clinical trials demonstrated a reduction in stroke with short-term anticoagulant therapy from 2.5% to 1.1% ($p < 0.01$) with heparin and phytonadione, 3.8% to 0.8% ($p = 0.001$) with heparin and warfarin, and 2.3% to 1.7% ($p =$ NS) with heparin and phenindione (75–77). If the patient is not a candidate for thrombolysis, then acute systemic anticoagulation with heparin is recommended in the setting of anterior wall Q-wave infarcts, severe left ventricular dysfunction, congestive heart failure, atrial fibrillation, evidence of mural thrombus on echocardiography, or a history of systemic or pulmonary embolism. Heparin anticoagulation may be accomplished by an intravenous bolus of 5,000 U followed by a continuous infusion of approximately 1,000 U/h adjusted to maintain the activated partial thromboplastin time at between 1.5 and 2.5 times the control value. If the patient receives coronary thrombolysis, heparin should be considered for prevention of systemic embolization in high-risk patients with congestive heart failure, large infarction, or atrial fibrillation when the activated partial thromboplastin time falls to within or below the therapeutic range (78).

The subsequent hospital course determines what adjuvant therapy is warranted at the time of discharge. Studies assessing longer-term anticoagulant therapy after acute myocardial infarction have demonstrated a reduction in embolic stroke that needs to be balanced by the increased risk of intracranial hemorrhage and is recommended for settings of increased embolic risk such as atrial fibrillation, prior systemic embolism, congestive heart failure, two-dimensional echo evidence of mural thrombus, or persistent left ventricular dysfunction with left ventricular ejection fraction values around 28% (53,79–81). The Warfarin–Aspirin Reduced Cardiac Ejection Fraction (WARCEF) Trial is comparing warfarin with aspirin for long-term stroke risk reduction in patients with reduced ejection fraction.

Valvular Heart Disease

On the basis of nonrandomized studies with historical controls, long-term anticoagulant therapy has been recommended for all patients with rheumatic mitral valve disease and paroxysmal or chronic atrial fibrillation (82). Even in the absence of atrial fibrillation, chronic anticoagulant therapy is warranted in certain subgroups such as mitral stenosis associated with enlargement of the left atrium of greater than 5.5 cm. Anticoagulation has also been recommended prior to balloon valvuloplasty of the mitral valve to reduce the embolic risk (83).

Thromboembolism is one of the most serious and feared complications of prosthetic heart valves. Many technical valve modifications have been designed to reduce thromboembolic potential and permit sufficient protection with lower-dose anticoagulation or antiplatelet therapy. Treatment recommendations are based upon the type of prosthetic valve and the presence of risk factors for thromboembolism such as prior thromboembolism, atrial fibrillation, coronary heart disease, large left atrium, left atrial thrombus, ball valve, more than one mechanical valve, or a mechanical valve in the mitral position.

The optimal intensity of anticoagulation that effectively prevents embolic complications while limiting hemorrhagic complications was refined in the 1990s. In 1992, the American College of Chest Physicians specified an INR range of 2.5 to 3.5 as optimal in the setting of mechanical heart valves. More recent studies have resulted in several U-shaped curves describing the relationship between the complication rate and intensity of anticoagulation depending upon such factors as the type of mechanical prosthetic valve and valve position. For example, patients with bileaflet valves are best treated with an INR of 3.0, whereas caged ball and tilting disc valves require a range of 4.0 to 4.9. Patients at higher risk, such as those with replacement of the mitral valve or a history of prior embolization, are best maintained at the higher end of the INR range, whereas those at lower risk are more safely treated at the lower end (84,85).

Patent Foramen Ovale and Mitral Valve Prolapse

Warfarin has been the usual therapy recommended in patients with PFO and presumed paradoxic or "cryptogenic" embolism. The choice of therapy in patients with "cryptogenic" stroke and a PFO has recently been obscured by the results of the Patent Foramen Ovale in Cryptogenic Stroke Study (PICSS) derived from the Warfarin–Aspirin Recurrent Stroke Study (WARSS) (86). PICSS found no significant difference between warfarin and aspirin for stoke prevention in patients with cryptogenic stroke and PFO, although the confidence intervals were wide (87). There are several subgroups of patients with PFO and stroke, and all may not require long-term warfarin. When a decision is made to close a PFO, it is now often done with an endovascular device (88). Typically, patients are maintained on aspirin and warfarin for 3 to 6 months after successful device closure, and then warfarin is discontinued.

Platelet dysfunction has been documented in patients with mitral valve prolapse. Antiplatelet therapy with aspirin is therefore the treatment of choice in patients with stroke due to mitral valve prolapse. As the absolute risk of stoke is low in asymptomatic patients discovered to have mitral valve prolapse, the routine use of antiplatelet therapy is not recommended.

REFERENCES

1. Webster MW, Chancellor AM, Smith HJ, et al. Patent foramen ovale in young stroke patients. *Lancet* 1988;2: 11–12
2. Cerebral Embolism Task Force. Cardiogenic brain embolism. *Arch Neurol* 1986;43:71–84.
3. Cerebral Embolism Task Force. Cardiogenic brain embolism: the second report of the Cerebral Embolism Task Force. *Arch Neurol* 1989;46:727.
4. Adams HP, Butler MJ, Biller J, et al. Nonhemorrhagic cerebral infarction in young adults. *Arch Neurol* 1986; 43:793.
5. Peterson P, Madsen EB, Brun B, et al. Silent cerebral infarction in atrial fibrillation. *Stroke* 1987;18: 1098–1100.
6. Okada Y, Yamaguchi T, Minematsu K, et al. Hemorrhagic transformation in cerebral embolism. *Stroke* 1989;20:598–603.
7. Minematsu K, Yamaguchi T, Omae T. "Spectacular shrinking deficit": major recovery from a major hemispheric syndrome by migration of an embolus. *Neurology* 1992;42:157–162.
8. Helgason C. Cardioembolic stroke topography and pathogenesis. *Cerebrovasc Brain Metab Rev* 1992;4: 28–58.
9. Caplan L. Top of the basilar syndrome: selected clinical aspects. *Neurology* 1980;30:72–79.
10. Rem JA, Hachinski VC, Boughner DR, et al. Value of cardiac monitoring and echocardiography in TIA and stroke patients. *Stroke* 1985;16:950.
11. Sirna S, Biller J, Skorton DJ, et al. Cardiac evaluation of the patient with stroke. *Stroke* 1990;21:14–23.
12. Amerenco P, Cohen A, Tzourio C, et al. Atherosclerotic disease of the aortic arch and the risk of ischemic stroke. *N Engl J Med* 1994;331:1474–1479.
13. Toyoda K, Yasaka M, Nagata S, et al. Aortogenic embolic stroke: a transesophageal echocardiographic approach. *Stroke* 1992;23:1056–1061.
14. Pop G, Sutherland GR, Koudstaal PJ, et al. Transesophageal echocardiography in the detection of intracardiac embolic sources in patients with transient ischemic attacks. *Stroke* 1990;21:560–565.
15. DeRook FA, Comess KA, Albers GW, et al. Transesophageal echocardiography in the evaluation of stroke. *Ann Intern Med* 1992;117:922.
16. Oppenheimer SM, Hachinski VC. The cardiac consequences of stroke. *Neurol Clin* 1992;10:167–176.
17. Tegeler CH, Downes TR. Cardiac imaging in stroke. *Stroke* 1991;22:1206–1211.
18. Ewy CA, Appleton CP, DeMaria AN, et al. ACC/AHA guidelines for the clinical application of echocardiography. *Circulation* 1990;82:2323.
19. Ringelstein EB, Koschorke S, Holling A, et al. Computed tomographic patterns of proven embolic brain infarction. *Ann Neurol* 1989;26:759–765.
20. Moulin T, Cattin F, Crepin-Leblond T, et al. Early CT signs in acute middle cerebral artery infarction: predictive value for subsequent infarct location and outcome. *Neurology* 1996;47:366–375.
21. Hart RG, Easton JD. Hemorrhagic infarcts. *Stroke* 1986;17:586.
22. Alberico RA, Patel M, Casey S, et al. Evaluation of the circle of Willis with three-dimensional CT angiography in patients with suspected in extracranial aneurysm. *AJNR Am J Neuroradiol* 1995;16:1571–1578.
23. Sorenson AG, Buonanno FS, Gonzales RG, et al. Hyperacute stroke: evaluation with combined multi-section diffusion-weighted and hemodynamically-weighted echoplanar MR imaging. *Radiology* 1996;199:391–401.
24. Caplan LR, Wolpert SM. Angiography in patients with occlusive cerebrovascular disease: a stroke neurologist and neuroradiologist's views. *AJNR Am J Neuroradiol* 1991;12:593–601.
25. Wolpert SM, Bruckmann H, Greenlee R, et al. Neuroradiologic evaluation of patients with acute stroke treated with recombinant tissue plasminogen activator. *AJNR Am J Neuroradiol* 1993;14:3–13.
26. Wolf PA, Dawber TR, Thomas HE, et al. Epidemiologic assessment of chronic atrial fibrillation and the risk of stroke: the Framingham Study. *Neurology* 1978;28: 973–977.
27. Wolf PA, Abbott RD, Kannel WB. Atrial fibrillation: a major contributor to stroke in the elderly. The Framingham Study. *Arch Intern Med* 1987;147:1561–1564.
28. Furberg CD, Psaty BM, Manolio TA, et al. Prevalence of atrial fibrillation in elderly subjects (the Cardiovascular Health Study). *Am J Cardiol* 1994;74:236–241.
29. European Atrial Fibrillation Trial Study Group. Secondary prevention in non-rheumatic atrial fibrillation after transient ischemic attack or minor stroke. *Lancet* 1993;324:1255–1262.
30. Atrial Fibrillation Investigators. Risk factors for stroke and efficacy of antithrombotic therapies in atrial fibrillation. Analysis of pooled data from five randomized controlled trials. *Arch Intern Med* 1994;154: 1449–1457.
31. Stroke Prevention in Atrial Fibrillation investigators. Predictors of thromboembolism in atrial fibrillation: clinical features in patients at risk. *Ann Intern Med* 1992;116:1–5.
32. Johannessen KA, Nordrehaug JE, von der Lippe G. Left ventricular thrombosis and cerebrovascular accident in acute myocardial infarction. *Br Heart J* 1984;51: 553–556.
33. Komrad MS, Coffey CE, Coffey KS, et al. Myocardial infarction and stroke. *Neurology* 1984;34:1403–1409.
34. Behar S, Tanne D, Abinader E, et al. Cerebrovascular accident complicating acute myocardial infarction: incidence, clinical significance, and short- and long-term mortality rates. *Am J Med* 1991;91:45–50.
35. Keating EC, Gross SA, Schlamowitz RA, et al. Mural thrombi in myocardial infarctions. *Am J Med* 1983;74: 989–995.
36. Weinreich DJ, Burke JF, Pauletto FJ. Left ventricular mural thrombi complicating acute myocardial infarction. *Ann Intern Med* 1984;100:789–794.
37. Meltzer RS, Visser CA, Fuster V. Intracardial thrombi and systemic embolization. *Ann Intern Med* 1986;104: 689–698.
38. Asinger RW, Mikell FL, Elsperger J, et al. Incidence of left ventricular thrombus after acute trans mural myocardial infarction: serial evaluation by two-dimen-

sional echocardiography. *N Engl J Med* 1981;305:297–302.

39. Schweizer P, Bardos P, Erbel R, et al. Detection of left atrial thrombi by echocardiography. *Br Heart J* 1984;51:553–556.

40. Maggiono AP, Franzosi MG, Santoro E, et al. The risk of stroke in patients with acute myocardial infarction after thrombolytic and antithrombotic treatment. *N Engl J Med* 1992;327:1–6.

41. Hess DC, D'Cruz IA, Adams RJ, et al. Coronary artery disease, myocardial infarction, and brain embolism. *Neurol Clin* 1993;11:399–417.

42. Vaitkus P, Barnathan ES. Embolic potential, prevention and management of mural thrombus complicating anterior myocardial infarction: a meta-analysis. *J Am Coll Cardiol* 1993;22:1004–1009.

43. Martin R, Bogousslavsky J. Mechanism of late stroke after myocardial infarct: the Lausanne Stroke Registry. *J Neurol Neurosurg Psychiatry* 1982;56:760–764.

44. Tanne D, Reicher-Reiss H, Boyko V, et al. Stroke risk after anterior wall acute myocardial infarction. *Am J Cardiol* 1995;76:825–826.

45. Coulshed N, Epstein EJ, McKendrick CS, et al. Systemic embolism in mitral valve disease. *Br Heart J* 1970;32:26–34.

46. Daly R, Mattingly TW, Holt CL, et al. Systemic arterial embolism in rheumatic heart disease. *Am Heart J* 1951;42:556–581.

47. Neilson GH, Galea EG, Hossack KF. Thromboembolic complications of mitral valve disease. *Aust NZ J Med* 1978;8:372–376.

48. Edmunds LH. Thromboembolic complications of current cardiac valvular prosthesis. *Ann Thorac Surg* 1982;34:96–106.

49. Stein PD, Alpert JS, Copeland J, et al. Antithrombotic therapy in patients with mechanical and biological prosthetic heart valves. *Chest* 1992;102[Suppl]:445S–455S.

50. Horstkotte D, Schulte HD, Bircks W, et al. Lower intensity anticoagulation therapy results in lower complication rates with the St. Jude Medical prosthesis. *J Thorac Cardiovasc Surg* 1994;107:1136–1145.

51. Rokey R, Rolak LA, Harati Y, et al. Coronary artery disease in patients with cerebrovascular disease: a prospective study. *Ann Neurol* 1984;16:50–53.

52. Hertzer NR, Young JR, Beven EG, et al. Coronary angiography in 506 patients with extracranial cerebrovascular disease. *Arch Intern Med* 1985;145:849–852.

53. Loh E, Sutton MSJ, Wun CCC, et al. Ventricular dysfunction and the risk of stroke after myocardial infarction. *N Engl J Med* 1997;336:251–257.

54. Dunkman WB, Johnson GR, Carson PE, et al. Incidence of thromboembolic events in congestive heart failure. *Circulation* 1993; 87[Suppl 6]:V194–V201.

55. Lechat P, Mas JL, Lascault G, et al. Prevalence of patent foramen ovale in patients with stroke. *N Engl J Med* 1988;318:1148–1152.

56. Chimowitz MI, Nemec JJ, Marwick TH, et al. Transcranial Doppler ultrasound identifies patients with right-to-left cardiac or pulmonary shunts. *Neurology* 1991;41:1902–1904.

57. Albert A, Muller HR, Hetzel A. Optimized transcranial Doppler technique for the diagnosis of cardiac right-to-left shunts. *J Neuroimag* 1997;7:159–163.

58. Hanna JP, Sun JP, Furlan AJ, et al. Patent foramen ovale and brain infarct: echocardiographic predictors, recurrence and prevention. *Stroke* 1994;25:782–786.

59. Homma S, DiTullio MR, Sacco RL, et al. Characteristics of patent foramen ovale associated with cryptogenic stroke. A biplane transesophageal echocardiographic study. *Stroke* 1994;25:582–586.

60. Nater B, Bogousslavsky J, Regli F, et al. Stroke patterns with atrial septal aneurysms. *Cerebrovasc Dis* 1992;2:342–346.

61. Cabanes L, Mas JL, Cohen A, et al. Atrial septal aneurysm and patent foramen ovale as risk factors for cryptogenic stroke in patients less than 55 years of age. A study using transesophageal echocardiography. *Stroke* 1993;24:1865–1873.

62. Barnett HJM, Boughner DR, Taylor DW, et al. Further evidence relating mitral valve prolapse to cerebral ischemic events. *N Engl J Med* 1980;302:139–144.

63. Lauzier S, Barnett HJM. Cerebral ischemia with mitral valve prolapse and mitral annular calcification. In: Furlan AJ, ed. *The heart and stroke: exploring mutual cerebrovascular and cardiovascular issues.* London: Springer-Verlag, 1987:63–100.

64. Cerebral Embolism Study Group. Immediate anticoagulation of embolic stroke: brain hemorrhage and management options. *Stroke* 1984;15:779–789.

65. International Stroke Trial (IST). A randomized trial of aspirin, subcutaneous heparin, both, or neither among 19435 patients with acute ischemic stroke. International Stroke Trial Collaborative Group. *Lancet* 1997;349:1569–1581.

66. Publications Committee for the Trial of ORG 10172 in Acute Stroke Treatment (TOAST) investigators. Low molecular weight heparinoid, ORG 10172 (danaproid), and outcome after acute ischemic stroke: a randomized controlled trial. *JAMA* 1998;279:1265–1272.

67. Sandercock P. Is there still a role for intravenous heparin in acute stroke? No. *Arch Neurol* 1999;56:1160–1161.

68. Moonis M, Fisher M. Considering the role of heparin and low-molecular weight heparins in acute ischemic stroke. *Stroke* 2002;33:1927–1933.

69. Albers GW, Sherman DG, Gress DR, et al. Stroke prevention in nonvalvular atrial fibrillation; a review of prospective randomized trials. *Ann Neurol* 1991;30:511–518.

70. Peterson P, Godtfredsen J, Boysen G, et al. Placebo-controlled, randomized trial of warfarin and aspirin for prevention of thromboembolic complications in chronic atrial fibrillation: the Copenhagen AFASAK Study. *Lancet* 1989;1:175–179.

71. Boston Area Anticoagulation Trial for Atrial Fibrillation investigators. The effect of low-dose warfarin on the risk of stroke in patients with nonrheumatic atrial fibrillation. *N Engl J Med* 1990;323:1505–1511.

72. Stroke Prevention in Atrial Fibrillation investigators. The Stroke Prevention in Atrial Fibrillation Study: final results. *Circulation* 1991;84:527–539.

73. Stroke Prevention in Atrial Fibrillation investigators. Warfarin versus aspirin for prevention of thromboembolism in atrial fibrillation. Stroke Prevention in Atrial Fibrillation II Study. *Lancet* 1994;343:687–691.

74. Stroke Prevention in Atrial Fibrillation investigators. Adjusted-dose warfarin versus low-intensity, fixed-dose warfarin plus aspirin for high-risk patients with atrial

fibrillation: Stroke Prevention in Atrial Fibrillation III randomised clinical trial. *Lancet* 1996;348:633–638.

75. Medical Research Council. Assessment of short-term anticoagulant administration after myocardial infarction. *Br Med J* 1969;1:335–342.

76. Veteran's Administration Cooperative Study: anticoagulants in acute myocardial infarction: results of a cooperative trial. *JAMA* 1973;225:724–729.

77. Drapkin A, Mersky C. Anticoagulant therapy after acute myocardial infarction: relation of therapeutic benefit to patient's age, sex, and severity of infarction. *JAMA* 1972;222:541–549.

78. Cairns JA, Lewis HD, Meade TW, et al. Antithrombotic agents in coronary artery disease. *Chest* 1995; 10[Suppl]:380S–400S.

79. Report of the 60+ Reinfarction Study Research Group. A double-blind trial to assess long-term anticoagulant therapy in elderly patients after myocardial infarction. *Lancet* 1980;2:989–994.

80. Smith P, Arnesen H, Holme I. The effect of warfarin on mortality and reinfarction after myocardial infarction. *N Engl J Med* 1990;323:147–152.

81. ASPECT Research Group. Effect of long-term oral anticoagulant treatment on mortality and cardiovascular morbidity after myocardial infarction. *Lancet* 1994;343: 499–503.

82. Levin HJ, Panker SG, Salzman EW. Antithrombotic therapy in valvular heart disease. *Chest* 1989; 95[Suppl]:98S–106S.

83. Levin HJ, Panker SG, Salzman EW. Antithrombotic therapy in valvular heart disease. *Chest* 1989; 95[Suppl]:98S–106S.

84. Stein PD, Kantrowitz A. Antithrombotic therapy in mechanical and bioprosthetic heart valves and saphenous vein bypass grafts. *Chest* 1989;95[Suppl]: 107S–117S.

85. Stein PD, Alpert JS, Copeland J, et al. Antithrombotic therapy in patients with mechanical and bioprosthetic heart valves. *Chest* 1995;95[Suppl]:371S–379S.

86. Warfarin Aspirin Recurrent Stroke Study (WARSS). *N Engl J Med* 2001;345:1444.

87. PFO in Cryptogenic Stroke Study (PICSS). Presented at the 27th International Stroke Conference, San Antonio, TX, U.S.A., February 2002.

88. Ende DJ, Chapra S, Rao S. Transcatheter closure of atrial septal defect or patent foramen ovale with the buttoned device for the prevention of recurrence of paradoxical embolism. *Am J Cardiol* 1996;78:233–236.

SUGGESTED READING

Bath PMW, Lindenstrom E, Boysen G, et al. Tinzaparin in acute ischaemic stroke (TAIST): a randomised aspirin-controlled trial. *Lancet* 2001;358:702–710.

Berge E, Abdelnoor M, Nakstad PH, et al. Low molecular-weight heparin versus aspirin in patients with acute ischaemic stroke and atrial fibrillation: a double-blind randomised study. *Lancet* 2000;355:1205–1210.

Chamorro A, Vila N, Ascaso C, et al. Heparin in acute stroke with atrial fibrillation clinical relevance of very early treatment. *Arch Neurol* 1995;56:1098–1102.

Collins R, MacMahon S, Flather M, et al. Clinical effects of anticoagulant therapy in suspected acute myocardial infarction: systematic overview of randomised trials. *Br Med J* 1996;313:652–659.

Coull BM, Williams LS, Goldstein LB, et al. Anticoagulants and antiplatelet agents in acute ischemic stroke: report of the Joint Stroke Guideline Development Committee of the American Academy of Neurology and the American Stroke Association (a Division of the American Heart Association). *Stroke* 2002;33:1934–1942.

Gilon D, Buonanno F, Joffe M. Lack of evidence of an association between mitral-valve prolapse and stroke in young patients. *N Engl J Med* 1999;341:8–13.

Mas J-L, Arquizan C, Lamy C, et al. Recurrent cerebrovascular events associated with patent foramen ovale, atrial septal aneurysm, or both. *N Engl J Med* 2001;345: 1740–1746.

Taylor FC, Cohen H, Ebrahim S. Systematic review of long term anticoagulation or antiplatelet treatment in patients with non-rheumatic atrial fibrillation. *Br Med J* 2001; 322:321–326.

Thomson R, Parkin D, Eccles M, et al. Decision analysis and guidelines for anticoagulant therapy to prevent stroke in patients with atrial fibrillation. *Lancet* 2000:355: 956–962.

Ischemic Stroke: Advances in Neurology, Vol. 92. Edited by
H.J.M. Barnett, Julien Bogousslavsky, and Heather Meldrum.
Lippincott Williams & Wilkins, Philadelphia © 2003.

23

Specifics of Patent Foramen Ovale

Jean-Louis Mas

*Department of Neurology, Paris V University; Department of Neurology, Sainte-Anne Hospital,
Paris, France*

Advances in cardiac imaging techniques have resulted in the recognition of several "new" potential cardioembolic sources. These findings, however, are often prevalent in individuals who have not suffered a stroke, and it is not always easy to differentiate between an incidentally associated abnormality or the direct cause of a stroke among affected individuals. A patent foramen ovale (PFO) is a typical example of a cardiac abnormality whose causal relation to stroke and prognostic and therapeutic implications are not clearly established (1).

ASSOCIATION OF PATENT FORAMEN OVALE WITH STROKE

The foramen ovale is a natural interatrial channel that normally closes after birth as pressure in the left atrium exceeds that in the right atrium. In about 30% of the population, however, the foramen stays patent throughout life, maintaining a potential channel through which blood may shunt from the right to the left atrium. The maximal size of the potential orifice ranges from 1 to 19 mm (mean 4.9 mm) (2). Transesophageal echocardiography with contrast material injection is considered the gold standard for diagnosing a PFO. A number of studies have recently shown that contrast-enhanced transcranial Doppler examination of the middle cerebral artery is highly sensitive and highly specific compared with contrast transesophageal echocardiography in detecting a right-to-left shunt, which, in the majority of cases, is due to a PFO (3).

During the last 15 years, several studies have shown that a PFO is detected much more frequently in patients with an otherwise unexplained ischemic stroke than in control subjects or patients with an identifiable cause of stroke (4–8). In a recent meta-analysis of case control studies (8) in which patients with ischemic stroke were compared with nonstroke control subjects, PFO was significantly associated with ischemic stroke in subjects younger than 55 years but not in older ones. The odds ratio of stroke in the former was 3.1 [95% confidence interval (CI): 2.3–4.2] (Table 23-1). Reported detection rates of PFOs in cryptogenic stroke patients, however, vary widely, ranging from 31% to 77% (8). Such disagreement may result partly from interobserver variability in the diagnosis of these septal abnormalities (9), different diagnostic techniques or criteria employed, or methodologic inconsistencies (8).

Cryptogenic stroke patients with PFO have been reported to be younger, less likely to have traditional risk factors for stroke (e.g., hypertension, diabetes, hypercholesterolemia, and smoking), and having, on average, a less severe stroke than patients without PFOs (10). These differences in stroke risk factors and stroke severity suggest different stroke mechanisms in patients with and without PFOs. They also indirectly suggest that PFOs play a role, whether causal or not, in the occurrence of stroke in young adults.

As PFOs are relatively common in patients without stroke, it is clinically useful to characterize PFOs into those conditions that, in varying degrees, are more likely to be associated with stroke. In this respect, several investigators have suggested that patients who have an atrial septal aneurysm (ASA) in addition to a PFO may constitute a subgroup of patients with a higher risk of stroke (7). Studies using transesophageal echocardiography have revealed that about 20% of patients with a PFO also had an ASA (10), a cardiac abnormality that itself was associated with cerebral emboli (7). Moreover, the prevalence of ASAs increased with the degree of shunting (10).

TABLE 23-1. *Comparison of prevalence of patent foramen ovale in patients with ischemic stroke and nonstroke control subjects according to age less than 55 years (A) and more than 55 years (B)*

Study	Stroke n/N	Control n/N	OR (95% CI Fixed)	Weight %	OR (95% CI Fixed)
Cabanes, 1993 (P)	43 / 100	9 / 50		13.8	3.44[1.51,7.83]
Chen, 1991 (P)	15 / 34	7 / 40		7.2	3.72[1.29,10.74]
Del Sette, 1998 (P)	26 / 73	8 / 50		12.3	2.90[1.19,7.11]
Job, 1994 (P)	38 / 74	27 / 63		28.6	1.41[0.72,2.77]
Jones, 1994 (P)	7 / 26	2 / 19		3.4	3.13[0.57,17.18]
Lechat, 1988 (P)	24 / 60	10 / 100		9.1	6.00[2.61,13.80]
Webster, 1988 (P)	20 / 40	6 / 40		6.0	5.67[1.95,16.46]
Zahn, 1995 (P)	50 / 120	11 / 55		17.7	2.86[1.34,6.07]
de Belder, 1992 (P)	5 / 39	1 / 39		1.8	5.59[0.62,50.25]
Total (95% CI)	228 / 566	81 / 456		100.0	3.10[2.29,4.21]

Chi-square 9.40 (df = 8) P: 0.31

A

Negative association   Positive association

Study	Stroke n/N	Control n/N	OR (95% CI Random)	Weight %	OR (95% CI Random)
Jones, 1994 (P)	28 / 194	29 / 183		45.4	0.90[0.51,1.57]
Zahn, 1995 (P)	15 / 68	4 / 26		28.4	1.56[0.46,5.22]
de Belder, 1992 (P)	13 / 64	3 / 56		26.2	4.50[1.21,16.74]
Total (95% CI)	56 / 326	36 / 265		100.0	1.60[0.63,4.06]

Chi-square 5.15 (df = 2) P: 0.08

B

Negative association   Positive association

From Overell JR, Bone I, Lees KR. Interatrial septal abnormalities and stroke. A meta-analysis of case-control studies. *Neurology* 2000;55:1172–1179, with permission.

Case control studies have shown that the presence of both cardiac abnormalities is consistently more strongly associated with ischemic stroke than is the presence of either factor alone (8). Several studies (11–16) have also suggested that a more severe right-to-left shunt, a larger opening of the PFO, or the presence of right-to-left shunting at rest (as opposed to shunting detected only during provocative maneuvers) may reflect a particular stroke risk. Most of these studies, however, did not focus on the association between concomitantly existing PFOs and ASAs, so that some of the demonstrated associations may involve both lesions in combination rather than a PFO alone, given the increasing prevalence of ASA with a greater extent of the shunt (10).

POTENTIAL MECHANISM(S) OF PATENT FORAMEN OVALE-ASSOCIATED STROKE

The mechanism of stroke in patients with a PFO remains ill defined. The shunt created by a PFO may allow the passage of thrombotic material from the venous bed into the arterial circulation, a condition defined as "paradoxic embolization." This mechanism has been well documented in isolated cases, both by autopsy and by echocardiographic studies, which demonstrated a thrombus caught in its passage through a PFO (1). Diagnosis based on such a stringent criterion, however, inherently underestimates the true frequency of paradoxic embolism because it depends upon a rather precise coincidence of the size of the thrombus and the orifice of the foramen ovale. Indirect criteria for paradoxic embolism include (a) an arterial embolism with no evidence of left-sided circulation source, (b) the potential for right-to-left shunting, and (c) the presence of venous thrombosis and/or pulmonary embolism (which not only provides evidence of the presence of venous thrombosis but also confirms that embolization has occurred).

Right-to-left shunting is common in the presence of a PFO. In fact, the normal pressure gradient across a PFO can be transiently reversed either spontaneously during early systole or by everyday Valsalva-inducing activities. In contrast, the presence of a venous source of thromboembolism (a key criterion for paradoxic embolism) is rarely demonstrated in stroke patients with a PFO (10,17). Failure to document a venous source of embolism may indicate that paradoxic embolism has not occurred, or alternatively, it may be due to underrecognition of venous thrombi. Indeed, there are many pitfalls in the diagnosis of venous thrombosis that may result in clinical underrecognition. The source of the emboli may

remain undetected because of its location or the size of the thrombus: Thrombi as small as 1 or 2 mm are undetectable by any imaging technique, but they may be sufficient to cause stroke, and the average size of a PFO easily allows their passage into the arterial circulation. Venous thrombi may disappear either spontaneously or after anticoagulation and do so before investigations are performed. Thus, failure to document venous thrombi does not necessarily exclude paradoxic embolism in a patient who has PFO. The problem of demonstrating venous thrombosis is made even more complex by the fact that when it occurs in a patient who has experienced a hemiplegic stroke, a venous thrombosis may be no more than the consequence of immobilization due to stroke rather than the cause of the stroke. On the other hand, the occurrence of stroke in a patient with recently diagnosed venous thrombosis or the simultaneous occurrence of pulmonary and systemic embolism should strongly suggest a paradoxic embolism, but these situations are uncommon. Thus, in a vast majority of patients with PFO-associated stroke, the clinical diagnosis of paradoxic embolism remains speculative.

Another potential mechanism of stroke is direct embolization from thrombi formed locally within the foramen or an associated ASA. Patency of the foramen may allow a thrombus formed on the right atrial side of the aneurysm to reach the systemic circulation. In single case reports, a thrombus within an aneurysm has been observed at autopsy (18), at surgical resection, or on echocardiography (19), but thrombi attached to an ASA and detected by echocardiography are apparently rare (20). Finally, atrial vulnerability has been found to be more frequent in patients with PFOs than in those without them (21), suggesting the potential role of transient atrial arrhythmias in thrombus formation.

RISK OF RECURRENT STROKE

In addition to the speculative nature of stroke mechanisms, therapeutic decisions have been hindered by the lack of precise data on the risk of recurrent stroke. Most available studies (12,16,22–26) were either retrospective, did not include a control group of patients with no septal abnormalities, involved small numbers of patients, or used heterogeneous treatments for secondary prevention. In the two studies that reported on stroke recurrence in relatively large series of young (under 60 years old) unselected stroke patients with PFO (23,24), the risks of experiencing a recurrent stroke were 1.2% and 1.9%, respectively. However, CIs of these estimates were large, and treatments were not controlled. In one of these studies (23), the combination of PFO and ASA was significantly associated with recurrent cerebral ischemia, with an average annual rate of recurrent stroke of 4.4%.

In the prospective, multicenter PFO-ASA Study (27), investigators used a standardized treatment (aspirin, 300 mg/day) to assess the absolute and relative risks of recurrent cerebrovascular events associated with a PFO, an ASA, or both abnormalities. The study cohort consisted of 581 consecutive patients aged between 18 and 55 years who had a recent ischemic stroke of unknown origin. At 4 years, the risk of recurrent stroke was 2.3% (95% CI: 0.3%–4.3%) in patients with isolated PFO (n = 216), 15.2% (95% CI: 1.8%–28.6%) in those with both PFO and ASA (n = 51), and 4.2% (95% CI: 1.8%–6.6%) in those with neither of these cardiac abnormalities (n = 304). Noteworthy was the finding that no recurrence occurred in patients with isolated ASA (n = 10). The presence of both cardiac abnormalities was the only septal disorder significantly associated with an increased risk of recurrent stroke (hazard ratio, 4.2; 95% CI: 1.5%–11.8%), whereas isolated PFO, whether small or large, was not (Table 23-2). This finding remained significant when the analysis was restricted to patients who had no traditional vascular risk factors.

SECONDARY PREVENTION

The optimal treatment strategy for secondary prevention in patients with PFOs or ASAs has not been determined. Therapeutic options include antiplatelet drugs, oral anticoagulants, transcatheter closure of the foramen, and open-heart surgery (28,29). All these therapeutic options bear risks that need to be weighed against the risk of spontaneous recurrent strokes. Unless we can delineate more stringent indications for these various therapeutic interventions, we may jeopardize some patients by exposing them to unnecessary complications of the treatment we have chosen for them. There are no published investigations showing the superiority of any one strategy over another.

In the rare case of an impending paradoxic embolism discovered at echocardiography, intracardiac embolectomy with correction of the intracardiac defect has been the preferred treatment. Thrombolytic therapy and anticoagulation with intravenous heparin have been reported to be effective in patients with impending paradoxic embolism in whom emergency surgery was not feasible (30). In the presence of a recent cerebral infarct, cardiopulmonary bypass might be hazardous because of the need for total-body heparinization and possible localized low-flow states, whereas thrombolytic

TABLE 23-2. *Cox proportional hazard models of predictors of recurrent cerebrovascular events*

Variable	Recurrent stroke		Recurrent stroke or TIA	
	Hazard ratio (95% CI)	p value	Hazard ratio (95% CI)	p value
Atrial septal abnormality		0.03[a]		0.03[a]
Neither[b]	1.0	—	1.0	—
Patent foramen ovale alone	0.86 (0.31–2.36)	0.77	1.34 (0.62–2.90)	0.45
Atrial septal aneurysm alone	—	0.98	—	0.97
Patent foramen ovale and atrial septal aneurysm	4.17 (1.47–11.84)	0.007	3.91 (1.59–9.59)	0.003
Age (per year of age)	1.06 (1.00–1.13)	0.04	1.02 (0.98–1.07)	0.25
Male sex	2.41 (0.91–6.37)	0.08	1.68 (0.81–3.48)	0.16
Number of vascular risk factors		0.81[a]		0.61[a]
0[b]	1.0	—	1.0	—
1	0.82 (0.32–2.10)	0.68	0.98 (0.46–2.08)	0.95
2	0.97 (0.28–3.37)	0.97	1.28 (0.46–3.55)	0.64
3	1.77 (0.37–8.44)	0.47	2.20 (0.61–7.89)	0.23

CI, confidence interval; TIA, transient ischemic attack.
[a]The p value is for the overall comparison.
[b]This group served as the reference group.
From Mas JL, Arquizan C, Lamy C, et al. Recurrent cerebrovascular events associated with patent foramen ovale, atrial septal aneurysm, or both. *N Engl J Med* 2001;345:1740–1746, with permission.

therapy may be hazardous because of the risk of cerebral hemorrhage.

In young patients (i.e., under 60 years old) who have an isolated PFO and who have had a single otherwise unexplained ischemic stroke, the PFO-ASA Study suggests that secondary prevention with aspirin is sufficient (27). If there is evidence for concomitant venous thrombosis and/or pulmonary embolism, anticoagulant therapy should be undertaken as long as the risk of venous thromboembolism persists. Long-term anticoagulation or PFO closure may be indicated in patients with high risk of recurrent venous thromboembolism or with recurrent cerebral ischemia on antiplatelet drugs. The potential benefit of surgical foramen closure is unclear. Whereas this procedure can prevent recurrent paradoxic embolism through a PFO, it does not prevent recurrent venous thromboembolism, with its potentially serious consequences.

The PFO-ASA Study also suggests that patients with both PFO and ASA who have had a cryptogenic stroke constitute a subgroup with a higher risk of stroke recurrence when they are on aspirin. Whether these patients would benefit from more aggressive therapeutic strategies such as a combination of antiplatelet drugs, long-term anticoagulation, or surgical correction of the cardiac abnormalities needs to be assessed in randomized clinical trials.

REFERENCES

1. Mas JL. Patent foramen ovale, atrial septal aneurysm and ischemic stoke in young adults. *Eur Heart J* 1994; 15:446–449.
2. Hagen PT, Scholz DG, Edwards WD. Incidence and size of patent foramen ovale during the first 10 decades of life: an autopsy study of 965 normal hearts. *Mayo Clin Proc* 1984;59:17–20.
3. Arquizan C, Coste J, Touboul PJ, et al. Is patent foramen ovale a family trait? A transcranial Doppler sonographic study. *Stroke* 2001;32:1563–1566.
4. Lechat P, Mas JL, Lascault G, et al. Prevalence of patent foramen ovale in patients with stroke. *N Engl J Med* 1988;318:1148–1152.
5. Webster MWI, Chancellor AM, Smith HJ, et al. Patent foramen ovale in young stroke patients. *Lancet* 1988;2: 11–12.
6. Di Tullio M, Sacco RL, Gopal A, et al. Patent foramen ovale as risk factor for cryptogenic stroke. *Ann Intern Med* 1992;117:461–465.
7. Cabanes L, Mas JL, Cohen A, et al. Atrial septal aneurysm and patent foramen ovale as risk factors for cryptogenic stroke in patients less than 55 years of age. A study using transesophageal echocardiography. *Stroke* 1993;24:1865–1873.
8. Overell JR, Bone I, Lees KR. Interatrial septal abnor-

9. Cabanes L, Coste J, Derumeaux G, et al., for the Patent Foramen Ovale and Atrial Septal Aneurysm Study Group. Inter- and intra-observer variability in detection of patent foramen ovale and atrial septal aneurysm with transesophageal echocardiography. *J Am Soc Eechocardiogr* 2002;15:441–447.
10. Lamy C, Giannesini C, Zuber M, et al., for the Patent Foramen Ovale and Atrial Septal Aneurysm Study Group. Clinical and imaging findings in cryptogenic stroke patients with and without patent foramen ovale: the PFO-ASA Study. *Stroke* 2002;33:706–711.
11. Homma S, Di Tullio MR, Sacco RL, et al. Characteristics of patent foramen ovale associated with cryptogenic stroke. A biplane transesophageal echocardiographic study. *Stroke* 1994;25:582–586.
12. Hausmann D, Mügge A, Daniel WG. Identification of patent foramen ovale permitting paradoxic embolism. *J Am Coll Cardiol* 1995;26:1030–1038.
13. Serena J, Segura T, Perez-Ayuso MJ, et al. The need to quantify right-to-left shunt in acute ischemic stroke. A case-control study. *Stroke* 1998;29:1322–1328.
14. Steiner MM, Di Tullio MR, Rundek T, et al. Patent foramen ovale size and embolic brain imaging findings among patients with ischemic stroke. *Stroke* 1998;29: 944–948.
15. Schuchlenz HW, Weihs W, Horner S, et al. The association between the diameter of a patent foramen ovale and the risk of cerebrovascular events. *Am J Med* 2000;109: 456–462.
16. De Castro S, Cartoni D, Fiorelli M, et al. Morphological and functional characteristics of patent foramen ovale and their embolic implications. *Stroke* 2000;31: 2407–2413.
17. Ranoux D, Cohen A, Cabanes L, et al. Patent foramen ovale: is stroke due to paradoxical embolism? *Stroke* 1993;24:31–34.
18. Silver MD, Dorsey JS. Aneurysms of the septum primum in adults. *Arch Pathol Lab Med* 1978;102:62–65.
19. Schneider B, Hanrath P, Vogel P, et al. Improved morphologic characterization of atrial septal aneurysm by transesophageal echocardiography: relation to cerebrovascular events. *J Am Coll Cardiol* 1990;16: 1000–1009.
20. Mügge A, Daniel WG, Angermann C, et al. Atrial septal aneurysm in adults patients. A multicenter study using transthoracic and transesophageal echocardiography. *Circulation* 1995;91:2785–2792.
21. Berthet K, Lavergne T, Cohen A, et al. Significant association of atrial vulnerability with atrial septal abnormalities in young patients with ischemic stroke of unknown cause. *Stroke* 2000;31:398–403.
22. Hanna JP, Sun JP, Furlan AJ, et al. Patent foramen ovale and brain infarct. Echocardiographic predictors, recurrence, and prevention. *Stroke* 1994;25:782–786.
23. Mas JL, Zuber M. Recurrent cerebrovascular events in patients with patent foramen ovale, atrial septal aneurysm, or both and cryptogenic stroke or transient ischemic attack. French Study Group on Patent Foramen Ovale and Atrial Septal Aneurysm. *Am Heart J* 1995;130:1083–1088.
24. Bogousslavsky J, Garazi S, Jeanrenaud X, et al. Stroke

recurrence in patients with patent foramen ovale. *Neurology* 1996;46:1301–1305.

25. Stone DA, Godard J, Corretti MC, et al. Patent foramen ovale: association between the degree of shunt by contrast transesophageal echocardiography and the risk of future ischemic neurologic events. *Am Heart J* 1996; 131:158–161.

26. Cujec B, Mainra R, Johnson DH. Prevention of recurrent cerebral ischemic events in patients with patent foramen ovale and cryptogenic strokes and transient ischemic attacks. *Can J Cardiol* 1999;15:57–64.

27. Mas JL, Arquizan C, Lamy C, et al. Recurrent cerebrovascular events associated with patent foramen ovale, atrial septal aneurysm, or both. *N Engl J Med* 2001;345:1740–1746.

28. Bridges ND, Hellenbrand W, Latson L, et al. Transcatheter closure of patent foramen ovale after presumed paradoxical embolism. *Circulation* 1992;86:1902–1908.

29. Devuyst G, Bogousslavsky J, Ruchat P, et al. Prognosis after stroke followed by surgical closure of patent foramen ovale: a prospective follow-up study with brain MRI and simultaneous transesophageal and transcranial Doppler ultrasound. *Neurology* 1996;47:1162–1166.

30. Mas JL. Diagnosis and management of paradoxical embolism and patent foramen ovale. *Curr Opin Cardiol* 1996;11:519–524.

Ischemic Stroke: Advances in Neurology, Vol. 92. Edited by
H.J.M. Barnett, Julien Bogousslavsky, and Heather Meldrum.
Lippincott Williams & Wilkins, Philadelphia © 2003.

24

Nonvalvular Atrial Fibrillation: An Important Cause of Stroke

Natan M. Bornstein and *Aleksandra M. Pavlovic

*Department of Neurology, Tel Aviv University—Sourasky Medical School and Department of
Neurology and Stroke Unit, Tel Aviv Sourasky Medical Center, Tel Aviv, Israel; *Department of
Cerebrovascular Diseases, Institute of Neurology, Belgrade, Serbia, Yugoslavia*

Atrial fibrillation (AF) is the most ubiquitous of arrhythmias, with a prevalence of 0.4% to 0.7% in the general population (1). The number of patients discharged from the hospital with this diagnosis has more than doubled over the last decade, and it has been described as one of the "epidemics" among the cardiovascular diseases (2). According to a recent cross-sectional study, approximately 2.3 million U.S. adults currently have AF, and this number has been projected to increase to more than 5.6 million by the year 2050, with more than 50% of affected individuals being 80 years of age or older (3). It is considered a disease of the elderly, as the prevalence of AF increases progressively after the age of 60 years: It is 0.5% in the 50- to 59-year age group, it rises to approximately 6% in the population older than 65 years, and it reaches up to 10% in people older than 75 years (4–6). The median age of individuals with AF is 75 years (6). The overall prevalence is greater in men than in women (1.1% versus 0.8%; $p < 0.001$) and in every age group (3). It also appears to be more common in white (2.2%) than in black (1.5%; $p < 0.001$) patients aged 50 years or older (3).

About 15% to 20% of all ischemic strokes are attributed to cardioembolism (7), and AF-related strokes comprise approximately 45% of all cardioembolic strokes (8,9). According to the results of several clinical trials, 91% of clinically evident embolic events in AF patients affect the brain.

A common cardiac arrhythmia, AF is a well-established independent risk factor for stroke, associated with about a 5-fold increased risk for stroke and a 1.5- to 1.9-fold higher risk of death (4). Its presence

increases the risk for recurrent stroke as well (10). Although the benefit of anticoagulation therapy in AF patients is well established, it is estimated that only 25% of AF patients worldwide actually receive this treatment.

ETIOLOGY

The causes of AF are multiple. Decline in the prevalence of rheumatic fever in developed countries made nonvalvular AF (NVAF) the more common condition, especially among the elderly. In addition to the background of rheumatic heart disease of AF—particularly with mitral stenosis—many other cardiac disorders including coronary heart disease, congestive or hypertrophic cardiomyopathy, mitral valve prolapse, and mitral valve annular calcification can lead to AF (11). In NVAF patients, there is often coexisting hypertension, diabetes mellitus, or coronary artery disease. In the setting of acute myocardial infarction or following cardiac surgery, AF is a common but usually self-limited problem, and it can be associated with cardiac and noncardiac surgery or diagnostic procedures as well. It is necessary to exclude treatable and potentially reversible noncardiac causes of AF, among which are thyrotoxicosis, acute alcohol intoxication, pulmonary embolism, acute hypoxia related to exacerbation of chronic pulmonary disease, pericarditis, and the use of drugs such as bronchodilators and cholinergics (11,12).

In up to 10% to 15% of cases, AF occurs in the absence of any apparent cardiac or systemic cause and is then referred to as being "lone" or "primary" AF (9,11). The majority of the affected patients is younger than 65 years, are believed to be at very low

Please also see Chapter 30.

risk for stroke, and have excellent prognosis, a status that can change with increasing age (13).

The danger of paroxysmal AF should not be underestimated, especially in the setting of other risk factors in which transition to chronic AF is more likely (in 25% patients after a 1-year period) (11). It has been reported that the risk of embolization in patients with paroxysmal AF is similar to that in chronic AF. With warfarin having been found to be an effective preventive agent, both of these groups should be treated in the same way (14–16).

MECHANISMS AND TYPES OF STROKE IN PATIENTS WITH ATRIAL FIBRILLATION

The onset and continuation of AF have been mapped in electrophysiologic studies, showing that multiple random intraatrial reentry circuits form the basis of the arrhythmia. In the setting of AF, the most important concern is embolization from left atrial intracavitary thrombi, although these patients can develop right atrial thrombi as well, with a risk for pulmonary embolization (12). Most of the ischemic strokes related to AF (70%) are due to embolism of stasis-induced thrombi forming in the left atrium and particularly its appendage (11). Cardioembolic strokes associated with AF are often considered to be massive and disabling. However, about 30% of AF-related strokes are caused by other mechanisms (17). Minor stroke and transient ischemic attacks (TIAs) frequently accompany AF (17,18), but small deep infarcts are relatively uncommon (17,19). There are data indicating that perhaps 25% to 30% of AF-related stroke is due to associated small-vessel disease, other cardiac sources of embolism, carotid atherosclerosis, aortic arch plaque, and other mechanisms (1,17). About one-half of elderly AF patients have chronic hypertension, and 12% have cervical carotid artery stenosis of at least moderate severity (1,18).

DIAGNOSIS

Approximately one-third of patients with AF are unaware of their condition (5). Transesophageal echocardiography, by being more sensitive, is superior to routine transthoracic echocardiography in detecting thrombi in the left atrium and in the left atrial appendage (12). One important finding is the detection of spontaneous echo contrast, which has been associated with the presence of a left atrium thrombus in 80% to 90% of patients (12). Spontaneous echo contrast can be related to other cardiac or systemic pathology. The use of transesophageal echocardiography in determining the type and timing of cardioversion in patients with AF lasting for more than 2 days has been proposed (11).

RISK FOR STROKE

AF is a well-established independent risk factor for stroke, leading to a 5.6-fold increase of risk according to data from the Framingham Study (4). About 16% to 25% of ischemic strokes are associated with AF, the percentage being higher in patients with large supratentorial infarcts (59%). It is the most common condition predisposing to thromboembolism in patients with and without valvular heart disease (8,12).

Randomized clinical trials of AF confirmed an overall annual stroke incidence of about 5% in the general population of patients with AF not treated with anticoagulation (8,18). Risk for recurrent stroke in AF patients without antithrombotic treatment is 12%/year (10), which is strikingly high compared with the annual rate of 5% after the first year for AF-free patients after first stroke or TIA (20). An ischemic stroke will occur during the lifetime of about 35% nonanticoagulated AF patients (12,18).

The importance of AF as a risk factor for stroke increases with age. The prevalence of AF increases with age, and the incidence of stroke in AF patients is similarly age related. The attributable risk of stroke from AF rises from 1.5% in individuals in their fifties to 15% in individuals in their seventies (4). AF is present in over one-third of individuals aged 80 to 89 years with acute ischemic stroke and is, thus, considered to be a leading cause of stroke in the elderly (4,8).

The risk of stroke is apparently similar between men and women (21). However, the prevalence of AF is strongly associated with advanced age in women (5). Results of the Stroke Prevention in Atrial Fibrillation (SPAF) Study III indicated female age older than 75 years to be a stroke risk factor (22).

NVAF is an independent risk factor for asymptomatic brain infarction (6,23–25). Computed tomography studies have shown that silent ischemic brain infarcts are present in 26% patients with NVAF (21). This raises the suspicion that the true frequency of stroke in AF patients may have been underestimated.

Increased stroke severity, disability, and mortality in AF patients have been well documented (11,21,24). AF portends a mortality rate double that of control subjects, due mostly to a predisposition to serious ventricular arrhythmias or fatal pulmonary embolism leading to sudden death but also due to stroke and its consequences (24,26).

RISK STRATIFICATION

There is a wide clinically important difference among subpopulations of AF patients in terms of risk rates, with risk varying 25-fold (i.e., from 0.5% to 12%/year) (21,27,28). The risk of stroke is not due solely to AF: It substantially increases with advancing age and in the presence of coexisting cardiovascular disease (18,21,29). For example, there is 17-fold increase in stroke risk in patients with mitral stenosis. Stratification of AF patients into subpopulations of those who are at relatively high and low risk for thromboembolism is an essential determinant of optimal antithrombotic prophylaxis, indicating which subgroup of patients will gain the greatest benefit from anticoagulant therapy (11).

Two prospective studies, Atrial Fibrillation Investigators and SPAF, provided the most reliable stratification schemes by addressing this issue with sufficient numbers of patients (18,22,28) (Table 24-1). Although the risk stratification schemes were not exactly the same, they were compatible with one another (27). Several clinical variables (e.g., age, history of hypertension, diabetes mellitus, prior stroke or TIA, coronary artery disease, impaired left ventricle function including recent congestive heart failure or ejection fraction of less than 25% by M-mode echocardiography), all of which were shown to be independently predictive of risk for thromboembolic events, are used clinically to characterize AF patients as at high or low risk for stroke (11,28). Among these factors, a past history of stroke and TIA predicted the highest risk factor for recurrent stroke whose annual

incidence rate was estimated to be approximately 10% to 12 %/year (1,10,18,26,27). Another stratification scheme, combining two existing ones, has been recently described [congestive heart failure, hypertension, age, diabetes, and stroke (CHADS2)] (30).

PREVENTION

AF is a modifiable risk factor, and it should be vigorously managed both in primary and in secondary prevention settings. The importance of general risk factor modification can never be overemphasized, and the identification of patients at particularly high risk, especially those who have reached the state when they need more specific therapies such as anticoagulations, is of greatest importance (31).

Primary Prevention Trials

The efficacy of anticoagulation for the primary prevention of stroke or TIAs in NVAF patients was established by five prospective, placebo-controlled, randomized trials, each of which had been terminated early since monitoring of the results showed significant efficacy of warfarin against placebo (14–16, 32–34) (Tables 24-2–4).

The pooled data from five primary prevention studies were analyzed and published in 1994 (18). An analysis of these results demonstrated that warfarin consistently decreased the risk of stroke with no significant increase in the frequency of major hemorrhage. The

TABLE 24-1. *Risk stratification schemes for patients with nonvalvular atrial fibrillation*

	High risk	Moderate risk	Low risk
AFI/ACCP Consensus Criteria	History of hypertension, diabetes, prior stroke or TIA, coronary artery disease, congestive heart failure	Age ≥65 yr, no high-risk features	Age <65 yr, no high-risk features
Stroke risk, no therapy	~6%/yr	~2%/yr	~1%/yr
SPAF III Study Criteria	Systolic BP >160 mm Hg, LV dysfunction, prior stroke or TIA, women >75 yr	History of hypertension, no high-risk features	No high-risk features or history of hypertension
Stroke risk with aspirin (95% CI)	~8%/yr	~3.5%/yr	~1%/yr

AFI, Atrial Fibrillation Investigators; ACCP, American College of Chest Physicians; TIA, transient ischemic attack; SPAF, Stroke Prevention in Atrial Fibrillation Study; BP, blood pressure; LV, left ventricle; CI, confidence interval.
Adapted from Hart RG, Sherman DG, Easton JD, et al. Prevention of stroke in patients with nonvalvular atrial fibrillation: views and reviews. *Neurology* 1998;51:674–681, with permission.

TABLE 24-2. *Antithrombotic treatment in atrial fibrillation: warfarin versus placebo*

Study	No. of patients	INR	RRR (%)	ARR [% (%/yr)]
AFASAK	671	2.8–4.2	58	2.6 (1.5)
SPAF I	421	2.0–4.5	65	4.7 (1.7)
BAATAF	420	1.5–2.7	86	2.6 (1.4)
CAFA	378	2.0–3.0	33	2.5 (—)
SPINAF	571	1.4–2.8	79	3.4 (5.8)
EAFT	439	2.5–4.0	66	8.4 (5.8)
Total	2,900	—	68 ($p < 0.001$)	—

INR, international normalized ratio; RRR, relative risk reduction; ARR, absolute risk reduction; AFASAK, Atrial Fibrillation, Aspirin, Anticoagulation; SPAF, Stroke Prevention in Atrial Fibrillation; BAATAF, Boston Area Anticoagulation Trial for Atrial Fibrillation; CAFA, Canadian Atrial Fibrillation Anticoagulation; SPINAF, Stroke Prevention in Nonrheumatic Atrial Fibrillation; EAFT, European Atrial Fibrillation Trial.

TABLE 24-3. *Antithrombotic treatment in atrial fibrillation: warfarin versus aspirin*

Study	No. of patients	INR	RRR (%)	ARR [% (%/yr)]
SPAF II	1,100	2.0–4.5	31	0.8 (0.3)
AFASAK	671	2.8–4.2	50	1.9 (0.5)
EAFT	455	2.5–4.0	62	6.4
PATAF	729	2.5–3.5	—	—
AFASAK II	339	2.0–3.0	13	—
Total	3,294	—	47 ($p < 0.001$)	—

INR, international normalized ratio; RRR, relative risk reduction; ARR, absolute risk reduction; SPAF, Stroke Prevention in Atrial Fibrillation; AFASAK, Atrial Fibrillation, Aspirin, Anticoagulation; EAFT, European Atrial Fibrillation Trial; PATAF, Primary Prevention of Arterial Thromboembolism in Patients with Nonvalvular Atrial Fibrillation.

TABLE 24-4. *Antithromobotic treatment in atrial fibrillation: aspirin versus placebo*

Study	No. of patients	Aspirin dose (mg/d)	RRR (%)	ARR [% (%/yr)]
AFASAK	672	75	18	0.7 (1.0)
SPAF I	1,120	325	44	2.5 (0.5)
EAFT	782	300	15	2.2 (2.5)
Total	2,785	—	21 ($p = 0.03$)	—

RRR, relative risk reduction; ARR, absolute risk reduction; AFASAK, Atrial Fibrillation, Aspirin, Anticoagulation; SPAF, Stroke Prevention in Atrial Fibrillation; EAFT, European Atrial Fibrillation Trial.

annual rate of stroke was 1.4% in patients on warfarin and 4.5% in the control subjects, with a risk reduction of 68% [95% confidence interval (CI) 50%–79%; $p <$ 0.01]. The rate of combined outcome of stroke, systemic embolism, or death was reduced with warfarin by 48% (95% CI 34%–69%). There was no significant difference in the rates of hemorrhage: 1% in the control subjects, 1% in the patients on aspirin, and 1.3% in the warfarin group. A very-low-risk group of patients under 65 years of age and without risk factors was identified: they had a stroke risk of 1%/year (95% CI 0.3%–3.1%) and probably should not receive warfarin (12,13).

These clinical trials used international normalized ratio (INR) ranges of approximately 1.8 to 4.2. The incremental risk of serious bleeding was less than 1%/year. Whether such low bleeding risk can be routinely achieved in clinical practice is an important question. In any event, low-intensity coagulation with maintenance of INR in the range of 2.0 to 3.0 clearly yields benefit (18,34).

Secondary Prevention Trials

The efficacy of adjusted-dose warfarin treatment for the secondary prevention of stroke has been demonstrated by two major randomized clinical trials. The European Atrial Fibrillation Trial (EAFT) group performed a multicenter, prospective, randomized trial in 1,007 patients with NVAF and a recent TIA or minor ischemic stroke to elucidate the preventive benefit of anticoagulant and aspirin (10,35). Patients were randomized to open anticoagulation with warfarin or double-blind treatment with either 300 mg/day of aspirin or placebo. During a mean follow-up of 2.3 years, the annual rate of stroke in patients receiving anticoagulation, aspirin, and placebo was 4%, 10%, and 12%, respectively. Anticoagulation was significantly more effective in reducing the risk of stroke than placebo, with a rate of 66% reduction hazard ratio (HR) of 0.34 (95% CI 0.20–0.57, $p < 0.0001$), whereas aspirin was not.

The on-treatment incidence of major bleeding was low: 2.8%/year in the group randomized to anticoagulation, 0.9% in the aspirin group, and 0.7% in the placebo group. Patients receiving warfarin experienced major or minor bleeding significantly more often than patients receiving aspirin (HR 2.8, 95% CI 1.7–4.8, $p < 0.001$) or placebo (HR 3.4, 95% CI 1.9–6.0, $p < 0.001$). However, none of the patients on warfarin had intracranial hemorrhage, whereas there were three cases of fatal cerebral bleeding: one in the placebo group and two in the aspirin group. The EAFT incidence rates for the occurrence of a first ischemic or hemorrhagic complication when analyzed by INR range indicated that the rate was lowest at INRs of 2.0 to 2.9, higher with INRs of 3.0 to 3.9, and much higher at INRs of 4.0 to 4.9 and those more than 5.0. The study showed that anticoagulation therapy reduced the risk of recurrent stroke by two-thirds in patients with NVAF and recent TIA or minor stroke. In absolute terms, 90 vascular events are prevented if 1,000 patients are treated for 1 year. In contrast, aspirin prevented 40 vascular events/1,000 patients/1 year.

The SPAF III Study compared the efficacy of adjusted-dose warfarin therapy (INR 2.0–3.0) with fixed-dose warfarin (INR 1.2–1.5 for initial dose adjustment) plus 325 mg/day of aspirin in stroke prevention in patients with NVAF (22,29). The investigators recruited 1,044 AF patients with at least one of the thromboembolic risk factors and assigned them randomly to these two groups. The mean INR during follow-up of 1.1 years was 2.4 in the adjusted-dose warfarin group and 1.3 in the fixed-dose warfarin plus aspirin group. The trial was stopped when an interim analysis showed that the rate of ischemic stroke and systemic embolism in patients on combination therapy (7.9%/year) was significantly higher ($p < 0.0001$) than in those given adjusted-dose warfarin (1.9%/year). A subgroup of 396 patients with

prior stroke was analyzed in the SPAF III trial. The incidence of ischemic stroke or systemic embolism in the adjusted-dose warfarin group was significantly lower (3.4%/year) than in the group receiving low-fixed-dose warfarin plus aspirin (11.9%/year). There was no difference in the incidence of major bleeding (2.4%/year versus 2.1%/year, respectively).

Warfarin is dramatically effective. According to the results of a meta-analysis that included six randomized clinical trials testing several antithrombotic agents to prevent stroke in AF patients, adjusted-dose warfarin reduced stroke by 62% (95% CI 48%–72%), with an absolute risk reduction of 2.7%/year for primary prevention and 8.4%/year for secondary prevention (36). Aspirin (six trials) reduced stroke by 22% (95% CI 2%–38%) with an absolute risk reduction of 1.5%/year for primary prevention and 2.5%/year for secondary prevention. Adjusted-dose warfarin was more efficacious than aspirin, with a relative risk reduction of 36% (95% CI 14%–52%), and the benefit of antithrombotic therapy was not offset by the occurrence of major hemorrhages (37).

Optimal Warfarin Dose

The optimal intensity of anticoagulation assessed in the EAFT Study showed that an anticoagulant therapy producing an INR between 2.0 and 2.9 reduced the combined incidence rate for ischemic and hemorrhagic events by 80% when compared with an INR of less than 2.0. On the other hand, an INR between 3.0 and 3.9 reduced the combined rate by 40%. When the INR was more than 5.0, the risk of bleeding complications became unacceptable. No significant reduction in thromboembolic evens was seen at an INR of less than 2.0 (35). However, this conclusion was obtained by comparing the event rate in a group of patients who had an INR between 1.0 and 1.9 with a group of patients who had an INR of more than 2.0. The efficacy was not assessed by further dividing the group of patients with INRs between 1.0 and 1.9 (25). Hylek and coworkers (38) investigated the lowest intensity of anticoagulation that was effective in preventing stroke in NVAF patients in a case control study. They found that anticoagulation prophylaxis was effective at an INR of greater than or equal to 2.0 and that the stroke risk rose as the INR decreased to less than 2.0. The SPAF III trial also suggested that INRs between 1.5 and 1.9 offer substantial protection against ischemic stroke (29). A prospective, randomized, multicenter Japanese study addressed the issue of low-target INR, allocating NVAF patients under the age of 80 years with previous stroke and TIA to a conventional-intensity group (INR 2.2–3.5) and a low-intensity group (INR 1.5–2.1) (39). The annual rate of ischemic stroke was low in both groups: 1.1%/year in the conventional-intensity group and 1.7%/year in the low-intensity group. Major hemorrhagic complications occurred with a significantly higher frequency in the conventional-intensity group (6.6%/year versus 0%/year; $p = 0.01$). The investigators concluded that the low-intensity warfarin protocol (INR 1.5–2.1) for secondary stroke prevention in NVAF patients, especially the elderly, appeared safer than the conventional-intensity therapy (INR 2.2–3.5) (39). In elderly people at risk of bleeding, an INR of 1.6 to 1.9 could be an option (38,39). The lowest effective dose of warfarin has not yet been identified.

Bleeding: The Main Therapy Complication

There are several factors that may increase risk of bleeding in warfarin treatment: age, uncontrolled hypertension (blood pressure of more than 180/100 mm Hg), alcohol excess, liver disease, bleeding lesions (gastrointestinal source, previous cerebral hemorrhage), tendency to bleeding (coagulation defects, thrombocytopenia), and concomitant use of aspirin with oral anticoagulants (21,25,39). It should be noted that 11% of patients with hemorrhagic stroke have AF, and therefore, intracranial hemorrhage should be excluded before treatment with anticoagulant agents.

Randomized trials with target INRs between 2.7 and 4.8 revealed a 10-fold increase in intracranial bleeding among patients given anticoagulation versus placebo (40). In a case control study of a relatively young cohort (one-half of the patients were under 65 years old), the risk of anticoagulation-associated brain hemorrhages was not substantially elevated until the INRs reached and exceeded 4.0, increasing exponentially above this level (41,42). The frequency of intracranial hemorrhage is age related, and it is usually a fatal complication (40,43).

Safe Anticoagulation

The patients who had been analyzed in reported studies were carefully selected and monitored so that bleeding risk could be minimized. It has been suggested that those patients were probably better-than-average candidates for safe anticoagulation and that risk of bleeding may be greater in a more generalized outpatient population (44).

Risk-versus-benefit balance of anticoagulation use has to be tailored for each patient individually (45).

Safe anticoagulation requires careful patient selection, assessment of bleeding risk and compliance, patient education, INR monitoring at least monthly, and regular medical supervision. Antiplatelet therapy may be selected as alternative treatment in patients who are unable to take warfarin properly because of cognitive decline or lack of caregiver supervision and in patients prone to falling and consequently at risk of head injury (25). The INR should be used in monitoring oral anticoagulation (1). Patients should be educated about drug interactions, the importance of compliance, and the early signs of bleeding.

Treatment in Elderly

AF-associated stroke is particularly a problem in patients older than 75 (11). About one-half of AF-associated strokes occur in this patient population, and it may be the most frequent cause of disabling stroke in elderly women (4). The safety and tolerability of long-term anticoagulation titrated to conventional levels have been less clear in the very elderly patients. Special consideration of stroke prevention in this age group is critical for successful prophylaxis. The risk of major hemorrhage among elderly AF patients who are on anticoagulation treatment is related to the intensity of anticoagulation, their age, and the fluctuations in INRs (1,42,43,46). The results of the SPAF II Study showed that the risk of major hemorrhage during anticoagulation substantially increased in AF patients older than 75 years compared with younger patients receiving anticoagulation of similar intensity (43,47). In patients older than 75, a mean INR of less than 3.0 was associated with a bleeding rate of 2.7%/year, whereas the bleeding rate was as high as 9.0%/year when the INR was more than 3.0. The overall yearly incidence of major bleeding complications was significantly higher in patients receiving warfarin treatment versus control subjects (2.8% versus 0.7%) (10).

A combined analysis of four clinical trials showed a low rate (0.3%/year) of intracranial bleeding among AF patients over 75 years of age when the target INR range was 2.0 to 3.0 (48). Nevertheless, the pooled data from five primary prevention trials demonstrated only one intracranial hemorrhage in 223 patients older than 75 years (compared with younger patients) who received warfarin (18). In the EAFT study, 63% of the patients receiving anticoagulation for secondary prophylaxis were 70 years old or older, and no intracranial bleeding occurred during warfarin therapy with a mean INR of 2.9 (10). There are data from a case control study suggesting that intracranial hemorrhage during anticoagulation treatment is not significantly increased until the INR exceeds 4.0 (42). These facts support the view of using a higher target INR in elderly patients. However, the INRs that had been achieved in patients over 75 years of age in the four clinical trials are unknown, and they are likely to be below an average of 2.5. In the only study that specifically focused on older patients, there was a mean achieved INR of 2.6 (target INR 2.0–4.5) during follow-up, which was associated with a substantial (1.8%/year) rate of intracranial bleeding (47).

The optimal intensity of anticoagulation in the elderly still remains unclear (25). Although the maximal degree of stroke prevention is probably obtained with INRs between 2.0 and 3.0, lower INRs (between 1.6 and 2.5) provide an efficacy that is estimated to be nearly 90% of the higher target intensities (49). The effects could be estimated as substantial although partial, and given the uncertainty about the safety of INRs higher than 2.5 in elderly AF patients, a target INR of 2.0 (range 1.6–2.5) may be a reasonable compromise. When this option for the elderly is chosen, special efforts to minimize the time spent below the target range are needed. However, a target INR range of 2.0 to 3.0 for providing maximal protection against ischemic stroke is also recommended because this range has been considered as being relatively safe (38,50).

Role of Aspirin and Other Agents

The efficacy of aspirin at a dosage between 75 and 325 mg/day was assessed in four double-blinded, placebo-controlled, randomized trials [Atrial Fibrillation, Aspirin, Anticoagulation (AFASAK); SPAF I; EAFT; European Stroke Prevention Study] and yielded a pooled risk reduction of 21% compared with placebo (10,32,33,51) (Tables 24-3–5). In two of these trials, aspirin was clearly less efficacious than warfarin (AFASAK, EAFT) (1,10,32). However, it should be borne in mind that aspirin and warfarin have equal efficacy in preventing noncardioembolic strokes. Other agents such as dipyridamole plus aspirin or ibuprofen also appear to be efficacious (1,52). This could offer an alternative for patients in whom anticoagulation is contraindicated, though AF patients are obviously not well protected unless they are anticoagulated (Tables 24-3 and 24-4). On the other hand, even low daily doses of aspirin increase the rate of major hemorrhage, with an average increase of about 0.5%/year in elderly people (1).

An important meta-analysis on long-term (1 year or longer) anticoagulation versus antiplatelet treatment in NVAF patients was conducted by Taylor and coworkers (53). The authors systematically reviewed randomized, controlled trials on this subject and identified five trials (AFASAK I, SPAF II, AFASAK II, Italian Study on Atrial Fibrillation (SIFA), Primary Prevention of Arterial Fibrillation (PATAF)] between 1989 and 1999 with a total of 3,298 patients. There was a borderline significant difference in nonfatal stroke in favor of anticoagulation [odds ratio (OR) 0.68, 95% CI 0.46–0.99]. The pooled ORs from the fixed effects model showed a nonsignificant trend in favor of anticoagulation in deaths from stroke (OR 0.74, 95% CI 0.39–1.46) and vascular death (OR 0.86, 95% CI 0.63–1.17). A random effects model that had been applied because of the heterogeneity between trials also showed no significant difference in combined fatal and nonfatal events (OR 0.79, 95% CI 0.61–1.02). The only trial to show a significant difference favoring anticoagulation was methodologically weaker in design than the others, with the lowest aspirin dose having been used compared with that

TABLE 24-5. *Prevention of stroke in nonvalvular atrial fibrillation: recommendations*

Risk group	Recommended treatment	Alternatives
Primary prevention		
"Lone" atrial fibrillation under age 60 yr	None	Aspirin 325 mg/d
Low risk	Aspirin 325 mg/d	Warfarin INR 1.6–3.0
Moderate risk	Aspirin or warfarin	—
High risk		
<75 yr of age	Warfarin INR 2.5 (range 2.0–3.0)	Aspirin if warfarin is contraindicated
>75 yr of age	Warfarin INR 2.5 (range 2.0–3.0) or warfarin INR 2.0 (range 1.6–2.5)	Aspirin if warfarin is contraindicated
Prior stroke or transient ischemic attack	Warfarin INR 3.0 (range 2.5–4.0)	Warfarin INR 2.5 (range 2.0–3.0), aspirin if warfarin is contraindicated

INR, international normalized ratio.

in other trials (75 mg) (AFASAK I). Major bleeding events were more common among patients treated with long-term anticoagulation (OR 1.45, 95% CI 0.92–2.27). There was marked clinical and methodologic heterogeneity between trials, and in all but one (AFASAK II), the ranges for the INR were higher than the recommended range of 2 to 3, although all trials stated that anticoagulation control was "adequate." Those authors implied that the evidence for current clinical practice in long-term anticoagulation for NVAF patients is not strong enough and that trials, both individual and pooled, are underpowered, giving the pooled data from 3,298 patients enrolled only 60% power to detect a difference. To detect a 25% superiority of anticoagulation over antiplatelet treatment with an event rate of 10%, a power of 80%, and a significance of 5%, trials would require 4,920 patients for each treatment group, a study that has not yet been performed (53).

RECOMMENDATIONS

According to class I evidence from previous trials, adjusted-dose warfarin reduces the risk of stroke in AF patients by about 70% (Table 24-5). Anticoagulation with warfarin is safe for patients who can be carefully monitored, preferably with INR or, if INR is unavailable, with prothrombin time tests. Although aspirin has some efficacy in reducing stroke risk in AF patients (by about 20%), it is clearly less efficacious than warfarin (which reaches an efficacy of 68%). For patients with AF aged 75 or younger who are at high risk for stroke and are considered to be safe candidates for anticoagulation, treatment with warfarin is recommended with a target INR of 2.5 (range 2.0–3.0). The warfarin dose in elderly AF patients (older than 75 years) is optional, as warfarin may be used with a lower INR target of 2.0 (target range 1.6–2.5) to decrease risk of hemorrhage; however, there are experts who disregard age and accept a higher INR target of 2.5 (target range 2.0–3.0), considering it as being appropriate and safe. Aspirin at 325 mg/day is recommended for patients with AF who are considered as being unable to receive anticoagulation therapy or as being at low risk of stroke. In AF patients at moderate risk of stroke, the decision between warfarin and aspirin should be made considering the individual patient's bleeding risk and preferences (28,52).

Decision-analysis models have been developed and can be used in making clinical decisions on anticoagulation treatment (54).

Implementation of Treatment in Clinical Practice

Although benefit from warfarin treatment in AF patients is clear, not all appropriate candidates for anticoagulation actually receive this treatment (45,54–56). Anticoagulation is underused in high-risk elderly patients, especially women; it is often used in low-risk patients; and it is frequently used in an inadequate dosage, with a peak of INR in a range lower than recommended (2.0–2.4), indicating that "the doctors were playing it safe" (45,55). The Stroke in Atrial Fibrillation Ensemble (SAFE) I was a pilot study with the aim of determining whether AF patients admitted for an acute stroke or TIA had been receiving prior antithrombotic treatment. The study analyzed 213 patients in three European centers, in 69.5% of whom AF was known prior to stroke. Only 34 (16%) of patients previously eligible for oral anticoagulation did receive treatment, and in only 6 of them was the INR between 2.0 and 3.5 (56). As an extension of a previous pilot study, the SAFE II trial had been designed to enroll 500 known AF patients from 40 centers in six European Union countries. Deplanque and coworkers (56) suggested several reasons for the gap between guidelines and practice, including contraindications, differences in patients' profiles between trials and real-life settings, different atmospheres and conditions of the trials, and poor application of the trials' results in clinical practice. Both physicians and patients wield influence in this situation, with risk-versus-benefit evaluation of anticoagulation use being the essential physician-related factor (45). Anticoagulation seems to be underused and misdirected in managing AF in different communities. Efforts to promote and support wider and more appropriate use of anticoagulation are needed.

CONCLUSION

AF is the most common clinically significant cardiac arrhythmia and a potent risk factor for ischemic stroke. The number of patients with AF is likely to increase 2.5-fold during the next 50 years. It has been established that anticoagulation treatment is capable of preventing more than two-thirds of cardioembolic events. The optimal intensity of anticoagulation for the prevention of both first and recurrent stroke seems to be an INR of between 2.0 and 3.0. Carefully selected and monitored NVAF patients at high risk for stroke have benefit from anticoagulation with very low associated risk. A target INR of between 1.6 and 2.6 may be an alternative for stroke prevention in elderly NVAF patients with a potential risk of hemorrhage. Antiplatelet treatment may be administered in patients who are at risk of bleeding or in whom anti-coagulation is contraindicated, although the efficacy of antiplatelets for secondary prevention of stroke in NVAF has not yet been established. Use of anticoagulants in clinical practice still lags considerably behind proved benefit-versus-risk data. Management of NVAF complications and the use of anticoagulants are still challenging issues, and further efforts are needed for resolving this matter.

ACKNOWLEDGMENT

Esther Eshkol is thanked for editorial assistance.

REFERENCES

1. Hart RG, Sherman DG, Easton JD, et al. Prevention of stroke in patients with nonvalvular atrial fibrillation: views and reviews. *Neurology* 1998;51:674–681.
2. Braunwald E. Shattuck Lecture. Cardiovascular medicine at the turn of the millennium: triumphs, concerns, and opportunities. *N Engl J Med* 1997;337:1360–1369.
3. Go AS, Hylek EM, Phillips KA, et al. Prevalence of diagnosed atrial fibrillation in adults. National implications for rhythm management and stroke prevention: the AnTicoagulation and Risk Factors in Atrial Fibrillation (ATRIA) Study. *JAMA* 2001;285:2370–2375.
4. Wolf PA, Abbott RD, Kannel WB. Atrial fibrillation as an independent risk factor for stroke: the Framingham study. *Stroke* 1991;22:983–988.
5. Furberg CD, Psaty BM, Manolio TA, et al. Prevalence of atrial fibrillation in elderly subjects (the Cardiovascular Health Study). *Am J Cardiol* 1994;74:236–241.
6. Feinberg W, Blackshear J, Laupacis A, et al. Prevalence, age distribution, and gender of patients with atrial fibrillation. *Arch Intern Med* 1995;155:469–473.
7. Wein TH, Bornstein NM. Stroke prevention. Cardiac and carotid-related stroke. In: Morgenstern LB, ed. *Neurologic clinics. Stroke.* Philadelphia: Saunders, 2000:321–341.
8. Sherman DG. Atrial fibrillation. In: Fieschi C, Fisher M, eds. *Prevention of ischemic stroke.* London: Martin Dunitz, 2000:137–145.
9. Rosenthal L. Atrial fibrillation. *E Med J* 2001;2(9) (*www. eMedicine.com*).
10. European Atrial Fibrillation Trial Study Group. Secondary prevention of vascular events in patients with nonrheumatic atrial fibrillation and recent transient ischemic attack or minor ischemic stroke. *Lancet* 1993; 342:1255–1262.
11. Prystowsky EN, Benson DW Jr, Fuster V, et al. A statement for healthcare professionals from the Subcommittee on Electrocardiography and Electrophysiology (American Heart Association, 1996, 1998). *Circulation* 1996;93:1262–1277.
12. Ezekowitz MD, Cohen IS, Gornick CG, et al. Atrial fibrillation. In: Daniel WG, Kronzon I, Mugge A, eds. *Cardiogenic embolism.* Baltimore: Williams & Wilkins, 1996:27–44.
13. Albers G. Atrial fibrillation and stroke: three new studies, three remaining questions. *Arch Intern Med* 1994; 154:1443–1448.
14. Stroke Prevention in Atrial Fibrillation Investigators. Design of a multicenter randomized trial for the Stroke Prevention in Atrial Fibrillation Study. *Stroke* 1990;21: 538–545.
15. Boston Area Anticoagulation Trial for Atrial Fibrillation Investigators. The effect of low-dose warfarin on the risk of stroke in nonrheumatic atrial fibrillation. *N Engl J Med* 1990;323:1505–1511.
16. Connolly SJ, Paupacis A, Gent M, et al. Canadian Atrial Fibrillation Anticoagulation (CAFA) Study. *J Am Coll Cardiol* 1991;18:349–355.
17. Miller VT, Rothrock JF, Pearce LA, et al. Ischemic stroke in patients with atrial fibrillation: effect of aspirin according to stroke mechanism: Stroke Prevention in Atrial Fibrillation Investigators. *Neurology* 1993; 43:32–36.
18. Atrial Fibrillation Investigators. Risk factors for stroke and efficacy of antithrombotic therapy in atrial fibrillation: analysis of pooled data from five randomized controlled trials. *Arch Intern Med* 1994;154:1449–1457.
19. Sandercock P, Bamford J, Dennis M, et al. Atrial fibrillation and stroke: prevalence in different types of stroke and influence on early and long-term prognosis. *Br Med J* 1992;305:1460–1465.
20. Whisnant JP. Natural history of transient ischemic attack and ischemic stroke. In: Whisnant JP, ed. *Stroke: populations, cohorts, and clinical trials.* Oxford: Butterworth-Heinemann, 1993:135–153.
21. Lip G, Lowe G. Antithrombotic therapy for atrial fibrillation. *Br Med J* 1996;312:45–49.
22. SPAF III Writing Committee for the Stroke Prevention in Atrial Fibrillation Investigators. Patients with nonalvular atrial fibrillation at low risk of stroke during treatment with aspirin. *JAMA* 1998;279:1273–1277.
23. Shinkawa A, Ueda K, Kiyohara Y, et al. Silent cerebral infarction in a community-based autopsy series in Japan: the Hisayama Study. *Stroke* 1995;26:380–385.
24. Jorgensen J, Nakayama H, Reith J, et al. Acute stroke with atrial fibrillation. The Copenhagen Stroke Study. *Stroke* 1996;27:218–224.
25. Yasaka M, Yamaguchi T. Secondary prevention of stroke patients with nonvalvular atrial fibrillation. Optimal intensity of anticoagulation. *CNS Drugs* 2001;15: 623–631.
26. Lin H, Kelly-Hayes M, Beiser A, et al. Stroke severity in atrial fibrillation: the Framingham Study. *Stroke* 1996;27:1760–1764.
27. Laupacis A, Albers G, Dalen J, et al. Antithrombotic therapy in atrial fibrillation. *Chest* 1998;114[Suppl]: S579–S589.
28. Report of the Quality Standards Subcommittee of the American Academy of Neurology. Practice parameter: stroke prevention in patients with nonvalvular atrial fibrillation. *Neurology* 1998;51:671–673.
29. Stroke Prevention in Atrial Fibrillation Investigators. Adjusted-dose warfarin versus low-intensity, fixed-dose warfarin plus aspirin for high-risk patients with atrial fibrillation: the Stroke Prevention in Atrial Fibrillation Trial III randomized clinical trial. *Lancet* 1996;348: 683–688.
30. Gage BF, Waterman AD, Shannon W, et al. Validation of clinical classification schemes for predicting stroke. Results from National Registry of Atrial Fibrillation. *JAMA* 2001;285:2864–2870.

31. Norrving B. Medical therapy to prevent ischemic stroke. In: Fisher M, ed. *Stroke therapy.* Boston: Butterworth-Heinemann, 1995:207–218.

32. Petersen P, Boysen G, Godtfredsen J, et al. Placebo-controlled, randomized trial of warfarin and aspirin for prevention of thromboembolic complications in chronic atrial fibrillation: the Copenhagen AFASAK Study. *Lancet* 1989;1:175–179.

33. Stroke Prevention in Atrial Fibrillation Investigators. Stroke Prevention in Atrial Fibrillation Study: final results. *Circulation* 1991;84:527–539.

34. Ezekowitz MD, Bridgers SL, James KE, et al., and SPINAF Investigators. Warfarin in the prevention of stroke associated with nonrheumatic atrial fibrillation. *N Engl J Med* 1992;327:406–412.

35. European Atrial Fibrillation Trial Study Group. Optimal oral anticoagulant therapy in patients with nonrheumatic atrial fibrillation and recent cerebral ischemia. *N Engl J Med* 1995;333:5–10.

36. Hart RG, Benavente O, McBride R, et al. Antithrombotic therapy to prevent stroke in patients with atrial fibrillation. *Ann Intern Med* 1999;131:492–501.

37. Parnetti L, Gallai V. Atrial fibrillation and stroke. *Cerebrovasc Dis* 2000;10[Suppl 4]:40–41.

38. Hylek EM, Skates SJ, Sheehan MA, et al. An analysis of the lowest effective intensity of prophylactic anticoagulation for patients with nonrheumatic atrial fibrillation. *N Engl J Med* 1996;335:540–546.

39. Yamaguchi T for Japanese NVAF–Embolism Secondary Prevention Cooperative Study Group. Optimal intensity of warfarin therapy for secondary prevention of stroke in patients with nonvalvular atrial fibrillation: a multicenter prospective randomized trial. *Stroke* 2000;31: 817–821.

40. Hart RG, Boop B, Anderson DC. Oral anticoagulants and intracranial hemorrhage: facts and hypothesis. *Stroke* 1995;26:1471–1477.

41. Fihn SD, McDonell M, Martin D, et al. Risk factors for complications of chronic anticoagulation. A multicenter study. Warfarin Optimized Outpatient Follow-up Study Group. *Ann Intern Med* 1993;118:511–520.

42. Hylek EM, Singer DE. Risk factors for intracranial hemorrhage in outpatients taking warfarin. *Ann Intern Med* 1994;120:897–902.

43. Stroke Prevention in Atrial Fibrillation Investigators. Bleeding during antithrombotic therapy for atrial fibrillation. *Arch Intern Med* 1996;156:411–416.

44. Gitter MJ, Jaeger TM, Petterson TM, et al. Bleeding and thromboembolism during anticoagulant therapy: a population-based study in Rochester, Minnesota. *Mayo Clin Proc* 1995;70:725–733.

45. Cohen N, Almoznino-Sarafian D, Alon I, et al. Warfarin for stroke prevention still underused in atrial fibrillation. Patterns of omission. *Stroke* 2000;31:1217–1222.

46. Fihn SD, Callahan CM, Martin DC, et al. The risk for and severity of bleeding complications in elderly patients treated with warfarin. *Ann Intern Med* 1996; 124:970–979.

47. Stroke Prevention in Atrial Fibrillation Investigators. Warfarin versus aspirin for prevention of thromboembolism in atrial fibrillation. Stroke Prevention in Atrial Fibrillation Study II. *Lancet* 1994;343:687–691.

48. Connolly SJ. Stroke Prevention in Atrial Fibrillation II Study [Letter]. *Lancet* 1994;343:1509.

49. Hart RG. Intensity of anticoagulation to prevent stroke in patients with atrial fibrillation [Letter]. *Ann Intern Med* 1998;128:408.

50. Hylek EM, Skates SJ, Singer DE. Anticoagulation for nonrheumatic atrial fibrillation [Letter]. *N Engl J Med* 1997;336:442.

51. Diener HC, Forbes C, Riekkinin PD, et al. European Stroke Prevention Study II. Efficacy and safety data. *J Neurol Sci* 1997;151:S13–S17.

52. Bogousslavsky J, Kaste M, Skyhoj Olsen T, et al., for the EUSI Executive Committee. Risk factors and stroke prevention. *Cerebrovasc Dis* 2000;10[Suppl 3]:12–21.

53. Taylor FC, Cohen H, Ebrahim S. Systematic review of long term anticoagulation or antiplatelet treatment in patients with non-rheumatic atrial fibrillation. *Br Med J* 2001;322:321–326.

54. Thomson R, Parkin D, Eccles M, et al. Decision analysis and guidelines for anticoagulant therapy to prevent stroke in patients with atrial fibrillation. *Lancet* 2000; 355:956–962.

55. Scott ME, Wallace WFM. Patients and doctors play it safe [Letter]. *Br Med J* 1996;312:51–52.

56. Deplanque D, Corea F, Arquizan C, et al. Stroke and atrial fibrillation: is stroke prevention treatment appropriate beforehand? SAFE I Study Investigators. *Heart* 1999;82:563–569.

Ischemic Stroke: Advances in Neurology, Vol. 92. Edited by
H.J.M. Barnett, Julien Bogousslavsky, and Heather Meldrum.
Lippincott Williams & Wilkins, Philadelphia © 2003.

25

Cardiac Rhythm Disorders and Muscle Changes with Cerebral Lesions

Raymond T.F. Cheung and *Vladimir Hachinski

*Department of Medicine, University of Hong Kong, Queen Mary Hospital, Pokfulam, Hong Kong; and
*University of Western Ontario; Stroke Program, Department of Clinical Neurologial Sciences,
London Health Sciences Centre, London, Ontario, Canada*

A variety of cerebral lesions are known to manifest cardiovascular disturbances, including cardiac arrhythmias, pathologic changes in the myocardium, marked fluctuations in arterial blood pressure, and neurogenic pulmonary edema (1). Electrocardiography (ECG) reveals cardiac arrhythmias and myocardial injuries. Serum levels of cardiac enzymes, echocardiography, and histologic examinations can also document myocardial damages. Variations in RR intervals and power spectral analysis can reflect heart rate variability that, in turn, measures the sympathetic and parasympathetic influences on the heart (2).

Clinicians often neglect these cardiovascular disturbances because they are not well described in the literature and textbooks and they do not assist in the diagnosis of the underlying cerebral lesions (3). More attention on the subject is warranted because these disturbances can be serious or even fatal and may worsen the prognosis of the primary condition. On the other hand, patients may present with prominent cerebrogenic cardiovascular disturbances to an internist or a cardiologist for suspected acute cardiac disorders (3). An unwary clinician may miss the underlying cerebral condition and fail to initiate relevant investigations and commence appropriate management with minimal delay.

Instead of cerebrogenic cardiovascular disturbances due to underlying neurologic disorders, other possible scenarios would include neurologic complications of cardiac disorders, multisystem diseases with neurologic and cardiac features, and coexisting neurologic and cardiac disorders (3). These possibilities are beyond the scope of this chapter.

We will briefly summarize the concept of brain–heart interactions; describe the clinical scenar-

ios of cardiac arrhythmias and myocardial changes seen in some common or important causes of cerebral lesions; outline the plausible peripheral and central neuroanatomic basis, as well as neurochemical mediators of cerebrogenic arrhythmias and cardiomyopathy; and suggest a pragmatic approach to cerebrogenic cardiovascular disturbances. Seizures, migraine, and strong emotions can also produce arrhythmias and myocardial damage; these conditions will not be discussed in this chapter because they are typically not associated with cerebral lesions.

BRAIN–HEART INTERACTIONS

The heart can function in an autonomous and isolated manner, but the ability to closely regulate cardiovascular functions is important, so that the cardiac output and tissue perfusion are appropriate to the body requirements under different circumstances or upon changes in the external and/or internal environment (3). The brain receives and integrates all external and internal stimuli to enable a proper control of the cardiovascular functions through the autonomic nervous system and endocrine–humoral system (Fig. 25-1). This brain–heart control enables second-to-second modulation of cardiac activity and vascular tone in response to physical activity, threats, stresses, and emotional changes (3). An integrated brain/autonomic system may be a cerebral defense system of evolutionary advantage to the survival of animals in the jungle because highly variable cardiovascular outputs are needed for different behaviors such as the attack of prey, escape from predators, and the quiet resting state (4). On the other hand, diseases of the central nervous system can disturb the

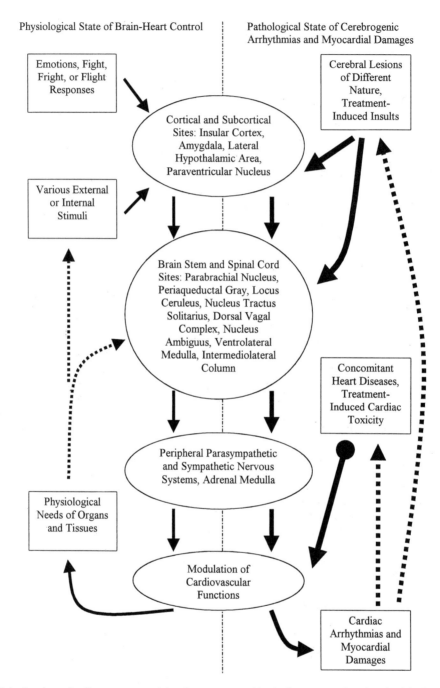

FIG. 25-1. A schematic diagram summarizing the concepts of brain–heart control under physiologic conditions **(left)** and of cerebrogenic arrhythmias and myocardial damages under pathologic states **(right)**. Thin filled arrows represent the direction of actions or influences originating from behavioral, emotional, or physiologic needs; thin dashed arrows represent the feedback interactions on the autonomic control of cardiovascular functions; thick filled arrows represent the proposed pathways of cerebrogenic cardiovascular disturbances; thick filled arrow with dotted origin emphasizes the relevance of concomitant heart diseases or treatment-induced cardiotoxicity; thick dashed arrows represent the vicious cycle of the effects of cerebrogenic disturbances on the cerebral and cardiac functions.

cardiovascular functions and produce serious consequences (Fig. 25-1).

The adult human brain constitutes only 2% of the total body weight but receives 15% of the total cardiac output at rest. The brain's high metabolic rate requires an uninterrupted blood supply, and various cardiac or vascular diseases can produce global or focal disturbances of cerebral functions (3). This heart–brain effect together with the aforementioned brain–heart control can lead to a vicious cycle ending up with significant mortality and morbidity.

COMMON OR IMPORTANT CEREBRAL LESIONS

Ischemic and Hemorrhagic Strokes

Historically, four acute stroke cases with ECG changes suggestive of acute myocardial ischemia were described in 1947; two patients had subarachnoid hemorrhage, but other neurologic details were not provided (5). In 1954, abnormal ECGs were reported from 17 stroke patients between 1 and 7 days after the stroke, and 14 of them had a bloody spinal tap, indicating intracerebral or subarachnoid hemorrhage. A triad of ECG changes was noted in the septal leads: prolongation of the QT interval, peaking and widening of T waves, and abnormal U waves (6). Subsequent studies indicated that similar ECG changes are observed in 40% to 70% of patients with subarachnoid hemorrhage, 60% to 70% of patients with intracerebral hemorrhage, and 15% to 40% of patients with ischemic stroke (7). Other reported ECG changes are depressed or elevated ST segments, flat or inverted T waves, peaked P waves, Q waves, and increased QRS amplitudes. Most of these changes reflect abnormal ventricular depolarization and/or repolarization (7). The ECG changes usually evolve for several days and disappear within 2 weeks, but QT prolongation and U waves may be permanent (8).

In addition, cardiac arrhythmias have been reported in 20% to 40% of patients with ischemic stroke or intracerebral hemorrhage (7). These arrhythmias included bradycardia, supraventricular tachycardias, atrial flutter, atrial fibrillation, ectopic ventricular beats, multifocal ventricular tachycardias, torsade de pointes, ventricular flutter, and ventricular fibrillation; supraventricular arrhythmias were more common than ventricular arrhythmias. Nevertheless, studies based on Holter data showed a higher incidence of ventricular arrhythmias (9,10). Practically all patients with subarachnoid hemorrhage have car-

diac arrhythmias of different forms, with multifocal ventricular premature beats in 54%, couplets in 40%, unsustained ventricular tachycardia in 29%, and torsade de pointes in 4% (11).

Elevation of creatine kinase (CK) was seen in 30% to 45% of stroke patients (12,13), but CK may be derived from skeletal muscles. Serum levels of the cardio-specific isoenzyme CK myocardial band (CK-MB) correlate well with the presence of ECG changes and/or cardiac arrhythmias (13). Serum CK-MB levels increase slowly and peak at a much lower value at 4 days after stroke rather than rapidly with a high peak as in acute myocardial infarction. Polypeptide subunits of the myofibrillar regulatory troponin complex such as troponin-T or troponin-I have been shown to be sensitive and specific markers of cardiac damage in myocardial ischemia (14). An increased troponin-T concentration initially after stroke has been found to be a powerful predictor of mortality during follow-up (15). It is interesting to investigate the time course of change in serum levels of troponin-T or troponin-I following stroke and correlate their levels with the location and size of stroke.

Ischemic heart disease and cerebrovascular disease often coexist in the same patient, and concomitant coronary heart disease may be the cause of ECG and cardiac myocardial changes following stroke (3,7). Direct evidence indicates that these changes may occur in the presence of normal coronary arteries and in the absence of acute coronary ischemia (1). Thus, concomitant cardiac diseases may further increase the risk of cerebrogenic arrhythmias and myocardial changes. In any case, the presence of cerebrogenic cardiovascular disturbances following stroke can worsen the prognosis because of hemodynamic consequences and/or cardiac damage. Among the stroke patients who had cardiac or sudden death, scattered cardiac myocytolysis, myofibrillar degeneration, subendocardial congestion or hemorrhage, lipofuscin deposition, and histiocytic infiltration rather than acute myocardial infarction were observed in the postmortem examination (16).

Head Injury

Head injury can produce diffuse axonal injury, focal cerebral hematoma, subdural or epidural hematoma, cerebral edema, hydrocephalus, raised intracranial pressure, and vascular injury. In addition, meningitis may complicate basal skull fracture or open-depressed skull fracture. Not surprisingly, ECG abnormalities related to head injuries have been reported on many occasions. In a study of 100 consecutive patients with acute subdural hematoma, dramatic ECG changes were noted, and 41 patients developed new cardiac arrhythmias (17) Reversible deep T-wave inversion and QT prolongation have been noted in the precordial leads of patients with head injury, and echocardiography may reveal reversible anterior or apical wall motion abnormality (18). Although these changes suggest coronary ischemia, coronary angiography or postmortem examination fails to document any significant coronary artery disease (18,19). Recognition of these cerebrogenic ECG changes following head injury is clinically important because neurosurgical intervention for the head injury should not be deferred and coronary angiography should not be undertaken.

Bizarre ECG changes indicative of ventricular tachycardia have been reported in an 18-year-old woman with subdural hematoma following head injury; the ventricular arrhythmia did not respond to intravenous antiarrhythmic drugs and electrical cardioversion (20). Torsade de pointes was reported in a 75-year-old man 1 day after blunt head injury in association with a left thalamic hematoma (21). Hypertension and bradycardia can complicate head or orbital injury; cerebral compression or intracranial hypertension may induce the Cushing response or oculocardiac reflex (22,23). An extreme scenario is traumatic cardiac arrest following head injury (24). Supraventricular tachyarrhythmia is also common, transient atrial fibrillation has been reported, but transient atrioventricular block due to vagal hyperactivity is rare (25–27).

Patients with severe head injury nearly always have raised plasma catecholamine concentration to indicate sympathetic hyperactivity, and elevated serum CK-MB level is seen in 30% of the cases (28). Focal cardiac myocytolysis with contraction band necrosis and subendocardial hemorrhage was found on postmortem examination. On the other hand, the accompanying bodily injuries, the act of cardiopulmonary resuscitation, the need for mechanical ventilation, and the use of medications such as sedatives, muscle relaxants, and anesthetic agents may contribute to the occurrence of cardiovascular disturbances following severe head injury. For example, long-term infusion of propofol at doses above 5 mg/kg for sedating head-injured patients in the intensive care unit may produce the propofol infusion syndrome with fatal cardiac arrests (29). Cardiac complications of head injury may be harmful or even fatal despite intensive care, supportive treatment, correction of anoxia, and raised intracranial pressure.

Multiple Sclerosis

Impaired autonomic nervous system is common in patients with multiple sclerosis; urinary, bowel, sexual, and sudomotor dysfunctions are the prominent autonomic features (30). Recent studies using standard noninvasive tests such as the Valsalva maneuver, rhythmic deep breathing, and sustained isometric handgrip have documented impairment of cardiovascular reflexes and suggested sympathetic dysfunctions to be predominant, and the severity of cardiovascular abnormalities does not correlate with the localization of brainstem lesions on neuroimaging (31). In a systematic study of 48 patients with multiple sclerosis (of both progressive and remitting types) who had no other diseases and who were not on medications affecting the autonomic nervous system, the mean corrected QT interval was prolonged in the patients when compared with the age- and sex-matched healthy control subjects (32). In addition, 27% of the patients compared with none of the control subjects had an abnormally prolonged corrected QT interval. Furthermore, abnormal T waves suggestive of prolonged repolarization were seen in some patients but not in the control subjects (32). Interestingly, similar observations were made in the rat experimental allergic encephalomyelitis model for multiple sclerosis (32). There are also case reports of paroxysmal atrial fibrillation associated with acute exacerbation of multiple sclerosis with active focal demyelination in the brainstem or precipitated by different courses of methylprednisolone at high dose in a 59-year-old man with chronic progressive multiple sclerosis (33).

Recent studies using echocardiography or cardiac magnetic resonance imaging and spectroscopy have documented that subclinical myocardial dysfunctions are common in patients with multiple sclerosis, especially at an advanced stage (34,35). Focal myocardial necrosis complicating multiple sclerosis has been reported in a patient with demyelinating lesion in the medulla (36). Recognition of myocardial dysfunctions is important because interferons can produce cardiac arrhythmias, myocardial ischemia, congestive heart failure, hypotension, and tachycardia (37) and the new immunosuppressive agent, mitoxantrone, is effective but cardiotoxic. Noninvasive assessment of cardiac sympathetic and parasympathetic control using heart rate variability performed in patients with multiple sclerosis during a stable phase revealed an enhanced sympathetic activity and a depressed parasympathetic activity (38,39). In addition, there is no correlation between the abnormal heart rate variability and the size or location of the demyelinating plaques on magnetic resonance imaging. Nevertheless, it would be interesting to examine for any correlation with demyelinating plaques adjacent to the insular cortex and amygdala.

Brain Tumors and Neurosurgical Procedures

Superficial brain tumors may present with repeated attacks of paroxysmal atrial tachycardia, bradycardia, or asystole during partial epileptic seizures (40,41). Studies using simultaneous ECG and intracranial depth electroencephalographic monitoring have shown that ictal involvement of the fronto-orbital cortex, the amygdalohippocampal complex, the fronto-central region, and the temporal neocortex can generate these arrhythmias (41). Neurosurgical procedures for brainstem tumors have substantial risks of perioperative cardiovascular disturbances; intensive monitoring and corticosteroids at high doses are recommended (42). Endoscopic third ventriculostomy for obstructive hydrocephalus in pediatric patients has a 40% incidence of bradycardia (43); other arrhythmias and cardiac arrest have been reported (44).

Meningitis and Encephalitis

Previously, Hersch (45) reported ECG repolarization changes in 15% and ventricular premature beats in 20% of cases of meningitis in a Bantu population. In a later study, Mehta and colleagues (46) reported notching of the T wave in 55% and QT prolongation in 13% of patients with meningitis. Other ECG changes include diffuse ST-segment elevation, other ST-T changes, sinoatrial block, and atrioventricular block (46–48). Sinus bradycardia is common, and atrioventricular dissociation is rare (46,48). Subclinical carditis may be an important mechanism of the ECG changes and cardiac arrhythmias in meningitis (48–51). ECG changes and cardiac arrhythmias are transient or intermittent and often asymptomatic without hemodynamic consequences (48). Continuous cardiac monitoring is recommended, and temporary pacing may rarely be needed for complete atrioventricular block or significant hypotension (52).

Patients with viral encephalitis may have cardiac manifestations due to concomitant viral myocarditis and/or pericarditis in the form of multisystem involvement (53–55). Not uncommonly, cardiac arrhythmias occur in patients with viral encephalitis without evidence of multisystem or cardiac involvement. For example, a patient with *Herpes simplex* encephalitis presented with sick sinus syndrome (56).

Temporary torsade de pointes or sinoatrial arrest has been reported as a complication of encephalitis, requiring intensive cardiac monitoring, temporary ventricular pacing, and/or magnesium infusion (57–59). In a clinicopathologic study, a 38-year-old woman presented initially with gastroduodenal dysmotility. She developed postoperative supraventricular tachyarrhythmia with hemodynamic disturbances and died in a few hours. Postmortem examination revealed brainstem encephalitis in the tegmental region with normal myocardium, including the cardiac conduction system, indicating cerebrogenic arrhythmias (60).

PATHOGENIC MECHANISMS OF CEREBROGENIC ARRHYTHMIAS AND CARDIOMYOPATHY

Neuroanatomic Mechanisms

Heart rate, cardiac rhythm, and contractility are modulated peripherally via the sympathetic and parasympathetic nervous systems. Interestingly, autonomic innervation of the heart is asymmetric (8). For example, the sinoatrial and atrioventricular nodes are more responsive to the parasympathetic influence, and the ventricular muscle is more sensitive to sympathetic control (8). In addition, the right vagus nerve affects predominately the sinoatrial node, and the left vagus nerve modulates mainly the atrioventricular node. Furthermore, arrhythmias can be induced more easily with stimulation of the left stellate ganglion or the left-sided cardiac sympathetic nerves than when the stimulation is made on the right cardiac sympathetic nerves (8).

Historically, the brainstem sympathetic and parasympathetic centers were thought to be the highest sites of autonomic control (61). Recent clinical observations and experimental studies have documented the importance of cortical and subcortical sites in autonomic control: the insular cortex and the amygdala (1). The insular cortex has been proposed to play a crucial role in cerebrogenic cardiovascular disturbances and sudden death (1). In addition to a viscerotopic sensory representation, the insular cortex receives taste, gastrointestinal, respiratory, chemoreceptor, and cardiovascular inputs and has rich reciprocal connections with the parabrachial nucleus, contralateral insular cortex, adjacent cortical regions, infralimbic cortex, thalamus, lateral hypothalamic area, and amygdala (62). Electrical or chemical stimulation of the rostral half of the posterior part of the dysgranular and agranular insular cortex elicits sympathetic responses, and parasympathetic responses are obtained with stimulation of the caudal part of the dysgranular and agranular insular cortex (63,64).

In a study of 24-h blood pressure recordings in 45 patients with cerebral infarction, circadian blood pressure variation was significantly increased after hemodynamic infarction but decreased after thromboembolic infarction (65). More importantly, involvement of the insular cortex was associated with a nocturnal rise of blood pressure, QT prolongation, and cardiac arrhythmias (65). In another systematic study of 52 patients with thromboembolic cerebral infarction, involvement of the insular cortex had a stronger association with the cardiovascular and autonomic disturbances than the infarction size (66). More recently, the effect of stroke location on cerebrogenic cardiac disturbances was examined in 62 patients with ischemic stroke and compared with that of 62 control subjects (67). Involvement of the right insular cortex was found to be associated with reduced heart rate variability and the occurrence of cerebrogenic sudden death (67). Most recently, the involvement of the insular cortex was an independent predictor of poor long-term outcome in 112 consecutive patients with their first unilateral thromboembolic cerebral infarction (68).

Biochemical or Neurochemical Mechanisms

Catecholamines, especially norepinephrine, mediate the peripheral effects of sympathetic activation at target tissues such as the myocardium (61). Intravenous infusion of norepinephrine reproduces the characteristic ECG and myocardial changes typical of cerebrogenic cardiac disturbances (8,14). Both experimental and clinical studies have confirmed an association between high serum norepinephrine levels and involvement of insular cortex (1).

In contrast, the central neurochemical mechanisms mediating the cerebrogenic cardiovascular disturbances are unknown. Direct and reciprocal ipsilateral connections exist between the insular cortex and the amygdala, and the amygdala directly mediates the cardiovascular responses to stressful stimuli (2). Immunoreactivities for neuropeptide Y, leucine-enkephalin, dynorphin, and neurotensin were found to increase within the amygdala on the side of damage after the insular cortex involvement by experimental stroke or excitotoxic injury (69,70). The amygdalar neurochemical change that follows a specific time course following experimental stroke (71) may mediate the cerebrogenic cardiovascular distur-

bances originating from the insular cortex. Cardiovascular responses to intermittent and continuous noise and air-jet stimulations were studied in rats at different times following right-sided experimental stroke or sham stroke (2). Cardiovascular responses to these stressful stimulations were exaggerated between days 5 and 7 following experimental stroke, and analyses of the heart rate variability confirmed significant increases in the sympathetic reactivity during the same period (2). Interestingly, this time period correlates well with the time course of amygdalar neurochemical changes (71).

CLINICAL IMPLICATIONS AND APPROACH TO CEREBROGENIC CARDIOVASCULAR DISTURBANCES

Monitoring of Patients

Recognition of cerebrogenic cardiovascular disturbances is important for making the correct diagnosis and initiating appropriate management (3). These disturbances can be severe or even life-threatening and may worsen the prognosis of the underlying cerebral conditions (3). A cardiocerebral approach may be advisable with monitoring of vital signs, cardiovascular functions, and neurologic status in patients with cerebral lesions of different nature. When cardiovascular disturbances such as ECG or myocardial changes are detected, intensive cardiocerebral monitoring and correction of any aggravating factors such as electrolyte disturbances become mandatory. Recent studies have consistently confirmed that insular cortex involvement is an independent risk factor of cerebrogenic cardiovascular disturbances (67). Other important factors include right-sided lesion, advancing age, coexisting hypertensive or ischemic heart disease, and presence of intense emotional stress (1).

Directions for Research

Much information on cerebrogenic cardiovascular disturbances has been gained from clinical observations and experimental studies in the last two decades, but wide gaps in knowledge remain. More research work should be conducted to enable us to predict the occurrence of serious or life-threatening cardiovascular disturbances and to identify the vulnerable period for the disturbances in various neurologic or neurosurgical conditions. More studies on the neurochemical mediators are needed to guide our search for effective interventions for cerebrogenic cardiovascular disturbances. Pilot studies should be conducted to evaluate the effectiveness of interventions in the treatment and prevention of cerebrogenic cardiovascular disturbances. Randomized, controlled trials are needed to confirm the benefit of the interventions.

REFERENCES

1. Cheung RTF, Hachinski V. The insula and cerebrogenic sudden death. *Arch Neurol* 2000;57:1685–1688.
2. Cheung RTF, Hachinski VC, Cechetto DF. Cardiovascular responses to stress following middle cerebral artery occlusion in the rat. *Brain Res* 1997;747:181–188.
3. Cheung RTF, Hachinski V. Cardiology. In: Samuels MA, ed. *Hospitalist neurology.* Boston: Butterworth–Heinemann, 1999:305–330.
4. Skinner JE. Neurocardiology. Brain mechanisms underlying fatal cardiac arrhythmias. *Neurol Clin* 1993;11: 325–351.
5. Byer E, Ashman R, Toth LA. Electrocardiogram with large upright T waves and long Q-T intervals. *Am Heart J* 1947;33:769–799.
6. Burch GE, Meyers R, Abildskov JA. A new electrocardiographic pattern observed in cerebrovascular accidents. *Circulation* 1954;9:719–723.
7. Oppenheimer SM, Hachinski VC. The cardiac consequences of stroke. *Neurol Clin* 1992;10:167–176.
8. Talman WT. Cardiovascular regulation and lesion of the central nervous system. *Ann Neurol* 1985;18:1–12.
9. Norris JW, Froggatt GM, Hachinski VC. Cardiac arrhythmias in acute stroke. *Stroke* 1978;4:392–396.
10. Rem JA, Hachinski VC, Boughner DR, et al. Value of cardiac monitoring and echocardiography in TIA and stroke patients. *Stroke* 1985;16:950–956.
11. Stober T, Anstatt T, Sen S, et al. Cardiac arrhythmias in subarachnoid hemorrhage. *Acta Neurochir* 1988;93: 37–44.
12. Dimant J, Grob D. Electrocardiographic changes and myocardial damage in patients with acute cerebrovascular accidents. *Stroke* 1977;8:448–455.
13. Norris JW, Hachinski VC, Myers MG, et al. Serum cardiac enzymes in stroke. *Stroke* 1979;10:548–553.
14. Bertinchant JP, Robert E, Polge A, et al. Comparison of the diagnostic value of cardiac troponin I and T determinations for detecting early myocardial damage and the relationship with histological findings after isoprenaline-induced cardiac injury in rats. *Clin Chim Acta* 2000;298:13–28.
15. James P, Ellis CJ, Whitlock RM, et al. Relation between troponin T concentration and mortality in patients presenting with an acute stroke: observational study. *Br Med J* 2000;320:1502–1504.
16. Oppenheimer SM, Cechetto DF, Hachinski VC. Cerebrogenic cardiac arrhythmias: cerebral electrocardiographic influences and their role in sudden death. *Arch Neurol* 1990;47:513–519.
17. VanderArk GD. Cardiovascular changes with acute subdural haematoma. *Surg Neurol* 1975;3:305–308.
18. Sharkey SW, Shear W, Hodges M, et al. Reversible myocardial contraction abnormalities in patients with an acute noncardiac illness. *Chest* 1998;114:98–105.
19. McLeod AA, Neil-Dwyer G, Meyer CH, et al. Cardiac sequelae of acute head injury. *Br Heart J* 1982;47: 221–226.
20. Loke YK, Lai VM, Tan MH, et al. Bizarre ECG in head injury mimicking ventricular tachycardia. *Singapore Med J* 1997;38:166–168.
21. Rotem M, Constantini S, Shir Y, et al. Life-threatening torsade de pointes arrhythmia associated with head injury. *Neurosurgery* 1988;23:89–92.
22. Shanlin RJ, Sole MJ, Rahimifar M, et al. Increased intracranial pressure elicits hypertension, increased sympathetic activity, electrocardiographic abnormalities and myocardial damage in rats. *J Am Coll Cardiol* 1988;12:727–736.
23. Hirjak D, Zajko J, Satko I. Bradycardia after orbital injury. Case report. *Int J Oral Maxillofac Surg* 1993;22: 26–27.
24. Fulton RL, Voigt WJ, Hilakos AS. Confusion surrounding the treatment of traumatic cardiac arrest. *J Am Coll Surg* 1995;181:209–214.
25. Marshall. Transient atrial fibrillation after minor head injury. *Br Heart J* 1976;38:984–985.
26. Cruickshank JM, Neil-Dwyer G, Degaute JP, et al. Reduction of stress/catecholamine-induced cardiac necrosis by beta 1-selective blockade. *Lancet* 1987;2: 585–589.
27. Wirth R, Fenster PE, Marcus FI. Transient heart block associated with head trauma. *J Trauma* 1988;28: 262–264.
28. Cruickshank JM, Neil-Dwyer G, Hayes Y, et al. Stress/catecholamine-induced cardiac necrosis. Reduction by beta 1-selective blockade. *Postgrad Med* 1988; 29:140–147.
29. Cremer OL, Moons KGM, Bouman EA, et al. Long-term propofol infusion and cardiac failure in adult head-injured patients. *Lancet* 2001;357:117–118.
30. Thomaides TN, Zoukos Y, Chaudhuri KR, et al. Physiological assessment of aspects of autonomic functions in patients with secondary progressive multiple sclerosis. *J Neurol* 1993;240:139–143.
31. Anema JR, Heijenbrok MW, Faes TJC, et al. Cardiovascular autonomic function in multiple sclerosis. *J Neurol Sci* 1991;104:129–134.
32. Drouin E, Nataf S, Lande G, et al. Abnormalities of cardiac repolarization in multiple sclerosis: relationship with a model of allergic encephalomyelitis in rat. *Muscle Nerve* 1998;21:940–942.
33. Moretti R, Torre P, Antonello RM, et al. Recurrent atrial fibrillation associated with pulse administration of high doses of methylprednisolone: a possible prophylactic treatment. *Eur J Neurol* 2000;7:130.
34. Ziaber J, Chmielewski H, Dryjanski T, et al. Evaluation of myocardial muscle functional parameters in patients with multiple sclerosis. *Acta Neurol Scand* 1997;95: 335–337.
35. Beer M, Sandstede J, Weilbach F, et al. Cardiac metabolism and function in patients with multiple sclerosis: a combined ^{31}P-MR-spectroscopy and MRI study. *Rofo Fortschr Geb Rontgenstr Neuen Bildgeb Verfahr* 2001; 173:399–404.
36. Raza-Ahmad A, Sangalang V, Klassen GA, et al. Focal myocardial necrosis associated with multiple sclerosis of the medulla. *Am J Cardiol* 1991;68:1542–1544.
37. Vial T, Descotes J. Clinical toxicity of the interferons. *Drug Saf* 1994;10:115–150.
38. Giubilei F, Vitale A, Urani C, et al. Cardiac autonomic dysfunction in relapsing–remitting multiple sclerosis during a stable phase. *Eur Neurol* 1996;36:211–214.

39. Monge-Argiles JA, Palacios-Ortega F, Vila-Sobrino JA, et al. Heart rate variability in multiple sclerosis during a stable phase. *Acta Neurol Scand* 1998;97:86–92.

40. Rush JL, Everett BA, Adams AH, et al. Paroxysmal atrial tachycardia and frontal lobe tumor. *Arch Neurol* 1977;34:578–580.

41. Kahane P, Di Leo M, Hoffmann D, et al. Ictal bradycardia in a patient with a hypothalamic hamartoma: a stereo-EEG study. *Epilepsia* 1999;40:522–527.

42. Mursch K, Buhre W, Behnke-Mursch J, et al. Perioperative cardiovascular stability during brainstem surgery. The use of high-dose methylprednisolone compared to dexamethasone. A retrospective analysis. *Acta Anaesthesiol Scand* 2000;44:378–382.

43. El-Dawlatly AA, Murshid WR, Elshimy A, et al. The incidence of bradycardia during endoscopic third ventriculostomy. *Anesth Analg* 2000;91:1142–1144.

44. Handler MH, Abbott R, Lee M. A near-fatal complication of endoscopic third ventriculostomy: case report. *Neurosurgery* 1994;35:525–527.

45. Hersch C. Electrocardiographic changes in subarachnoid haemorrhage, meningitis, and intracranial space-occupying lesions. *Br Heart J* 1964;26:785–793.

46. Mehta SS, Kronzon I, Laniado S. Electrocardiographic changes in meningitis. *Isr J Med Sci* 1974;10:748–752.

47. Vitris M, Charriere JM, Aubert M. Acute auriculoventricular block in cerebrospinal meningitis. *Dakar Med* 1983;28:337–342.

48. Shapira MY, Hirshberg B, Ben-Yehuda A. Asymptomatic temporary atrioventricular dissociation complicating meningococcal meningitis. *Int J Cardiol* 1997; 62:277–278.

49. Detsky AS, Salit IE. Complete heart block in meningococcemia. *Ann Emerg Med* 1983;12:391–393.

50. Patial RK, Kashyap S, Bansal SK, et al. Lyme disease in a Shimla boy. *J Assoc Physicians India* 1990;38: 503–504.

51. Etherington J, Salmon J, Ratcliffe G. Atrio-ventricular dissociation in meningococcal meningitis. *J R Army Med Corps* 1995;141:169–171.

52. Morriss JH, Gillette PC, Barrett FF. Atrioventricular block complicating meningitis: treatment with emergency cardiac pacing. *Pediatrics* 1976;58:866–868.

53. Young EJ, Killam AP, Greene JF Jr. Disseminated herpesvirus infection. Association with primary genital herpes in pregnancy. *JAMA* 1976;235:2731–2733.

54. Nigro G, Pacella ME, Patane E, et al. Multi-system Coxsackie virus B-6 infection with findings suggestive of diabetes mellitus. *Eur J Pediatr* 1986;145:557–559.

55. Duppenthaler A, Pfammatter JP, Aebi C. Myopericarditis associated with central European tick-borne encephalitis. *Eur J Pediatr* 2000;159:854–856.

56. Pollock S, Reid H, Klapper P, et al. Herpes simplex encephalitis presenting as the sick sinus syndrome. *J Neurol Neurosurg Psychiatry* 1986;49:331–332.

57. De Keyser J, De Boel S, Ceulemans L, et al. Torsade de pointes as a complication of brainstem encephalitis. *Intensive Care Med* 1987;13:76–77.

58. Alehan D, Ceviz N, Celiker A. Torsade de pointes associated with encephalitis. *Turk J Pediatr* 1999;41: 395–398.

59. Alsolaiman MM, Alsolaiman F, Bassas S, et al. Viral encephalitis associated with reversible asystole due to sinoatrial arrest. *South Med J* 2001;94:540–541.

60. Alampi G, Bortolotti M, Mattioli S, et al. Brain stem encephalitis in a patient with gastroduodenal and cardiovascular dysfunction: a case report. *Clin Neuropathol* 1990;9:16–20.

61. Samuels MA. Neurally induced cardiac damage. *Neurol Clin* 1993;11:273–291.

62. Cechetto DF, Saper CB. Role of the cerebral cortex in autonomic function. In Loewy AD, Spyer KM, eds. *Central regulation of autonomic functions.* New York: Oxford University Press, 1990:208–223.

63. Oppenheimer SM, Cechetto DF. Cardiac chronotropic organization of the rat insular cortex. *Brain Res* 1990; 533:66–72.

64. Yasui Y, Breder CD, Saper CB, et al. Autonomic responses and efferent pathways from the insular cortex in the rat. *J Comp Neurol* 1991;303:355–374.

65. Sander D, Klingelhofer J. Changes of circadian blood pressure patterns after hemodynamic and thromboembolic brain infarction. *Stroke* 1994;25:1730–1737.

66. Sander D, Klingelhofer J. Stroke-associated pathological sympathetic activation related to size of infarction and extent of insular damage. *Cerebrovasc Dis* 1995;5: 381–385.

67. Tokgözoglu SL, Batur MK, Topçuoglu MA, et al. Effects of stroke localization on cardiac autonomic balance and sudden death. *Stroke* 1999;30:1307–1311.

68. Sander D, Winbeck K, Klingelhofer J, et al. Prognostic relevance of pathological sympathetic activation after acute thromboembolic stroke. *Neurology* 2001;57: 833–838.

69. Allen GV, Cheung RTF, Cechetto DF. Neurochemical changes following chronic occlusion of the middle cerebral artery in rats. *Neuroscience* 1995;68:1037–1050.

70. Cheung RTF, Cechetto DF. Neuropeptide changes following excitotoxic lesion of the insular cortex in rats. *J Comp Neurol* 1995;362:535–550.

71. Cheung RTF, Diab T, Cechetto DF. Time-course of change in neuropeptides over peri-ischemic zone and amygdala following focal ischemia in rats. *J Comp Neurol* 1995;360:101–120.

Ischemic Stroke: Advances in Neurology, Vol. 92. Edited by
H.J.M. Barnett, Julien Bogousslavsky, and Heather Meldrum.
Lippincott Williams & Wilkins, Philadelphia © 2003.

26

Sudden Death

Ale Algra

*Departments of Neurology and Clinical Epidemology, Julius Center for Health Sciences and Primary
Care, University Medical Center Utrecht, Utrecht, The Netherlands*

Even in the Bible, cases of sudden death are mentioned: For example, Ananias and Saffira, charged by
Peter to have lied to God, dropped dead (1). Often,
extreme grief or anger plays a role, relating extremes
of brain function with almost instantaneous fatal cardiac sequelae. Such input from the brain may be particularly threatening in patients who have a cardiac
substrate that is at increased risk by scarring after
myocardial infarction (2). In this chapter, the relationship between ischemic lesions of the brain and the
occurrence of sudden death is described.

DEFINITION OF SUDDEN DEATH

A definition of sudden cardiac death could be the following: unexpected natural death due to cardiac
causes in an individual with or without known preexisting heart disease within 1 h of the onset of the terminal event; in the case of unwitnessed death, the vic-
tim has been seen to be well within the preceding 24
h. This definition includes patients dying unexpectedly during sleep. Essential elements in the definition
are (a) natural death, (b) unexpected occurrence, (c)
rapid development, and (d) cardiac cause.

Deaths from unnatural causes such as accidents,
homicide, and suicide are not included in this definition. The unexpectedness of the sudden death is crucial and is related to the history of disease and the
presence of disability prior to death. Deaths in individuals who have severe limitations of activities
because of physical or mental illness are usually not
considered as sudden, unexpected deaths (3). The
above definition uses a time interval of 1 h between
onset of complaints and death. A problem with this
definition is the fact that the death may not have been
witnessed and therefore formally should be excluded.
This exclusion, however, leads to the neglect of an

important number of deceased who die within a short
time after the onset of complaints, for the faster the
demise, the smaller the opportunity of witnessing. To
include this latter group of often-instantaneous
deaths, the above definition is extended to those victims in whom death was unwitnessed but who were
seen to be well in the preceding 24 h. Although not
always specified as such, in most definitions of sudden death, it is sudden *cardiac* death that is aimed at;
thus, in the definition of sudden cardiac death, natural, noncardiac causes of death are excluded (e.g.,
pulmonary embolism, aortic dissection, stroke).
Stroke, although generally believed to account for
10% to 20% of sudden deaths, does not fit the definition of sudden cardiac death for two reasons: First,
only very few stroke patients die within 1 h after
onset of complaints (4). Second, the cause of death is
noncardiac.

Several definitions of sudden cardiac death are
faced in the literature. Differences regard mostly the
time interval from onset of complaints to death. In
large community-based studies, one often uses a 24-
h definition because of difficulties in obtaining
detailed information on the terminal process. In
smaller studies aimed at the pathology of sudden cardiac death and with more detailed clinical observations, frequently a more strict time criterion is used.

BRAIN, AUTONOMIC NERVOUS SYSTEM,
AND HEART

Several observations from animal studies and careful studies in series of limited size in humans point to
a direct interaction of brain and heart by way of the
autonomic nervous system. Experiments in dogs have
shown that the threshold for ventricular fibrillation
may be influenced by stimulation of neural pathways

in the brain (5). Occlusion of the middle cerebral artery in rats demonstrated a differential effect on sympathetic activity according to the side of occlusion (6). The insular cortex has specifically been designated as a critical area in arrhythmogenesis (7). In another study, Oppenheimer and colleagues (8) found that stroke involving the left insular cortex was accompanied by augmented sympathetic and decreased parasympathetic cardiac tone while cardiac arrhythmias occurred. Barron et al. (9) reported from a study with 20 patients with a right-sided hemispheric stroke and 20 patients with such a lesion on the left side that cardiac parasympathetic innervation was reduced most in the patients with right-sided lesions. Parasympathetic activity was assessed by means of the respiratory-related activity of the power spectrum analysis of the beat-to-beat variation in 250 consecutive RR intervals obtained from a chest lead electrocardiogram (ECG).

The effect of brain lesions on the risk of sudden death may be studied by way of an intermediate characteristic: heart rate variability. On the one hand, brain lesions influence several components of heart rate variability, as exemplified by the study of Barron et al. (9). On the other, decreased heart rate variability is strongly associated with the risk of sudden death (10,11). Hence, heart rate variability may be viewed as a proxy for sudden death.

So far, however, there have been studies of only limited size on the direct relationship between brain infarction and the occurrence of sudden death.

BRAIN INFARCTION AND SUDDEN DEATH

Naver and colleagues (12) studied 23 Swedish patients with monofocal stroke (including three hemorrhages). Thirteen patients had right-sided lesions and 10 a lesion on the left side. These patients were compared with 21 age- and sex-matched control subjects and 11 patients who had had a transient ischemic attack (TIA) 6 to 24 months previously. Heart rate variability during deep breathing was significantly smaller in patients with right-sided lesions than in patients with left-sided lesions. The difference remained present if the analysis was restricted to the 14 patients with hemispheric lesions. During 3 years of follow-up, five patients with a right-sided lesion died, whereas one patient with a left-sided lesion died. However, no information on the timing of the terminal events was provided.

In a Finnish study, Korpelainen et al. (13) studied 31 patients with a hemispheric brain infarction and 31 age- and sex-matched control subjects. There were 19 patients with right hemispheric lesions and 12 with a left hemispheric lesion. All measures of heart rate variability were lower in stroke patients than in control subjects at the acute stage and 1 and 6 months after the stroke. The suppression of heart rate variability "did not depend" on the side of infarction; however, their article did not provide the actual data. No mention was made about patients dying suddenly during the study period.

In a prospective study from Turkey, 62 patients with a single acute middle cerebral artery infarct with a minimal diameter of 3 cm were included (14). The patients were compared with 62 age- and sex-matched control subjects. There were 32 patients with a left-sided brain infarct (25 infarcts included the insula) and 30 with a right-sided infarct (23 included the insula). Both low- and high-frequency components of the power spectrum analysis of the heart rate variability were lower in patients with right-sided stroke (Table 26-1). Seven patients who were previously clinically stable died suddenly in the hospital. At their death, three of these patients were on ECG monitoring that showed ventricular tachycardia deteriorating into ventricular fibrillation. Remarkable was that all sudden death patients had insular lesions, five of which were on the right side.

TABLE 26-1. *Power spectrum analysis of heart rate variability*

	Side of stroke		Difference	95% CI
	Left (n = 32)	Right (n = 30)		
LF (0.04–0.015 Hz)	314 ± 188	166 ± 120	148	67–299
HF (0.15–0.40 Hz)	113 ± 109	51 ± 30	62	21–103

Values are means ± SD.
CI, confidence interval; HF, high frequency; LF, low frequency.
Adapted from Tokgözoglu SL, Batur MK, Topçuoglu MA, et al., Effects of stroke localization on cardiac autonomic balance and sudden death. *Stroke* 1999;30:1307–1311.

SUDDEN DEATH IN THE NORTH AMERICAN SYMPTOMATIC CAROTID ENDARTERECTOMY TRIAL

Within the North American Symptomatic Carotid Endarterectomy Trial (NASCET), the influence of the presence and side of ischemic stroke on the long-term risk of sudden death was assessed in 2,778 patients with a TIA or minor ischemic stroke and carotid artery disease (15,16). Location of any ischemic stroke was centrally evaluated by an experienced neuroradiologist at a baseline brain scan. Vascular deaths were rereviewed to assess the timing of the terminal event. Three definitions of sudden death were used: (a) death within 10 min after onset of symptoms (witnessed and with reliable information), (b) death within 1 h of symptom onset (also witnessed and with reliable information), and (c) death within 24 h of symptom onset (witnessed without reliable data on the timing of events or the patient found dead unexpectedly). In the event of an acute noncardiac cause, the case was not counted as sudden death. Death within 24 h was used for the primary analyses.

A total of 217 patients had died within 24 h of symptom onset, 91 deaths were within 1 h, and 65 within 10 min of onset. At least one brain infarction was present in 1,483 (53.4%) patients; 471 (17.0%) had one or more left-sided lesions; 477 (17.2%) had one or more right-sided lesions; and 535 (19.3%) had an infarction on both sides. Patients with brain infarction had more risk factors for sudden death.

The 5-year risk of sudden death with 24 h after onset of symptoms was 5.3% in the patients without brain infarction, 6.0% with a right-sided lesion, 8.8% with a left-sided lesion, and 9.7% for patients with infarctions on both sides. The crude relative risk of right-sided brain infarction versus no infarction was 1.06 [95% confidence interval (CI) 0.69–1.63], that for left-sided brain infarction 1.67 (95% CI 1.16–2.41), and that for bilateral brain infarction 1.91 (95% CI 1.35–2.71). If the differences between the patients with and without brain infarction with regard to age, history of angina, diabetes mellitus, hypertension, myocardial infarction, and left ventricular hypertrophy were taken into account, the adjusted relative risks were 0.96 (95% CI 0.62–1.47), 1.45 (95% CI 1.00–2.10), and 1.40 (95% CI 0.98–2.00), respectively. Additional adjustment for other patient characteristics did not influence the relative risks. Death within 24 h was 1.44 times more frequent (adjusted relative risk) for patients with any left-sided lesion than in those without a left-sided lesion (95% CI 1.09–1.90). For death within 1 h and death within 10

min, similar observations were made; however, the relative risks for left-sided lesions tended to be higher with these stricter outcome definitions.

CONSIDERATIONS

The finding in the NASCET substudy of an increased long-term risk of sudden death of left-sided brain infarction, irrespective of right-sided infarction, is at odds with the studies discussed above. Several explanations for these differences might be offered. First, virtually all previous observations pertained to the effects of acute interventions (5–8) or to the acute phase of stroke (12–14,17), whereas the NASCET substudy dealt with the long-term effects of brain infarction. It is quite possible that the acute effects of brain infarction differ from its chronic effects. In the weeks or months after the event, a new balance between parasympathetic and sympathetic nervous system activity may develop, as well as between the left and right side of the sympathetic nervous system. Recently, Oppenheimer (18) suggested that strokes involving the left insula are associated with increased sympathetic and decreased parasympathetic cardiac tone, creating a proarrhythmic state in the ventricular myocardium. This suggestion, however, again was based on data obtained in the acute phase (8). A second, partly related explanation could be the selection of patients into the NASCET. If right-sided infarction is associated with a higher incidence of sudden death in the acute phase of brain ischemia (8,12–14), only survivors of right-sided brain infarction would have entered NASCET. Third, the findings may be ascribed to the definition of sudden death used. This, however, is improbable because the findings of the study were consistent over three different outcome definitions. Finally, the results may be a chance finding, even if the 95% CI of the relative risk of any versus no left-sided lesion did not include the neutral value. Because the findings from NASCET eventually may have clinical implications, for example, the use of β-blocking drugs in patients with left-sided brain infarction, these findings need to be corroborated in other clinical studies.

REFERENCES

1. Engel GL. Sudden and rapid death during psychological stress. Folklore or folk wisdom? *Ann Intern Med* 1971; 74:771–782.
2. Myerburg RJ, Kessler KM, Bassett AL, et al. A biological approach to sudden cardiac death: structure, function and cause. *Am J Cardiol* 1989;63:1512–1516.

3. Kuller LH. Sudden death—definition and epidemiologic considerations. *Prog Cardiovasc Dis* 1980;23:1–12.

4. Phillips LH, Whisnant JP, Reagan TJ. Sudden death from stroke. *Stroke* 1977;8:392–395.

5. Lown B, Verrier RL. Neural activity and ventricular fibrillation. *N Engl J Med* 1976;294:1165–1170.

6. Hachinski VC, Oppenheimer SM, Wilson JX, et al. Asymmetry of sympathetic consequences of experimental stroke. *Arch Neurol* 1992;49:697–702.

7. Oppenheimer SM, Wilson JX, Guiraudon C, et al. Insular cortex stimulation produces lethal cardiac arrhythmias: a mechanism of sudden death? *Brain Res* 1991;550:115–121.

8. Oppenheimer SM, Kedem G, Martin WM. Left-insular cortex lesions perturb cardiac autonomic tone in humans. *Clin Auton Res* 1996;6:131–140.

9. Barron SA, Rogovski Z, Hemli J. Autonomic consequences of cerebral hemisphere infarction. *Stroke* 1994;25:113–116.

10. Kleiger RE, Miller JP, Bigger JT Jr, et al. Decreased heart rate variability and its association with increased mortality after acute myocardial infarction. *Am J Cardiol* 1987;59:256–262.

11. Algra A, Tijssen JGP, Roelandt JRTC, et al. Heart rate variability from 24-hour electrocardiography and the 2-year risk for sudden death. *Circulation* 1993;88:180–185.

12. Naver HK, Blomstrand C, Wallin BG. Reduced heart rate variability after right-sided stroke. *Stroke* 1996;27:247–251.

13. Korpelainen JT, Sotaniemi KA, Huikuri HV, et al. Abnormal heart rate variability as a manifestation of autonomic dysfunction in hemispheric brain infarction. *Stroke* 1996;27:2059–2063.

14. Tokgözoglu SL, Batur MK, Topçuoglu MA, et al. Effects of stroke localization on cardiac autonomic balance and sudden death. *Stroke* 1999;30:1307–1311.

15. Barnett HJ, Taylor DW, Eliasziw M, et al. Benefit of carotid endarterectomy in patients with symptomatic moderate or severe stenosis. *N Engl J Med* 1998;339:1415–1425.

16. Algra A, Gates PC, on behalf of the NASCET Group. Side of brain infarction and handedness as predictor of sudden death in patients with cerebral ischaemia. *Cerebrovasc Dis* 2000;10:104(abst).

17. Oppenheimer SM, Gelb A, Girvin JP, et al. Cardiovascular effects of human insular cortex stimulation. *Neurology* 1992;42:1727–1732.

18. Oppenheimer S. Forebrain lateralization of cardiovascular function: physiology and clinical correlates. *Ann Neurol* 2001;49:555–556.

Ischemic Stroke: Advances in Neurology, Vol. 92. Edited by
H.J.M. Barnett, Julien Bogousslavsky, and Heather Meldrum.
Lippincott Williams & Wilkins, Philadelphia © 2003.

27

Cerebral Venous and Sinus Thrombosis: Incidence and Causes

Jan Stam

Department of Neurology, University of Amsterdam; Department of Neurology, Academic Medical Centre, Amsterdam, The Netherlands

INCIDENCE

The exact incidence of cerebral venous and sinus thrombosis (CVST) is unknown, but indirect data may give an approximate estimate. Kalbag and Woolf (1), in their classic study of cerebral venous thrombosis, give mortality figures from the British Registrar General. From 1952 to 1961, on average, 21.7 deaths from "phlebitis and thrombophlebitis of the intracranial venous sinuses" were reported annually in a population of 56 million at that time (0.39 deaths per million). The mortality of CVST during that period of time is not known but probably varied between 20% and 50%. This would yield an estimated incidence of about one to two cases per million.

In our clinical trial, we recruited, on average, 13 adult patients annually from 1992 to 1996 (2,3). We estimate that we recruited about 25% to 50% of all cases in the Netherlands, with a population of 16 million. If our assumption is correct, this gives an annual incidence of approximately 1.5 to 3 per million (adults).

A recently published study of 160 cases from the Canadian Pediatric Ischemic Stroke Registry calculated an annual incidence among children (up to 18 years) of 6.7 per million. Almost 50% of the sample were neonates (younger than 3 months), which indicates a higher incidence in that age group. Many authors suggest that CVST is underdiagnosed and underreported, but this assumption has not been proven.

Towbin (4) reported a high incidence in consecutive postmortem examinations. He found 17 cases in 182 autopsies (9.3%). In elderly patients, the incidence was even higher. This high incidence has never been confirmed, to our knowledge, and seems exceptional. In a recent series of 102 consecutive postmortem examinations, the sinuses were carefully examined for thrombosis according to a predefined protocol. Only two cases of CVST were found. Both were patients who died from other brain diseases and probably developed sinus thrombosis as a complication during the terminal phase of their disease [H.P. Bienfait (in press: *J Neurol*)].

Sex Ratio

In recent studies, a significant predominance of female patients has become apparent (2). In older series, the numbers of men and women were approximately equal. The above-mentioned British mortality registry reported 104 male and 113 female deaths from sinus thrombosis from 1952 to 1961 (52% women) (1). As an example of the increasing percentage of females, we give data from our own studies in the Netherlands (Table 27-1) (3,5). The data by Ferro et al. (6) point in the same direction: In their retrospective cases up to 1995, 33% of the patients were female, but in the prospective study from 1995 to 1998, the number was 74%. In children, the sex ratio is close to 50% (46% females in the Canadian registry, Table 27-2). We postulated that the shift in sex ratio that started in the mid-1980s was caused by the increased use of contraceptive pills, which are an established risk factor of CVST (see below) (2).

CAUSES AND RISK FACTORS

More than 100 putative causes, risk factors, and conditions associated with sinus thrombosis have been described. Bousser and Ross Russell (7) give an

TABLE 27-1. *Sex ratio in adults with sinus thrombosis from 1970 to 1996: retrospective and trial data from the Netherlands*

Series	Years	n	% Female	p^a
Retrospective 1	1970–1985	24	50	—
Retrospective 2	1986–1991	27	74	0.01
CVST Trial	1992–1996	59	85	<0.0001

CVST, cerebral venous and sinus thrombosis.
[a]p: Likelihood that the observed deviation from 50% is due to chance.
From de Bruijn SF, Stam J. Randomized, placebo-controlled trial of anticoagulant treatment with low-molecular-weight heparin for cerebral sinus thrombosis. *Stroke* 1999;30:484–488; and Bienfait HP, Stam J, Lensing AW, et al. [Thrombosis of the cerebral veins and sinuses in 62 patients.] *Ned Tijdschr Geneeskd* 1995;139: 1286–1291, with permission.

extensive review of many causes of CVST in their monograph. As CVST is a rare condition, much knowledge of possible causes is based upon case reports and—often retrospective—case series. These studies have many limitations and do not permit reliable, quantitative conclusions about risk and causation. One obvious problem with single case reports is the likelihood that an observed association is due to chance. Several case reports, for instance, have been published about CVST in patients with multiple sclerosis. As multiple sclerosis often is a chronic disease, which is not infrequent in young women, the association may be due to chance, or the real "cause," or rather risk factor, may not be multiple sclerosis but the use of oral contraceptives. On the other hand, repeated observations in small case series by carefully observing clinicians may well be the first signal of a new association that is later confirmed and even

understood. In the case of multiple sclerosis, two independent case reports concluded that the cause of sinus thrombosis in patients with this condition might have been the lumbar puncture combined with steroid treatment (8,9). Interestingly, lumbar puncture has also been described as a possible cause of CVST, independently of multiple sclerosis (10).

Another example is the role of oral contraceptives. Already in 1970, an association between oral contraceptive use and sinus thrombosis was suspected, and many case reports followed (11). Only recently the association became more firmly based upon case control studies, which also demonstrated the interaction with the genetic procoagulant factors that have been discovered in the last decades (12,13). Also, much progress has been made in understanding the complex interactions of oral contraceptives with the hemostatic system (14).

TABLE 27-2. *Major causes and risk factors as reported in some large retrospective and prospective studies*

	Country and time period					
	France,* 1975–2001 (7)	Portugal, 1980–1998 (6)		Netherlands, 1992–1996 (3)	Canada, 1992–1997 (22)[a]	
		Retro.	Prosp.		A	B
No. of cases	200	51	91	59	69	91
% female	62	33	74	85	46	
Regional infections	16	16[b]	18[b]	0	10	23
Oral contraceptive[c]	41	56	35	70	—	3
Pregnancy/puerperium[c]	17	18	7	14	—	—
Genetic prothrombotic conditions	23	2	9	18	16	
Mechanical[d]	6	4	3	3	0	
Systemic disease[e]	21	20	14	7	88	91
Unknown	23	27	27	17	1	3

Values are percentages.
[a]A, neonates; B, older children up to 18 yr.
[b]Includes cases of meningitis.
[c]Percentage of female patients.
[d]Trauma, neurosurgery, lumbar puncture.
[e]Vasculitis, cancer, hematologic disorders.
*M.G. Bousser: personal communication.

The aim of the present review is not to give an exhaustive list of all possible causes that have been reported but to present a brief summary of the best available evidence, with emphasis on the larger, preferably prospective, case series and case control studies.

Genetically Based Prothrombotic Conditions

During the last decades, a number of genetic conditions have been identified that interfere with normal coagulation and increase the risk of thrombosis. These "procoagulant conditions," also called "genetic thrombophilias," were mostly discovered in groups of patients with the more frequent leg-vein thrombosis (15). Later, the presence of these factors was also found in cerebral sinus thrombosis, often in case reports and small case series but also increasingly in case control studies. At present, it seems that none of these genetic procoagulant conditions is specifically related to sinus thrombosis. Rather, these thrombophilias imply a systemically increased risk of thrombosis that may either cause leg-vein thrombosis or—more rarely—sinus thrombosis. Often, an additional environmental factor is present that is the direct cause of thrombosis in an individual with a genetically increased risk.

Antithrombin

Deficiency of antithrombin (formerly called antithrombin III) is the earliest known cause of hereditary thrombophilias. Now, more than 250 mutations of the AT gene have been discovered (15,16). Nevertheless, the prevalence in the general population is low, far less than 1% in most populations. Although antithrombin deficiency is associated with an increased risk of thrombosis, cases of CVST are rare. Bousser and Ross Russell (7) listed only 1 case in their series of 135. Acquired antithrombin deficiency, often caused by nephrotic syndrome, seems more frequent.

Protein C and S Deficiency

Protein C is a natural anticoagulant. In the activated state, it inhibits normal coagulation by cleaving clotting factors Va and VIIIa. Protein S acts as a cofactor of protein C. Hundreds of different mutations in the genes of these proteins have been found (15). Heterozygotes for protein C or S deficiency have an approximately 10-fold increased risk of leg-vein thrombosis. In addition, acquired deficiencies of these proteins occur.

Protein C deficiency has been reported in a number of patients with sinus thrombosis (17,18). Deschiens et al. (17) found 1 case among 40 patients. In the Dutch sinus thrombosis trial, we found 2 cases among the 59 patients enrolled (2). Protein S deficiency in patients with CVST seems even more rare. It has been described in occasional case reports, often in children or young adults (19–21). Bousser and Ross Russell, in a large series of 135 cases (collected from 1975 to 1995), identified 1 patient with protein S deficiency. Deschiens et al. (17) found 1 case in their series of 40. We did not find any cases in the CVST Trial (2). In a large study of children with CVST, low levels of protein C and S were more frequent (7% and 4%, respectively), but most of these cases were acquired and not hereditary (22).

Factor V Mutation

The most frequently occurring mutation in coagulation factor V is the G1691→A mutation, also called "factor V–Leiden mutation." It renders factor V resistant to neutralization by activated protein C and consequently causes a procoagulant state, also called "activated protein C resistance." It is variably prevalent in healthy white populations, with frequencies ranging from 1% to 15%, and is far more frequent in patients with leg-vein thrombosis (10%–50%) (15).

In a number of case control studies, the factor V–Leiden mutation was more frequent in patients with CVST than control subjects. Zuber et al. (16) found it in 4 of 19 patients and in 1 of 57 control subjects [odds ratio (OR) 14.9]. Lower ORs of 7.8 and 2.5 were found in later case control studies (13,23). Part of these variations can be explained by the different prevalences of the mutation in the control populations. Weih et al. (24) performed a meta-analysis of the available case control studies of the association between factor V–Leiden and CVST. They calculated an estimated pooled OR of 4.3 (95% CI 2.4–7.6).

Interestingly, one study demonstrated the co-occurrence of the factor V–Leiden mutation and the plasminogen activator inhibitor-1 4G/4G genotype in patients with CVST (25). The combination was significantly more frequent in patients than in control subjects. The 4G allele is associated with increased levels of plasminogen activator inhibitor-1, which leads to decreased fibrinolysis.

Prothrombin Mutation

The G→A transition at nucleotide position 20210 in the prothrombin gene, discovered in 1996, is associated with elevated plasma prothrombin levels and an increased risk of venous thrombosis. In a case control study, this polymorphism was present in 4 of 45 (8.9%) patients with CVST and in 2.3% of control subjects (age-adjusted OR 5.7, 95% CI 1.5–21.5) (26). Martinelli et al. (13) found this mutation in 8 of 40 (20%) patients with CVST and in 3% of healthy control subjects (OR 10.2, 95% CI 2.3–31.0). In their meta-analysis of three studies, Weih et al. (24) calculated a pooled OR of 5.8 (95% CI 2.5–13.8).

Hyperhomocystinemia

Several mutations in genes coding for enzymes involved in the metabolism of homocysteine cause mildly elevated serum levels of homocysteine in heterozygotes. Also, a number of acquired causes of hyperhomocystinemia are known, notably deficiencies of vitamins B_6 and B_{12} and folate. Hyperhomocystinemia is a risk factor for leg-vein thrombosis. In a meta-analysis of case control studies of leg-vein thrombosis, an OR of 2.5 (95% CI 1.6–4.4) was found, closely matching the odds ratio in an earlier large case control study (27,28). Therefore, it is likely that this factor is also causally involved in sinus thrombosis, but adequate case control studies are not available. In our series of 59 cases, homocysteine was measured in 15 patients, 6 of whom had hyperhomocystinemia (2).

A mutation of the 5,10-methylene tetrahydrofolate reductase (MTHFR) gene (the C677→ T mutation) causes mild homocystinemia. In a small retrospective study, Hillier et al. (29) found the 5 homozygotes for the MTHFR C677→T mutation among 15 patients with CVST (30%) compared with 3.2% in a healthy reference population.

Acquired Prothrombotic Conditions

The definition of an acquired prothrombotic condition varies in different publications. The term may be used to describe all diseases, conditions, or drugs that are known to increase the risk of thrombosis, such as cancer, pregnancy, etc. In this review, the concept is limited to conditions in which the thrombotic mechanism is mostly or exclusively attributable to changes in clotting factors or antibodies. Hyperhomocystinemia can be grouped under both the genetic and the acquired prothrombotic conditions.

Nephrotic Syndrome

Many case reports describe the development of CVST in patients with nephrotic syndrome. In two large case series of CVST, the percentage varied from 1% to 3% (2,7). The development of thrombosis in patients with nephrotic syndrome is usually ascribed to renal loss of anticoagulant proteins such as antithrombin and proteins C and S, but other changes in clotting factors have also been found.

Antiphospholipid Antibodies

Antiphospholipid antibodies give rise to an increased thrombotic risk. Variably increased frequencies of antiphospholipid antibodies have been found in groups of patients with CVST. Anticardiolipin antibodies were present in 10 of 123 (8%) children in a Canadian study (22). One study found 8 anticardiolipin-positive patients in a group of 15 cases of CVST (30). Another study of 40 patients with CVST found only 3 anticardiolipin-positive cases (8%), but many of these patients were examined long after the acute phase of the disease (17). In the 34 patients tested for anticardiolipin antibodies in our study, 4 (12%) were positive (2). In addition, we also found 4 of 41 patients with CVST (10%) positive for the lupus anticoagulant. In two patients, the lupus anticoagulant and anticardiolipin antibodies co-occurred.

Sussman et al. (31), in an interesting study of 38 cases of benign intracranial hypertension, found a high incidence of antiphospholipid antibodies (32%) and other indications of a procoagulant state. This indicates that occult CVST might be involved in the pathogenesis of benign intracranial hypertension in a number of cases.

Pregnancy and Puerperium

The increased thrombotic tendency at the end of pregnancy, and especially after delivery, may give rise to leg-vein thrombosis and, less frequently, to cerebral sinus thrombosis. In the large case series of CVST, about 7% to 18% of all cases are pregnancy related or puerperal (Table 27-2). A study from the United States, based upon a very large database, estimated the frequency of peri- and postpartum CVST to be 11.6 cases/100,000 deliveries, which is slightly below the estimated incidence of peri- and postpartum arterial stroke (13.1 cases/100,000 deliveries). Factors significantly associated with peri- and postpartum CVST were cesarean delivery, hypertension, and infections (32). Cantu and Barinagarrementeria (33) published a large retrospective series of obstetric CVSTs from Mexico, consisting of 67 women, and compared them with nonobstetric cases. They concluded that the prognosis in pregnancy-related CVST is better, but still the mortality in their study was 9%.

Oral Contraceptives

An increased risk of venous thrombosis, including CVST, in women who use oral contraceptives has long been suspected (11). The subject has been controversial, but most experts now agree that oral contraceptives increase the risk of venous thrombosis. In addition to epidemiologic evidence, understanding of the mechanisms of the prothrombotic effects induced by oral contraceptives has increased significantly in recent years (14). In 1998, we demonstrated the association between oral contraceptives and sinus thrombosis in a case control study (12). Thirty-four of 40 (85%) women with cerebral sinus thrombosis used oral contraceptives. In a reference population in the Netherlands, oral contraceptive use was 45%. The age-adjusted OR was 13 (95% CI 5–37). In women who used oral contraceptives and who were also carriers of a hereditary prothrombotic condition, the risk of CVST was increased about 30-fold, which indicates that both factors interact in the development of cerebral sinus thrombosis. Also, it appeared that the risk of CVST associated with third-generation oral contraceptives (containing gestodene or desogestrel) was larger than that of other oral contraceptive preparations (34). Martinelli et al. (13) obtained similar findings. In their study, the use of oral contraceptives was also more frequent among women with CVST than among control subjects (OR 22.1, 95% CI 5.9–84.2). They showed an interaction between oral contraceptive use and the prothrombin gene mutation (13).

Other Drugs

L-Asparaginase is used in the treatment of leukemia and interferes with the synthesis of various proteins involved in hemostasis and thrombosis. Both thrombotic and hemorrhagic complications occur. CVST after treatment with L-asparaginase has been reported in multiple case reports. It was applied to 11 of 160 (7%) children who developed CVST in the Canadian pediatric study (22). In a large study of 288 children with acute lymphatic leukemia, CVST occurred in 6%, mostly related to the start of induction therapy (35). However, CVST does also occur in leukemic patients independently of induction therapy. Tamoxifen increases the risk of thrombosis and has been associated with CVST in case reports.

Mechanical Causes

All large case series report a number of patients who develop CVST after closed head injury, direct injuries to the sinuses, neurosurgical interventions, or lumbar puncture, varying from 3% to 6% of the CVST cases (Table 27-2). In the Canadian pediatric study, head injury was not reported as a separate category. Recently, it has become clear that lumbar puncture may occasionally cause sinus thrombosis. Wilder-Smith et al. (10) described five patients who developed CVST after a lumbar puncture. Three patients had the factor V–Leiden mutation. In a retrospective series of 66 cases of CVST, they found that in 8%, a lumbar puncture had been performed recently. De Bruijn et al. (36) described six patients with CVST after a lumbar puncture, among a series of 89 cases (7%). The most likely explanation is that the low cerebrospinal fluid pressure after a lumbar puncture causes a slight downward shift of the brain and traction on the cortical veins and sinuses. Deformation of the venous walls may induce thrombosis in susceptible individuals. The diagnosis is not easy, as the headache of sinus thrombosis may be confused with the frequent postural headache after a lumbar puncture (8).

Infections

Infectious disease has long been recognized as a cause of sinus thrombosis. CVST related to regional infections in the head and neck areas was more frequent in the preantibiotic era. Especially otitis and mastoiditis might be complicated by sigmoid and lateral sinus thrombosis. The ensuing intracranial hypertension and papilledema even prompted the classic concept of "otitic hydrocephalus," which is also a classic misnomer, because the ventricles are usually normal in CVST. The incidence of CVST as a complication of regional infections has declined significantly. In more recent case series from France and The Netherlands, the percentage of regional infections was only 4% and 0%, respectively, but the Dutch cases were only adults (Table 27-2). The percentage of regional infections is still high in children (18%; Table 27-2). Meningitis without a regional source of infection is a rare cause of sinus thrombosis. Systemic infectious disease without meningitis has also been observed in patients with sinus thrombosis. This cause of CVST is rare in adults but is frequently observed in children under 3 months old. In the Canadian Pediatric Stroke Registry, "bacterial sepsis" was reported in 11 of 69 (16%) neonates with CVST (22).

Noninfectious Inflammatory Disease

A number of generalized inflammatory or autoimmune disorders are occasionally complicated by CVST, mostly published in case reports. Systemic lupus erythematosus is rarely complicated by CVST. The development of sinus thrombosis in systemic lupus erythematosus can sometimes be attributed to nephrotic syndrome, and often to the presence of antiphospholipid antibodies, but it may also occur without these additional risk factors (37).

Granulomatous inflammatory disease such as Wegener's granulomatosus and sarcoidosis has rarely been complicated by sinus thrombosis. Also, inflammatory bowel disease (ulcerative colitis and Crohn's disease) is known to increase the risk of thrombosis, and a number of cases with cerebral sinus thrombosis have been published (38). Changes in the levels of pro- and anti-thrombotic proteins probably explain the thrombosis in inflammatory bowel disease.

Behçet's Disease

A special position is taken by Behçet's disease, owing to its close association with cerebral sinus thrombosis. The hallmarks of Behçet's disease are uveitis, oral and genital ulcerations, and often arthritis, chronic aseptic meningitis, and venous thrombosis. The disease is more frequent in Turkish, Arab, and Asian populations. In one series of 40 adult patients with CVST from Saudi Arabia, 10 had Behçet's disease (39). In the French series of 135 patients with CVST, 18 had Behçet's disease (13%) (7). This high percentage may be related to the presence of a large North African immigrant community in Paris. Conversely, in many patients with Behçet's disease and neurologic symptoms, especially intracranial hypertension, the cause is sinus thrombosis. From 41 patients with Behçet's disease from Kuwait, 11 had intracranial hypertension, of whom 10 had proven sinus thrombosis (40). In a large study of 250 cases of Behçet's disease, 10% had sinus thrombosis, mostly presenting as intracranial hypertension (41).

Other Systemic Diseases

Cancer

An association between leg-vein thrombosis and cancer has been observed in many studies. A recent meta-analytic review concluded that the risk of a new diagnosis of cancer is increased about four- to sevenfold in patients within 6 to 12 months of the diagnosis of idiopathic venous thrombosis (42). Also, patients with cancer have an increased risk to develop thrombosis. Therefore, it is not surprising that cancer is occasionally reported in patients with CVST. Bousser and Ross Russell (7) report only 4 cases (3%, excluding 2 cases of leptomeningeal metastasis) among 135 patients with CVST. The frequency of cancer (excluding hematologic malignancies) in children with CVST is probably higher. DeVeber and Andrew (22) report cancer in 8% of 160 children with CVST, but some of these cases may have been caused by antineoplastic drugs.

Hematologic Disorders

Pathologic changes in the cellular composition of the blood can increase the risk of thrombosis. Increased numbers of thrombocytes, erythrocytes, or leukocytes are all occasionally associated with sinus thrombosis. Thus, CVST is reported in cases of polycythemia (both primary and secondary), thrombocythemia, and leukemia (7). The study by Wermes et al. (35) in childhood leukemia has already been mentioned. They found CVST in 6% of 288 children with acute lymphatic leukemia, usually related to the start of induction therapy. The Canadian Pediatric Registry recorded a hematologic disorder in 12% of children with CVST (22).

Anemia can also cause thrombosis. At least 10 case reports have been published of CVST in relation to paroxysmal nocturnal hemoglobinuria. From a cohort of 80 patients with paroxysmal nocturnal hemoglobinuria, 31 developed some kind of venous thrombosis, of whom 4 had CVST (43).

Dehydration and Congestive Heart Failure

Both dehydration and congestive heart failure, when severe, may impair blood flow in the cerebral venous system sufficiently to cause thrombosis in some cases. Dehydration as a cause of CVST was probably more frequent before the widespread use of intravenous fluid replacement. Today, these causes of CVST are reported mainly in severely ill patients at both extremes of life: the very young and the very old. The high incidence in the autopsy series by Towbin (4) has already been mentioned. He found 10% CVST in consecutive autopsies in patients older than 60 years and attributed many cases to congestive heart failure. This high incidence was not confirmed in a recent study, with only 2 cases in 102 autopsies (H.P. Bienfait; in press, *J Neurol*). In children, dehydration was reported in 25%, and even more frequently in neonates (30%) with CVST (22). The same study reported "heart disease" in 5% of the children with CVST.

Unknown Causes

Despite the increased knowledge of risk factors and causes of CVST, in a number of patients the cause of CVST remains elusive, even after extensive diagnostic investigations. The number of cases without identified cause or risk factor in different studies varies according to the extent of workup and also depends heavily on the definition of cause or risk factor. In adult cases, the fraction of "unknown" varies between 17% and 27%. In children, no risk factor was identified in only in 2% of all cases (see deVeber and Andrew, Canadian registry, Table 27-2).

REFERENCES

1. Kalbag RM, Woolf AL. *Cerebral venous thrombosis.* London: Oxford University Press, 1967.
2. de Bruijn SF. *Cerebral venous sinus thrombosis: clinical and epidemiological studies* [Dissertation]. Amsterdam: Thesis Publishers, 1998.
3. de Bruijn SF, Stam J. Randomized, placebo-controlled trial of anticoagulant treatment with low-molecular-weight heparin for cerebral sinus thrombosis. *Stroke* 1999;30:484–488.
4. Towbin A. The syndrome of latent cerebral venous thrombosis: its frequency and relation to age and congestive heart failure. *Stroke* 1973;4:419–430.
5. Bienfait HP, Stam J, Lensing AW, et al. Trombose van de cerebrale venen en sinussen bij 62 patienten [Thrombosis of the cerebral veins and sinuses in 62 patients]. *Ned Tijdschr Geneeskd* 1995;139:1286–1291.
6. Ferro JM, Correia M, Pontes C, et al. Cerebral vein and dural sinus thrombosis in Portugal: 1980–1998. *Cerebrovasc Dis* 2001;11:177–182.
7. Bousser M-G, Ross Russell RW. *Cerebral venous thrombosis.* London: Saunders, 1997.
8. Aidi S, Chaunu MP, Biousse V, et al. Changing pattern of headache pointing to cerebral venous thrombosis after lumbar puncture and intravenous high-dose corticosteroids. *Headache* 1999;39:559–564.
9. Stadler C, Vuadens P, Dewarrat A, et al. [Cerebral venous thrombosis after lumbar puncture and intravenous steroids in two patients with multiple sclerosis]. *Rev Neurol (Paris)* 2000;156:155–159.
10. Wilder-Smith E, Kothbauer-Margreiter I, Lammle B, et al. Dural puncture and activated protein C resistance: risk factors for cerebral venous sinus thrombosis. *J Neurol Neurosurg Psychiatry* 1997;63:351–356.
11. Buchanan DS, Brazinsky JH. Dural sinus and cerebral venous thrombosis. Incidence in young women receiving oral contraceptives. *Arch Neurol* 1970;22:440–444.
12. de Bruijn SF, Stam J, Koopman MM, et al. Case-control study of risk of cerebral sinus thrombosis in oral contraceptive users and in carriers of hereditary prothrombotic conditions. The Cerebral Venous Sinus Thrombosis Study Group. *Br Med J* 1998;316:589–592.
13. Martinelli I, Sacchi E, Landi G, et al. High risk of cerebral-vein thrombosis in carriers of a prothrombin-gene mutation and in users of oral contraceptives. *N Engl J Med* 1998;338:1793–1797.
14. Vandenbroucke JP, Rosing J, Bloemenkamp KW, et al. Oral contraceptives and the risk of venous thrombosis. *N Engl J Med* 2001;344:1527–1235.
15. Franco RF, Reitsma PH. Genetic risk factors of venous thrombosis. *Hum Genet* 2001;109:369–384.
16. Zuber M, Toulon P, Marnet L, et al. Factor V Leiden mutation in cerebral venous thrombosis. *Stroke* 1996;27:1721–1723.
17. Deschiens MA, Conard J, Horellou MH, et al. Coagulation studies, factor V Leiden, and anticardiolipin antibodies in 40 cases of cerebral venous thrombosis. *Stroke* 1996;27:1724–1730.
18. Wintzen AR, Broekmans AW, Bertina RM, et al. Cerebral haemorrhagic infarction in young patients with hereditary protein C deficiency: evidence for "spontaneous" cerebral venous thrombosis. *Br Med J (Clin Res Ed)* 1985;290:350–352.
19. Koelman JH, Bakker CM, Plandsoen WC, et al. Hereditary protein S deficiency presenting with cerebral sinus thrombosis in an adolescent girl. *J Neurol* 1992;239:105–106.
20. Enevoldson TP, Russell RW. Cerebral venous thrombosis: new causes for an old syndrome? *Q J Med* 1990;77:1255–1275.
21. Cros D, Comp PC, Beltran G, et al. Superior sagittal sinus thrombosis in a patient with protein S deficiency. *Stroke* 1990;21:633–636.
22. deVeber G, Andrew M. Cerebral sinovenous thrombosis in children. *N Engl J Med* 2001;345:417–423.
23. Ludemann P, Nabavi DG, Junker R, et al. Factor V Leiden mutation is a risk factor for cerebral venous thrombosis: a case-control study of 55 patients. *Stroke* 1998;29:2507–2510.
24. Weih M, Junge-Hulsing J, Mehraein S, et al. Hereditare Thrombophilien bei ischamischem Schlaganfall und Sinusvenenthrombosen. Diagnostik, Therapie und Meta-Analyse [Hereditary thrombophilia with ischemic stroke and sinus thrombosis. Diagnosis, therapy and meta-analysis]. *Nervenarzt* 2000;71:936–945.
25. Junker R, Nabavi DG, Wolff E, et al. Plasminogen activator inhibitor-1 4G/4G-genotype is associated with cerebral sinus thrombosis in factor V Leiden carriers. *Thromb Haemost* 1998;80:706–707.
26. Reuner KH, Ruf A, Grau A, et al. Prothrombin gene G20210→A transition is a risk factor for cerebral venous thrombosis. *Stroke* 1998;29:1765–1769.
27. den Heijer M, Rosendaal FR, Blom HJ, et al. Hyperhomocystinemia and venous thrombosis: a meta-analysis. *Thromb Haemost* 1998;80:874–877.
28. den Heijer M, Koster T, Blom HJ, et al. Hyperhomocystinemia as a risk factor for deep-vein thrombosis. *N Engl J Med* 1996;334:759–762.
29. Hillier CE, Collins PW, Bowen DJ, et al. Inherited prothrombotic risk factors and cerebral venous thrombosis. *Q J Med* 1998;91:677–680.
30. Carhuapoma JR, Mitsias P, Levine SR. Cerebral venous thrombosis and anticardiolipin antibodies. *Stroke* 1997;28:2363–2369.
31. Sussman J, Leach M, Greaves M, et al. Potentially prothrombotic abnormalities of coagulation in benign

intracranial hypertension. *J Neurol Neurosurg Psychiatry* 1997;62:229–233.

32. Lanska DJ, Kryscio RJ. Risk factors for peripartum and postpartum stroke and intracranial venous thrombosis. *Stroke* 2000;31:1274–1282.

33. Cantu C, Barinagarrementeria F. Cerebral venous thrombosis associated with pregnancy and puerperium. Review of 67 cases. *Stroke* 1993;24:1880–1884.

34. de Bruijn SF, Stam J, Vandenbroucke JP. Increased risk of cerebral venous sinus thrombosis with third-generation oral contraceptives. Cerebral Venous Sinus Thrombosis Study Group. *Lancet* 1998;351:1404.

35. Wermes C, Fleischhack G, Junker R, et al. Cerebral venous sinus thrombosis in children with acute lymphoblastic leukemia carrying the MTHFR TT677 genotype and further prothrombotic risk factors. *Klin Padiatr* 1999;211:211–214.

36. de Bruijn SF, Stam J, Kappelle LJ. *Headache after dural puncture caused by cerebral venous sinus thrombosis: a report of six cases*. In: *Cerebral venous sinus thrombosis: clinical and epidemiological studies*. Amsterdam: Thesis Publishers, 1998:35–42.

37. Vidailhet M, Piette JC, Wechsler B, et al. Cerebral venous thrombosis in systemic lupus erythematosus. *Stroke* 1990;21:1226–1231.

38. Musio F, Older SA, Jenkins T, et al. Cerebral venous thrombosis as a manifestation of acute ulcerative colitis. *Am J Med Sci* 1993;305:28–35.

39. Daif A, Awada A, al Rajeh S, et al. Cerebral venous thrombosis in adults. A study of 40 cases from Saudi Arabia. *Stroke* 1995;26:1193–1195.

40. Farah S, Al Shubaili A, Montaser A, et al. Behçet's syndrome: a report of 41 patients with emphasis on neurological manifestations. *J Neurol Neurosurg.Psychiatry* 1998;64:382–384.

41. Wechsler B, Vidailhet M, Piette JC, et al. Cerebral venous thrombosis in Behçet's disease: clinical study and long-term follow-up of 25 cases. *Neurology* 1992; 42:614–618.

42. Rickles FR, Levine MN. Epidemiology of thrombosis in cancer. *Acta Haematol* 2001;106:6–12.

43. Hillmen P, Lewis SM, Bessler M, et al. Natural history of paroxysmal nocturnal hemoglobinuria. *N Engl J Med* 1995;333:1253–1258.

Ischemic Stroke: Advances in Neurology, Vol. 92. Edited by
H.J.M. Barnett, Julien Bogousslavsky, and Heather Meldrum.
Lippincott Williams & Wilkins, Philadelphia © 2003.

28

The Treatment of Cerebral Venous Sinus Thrombosis

Jan Stam

Department of Neurology, University of Amsterdam; Department of Neurology, Academic Medical Centre, Amsterdam, The Netherlands

PATHOPHYSIOLOGIC CONSIDERATIONS

Two often simultaneously present processes explain the symptoms in patients with cerebral venous sinus thrombosis (CVST) and form the background of the treatment options. First, thrombosis of one or more cerebral veins causes cerebral edema, nonhemorrhagic venous infarcts, or hemorrhagic infarcts. Venous infarcts cause neurologic deficits depending on their location and often partial or generalized epileptic seizures. Small cortical venous infarcts may be asymptomatic and can be seen on computed tomography (CT) or magnetic resonance imaging (MRI) scans of patients with CVST. Centrally located edema or infarcts, especially bilateral thalamic lesions, are caused by thrombosis of the deep cerebral sinuses and veins (straight sinus, internal cerebral vein) (Fig. 28-1). These lesions may cause severe behavioral symptoms as the only clinical manifestation of CVST. Studies with diffusion MRI have shown that vasogenic and cytotoxic edema coexist in CVST. Vasogenic edema seems to be more prominent and to develop earlier than in arterial ischemia (1,2).

Second, thrombosis of the sinuses impairs absorption of cerebrospinal fluid (CSF) and may cause intracranial hypertension. If there is no additional thrombosis of the cerebral veins, intracranial hypertension may be the only manifestation of CVST. Patients typically present with headache and sometimes diplopia, caused by abducens nerve paresis. Occasionally, they have visual symptoms due to optic

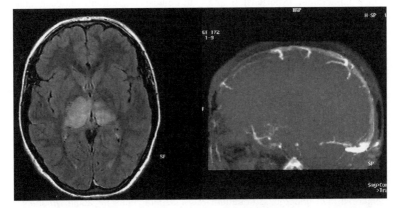

FIG. 28-1. A 19-year-old woman using a third-generation contraceptive experienced headache for 1 week, vomiting, then apathy and left-sided paresis, followed by rapid loss of consciousness and fixed pupils. **Left:** Magnetic resonance image shows bilateral thalamic edema or infarction. **Right:** Magnetic resonance angiography shows patent superior sagittal sinus but absent flow in deep venous sinuses.

nerve papilledema, which may herald severe visual loss or even blindness.

ACUTE TREATMENT: GENERAL MEASURES

Treatment in the acute phase should be directed at arresting the thrombotic process and preventing further deterioration. Anticoagulant treatment and thrombolysis will be discussed below. Even though the diagnosis of CVST is usually made easily by MRI and MR angiography, the average delay between onset of symptoms and diagnosis still is about 10 days in recent studies (3,4). Therefore, even if effective antithrombotic therapy is installed immediately, a number of patients will already present with local cerebral edema, venous infarcts, hemorrhages, and intracranial hypertension. Especially the combination of acutely elevated CSF pressure with one or more large venous infarcts can be dangerous, and these patients may die within hours from herniation (Fig. 28-2). In addition, both focal and generalized seizures occur frequently (in about 40%). The combination of impaired consciousness and intracerebral hemorrhages in patients with CVST is statistically associated with a poor outcome (5), but remarkable recovery may occur.

Therapeutic measures in the acute phase are aimed at stabilizing the patient, preventing new infarcts, and preventing or reversing herniation. The latter may require intravenous mannitol or even surgical removal of the hemorrhagic infarct (6). It is not known whether administration of corticosteroids in the acute phase improves outcome. As early vasogenic edema in acute CVST may be important (1), treatment with corticosteroids (such as 10 mg i.v. dexamethasone) may help to reduce intracranial hypertension and brain shift in severe cases. Prophylactic antiepileptic treatment may be considered. Possible causes of CVST, such as infections, should be sought actively in the acute phase and treated when possible.

ANTICOAGULANT TREATMENT: HEPARIN

Much controversy about the treatment of CVST has concerned the application of heparin. Anticoagulant treatment for CVST may arrest the thrombotic process and prevent extension of thrombus from the sinuses to the cortical veins. Also, anticoagulants may prevent pulmonary embolism that may complicate sinus thrombosis (7). On the other hand, it may be argued that in patients with CVST limited to the sinuses with only intracranial hypertension, the prognosis is good, and taking the inevitable risk of heparin treatment [about 2% major hemorrhages (8)] may not be justified.

Those reluctant to use anticoagulant treatment emphasized the risk of bleeding induced by heparin, especially in the brain in patients with CVST. About 50% of CT scans of patients with CVST may show evidence of (venous) infarction, about half of which are hemorrhagic, and bleeding into those areas may be promoted by anticoagulants. Nevertheless, reports of intracranial hemorrhage in patients with CVST who are treated with heparin are rare. Neurologic deterioration due to intracerebral hemorrhage after anticoagulant treatment for sinus thrombosis has been described in two patients (9). These cases have been criticized: One patient received urokinase in addition to heparin, and the other developed CVST while on prophylactic subcutaneous heparin (10). In a study from Portugal, new intracranial hemorrhages developed in 4 of the 112 (3.6%) patients with sinus thrombosis treated with anticoagulants and in 2 of 30 (6.7%) patients who did not receive anticoagulants

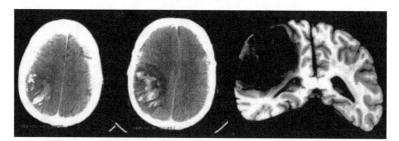

FIG. 28-2. A 36-year-old man undergoing treatment with L-asparaginase for acute lymphatic leukemia. **Left:** Right-sided parietal hemorrhagic infarct was caused by sinus thrombosis (confirmed by angiography; not shown). He underwent immediate treatment with heparin. **Middle:** Enlargement of hemorrhagic infarct is seen after treatment with heparin. **Right:** Rapid deterioration and death by herniation due to large right parietal hematoma occurred.

(4). Einhäupl et al. (11) report 3 new intracranial hemorrhages in an uncontrolled series of 56 patients (5.4%) treated with dose-adjusted intravenous heparin.

A number of studies suggest that the neurologic outcome after cerebral sinus thrombosis could improve with anticoagulant treatment, without an increase in hemorrhagic complications, but these are uncontrolled case series (4,12–14). Because the presentation and the prognosis of CVST are so variable, case reports, case series, and personal experience will not help to decide the best policy. Only randomized, controlled trials can solve the dilemma, but owing to the rarity of the disease, only limited evidence from trials is available.

RANDOMIZED TRIALS OF ANTICOAGULANT TREATMENT

Einhäupl et al. (11) performed the first clinical trial of heparin in CVST. They used intravenous high-dose unfractionated heparin, 25,000 to 65,000 IU/day, after a bolus of 3,000 IU. The treating physician was not blinded, but the patients and the physicians who assessed the outcomes were. After 10 patients in each treatment group, the study was stopped because the investigators concluded a statistically significant effect in favor of heparin. In the placebo group, three patients died, six survived with a minor deficit, and one recovered completely. In the heparin group, two patients had minor deficits and eight recovered completely. The statistical analysis was based upon scores on a CVST severity scale, a composite rating scale that contains scores for headache, paresis, seizures, and consciousness. By using the scores on this scale, statistical significance was demonstrated, due mainly to five patients with "slight" paresis in the control group. This paresis must have been very slight because the scale has three categories of more severe paresis (mild, moderate, and severe). If all surviving patients with a minor deficit (slight or mild paresis) are considered independent, the main result of the trial is not significant ($p = 0.21$, Fisher's exact test, two sided). The difference in mortality between the heparin and placebo groups suggests that heparin is effective, but the difference may well be due to chance.

There was a large delay before the treatment was started (means of 33 and 25 days for the heparin and placebo groups, respectively). A diagnostic delay of about 1 month for sinus thrombosis is very long, even before the advent of MRI. Patients might have been selected who deteriorated after an initial favorable course without anticoagulant treatment, although the article does not mention such selection. A protracted course might be explained by ongoing thrombosis, possibly equilibrated by natural thrombolysis, or by early rethrombosis. This is very rare in our experience and in the literature and would make the generalization of the results of this trial questionable.

Although this trial did not show convincingly that heparin is significantly better than placebo, it at least showed that heparin could be applied safely in the 10 patients who received it. No intracranial hemorrhages occurred. Moreover, there was a clear, though nonsignificant, trend of reduced mortality in the heparin-treated patients.

A second trial used subcutaneous low-molecular-weight heparin (nadroparin) in a therapeutic dose (3). Randomized trials in patients with leg-vein thrombosis or pulmonary embolism show that low-molecular-weight heparin is as effective as unfractionated heparin and causes fewer hemorrhagic complications (8). An additional advantage is that low-molecular-weight heparin can be given in fixed doses, adjusted only for body weight, without the need of laboratory monitoring.

Sixty patients (30 in each group) were included in this randomized, double-blind, multicenter trial. Treatment consisted of nadroparin, 180 anti-factor Xa U/kg/24 h, or placebo for 3 weeks, followed by warfarin for 10 weeks in the patients allocated to nadroparin. Outcomes were assessed with a well-validated scale for activities of daily living (Barthel index) and with a commonly used stroke handicap scale (modified Rankin scale). There were two assessments: one early, double-blind assessment after 3 weeks, at the end of the nadroparin (or placebo) treatment, and one after 12 weeks, the end of the open-label warfarin treatment.

Both after 3 weeks and after 12 weeks, the group on anticoagulant treatment had a slightly lower proportion of poor outcomes than the placebo group. After 12 weeks, 4 of 30 (13%) in the nadroparin group had a poor outcome, defined as death or dependence (Rankin score of 3 to 5). In the placebo group, 6 of 29 (21%) had a poor outcome. This difference is not statistically significant (Fisher's exact test, $p = 0.51$). One patient was withdrawn after randomization because of a wrong diagnosis. Inclusion of this patient in an intention-to-treat analysis did not essentially alter the results.

The delay between onset of symptoms and treatment in this trial (mean 10.5 days) was much shorter than in the first trial. The proportion of patients in coma was similar in both studies. The second trial included more patients with some degree of cerebral hemorrhage (49% versus 25%). As in Einhaupl's study, we did not observe any intracranial hemorrhagic complications, but one patient in the nadroparin group had a major gastrointestinal hemorrhage. One patient on placebo died suddenly from suspected pulmonary embolism.

In addition to the two European trials, there are reports of two randomized trials from India. The first trial included 57 women with puerperal CVST (15). The diagnosis was not confirmed by angiography or MRI/MR angiography but by CT only. Patients with signs of cerebral hemorrhage on CT were excluded. Patients were initially treated with intravenous unfractionated heparin, 5,000 IU every 6 h, which was then dose-adjusted to reach an activated partial thromboplastin time of 1.5 times the baseline value. Details of the randomization procedure, allocation concealment, and predefined outcome measures are not available. Assessment was not blinded. Twenty-nine patients received heparin, and 28 were controls. In the heparin group, all patients recovered. Two patients in the control group died, and one had a residual paresis at 6 months. This result is in agreement with the European trials, showing a nonsignificant trend of reduced mortality in patients treated with heparin (Fisher's exact test, $p = 0.24$).

Another study from India reported a randomized, blinded, placebo-controlled trial of 40 patients (20 heparin, 20 placebo). This study has been published only as an abstract (16). Details of diagnostic confirmation, randomization procedure, allocation concealment, and predefined outcome measures are not available. According to the abstract, mortality was 15% in the heparin group and 40% in the placebo group. This difference is statistically not significant (χ^2, $p = 0.16$).

META-ANALYSIS OF HEPARIN TRIALS

The validity of a meta-analysis of the few available trials has been questioned, as different kinds of heparin and different outcome scales were used (17). It may be argued, however, that conventional heparin and low-molecular-weight heparin have similar anticoagulant effects in patients, at least in leg-vein thrombosis: A Cochrane meta-analysis of 14 randomized trials of leg-vein thrombosis showed similar efficacy of low-molecular-weight and conventional heparin treatment but fewer hemorrhages after the former (8). Therefore, lumping together both European CVST trials seems justified as far as treatment is concerned. The problem of the different outcome scales can be overcome by analyzing only mortality and the dichotomy: independent survival versus death or dependence. Both trials give sufficient details to make that distinction. In addition, both European trials apply standard diagnostic confirmation (angiography or MRI/MR angiography) and meet minimal methodologic standards. Meta-analysis shows a nonsignificant relative risk of 0.46 [95% confidence interval (CI) 0.16–1.31] of death or dependency associated with anticoagulant therapy (18). The absolute reduction in the risk of death or dependency at follow-up is −13% (95% CI −30%–+3%). Similar results are obtained for the outcome death: Anticoagulant treatment was associated with a relative risk of death of 0.33 (95% CI 0.08–1.21). The absolute reduction in the risk of death was −13% (95% CI −27%–+1%). In conclusion, meta-analysis of both trials does not show a significant benefit of heparin treatment for sinus thrombosis, but there is a nonsignificant trend in favor of heparin treatment.

Inclusion of the Indian trials in a meta-analysis is even more controversial. The first trial included only puerperal cases and excluded patients with baseline intracerebral hemorrhage, and the diagnosis was made by clinical examination and CT scan (15). From the second trial, only the crudest results are available from the abstract (16). Nevertheless, both trials confirm the trend of a small benefit of heparin. If we tentatively combine the most robust (mortality) data of all four known trials of anticoagulant treatment for CVST, then the pooled relative risk for death would be 0.33 (95% CI 0.14–0.78).

In the European trials, no confirmed cases of pulmonary embolism occurred, but both studies report one probable case in each control group. The trials were not powered to demonstrate a reduction of pulmonary embolism. However, as in leg-vein thrombosis, the prevention of this potentially lethal complication may be an important benefit of anticoagulant treatment for patients with CVST.

SAFETY OF HEPARIN

As mentioned before, an important reason to withhold anticoagulant treatment in CVST was the fear of (new) intracranial hemorrhages. In both European trials, no such hemorrhages occurred in the 40 patients treated. This suggests that the risk of intracranial hemorrhage in patients with sinus thrombosis who are treated with anticoagulants is small. However, an incidence of 0/40 is associated with a 95% CI of 0% to 9%; thus, an incidence of up to 9% new intracranial hemorrhages cannot be excluded by the trial data.

In two case series treated with heparin, no new intracerebral hemorrhages occurred (13,14), but in two other studies, new intracerebral hemorrhages occurred in 3.6% to 5.4% of the anticoagulated patients, respectively (4,11).

Extracranial major hemorrhage occurred in only 1 of the 40 patients with CVST treated in the European trials (3.3%). This is within the range to be expected in any group of patients treated with heparin. Van den Belt et al. (8), in their meta-analysis, report 1.3% major hemorrhages in patients treated with low-molecular-weight heparin and 2.1% in those treated with unfractionated intravenous heparin (odds ratio 0.60, 95% CI 0.39–0.93).

THROMBOLYSIS: CASES AND CASE SERIES

Because the randomized trials and their combined analysis have shown that heparin is probably effective, but not a panacea, for sinus thrombosis, it seems justified that other, more aggressive treatments are tried in some patients in some centers. Direct thrombolysis aims to dissolve the thrombus by application of a thrombolytic substance within the sinus. The theoretical advantage of this approach is that the drug is delivered where needed, and not systemically, and "downstream" from any cerebral infarcts that may be or become hemorrhagic. One of the problems is how to get the drugs into the thrombosed sinus, and, of course, there is the ever-present danger of hemorrhagic complications. To get the drug where it should work, a catheter has to be pushed into the thrombus and gradually worked to a more distal position while the thrombus is dissolved (Fig. 28-3). Some of the published procedures are long, cumbersome, and

expensive: Patients remain with catheters in their sinuses on intensive care units for days, with daily radiologic assessments and frequent applications of the thrombolytic agent.

The published experience so far consists only of case reports and small case series. The interpretation is difficult because of the variability of drugs applied, of routes of application and dosage, and of patient selection. Moreover, from some studies, especially from radiology departments, it is almost impossible to infer the clinical condition of the patient before thrombolysis or the clinical outcome after the procedure.

Canhão et al. (19) performed a very useful systematic review of all published cases up to July 2001. They identified 72 publications about a total of 169 patients, all single case reports or uncontrolled case series. Most patients were treated with urokinase, usually infused directly into the thrombosed sinus. One hundred forty-six patients were treated with local thrombolysis. One-third of the patients had some hemorrhage on their pretreatment (CT or MR) scans, and 32% were comatose. New symptomatic intracranial hemorrhages were reported in 5% of the cases. Mortality at the end of follow-up was 9%, and 4% of the patients were dependent (Rankin scores of 3 to 5). As these studies are all uncontrolled, it is hard to make any conclusions on the efficacy of local thrombolysis for CVST. However, the amount of patients in coma (32%) suggests that the clinical spectrum in these 72 studies included many severe cases. Yet, the mortality is comparable with that of the European trial with low-molecular-weight heparin: 9% in the thrombolysis cases and 7% in the heparin group of the trial. This suggests that local thromboly-

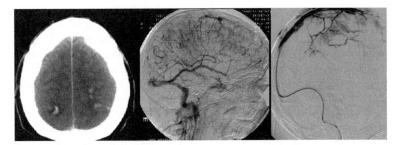

FIG. 28-3. Thrombosuction in a 29-year-old man with headache and clinical deterioration after seizures due to sinus thrombosis. **Left:** Computed tomography scan shows bilateral cortical hemorrhagic infarcts. **Middle:** Digital subtraction angiography demonstrates extensive thrombosis of the superior sagittal sinus. The deep system (straight sinus) is patent. **Right:** Thrombosuction in progress. The catheter is visible in the sigmoid, transverse, and superior sagittal sinuses, beginning recanalization of the latter. Mechanical thrombosuction was performed with a hydrolyzer catheter followed by local thrombolysis with urokinase. Duration was 4 h. (Courtesy of Dr. C.B.L.M. Majoie.)

sis may be an effective treatment for sinus thrombosis. However, the apparently good results may also be explained by publication bias. A randomized trial to compare heparin and local thrombolysis is justified and needed.

Until better evidence becomes available, local thrombolysis may be applied in centers with sufficient experience in interventional radiology and should probably be restricted to patients with a poor prognosis.

POSTACUTE TREATMENT: ORAL ANTICOAGULANTS

There are no studies available on how long patients should continue with (oral) anticoagulant treatment after CVST. Estimates of the rate of recurrent CVST after a first episode vary widely. The risk of recurrence was almost 12% in one study, with most recurrences in the first year, and 14% of the patients suffered extracranial thrombotic events (20). In another study, no recurrences were observed in a prospective cohort of 91 patients, but 5% suffered extracranial thrombotic events, during an average follow-up of 1 year (21). A randomized, double-blind trial of leg-vein thrombosis showed that recurrent thromboembolism in patients who stopped anticoagulant treatment after 3 months was significantly higher than in those who continued with anticoagulants (22). The optimal duration of anticoagulant treatment is unknown, and an increased rate of bleeding is inevitable with longer anticoagulant treatment. In our trial, we treated patients for at least 3 months, corresponding with the policy for leg-vein thrombosis at that time (3). We now prefer treatment with vitamin K antagonists for 6 to 12 months after a first episode of CVST in patients without known risk factors and without increased hemorrhagic risk. The target international normalized ratio range is 2 to 3.5 (intermediate intensity).

In patients with an increased risk by inherited thrombophilia (antithrombin C or S, factor V–Leiden, or prothrombin 20210 mutations, hyperhomocystinemia) or acquired prothrombotic conditions, we follow the recommendations of Middeldorp et al. (23): After vitamin K antagonists for 1 year after the first episode, those patients need anticoagulant protection in high-risk situations (surgery, trauma, immobilization, pregnancy, postpartum). Prophylaxis during pregnancy is most conveniently achieved by subcutaneous low-molecular-weight heparin. In addition, we discourage oral contraception containing estrogens for those patients, because they are associated with an increased risk of CVST (24). These women need consultation on alternative contraception. Intrauterine devices with local hormone release seem a safe and effective solution for a number of women.

SUBACUTE OR CHRONIC INTRACRANIAL HYPERTENSION

In about 20% of patients with CVST, the only symptoms are those of raised intracranial pressure, caused by a diminished absorption of CSF from the thrombosed sinuses. The main symptom is daily headache, sometimes with diplopia caused by abducens nerve palsy. Ophthalmologic examination reveals optic nerve papilledema, which may cause transient visual obscuration. A CT scan is sufficient to rule out tumors or other space-occupying processes, but MRI and MR angiography are the preferred imaging techniques to diagnose sinus thrombosis. In the absence of a space-occupying process, a lumbar puncture to measure the pressure can be performed safely. This diagnostic puncture is also the start of treatment, with the objectives to lower the intracranial pressure, to relieve headache, and to prevent blindness. If the symptoms are limited to those of chronic intracranial hypertension without evidence of cortical vein thrombosis, we avoid anticoagulants because repeated lumbar punctures or surgery may be needed to lower the pressure.

After the diagnostic lumbar puncture, acetazolamide, 500 mg twice daily, should be started. Some patients cannot tolerate acetazolamide, mainly because of paresthesias; in those cases, diuretics can be tried (furosemide, 2 mg/kg, three times daily). In patients who do not respond and who have severe papilledema, repeated lumbar punctures should be done to keep the pressure low. Alternatively, an external lumbar drain may be applied for a couple of days. If, in spite of these measures, the vision is deteriorating or after acute visual loss, high-dose intravenous methylprednisolone (1,000 mg daily for 5 days) should be tried. It has been used successfully in cases of severe papilledema caused by idiopathic intracranial hypertension (25).

These measures are often sufficient to control the intracranial pressure during the time period of diminished absorption of CSF. However, in some patients, CSF pressure remains elevated, although the thrombosed sinuses apparently have recanalized. These patients continue to have headaches and papilledema and may suffer progressive visual loss from peripheral constriction of the visual fields. In those cases, a lumboperitoneal shunt may be needed to drain the

CSF. Alternatively, fenestration of the optic nerve sheet should be considered in patients with papilledema and progressive visual loss (26). Both procedures have complications and adverse effects, and it has not yet been established which procedure gives the best long-term results.

SUMMARY: PROPOSED TREATMENT POLICY

Clearly, more research is needed to answer the many remaining questions about the best treatment of CVST. In the meantime, we have to make treatment decisions based upon the best available evidence. Our current policy depends on the clinical presentation.

Patients with Chronic Intracranial Hypertension by Cerebral Venous Sinus Thrombosis

These patients have no other neurologic symptoms except those caused by increased intracranial pressure. They usually have sinus thrombosis without cortical vein thrombosis. If these symptoms last longer than 2 to 3 weeks, the risk of new venous infarcts is virtually absent, in our experience. The main risk is visual deterioration or even blindness if there is severe papilledema. The priority is lowering the intracranial pressure. Therefore, we do not anticoagulate those patients, but first do a lumbar puncture, repeated if needed. In addition, we try acetazolamide. If this is not successful, a surgical procedure to drain the CSF is needed (lumboperitoneal shunt). If severe papilledema threatens the vision, optic nerve sheet fenestration can be offered. For patients with an increased risk of recurrent thrombosis, we prescribe prophylactic vitamin K antagonists after the intracranial pressure has been controlled.

Patients With Acute or Subacute Cerebral Venous Sinus Thrombosis, With or Without Venous Infarcts or Hemorrhages

We prefer low-molecular-weight heparin in high ("therapeutic") doses, such as nadroparin, approximately 180 anti-factor Xa U/kg/24 h, to be followed by oral anticoagulant treatment (vitamin K antagonists) for 6 to 12 months. Many experts prefer intravenous unfractionated heparin, but the therapeutic response, as assessed by activated partial thromboplastin time measurements, is unpredictable. The theoretical advantage of a more rapid anticoagulant effect is offset by the problem of finding the right dose of heparin.

Patients with a Poor Prognosis (Coma and Severe or Expanding Hemorrhages)

These patients are severely endangered and may deteriorate from cerebral herniation. Especially multiple hematomas or large temporoparietal hemorrhagic infarcts may cause cerebral herniation within hours. In these patients, who usually have extensive sinus thrombosis and cortical vein thrombosis, we try mechanical thrombosuction and thrombolysis. Intravenous dexamethasone may help to reduce vasogenic edema. Occasionally, the only way to prevent fatal herniation is administration of mannitol, followed by surgical removal of the hemorrhagic infarct.

REFERENCES

1. Chu K, Kang DW, Yoon BW, et al. Diffusion-weighted magnetic resonance in cerebral venous thrombosis. *Arch Neurol* 2001;58:1569–1576.
2. Yoshikawa T, Abe O, Tsuchiya K, et al. Diffusion-weighted magnetic resonance imaging of dural sinus thrombosis. *Neuroradiology* 2002;44:481–488.
3. de Bruijn SF, Stam J, CVST Study Group. Randomized, placebo-controlled trial of anticoagulant treatment with low-molecular-weight heparin for cerebral sinus thrombosis. *Stroke* 1999;30:484–488.
4. Ferro JM, Correia M, Pontes C, et al. Cerebral vein and dural sinus thrombosis in Portugal: 1980–1998. *Cerebrovasc Dis* 2001;11:177–182.
5. de Bruijn SF, de Haan RJ, Stam J. Clinical features and prognostic factors of cerebral venous sinus thrombosis in a prospective series of 59 patients. For the Cerebral Venous Sinus Thrombosis Study Group. *J Neurol Neurosurg Psychiatry* 2001;70:105–108.
6. Nagpal RD. Dural sinus and cerebral venous thrombosis. *Neurosurg Rev* 1983;6:155–160.
7. Diaz JM, Schiffman JS, Urban ES, et al. Superior sagittal sinus thrombosis and pulmonary embolism: a syndrome rediscovered. *Acta Neurol Scand* 1992;86:390–396.
8. van den Belt A, Prins MH, Lensing A, et al. *Fixed dose subcutaneous low molecular weight heparins versus adjusted dose unfractionated heparin for venous thromboembolism (Cochrane review).* Oxford: Cochrane Library, Update Software, 2002.
9. Gettelfinger DM, Kokmen E. Superior sagittal sinus thrombosis. *Arch Neurol* 1977;34:2–6.
10. Bousser M-G, Ross Russell RW. *Cerebral venous thrombosis.* London: Saunders, 1997.
11. Einhäupl KM, Villringer A, Meister W, et al. Heparin treatment in sinus venous thrombosis. *Lancet* 1991;338:597–600.
12. Bousser M-G, Chiras J, Bories J, et al. Cerebral venous thrombosis—a review of 38 cases. *Stroke* 1985;16:199–213.
13. Ameri A, Bousser M-G. Cerebral venous thrombosis. *Neurol Clin* 1992;10:87–111.
14. Brucker AB, Vollert-Rogenhofer H, Wagner M, et al. Heparin treatment in acute cerebral sinus venous thrombosis: a retrospective clinical and MR analysis of 42 cases. *Cerebrovasc Dis* 1998;8:331–337.

15. Nagaraja D, Rao B, Taly AB, et al. Randomized controlled trial of heparin in puerperal cerebral venous/sinus thrombosis. *Nimhans J* 1995;13:111–115.
16. Maiti B, Chakrabarti I. Study on cerebral venous thrombosis with special reference to efficacy of heparin. *J Neurol Sci* 1997;150[Suppl]:S147(abst).
17. Benamer HT, Bone I. Cerebral venous thrombosis: anticoagulants or thrombolytic therapy? *J Neurol Neurosurg Psychiatry* 2000;69:427–430.
18. Stam J, de Bruijn SF, deVeber G. Anticoagulation for cerebral sinus thrombosis. (Cochrane review). In: The Cochrane library, Issue 4, 2002. Oxford: Update software.
19. Canhão P, Falcao F, Ferro JM. Thrombolytics for cerebral sinus thrombosis: a systematic review. *Cerebrovasc Dis* (*in press*).
20. Preter M, Tzourio C, Ameri A, et al. Long-term prognosis in cerebral venous thrombosis. Follow-up of 77 patients. *Stroke* 1996;27:243–246.
21. Ferro JM, Lopes MG, Rosas MJ, et al. Long-term prognosis of cerebral vein and dural sinus thrombosis.

Results of the Venoport Study. *Cerebrovasc Dis* 2002; 13:272–278.
22. Kearon C, Gent M, Hirsh J, et al. A comparison of three months of anticoagulation with extended anticoagulation for a first episode of idiopathic venous thromboembolism. *N Engl J Med* 1999;340:901–907.
23. Middeldorp S, Buller R, Prins MH, et al. Approach to the thrombophilic patient. In: Colman RWHJ, ed. *Hemostasis and thrombosis—basic principles and clinical practice.* Philadelphia: Lippincott Williams & Wilkins, 2000.
24. de Bruijn SF, Stam J, Koopman MM, et al., Cerebral Venous Sinus Thrombosis Study Group. Case-control study of risk of cerebral sinus thrombosis in oral contraceptive users and in carriers of hereditary prothrombotic conditions. *Br Med J* 1998;316:589–592.
25. Liu GT, Glaser JS, Schatz NJ. High-dose methylprednisolone and acetazolamide for visual loss in pseudotumor cerebri. *Am J Ophthalmol* 1994;118:88–96.
26. Tse DT, Chang WJ. Surgery of the orbit and optic nerve. In: Glaser JS, ed. *Neuroophthalmology.* Philadelphia: Lippincott Williams & Wilkins, 1999:520–523.

Ischemic Stroke: Advances in Neurology, Vol. 92. Edited by
H.J.M. Barnett, Julien Bogousslavsky, and Heather Meldrum.
Lippincott Williams & Wilkins, Philadelphia © 2003.

29

Reflections on the Conduct of Multicenter Stroke Prevention Studies

H.J.M. Barnett and Heather Meldrum

John P. Robarts Research Institute, London, Ontario, Canada

During the last half of the twentieth century, new evidence of disease mechanisms, outlook, and treatment poured at full flood from hospitals, basic science departments, and pharmaceutical laboratories. Defining what these advances in knowledge mean for patients has been dependent on many things, but none more important than the perfection of the randomized clinical trial. Nowhere has this been more evident than in the validation or rejection of treatments aimed at preventing stroke.

The earliest randomized trials in stroke prevention evaluated warfarin and were published between 1961 and 1966. They had methodologic problems and were small, with a total of 185 patients, and the results were inconclusive. The first randomized trial involving platelet inhibitors for patients with cerebral vascular disease was published in 1969. It was a small and negative evaluation of dipyridamole. In 1970, the first surgical trial studied carotid endarterectomy and reported a negative benefit in stroke prevention.

Positive and negative lessons were learned from the early randomized trials. On the positive side, neurologists, surgeons, and family physicians agreed, reluctantly at first, to accept random assignment of putatively beneficial treatment for their patients with stroke-threatening symptoms. Despite the protean presentation of threatened stroke, protocols could be designed clearly defining eligible patient characteristics and identifying existing or potential comorbid conditions that would exclude entry. On the negative side, mistakes were made that were important in defining the requirements for subsequent trials. These involved problems in design, execution, analysis, and reporting. The design of the first carotid endarterectomy trial, the Joint Study, was flawed when patient entry accepted not only focal symptoms in the carotid territory but also vertebral–basilar territory symptoms and nonspecific so-called "diffuse non-hemispheric symptomology" (1). In the execution of this and other early trials, crossovers and loss to follow-up were too frequent to conform to acceptable modern standards (2). Five percent is the desirable limit, and at 20% a trial is considered flawed. In the Joint Study, the primary analysis was conducted using the condition of the patients at the time of hospital discharge, omitting deaths that occurred in hospital. Scrupulous modern trials require the inclusion of all outcomes from the moment of randomization in the primary analysis.

The beneficiary of these lessons was the next generation of trials, with positive evaluations of platelet inhibitors in noncardiac transient ischemic attack and stroke patients and of warfarin in six nonvalvular atrial fibrillation trials. A trial evaluating cerebral bypass surgery did not find benefit, whereas the endarterectomy trials did find benefit, favoring surgery for symptomatic patients. Soon, cerebral endovascular procedures will be joining the list of treatments evaluated by randomized, controlled clinical trials.

This chapter is not about the methodology, design, and analysis of randomized trials. This methodology already has a rich literature. Rather, it is a reflection by the authors about the lessons learned by conducting four large multicenter stroke prevention trials: a drug trial [Canadian Cooperative Stroke Study (3)]; two surgical trials [North American Symptomatic Carotid Endarterectomy Trial (NASCET) (4,5) and Cooperative Study of Extracranial/Intracranial (EC/IC) Arterial Anastomosis (6)]; and a combined drug and surgical trial [ASA (Acetylsalicylic Acid) and Carotid Endarterectomy Trial (ACE) (7)]. We will use our experience with these trials and refer to others to illustrate some of the usual and some of the unexpected requirements needed to bring a trial to a credible conclusion. The following description of 10 requirements to conduct a credible stroke prevention trial is not prioritized by order of importance (Table 29-1).

1. **A burning issue must be the motivation for the trial.** This issue cannot be settled by any other strategy. Large amounts of time, energy, money, and patient and investigator dedication are required to conduct a credible trial. The issue must be clinically relevant and should impact a great number of patients to persuade neurologists and other clinicians to change established practice patterns. The treatment under evaluation must have a reasonable chance of being effective, must be less hazardous than the disease it seeks to prevent, and cannot be tested by any other strategy. The test and control treatments must be justifiable on medical and ethical grounds.

2. **Equipoise must exist in the minds of all participants.** Equipoise is the knowledge that either treatment in the study may turn out to be superior. Alternatively, an investigator may have a bias for one treatment over the other but remains uncertain if the preferred treatment is useful or harmful. Either belief makes it acceptable to participate in a trial.

3. **The patients must be the centerpiece of the study.** The patients are the heart and the soul of any trial. The design and conduct must be sensitive to the patients' best interests, safety, and understanding of the trial. All patients must know that a particular doctor and research coordinator are available to them at all times during the study and that they will never be denied the best-known medical care. At the end of the

TABLE 29-1. *Ten requirements for the conduct of a credible stroke prevention trial*

- A burning issue must be the motivation for the trial.
- Equipoise must exist in the minds of all participants.
- The patients must be the centerpiece of the study.
- The protocol must be a multidisciplinary effort.
- Outcome events must be identified in advance and clearly defined.
- Impeccable data management is essential.
- Full access to the data and all analyses is necessary.
- The patients in the trial—not outside the trial—matter.
- The right team of participants must be selected.
- The principal investigator must be an expert stroke neurologist.

study, the patients must know that they will immediately be informed of the trial results and what it means to their future care.

When neither physician nor coordinator is able to establish good rapport, patients may seek medical advice elsewhere and may get unproven treatment that violates the protocol. Patients well bonded to the study physician and coordinator will advise of a move and can be transferred to a center near their new home. Forms that contain other relatives' and friends' addresses can be used to help locate lost patients.

The EC/IC Bypass Study followed patients twice through federal prison sentences and once restored contact with a news reporter whose follow-up was lost during imprisonment by an Ethiopian guerrilla group. This patient knew of the importance attached to the trial by his caring physician. When all else fails in attempts to locate missing patients, private detective agencies may be hired to locate them, taking care that rights to privacy are not violated. In our experience, patients totally unwilling to be traced were avoiding a spouse, a creditor, or the law. When patients understand their relevance to the study and its importance, disappearances can be reduced to a minimum. With determination to lose no patients set out as a goal from the beginning of NASCET, this study, conducted on five continents over 10 years, reduced loss to follow-up from the usual 15% down to 0.2%.

Diligent and committed participating investigators will accept the challenge to lose no patients. This commitment was shown in NASCET when one investigator ventured into the hostile environment of a drug- and crime-infested neighborhood three times a year to follow a patient. Another investigator drove into Mexico to find the details of the cause of death of one patient. Constant surveillance of patients by a caring team will reduce patients lost to follow-up to a minimum.

4. **The protocol must be a multidiscipline effort.** It must be designed and agreed upon by senior members of all the disciplines required to conduct the study. For stroke prevention trials, the disciplines will include neurologists, biostatisticians, and research coordinators and will also commonly include surgeons, neuroradiologists, cardiologists, epidemiologists, methodologists, internists, and pharmacologists.

In its design stage, the protocol must be shared with the potential investigative collaborators at the centers. If they are not comfortable with it, they will not join; or if they join with reluctance, their contributions will be spotty or even negligible, and worst of all, they may follow and document their patients with indifference.

The funding source, the patients, and all participants must recognize that the protocol may be modified, but only under compelling circumstances. Should new methods of managing the patients' illnesses or comorbid conditions be proven during a study, this strategy cannot be denied to the patients. An example in NASCET was an age restriction when the study was launched. Anecdotal evidence recommended against endarterectomy in the elderly, and an upper age limit of 80 years was mandated. At the end of the second year when the "stopping rules" determined that the patients with severe stenosis (greater than 70%) were benefited by endarterectomy, separate analysis determined that patients over 65 years fared equally well as, if not better than, those less than 65 years. With these new data, the investigators agreed that the age limit of 80 years should be abandoned for the remaining 6 years of patient entry. This adjustment was applied equally to both treatment arms, so bias was not introduced by this change. As Chapter 38 discloses, the elderly with symptomatic carotid disease are truly at the highest risk treated medically, but when they are without comorbid conditions, the operative risk is not increased and therefore they enjoy the greatest benefit from carotid endarterectomy. If the NASCET protocol had not allowed important changes, this knowledge would not have been acquired.

5. **Outcome events must be identified in advance and clearly defined.** Stroke and death sound like obvious descriptions of outcomes, but for each stroke, a lot more than a simple notation of the event needs to be ascertained and put into the record. Type (ischemic, hemorrhagic); cause (large artery, lacunar, cardioembolic, aortoembolic); anatomic location (within or outside the original arterial territory, side and laterality of intervention); and disability both immediate and long term are essential in the gathering of outcome data. This requires the meticulous attention of a multidiscipline team of investigators. The source documents must allow for all of these data to be recorded and appropriate confirmatory data to be verified. Outcomes of death need to be scrupulously examined because of the importance of identifying deaths due to stroke and to other vascular or nonvascular causes.

NASCET, a trial in which the participating investigators could not be blinded to an endarterectomy scar, devised a four-tier system of confirming, evaluating, and classifying stroke outcomes. The neurologist and surgeon at the participating center together filled out the outcomes form. Its completeness was then confirmed by the central office research coordinator. The decision concerning the type, cause, location, etc., of the stroke was made by the stroke research neurologist (fellow). The senior investigators of neurology, surgery, and neuroradiology at the central office were then presented with all details, except for the treatment category, and a final decision was made. The outcome event documents were then forwarded to independent adjudicators, expert in stroke, for their evaluation, again deprived only of the treatment category. Rare differences between central office investigators and adjudicators were sent to other external adjudicators, and the final decision was entered into the database. This process made use of all possible expertise in the interpretation of the nuances of stroke neurology, with no breach of confidentiality of the treatment arm. It would be difficult for this four-tier system to misidentify a stroke mimic and erroneously label it a stroke. The experts at the first two levels of judgment were not blinded, but the experts in the final two levels were totally shielded from awareness of the treatment arm. At all four levels, there was complete understanding of the design and goals of the trial.

Some trials place the outcome events under the external data management team as soon as their occurrence is known. In stroke studies, it is desirable to be more searching to ensure that accurate allocation of site, laterality, severity, cause, and type of stroke will be recorded. Seasoned stroke neurologists, aided by neuroradiologists and other experts, are better able to ensure the completeness and accuracy of the preadjudication database.

Surgical trials in stroke prevention will logically have as the most important outcome events strokes that occur on the side of sufficient disease to warrant the procedure, whether it be bypass surgery, endarterectomy, or endovascular angioplasty/stenting. Detailed evaluation of deaths due to any cause that occur in the perioperative (30-day) period will be required. Secondary analyses will require inclusion of stroke from any cause.

Drug trials do not include laterality but must include death. Some recent drug trials have ventured into a realm of uncertain consequence by entering patients with vascular disease in any area (specifically, the vessels to the lower limbs, the heart, and the brain). Claims are being made that because the combined outcomes in any of these arterial territories gave a positive result, the benefit can be claimed for them all. The fallacy here is that patients who present with stroke symptoms are at much greater risk of subsequent stroke than of an outcome in the other territories. Patients in stroke prevention studies are much more likely to be patients who have recently experienced stroke-threatening symptoms or minor stroke. The outcome of prime consequence must be stroke, and if stroke is not reduced significantly, we do not agree that claims can be made about the value of a new drug based on a combined outcome.

6. **Impeccable data management is essential.** Impeccable data management is a *sine qua non*. Its integrity cannot be subject to any degree of compromise. Mechanisms must be built into multicenter trials to avoid scientific fraud that may creep into any study where hundreds of participants in scores of centers will be involved. The outcomes of NASCET and the EC/IC Study were signed off by both neurologist and surgeon. NASCET required a brief written synopsis of the details of a stroke outcome. Additionally, the checking off normal or abnormal neurologic symptoms or signs was required during clinic visits every 4 months and after every outcome. The design of the forms allowed this to be done quickly when abnormalities were absent. A final question about any change ("Yes" or "No") served as an additional final written check. The type, cause, disability, laterality, and territory of every stroke had to be on the record. All forms were scrutinized on arrival by critical and searching staff at the central office. Irregularities in the completion of the forms led to immediate inquiries, and honest errors were corrected.

Such irregularities disclosed one deliberate attempt in the EC/IC Study to add fake outcomes to one of the treatment arms. This distortion involved 12 medically treated patients over an 18-month period. In the surgical arm, outcomes in some patients had been clumsily removed from the case report forms. As soon as this discrepancy in outcomes was detected, the principal investigator insisted that all patients in this center be reexamined by an outside expert, all details corrected, and all of the patients followed by this expert until the end of the trial. Adequate documentation with crosschecks obviated the persistence of fraudulent information in the database. The final results might otherwise have been distorted. Recent incidents of fraud have been exposed in other trials when financial gain or kudos altered the behavior of individual investigators (8,9).

Timeliness of documentation is crucial to the credibility of data. Indolence and failure to be diligent with patient follow-up occur occasionally as investigators become overcommitted. The central office staff needs to keep this in focus or data may be lost. This indifference in the EC/IC Study led one investigator, after considerable prodding from staff at the central office, to finally fill out late forms. Further persistent slowness by this investigator led a sleuthing central office coordinator to discover that to prevent annoying phone calls, forms were submitted on two patients who had previously died. This dishonest collaborator was dismissed, and the department chairperson completed the forms for the remainder of the study. Human frailties cannot be allowed to skew results of important trials. Data retrieval and review must be designed to ensure the impeccability of the information on each patient.

7. **Full access to the data and all analyses is necessary.** Full access to the data and all analyses by the investigators at the end of the study is a prerequisite to the credible conduct of any trial. The major medical journals recently decreed that they will publish no clinical trial results from which full transparency in the design, execution, data management, and analyses is not ensured (10). The market, and not necessarily scientific accuracy, has been a motivating force in some clinical studies. New regulations by the journals will help restore confidence in trials testing new drugs or trials seeking modification of old treatments or trials testing new technology. The patents of new pharmaceuticals and technologies belong to industry, and unhappily, attempts are made at times to manipulate trial design and execution with market forces taking precedence over scientific pursuit. The complete data should belong to the investigators as well as industry.

All committed investigators on the study team need to know that at the end of the collaborative trial, they are entitled to use "their data" in conjunction with the principal investigator to make important preplanned secondary and subgroup studies. Authorship of the primary and secondary publications must be decided in advance. Courtesy authorships are to be discouraged.

Secondary analyses and subgroup observations beyond the primary outcomes are regarded by some as being outside the scope of a randomized trial. We disagree. Opportunities present themselves in any stroke prevention trial to add to knowledge about the many variables that constitute a population of patients afflicted with stroke. These variables must be identified in advance and pertinent prospective data recorded in detailed source documents, including follow-up forms completed at frequent regularly scheduled clinic visits. Scrupulous databases do not ensure that statistically significant subsets will be achievable but bring this goal within reach. Chapter 39 outlines the main secondary and subgroup analyses and observations that were feasible, planned, and published from the NASCET data.

From secondary and subgroup analyses, claims will not be made that involve decisions about efficacy unless the protocol planned such analyses. Frequently, subgroup studies provide observations that will lead to future randomized trials or will be linked to other similar studies that will add to the study in question and together have sufficient power to make definitive statements. For example, an observation in the first phase of NASCET directed attention to the possibility of an optimum dose of aspirin in the perioperative period. Accordingly, a parallel, randomized trial to determine the optimum dose, the ACE Trial, was started in NASCET centers.

Combined analyses from similar trials may add to the strength and validity of subgroup analyses. Care must be taken that the data of the combined analyses are equally scrupulous and have identical or nearly identical descriptions of expected characteristics and outcomes.

Interpretation of analyses must distinguish between benefit that is statistically significant but of dubious clinical importance. An example of this is the statistically significant relative risk reduction of 53% favoring carotid endarterectomy in the Asymptomatic Carotid Atherosclerosis Study (11). Because the medical risk was low, this reduction translated into only a 1% annual absolute risk reduction. The number needed to treat to prevent one stroke at 2 years is 83 subjects. Some, including the authors, consider this a clinically unimportant result.

8. **The patients in the trial—not outside the trial—matter.** Acceptance of clinical trial results depends heavily on the ability to be certain that the patients requiring investigation as described in the protocol were the patients who were randomized. Failure to identify the entry of patients not eligible constitutes a flaw in the execution of a study. NASCET's central office coordinators scrutinized the documents for each entrant and marked all entries that breached the protocol. Examples were a brain tumor presenting with mimics of transient ischemic attacks, a moderate (asymptomatic) carotid stenosis and a computed tomography (CT) examination that was misinterpreted and missed the infiltrating glioma, another patient with a brain tumor that was a parasagittal meningioma presenting with apparent ischemic events in whom the CT was erroneously obtained after randomization, a patient mistakenly believed to have ocular ischemia but proved to have

serious glaucoma, a filling defect appearing to be a severe stenosis when the "lesion" proved to be a dental filling that by chance was superimposed over the contrast material in the internal carotid artery, two patients whose transient "numb attacks" were best explained by carpal tunnel syndrome, and two patients who, in subsequent visits, were properly assigned to the classic migraine group. In accepting 2,885 *bona fide* examples of the type of patients that were desired for NASCET, 26 patients proved not to have the disease under study. In conformance with the demands of analysis by intention to treat of all patients after randomization, these 26 were followed annually, their outcomes were known, and the analysis including them had no impact on the results. Proper identification of exclusions is important, so the reputation, especially among clinical critics, of the scrupulous nature of the trial will not be spoiled.

At the completion of the EC/IC Bypass Trial, an outcry erupted from a group that was distressed because the procedure that "should have worked" was not validated by the analyses. Phone calls to participating surgeons, by one of the disappointed, revealed that a small number of surgeons had selected some of their patients for EC/IC bypass surgery without randomization (12). This breach of intent to randomize all eligible patients involved 10 of the 71 centers. When the analyses were repeated, both omitting and including these centers, the results were the same. The claim of skewing of the results was hollow because patients in all potential treatment categories, which had been proposed as potentially benefiting from the procedure, were fully represented in the database (13). The concept held that unless a group that is unique is withheld from a trial, the results are generalizable to the type of patient defined in a trial's protocol. It is the patients who are within, not without, a trial that are of importance in any analyses.

In some European trials, discretionary selection of patients has allowed the investigators to state that it is their belief that certain patients within the protocol definitions may be given the putative treatment under study or may be withheld from the trial and not entered. This is called the "uncertainty principle," and only patients in the "gray zone," where the investigator is unsure of the best treatment, are randomized. This presumption of a belief in the need for or the denial of a need for the treatment based on "personal experience" suggests that there is firm knowledge when, in fact, it does not exist. The uncertainty principle does nothing to help prove for all patients without equivocation that the treatment is effective or ineffective, prolongs the duration of trials, and has been shown by the recruitment record of North American trials to be an unnecessary acquiescence to traditional experiential decision-making.

Entry data, including all baseline characteristics, the exact details of the entry event, and the condition of the patient at entry, are on record in the hospital charts, the participating physicians' offices, and the study documents. So, too, are the details of the outcome events. Auditing of the primary documents and their comparison with the data submitted in the trial documents are the most accurate way of validating the correctness of the trial data. From experience, we believe that visits by the principal investigator or appointed representatives are the best way to achieve these validations. It is an undertaking that is costly of time, energy, and money but leaves no doubt about the validity of the data. Audit by an outside auditor is an alternative strategy, but these outsiders lack the opportunities for personal contact, important in the pursuit of multicenter trials, nor do they have the expertise in stroke required by the protocol to verify eligibility and outcome events.

9. **The right team of participants must be selected.** Selection of committed participants can affect study recruitment and timeliness of the receipt of the data. Investigators must be committed and be experts in stroke neurology who understand the methodology and conduct of randomized stroke prevention trials. The success of the trial rests with the investigators so their interest must be high. Academic centers, as well as dedicated private practitioners can make valuable contributions. The best and worst performances from recruiting centers cannot always be predicted. Some of the most prestigious academic institutions produced disappointingly few patients in our studies and had higher than the usual numbers of dropouts. Conversely, some private clinics had enviable records. The roster of recruiting centers and investigators may change during the course of a study because of an alteration in local conditions, such as a change in referral patterns or a key investigator moving to another institution. At the time of center recruitment, participants need to examine their plans for other research projects that could siphon eligible patients from the proposed study under review or introduce a contaminating treatment or investigation to the population under study.

When the performance at a center does not meet expectations, a new center needs to be recruited to replace it. Our experience was of the need to expand the number of centers to at least double that anticipated initially to meet patient recruitment goals. The

time it took to recruit all of the patients was doubled as well. The NASCET was originally designed to have 50 centers in North America; when it finished, it had 103 centers worldwide. Instead of taking 5 years to enter all of its patients, it took 9 years to meet the sample size. Unfortunately, ours is not an uncommon experience, making it important to have alternative centers and recruitment strategies available.

10. **The principal investigator must be an expert stroke neurologist.** The leadership of a trial deserves comment in the context of designing and executing a study. The principal investigator, or "captain on the bridge," should be an authority on all aspects of the disorder under investigation. Key to a results paper that will withstand critical scrutiny are the certainty that the appropriate patients have the disorder that is under putative therapeutic modification, that the exclusions are clearly described, and that all aspects of outcomes are documented with clarity, accuracy, and completeness. These prerequisites indicate that a stroke neurologist is the appropriate leader for a stroke prevention trial. In a drug or a device trial, the principal investigator must have no conflict of interest resulting from remuneration from the manufacturers of drugs or devices and certainly must be without any financial interest in a patent on a drug or device. Surgeons must be closely involved in the evaluation of surgical procedures, but their involvement should be collaborative and advisory rather than as the principal investigator. In many respects, a surgeon's interest in a trial testing surgical efficacy is comparable with a pharmaceutical manufacturer's interest in a drug trial. Conflict of interest is best avoided by seeking surgeons' collaboration as coinvestigators rather than in the role of principal investigator. Conflicts of interest will be perceived otherwise, even if they are not real. Radiologists, interventionalists, biostatisticians, and pharmacologists are required as senior collaborators and coinvestigators in stroke trials.

The principal investigator of a multicenter trial must have time, energy, and commitment to initiate, complete, and publish the trial. Diplomacy is required in dealing with the aspirations, prejudices, and egocentric tendencies of fellow investigators. The leader of the trial must be sensitive to the fact that the patient and the patient's needs are central to the study. The principal investigator must never lose sight of the fact that "good doctoring" is vital to the pursuit of excellence in the trial and must ensure that this is being achieved in every center.

A randomized trial will not succeed without a close association with an experienced, clinically oriented biostatistician, preferably with expertise in trial methodology. A biostatistician is essential in designing any trial and ensuring reasonable estimates of sample size requirements. The appropriate sample size needs to be estimated in collaboration with clinicians fully acquainted with all the reports relating to the prognosis of the condition being studied. The number of patients to be recruited in the trial should be anticipated using the expected risk of outcomes rather than using the total number of patients at risk.

An expert neuroradiologist is essential in a stroke prevention trial. The uniformity and accuracy of the images of the brain or arteries are an important part of confirming the eligibility of patients as well as the exclusions in any stroke trial. Differences of opinion between the central office neuroradiologist and counterparts in participating centers are best resolved by personal discussion between the two. In NASCET, when there were differences of opinion, a leading expert from a nonparticipating center was consulted to make the final determination.

FINAL COMMENT

At stake in the conduct of clinical trials is the introduction or rejection of a therapy that will, at times, alter the practice of medicine. This challenge is a worthy one, and the reward is the recognition that the care of patients has been improved.

REFERENCES

1. Fields WS, Maslenikov V, Meyer JS, et al. Joint study of extracranial occlusion. V. Progress report of prognosis following surgery or nonsurgical treatment for transient cerebral ischemic attacks and cervical carotid artery lesions. *JAMA* 1970;211:1993–2003.
2. Sackett DL, Richardson WS, Rosenberg W, et al. *Evidence-based medicine: how to practice and teach EBM.* New York: Churchill Livingstone, 1997.
3. Canadian Cooperative Stroke Study Group. Randomized trial of therapy with platelet anti-aggregants for threatened stroke. 1. Design and main results of the trial. *Can Med Assoc J* 1980;122:293–296.
4. North American Symptomatic Carotid Endarterectomy Trial Collaborators. Beneficial effect of carotid endarterectomy in symptomatic patients with high-grade stenosis. *N Engl J Med* 1991;325:445–453.
5. Barnett HJM, Taylor DW, Eliasziw M, et al., for the North American Symptomatic Carotid Endarterectomy Trial Collaborators. Benefit of carotid endarterectomy in symptomatic patients with moderate and severe stenosis. *N Engl J Med* 1998;339:1415–1425.
6. EC/IC Bypass Study Group. Failure of extracranial–intracranial arterial bypass to reduce the risk of ischemic stroke. *N Engl J Med* 1985;313:1191–1200.
7. Taylor DW, Barnett HJM, Haynes RB, et al., for ASA and Carotid Endarterectomy (ACE) Trial Collaborators. Low-dose and high-dose acetylsalicylic acid for patients undergoing carotid endarterectomy: a randomized controlled trial. *Lancet* 1999;353:2179–2184.
8. Enserink M. Fraud and ethics charges hit stroke drug trial. *Science* 1996;274:2004–2005.
9. Angell M, Kassirer JP. Setting the record straight in the breast cancer trials. *N Engl J Med* 1994:330:1448–1450.
10. Davidoff F, DeAngelis CD, Drazen JM, et al. Sponsorship, authorship and accountability. *JAMA* 2001;286:1232–1234.
11. Executive Committee for the Asymptomatic Carotid Atherosclerosis Study. Endarterectomy for asymptomatic carotid artery stenosis. *JAMA* 1995;273:1421–1428.
12. Sundt TM Jr. Was the international randomized trial of extracranial–intracranial arterial bypass representative of the population at risk? *N Engl J Med* 1987;316:814–816.
13. Barnett HJM, Sackett D, Taylor DW, et al. Are the results of the Extracranial–Intracranial Bypass Trial generalizable? *N Engl J Med* 1987;316:820–824.

Ischemic Stroke: Advances in Neurology, Vol. 92. Edited by
H.J.M. Barnett, Julien Bogousslavsky, and Heather Meldrum.
Lippincott Williams & Wilkins, Philadelphia © 2003.

30

Antithrombotic Therapies for Stroke Prevention in Atrial Fibrillation

Robert G. Hart

*Department of Medicine/Neurology, University of Texas Health Science Center,
San Antonio, Texas, U.S.A.*

Atrial fibrillation (AF) is a supraventricular cardiac tachyarrhythmia characterized by uncoordinated atrial activity leading to stasis-precipitated thrombi in the left atrial appendage. About one of six ischemic strokes occurs in patients with nonvalvular AF. The usual mechanism of stroke is embolism of left atrial appendage thrombi, but perhaps one-quarter are due to coexistent noncardioembolic causes of ischemic stroke (1,2). Because the diagnosis of AF usually precedes stroke by many months to years and because antithrombotic drugs are efficacious for stroke prevention, most AF-associated strokes are potentially preventable, challenging clinicians and health care systems/organizations to implement effective preventive strategies. It is worth emphasizing that warfarin does not substantially benefit many unselected AF patients over treatment with aspirin but offers large reductions in stroke to high-risk AF patients. Optimal prevention involves selecting antithrombotic prophylaxis after stratifying stroke risk, choosing an appropriate target international normalized ratio (INR), and considering individual patient preferences.

More than a score of randomized clinical trials and many hundreds of case control studies, case series, and population-based studies have addressed stroke prevention in AF and have been reviewed (3–6). Here, recent data and new ideas are considered, focusing on secondary prevention issues of particular relevance to neurologists.

EPIDEMIOLOGY: RECENT STUDIES

A survey from a large health maintenance organization (7) confirmed population-based evidence (8)

about the prevalence of AF: AF affects about 1% of adults, about one in 25 people over age 60, and nearly 10% of those aged 80 years or older. About half of people with AF are over age 75, and nearly half are women. Adjusted for age, AF appears to be more frequent in whites than in blacks (7,9). About 2.3 million U.S. adults have AF; this number is expected to increase substantially in the next two decades owing to growing numbers of the very elderly, and the importance of AF-associated stroke will likely increase. In the U.S.A., AF is a more frequent and important risk factor for stroke for whites than for blacks or for Caribbean Hispanics (10). This probably holds for whites versus Chinese (11) and Mexican Americans (12).

RANDOMIZED CLINICAL TRIALS

Results from 19 randomized clinical trials testing antithrombotic therapies involving 10,403 participants have been published to date (3,13). By meta-analysis, adjusted-dose warfarin with achieved INRs between 2 and 3 is highly efficacious for stroke prevention (60% reduction in all stroke), aspirin is modestly efficacious (20% reduction), and warfarin is much more efficacious than aspirin (Table 30-1) (14).

The effect of antithrombotic therapy varies according to the ischemic stroke mechanism in AF patients (Fig. 30-1). Aspirin reduces noncardioembolic strokes more than cardioembolic strokes in AF patients, whereas adjusted-dose warfarin is much more efficacious than aspirin for prevention of cardioembolic strokes. Cardioembolic strokes in AF patients are particularly disabling and frequent among AF patients at high risk for stroke. Warfarin reduces cardioembolic stroke in AF patients by about 85%

TABLE 30-1. *Randomized trials of antithrombotic therapies in atrial fibrillation: metaanalysis*

	No. of trials	No. of participants	Risk reduction [% (95% CI)]	p
Adjusted-dose warfarin vs. placebo	6	2,900	62 (48, 72)	<0.001
Aspirin vs. placebo	6	3,119	22 (2, 38)	0.03
Antiplatelet vs. placebo[a]	6	3,337	24 (7, 39)	0.01
Adjusted-dose warfarin vs. aspirin	5	2,837	36 (14, 52)	0.003

Stroke includes both ischemic and hemorrhagic stroke.
CI, confidence interval.
[a]Includes 218 participants given dipyridamole alone or combined with aspirin.
From Hart RG, Benavente O, McBride R, Pearce LA. Antithrombotic therapy to prevent stroke in patients with atrial fibrillation: a meta-analysis. *Ann Intern Med* 1999;131:492–501, with permission.

during therapeutic anticoagulation, whereas the effect of aspirin on this stroke subtype is about 15% (1).

Put simply, the major effect of aspirin in AF patients is on small noncardioembolic strokes, whereas warfarin prevents the typically larger cardioembolic events.

Although adjusted-dose warfarin reduces stroke for all AF patients, anticoagulation of unselected AF patients offers only modest absolute reductions in stroke rate. This is explained by the relatively low absolute rate of stroke among unselected AF patients taking aspirin, averaging between 3 and 4%/year (15,16). This translates into 50 to 67 AF patients needed to be treated with anticoagulants instead of aspirin for 1 year to prevent one stroke. (This is anal-

ogous to the benefits of carotid endarterectomy for asymptomatic versus symptomatic carotid artery stenosis: The relative risk reduction is large for both, but the absolute benefits are radically different.) Stratification of stroke risk with subsequent anticoagulation of high-risk AF patients, aspirin for low-risk AF patients, and selective anticoagulation of moderate-risk AF patients depending on bleeding risks and individual patient preferences is a more sensible approach, in my view.

Results of three small, randomized trials of antithrombotic therapy in AF have recently been published and provide useful nuances to antithrombotic management. The Japanese secondary prevention trial randomized 115 AF patients under age 80 years

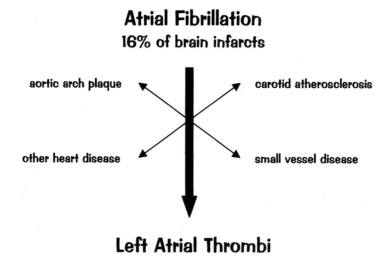

Atrial Fibrillation
16% of brain infarcts

aortic arch plaque   carotid atherosclerosis

other heart disease   small vessel disease

Left Atrial Thrombi
10% of brain infarcts

FIG. 30-1. The mechanisms of ischemic stroke in patients with atrial fibrillation. Whereas most are cardioembolic, an important minority are due to other coexistent cerebrovascular diseases in these typically hypertensive elderly patients. (From Hart RG, Halperin JL. Atrial fibrillation and thromboembolism: a decade of progress in stroke prevention. Ann Intern Med 1999;131:688–695, with permission).

(mean age 67 years) with recent ischemic stroke or transient ischemic attack (TIA) to two different target intensities of warfarin anticoagulation: 1.5 to 2.1 (achieved 1.9) versus 2.2 to 3.5 (achieved 2.3) (17). This unblinded trial was stopped at an interim analysis owing to a perceived excess of major bleeding in those assigned more intensive anticoagulation (6 versus 0; $p = 0.01$). The risk of major hemorrhage was unusually high (6.6%/year) in those given conventional-intensity anticoagulation and was associated with advancing patient age and INR. Too few strokes occurred to assess the relative effects of the two target anticoagulation intensities, although the observed rate was low in both arms during nearly 2 years of mean follow-up. This trial showed that lower-intensity anticoagulation is probably safer than the higher intensity in Japanese AF patients, but no firm conclusions can be made about overall benefit versus risk owing to the small number of strokes.

A French Trial compared anticoagulation alone (achieved INR 2.3) versus anticoagulation plus aspirin in 157 AF patients (mean age 74) with one or more additional stroke risk factors (18). The trial was stopped for logistical reasons (poor recruitment, lack of funding) after about 1-year mean follow-up. Only a handful of strokes and major hemorrhages were observed; minor hemorrhages were significantly more frequent in those receiving aspirin combined with anticoagulation. The observed rate of major bleeding (1.4%/year) was lower than that reported in the Japanese secondary prevention trial, despite comparable achieved INRs, although confidence intervals for the rates overlapped owing to the relatively small number of bleeding events.

A recent pilot trial randomized 257 AF patients to three dosages of a novel oral direct thrombin inhibitor, ximelagatran, versus adjusted-dose warfarin for 12 weeks (13). Ximelagatran was well tolerated, and this initial experience prompted large Phase III trials now underway that have enrolled over 7,500 high-risk AF patients worldwide (with results expected in mid-2003).

Other ongoing trials include the Birmingham Atrial Fibrillation Treatment in the Aged (BAFTA), which plans to randomize 1,200 AF patients aged 75 years or older to receive either warfarin (target INR 2.5) or aspirin (75 mg/day) to define better the benefit/risk in the very elderly, among whom most AF-associated strokes occur. The Japanese Atrial Fibrillation Stroke Prevention Trial proposes to randomize 1,000 AF patients without prior stroke/TIA to aspirin 162 mg/day versus placebo, justified by the paucity of Japanese participants in randomized trials to date,

by concern that Japanese patients may have a particular propensity to bleeding during antithrombotic therapies, with the hypothesis that stroke rates and factors predictive of initial stroke in Japanese AF patients may be unique.

It has been a longstanding controversy whether iatrogenic interventions to restore and maintain sinus rhythm (thereby reducing atrial appendage stasis and thrombus formation) are of overall benefit, improving quality of life and obviating the need for lifelong anticoagulation. Preliminary results of the large, randomized Atrial Fibrillation Follow-up Investigation of Rhythm Management (AFFIRM) Trial showed no benefits on mortality or quality of life by efforts to maintain sinus rhythm, but the trial design does not permit firm conclusions regarding the need for continuing anticoagulation if sinus rhythm is restored.

As almost all emboli in nonvalvular AF originate in the atrial appendage (rather than in the body of the left atrium proper), obliteration of the left atrial appendage could reduce embolism risk, potentially obviating the need for anticoagulation in high-risk AF patients. Appendage obliteration can be achieved at open thoracotomy (as often done at the time of coronary bypass surgery), thoracoscopically, or via a percutaneous occlusion device. The efficacy and cardiac/hemodynamic consequences of appendage obliteration for stroke prevention await long-term follow-up studies.

MAJOR HEMORRHAGE DURING ANTICOAGULATION THERAPY

Elderly patients with AF tolerate carefully administered anticoagulation with oral vitamin K inhibitors (i.e., warfarin and its congeners) surprisingly well compared with patients with intrinsic cerebrovascular disease (19). According to pooled data from the last seven published clinical trials with target INRs of 2 to 3, 1,567 warfarin-treated participants (mean age 72 years) with a mean achieved INR of 2.5 had an observed rate of intracerebral hemorrhage of 0.5%/year during an average follow-up of 1.3 years/patient (3,18). Upon pooling of two recently published nontrial cohorts, 574 warfarin-treated patients (mean age 72 years) with a mean achieved INR of 2.5 had an observed rate of intracerebral hemorrhage of 0.6%/year during an average follow-up of 1.5 years/patient (2,20). Lower rates of intracerebral hemorrhage reported from the first-generation clinical trials (0.3%/year) probably reflect the lower average age patient age (67 years) and lower achieved INRs (21). Rates of non–central nervous system major hemorrhage are more difficult to analyze owing to the varying nonstandard criteria, but rates from clinical practice appear to be similar to those reported in clinical trials: about 2%/year and mostly gastrointestinal hemorrhage (22). In recent clinical series of AF patients with target INRs of 2 to 3, about two-thirds of INRs during long-term follow-up after initial dose titration were within the target range (2,20), representing good-quality anticoagulation. In short, recent clinical trials and case series are reassuring that warfarin can be administered with tolerable bleeding complications that do not offset benefits for most AF patients (assuaging concerns initially raised by the Stroke Prevention in Atrial Fibrillation II Trial, which tested higher INRs in very elderly AF patients) (23). On the other hand, rates of serious bleeding and particularly intracerebral hemorrhage during anticoagulation are sensitive to patient age and to the intensity of anticoagulation. More data are needed to compare benefits and risks of anticoagulation in AF patients over age 75 (about half of all AF patients), and the results of BAFTA will be important. Targeting an INR of 2.0 (target range 1.6 to 2.5) may be sensible for primary prevention in very elderly AF patients (3,6,17).

Recent studies have linked apolipoprotein E genotype (as a marker of amyloid angiopathy) and leukoaraiosis detected by computed tomography to the risk of intracerebral bleeding during anticoagulation therapy (19,24). Diffusion tensor magnetic resonance imaging techniques can detect the presence of microhemorrhages in elderly people without prior clinical brain hemorrhages, postulated to be a risk factor for subsequent clinical bleeding. The positive and negative predictive values of these markers have not been adequately established overall or for AF patients (who may differ from those with primary cerebrovascular causes of ischemia), and at present, these markers are not ready for routine clinical use.

STRATIFYING RISK FOR PRIMARY PREVENTION OF STROKE IN ATRIAL FIBRILLATION PATIENTS

The stroke rate varies more than 20-fold among AF patients, from 0.5%/year for young (under age 65) AF patients without organic heart disease or hypertension (i.e., "lone" AF) to 12%/year for AF patients with prior stroke or TIA. Clinical features independently associated with high stroke rates in AF patients have been defined and integrated into several risk stratification schemes (25–28). Advancing age, hypertension, left ventricular dysfunction, and prior stroke/TIA are consistent independent stroke risk factors in AF patients, with diabetes, coronary artery disease, and female gender less consistently emerging from multivariate models. Although it has been demonstrated that transesophageal echocardiographic measures of stasis (i.e., appendage ejection fraction and flow velocity, dense spontaneous echo contrast) are predictors of embolic risk in AF patients, whether results of transesophageal echocardiography add to clinical risk stratification schemes has yet to be defined (29).

AF patients with relatively low rates of stroke who do not benefit substantially from anticoagulation can be identified. In a large prospective study, the Stroke Prevention in Atrial Fibrillation Investigators identified AF patients with a low risk for stroke during treatment with aspirin using specific clinical criteria (Table 30-2) (25). During a mean 2-year follow-up of

TABLE 30-2. *SPAF Study risk stratification scheme*

Criteria	% of cohort	Observed stroke (%/yr) rate[a]
Secondary prevention (prior stroke/TIA)	9	11
Primary prevention		
High risk	15	7
Women >75 yr		
Systolic BP >160 mm Hg		
LV dysfunction		
Moderate risk	35	3
Hypertension but BP <160 mm Hg		
Low risk	41	1
No high-risk features		
No hypertension		

SPAF, Stroke Prevention in Atrial Fibrillation; TIA, transient ischemic attack; BP, blood pressure; LV, left ventricular (LV dysfunction includes clinical heart failure and abnormal echocardiography).
[a]During aspirin therapy in 2,012 patients with atrial fibrillation from the SPAF Study cohort.
From Pearce LA, Hart RG, Halperin JL. Assessment of three schemes for stratifying stroke risk in patients with nonvalvular atrial fibrillation. *Am J Med* 2000;109:45–51, with permission.

892 AF patients, the observed stroke rates were 2.0%/year for stroke of any severity and 0.8%/year for disabling stroke (Rankin level 2 or worse). These criteria for identifying low-risk AF patients have been validated in a population-based AF cohort (16) and a hospital-based AF cohort (26). Additional studies of the reliability and durability of stroke risk stratification schemes for AF patients, validating their application in clinical practice, are needed. Reliable risk stratification to identify AF patients who benefit most and least from lifelong anticoagulation is an important precursor to selection of antithrombotic prophylaxis.

IMMEDIATE ANTITHROMBOTIC THERAPY FOLLOWING STROKE IN ATRIAL FIBRILLATION PATIENTS

Recent studies confirm that patients with AF-associated stroke are, on average, older and more often women, with larger hemispheric strokes and higher early mortality than other ischemic stroke patients (30–32). Given the typically advanced patient age (averaging in the late seventies) and large infarct size coupled with the threat of early, recurrent cardiogenic embolism, the benefit versus risk of immediate antithrombotic therapies in acute AF-associated stroke merits special consideration (33).

Early recurrent ischemic stroke appears to be only modestly more frequent in patients with AF versus non-AF patients (30,34), occurring in about 5% over 14 days in AF patients given early aspirin therapy (33). The effects of aspirin use on early recurrent ischemic stroke in AF patients were quantitatively different in the two large randomized trials testing aspirin in this setting, with their pooled results showing a nonstatistically significant reduction of about 20% (95% confidence interval -5,41) (11,33,35). The two clinical trials testing heparins [unfractionated heparin given subcutaneously in the International Stroke Trial, a low-molecular-weight heparin given intravenously in the Heparin in Acute Embolic Stroke Trial (HAEST)] reported different effects on early recurrent ischemic stroke (30,36). Methodologic vagaries that could explain the discrepant results have been discussed (33), but importantly, neither trial showed a benefit of anticoagulation on functional outcome 3 to 6 months later, nor have other randomized trials of low-molecular-weight heparins in patients with mixed cardioembolic sources (37–39).

In summary, data from randomized trials show that early recurrent ischemic stroke is less frequent than commonly estimated a decade ago, but that it is not trivial. Owing to the methodologic vagaries of these trials, it is uncertain whether heparin reduces early recurrent stroke, but it seems clear that heparin and low-molecular-weight heparins offer no overall benefit for the majority of patients with AF-associated stroke. Subgroups with particularly high risks of early recurrent embolism have been hypothesized (e.g., appendage thrombi present on transesophageal echocardiography done after stroke) but not validated. Given the available evidence, it seems reasonable to administer aspirin immediately, along with subcutaneous heparin 5,000 U twice daily if leg weakness is present. Warfarin for long-term secondary prevention can be initiated as soon as the patient is medically and neurologically stable, typically after 1 or 2 days (discontinuing aspirin when the INR is therapeutic) (33).

LONG-TERM SECONDARY PREVENTION OF STROKE IN ATRIAL FIBRILLATION PATIENTS

By all accounts, AF patients with TIA or initial ischemic stroke are at high risk for recurrent stroke, averaging 12%/year in the absence of antithrombotic therapy (14). For these AF patients, adjusted-dose warfarin dramatically reduces the rate of recurrent stroke (by nearly 70%), whereas antiplatelet agents offer only modest reductions (14). All published guidelines presently recommend adjusted-dose warfarin (target INR 2.5) for secondary prevention of stroke in patients with AF who can safely receive it (40).

Although most ischemic strokes and TIAs in AF patients are cardioembolic, a subset are due to other cerebrovascular mechanisms, for which warfarin is not more efficacious than aspirin (1,41). A recent case series prospectively classified ischemic stroke subtypes in AF patients and found no apparent reduction in recurrent stroke by warfarin versus aspirin for the 20% of AF patients with initial lacunar stroke (2). In this study, the rate of recurrent stroke was high (9%/year) in AF patients with lacunar stroke treated with either warfarin or aspirin; most recurrent strokes in this subset were also lacunar. Should AF patients presenting with lacunar strokes be treated with antiplatelet therapy? This is tempting and a logical extrapolation of mechanistic constructs, but available clinical data are insufficient to withhold anticoagulation, in my view. Reproducibility of classification of ischemic stroke subtypes in clinical practice is uncertain, recurrent rates are based on small numbers from nonrandomized comparisons, and some fraction of lacunar strokes in AF patients is undoubtedly cardioembolic (42).

About 5% to 10% of AF patients with ischemic stroke/TIA have severe ipsilateral cervical carotid artery stenosis. Estimates based on attributable risk support the likelihood of the stenosis as the cause of ischemia if the severity of stenosis is 70% or greater. Carotid endarterectomy seems reasonable for AF patients with high-grade ipsilateral stenosis, followed by anticoagulation (although data supporting this strategy are lacking), favoring the use of carotid imaging for AF patients with anterior circulation ischemia.

Hypertension increases the risk of cardioembolic stroke in AF patients by promoting left atrial appendage stasis, probably mediated by left ventricular diastolic abnormalities. However, it is uncertain whether reducing blood pressure in established hypertensive heart disease improves appendage stasis and lowers the risk of cardioembolic stroke in AF patients. Aggressive, prolonged control of hypertension following stroke in AF patients appears likely to reduce stroke risk in AF, but this has not been established. The recent PROGRESS (Perindopril Protection Against Recurrent Stroke Study) Trial demonstrated the benefits of aggressive blood pressure control following stroke and TIA in noncardioembolic ischemia (43), and a target systolic blood pressure of less than 130 mm Hg is an aggressive, empiric approach. Whether specific types of antihypertensive agents offer greater protection against stroke is controversial and unstudied to date in AF patients. Based on aggregate results of PROGRESS (43), the Veterans Affairs Cooperative Study (44), and the Losartan Intervention for Endpoint Reduction in Hypertension (LIFE) Trial (45) (although these three trials were not restricted to AF patients), initiating treatment with a low-dose thiazide diuretic and angiotensin-converting enzyme inhibitors is recommended, unless there are contraindications or indications for use of other classes of antihypertensive agents.

Should patients presenting with ischemic stroke who are in sinus rhythm routinely undergo prolonged electrocardiographic monitoring to detect paroxysmal AF? The yield appears to be low (1%–3%), but the data are sparse and inconclusive (46). In those with cortical ischemia without other identified etiologies, particularly if bilateral cortical ischemia is evident clinically or by neuroimaging, monitoring to detect occult paroxysmal AF seems reasonable.

CONCLUSIONS

AF-associated stroke is an important cause of brain ischemia and will be an even larger problem in the near future, as the number of elderly people with AF burgeons. Quite a lot is now known about stroke in AF patients and its prevention. Do the range of ideas described above make management decisions too complicated for most physicians, causing more confusion than good? Some advocate that "AF = give warfarin" has the virtue of simplicity, without requiring knowledge of the nuances needed to individualize therapy. Reliable data are available to allow patient-specific strategies for stroke prevention, avoiding or postponing anticoagulation for many hundreds of thousands of low-risk AF patients. New antithrombotic agents are on the near horizon; other management options include attempts to restore sinus rhythm, appendage obliteration, and aggressive control of blood pressure, but these have not been proven to reduce stroke risk. The complexities of management reflect the explosion of useful clinical information developed over the last 15 years. Other areas of stroke prevention are likely to become similarly complex as more is known.

Prevention of stroke in AF patients has been a triumph of clinical research over the last decade, carried out by investigators around the world. Efficacious preventive therapies tailored to the individual's risks and preferences are now available for most patients with AF. Many important clinical questions are yet to be answered, and the challenge remains to apply these advances in stroke prevention optimally.

REFERENCES

1. Hart RG, Pearce LA, Miller VT, et al. Cardioembolic vs. noncardioembolic strokes in atrial fibrillation: frequency and effect of antithrombotic agents in the Stroke Prevention in Atrial Fibrillation studies. *Cerebrovasc Dis* 2000;10:39–43.
2. Evans A, Perez I, Yu G, et al. Should stroke subtype influence anticoagulation decisions to prevent recurrence in stroke patients with atrial fibrillation? *Stroke* 2001;32:2828–2832.
3. Hart RG, Halperin JL. Atrial fibrillation and stroke. Concepts and controversies. *Stroke* 2001;32:803–808.
4. Anderson DC, Koller RL, Asinger RW, et al. Atrial fibrillation and stroke: epidemiology, pathophysiology, and management. *Neurologist* 1998;4:235–258.
5. Hart RG, Halperin JL. Atrial fibrillation and thromboembolism: a decade of progress in stroke prevention. *Ann Intern Med* 1999;131:688–695.
6. Hart RG, Sherman DG, Easton JD, et al. Prevention of stroke in patients with nonvalvular atrial fibrillation. *Neurology* 1998;51:674–681.
7. Go AS, Hylek EM, Phillips KA, et al. Prevalence of diagnosed atrial fibrillation in adults. *JAMA* 2001;285: 2370–2375.
8. Feinberg WM, Blackshear JL, Laupacis A, et al. Prevalence, age distribution, and gender of patients with

atrial fibrillation: analysis and implications. *Arch Intern Med* 1995;155:469–473.

9. Psaty BM, Manolio TA, Kuller LH, et al. Incidence of and risk factors for atrial fibrillation in older adults. *Circulation* 1997;96:2455–2461.

10. Sacco RL, Boden-Albala B, Abel G, et al. Race–ethnic disparities in the impact of stroke risk factors. The Northern Manhattan Stroke Study. *Stroke* 2001;32:1725–1731.

11. Chen ZM, Sandercock P, Pan HC, et al., on behalf of the CAST and IST Collaborative Groups. Indications for early aspirin use in acute ischemic stroke: a combined analysis of 40,000 randomized patients from the Chinese Acute Stroke Trials and the International Stroke Trial. *Stroke* 2000;31:1240–1249.

12. Worley KL, Lalonde DR, Kerr DR, et al. Survey of the causes of stroke among Mexican Americans in South Texas. *Texas Med* 1998;94:62–67.

13. Petersen P. Long-term treatment of patients using the new oral direct thrombin inhibitor ximelagatran versus warfarin in moderate to high stroke risk patients with atrial fibrillation. *J Neurol Sci* 2001; 187[Suppl I]:S124–S125.

14. Hart RG, Benavente O, McBride R, et al. Antithrombotic therapy to prevent stroke in patients with atrial fibrillation: a meta-analysis. *Ann Intern Med* 1999;131:492–501.

15. Pearce LA, Hart RG, Halperin JL. Assessment of three schemes for stratifying stroke risk in patients with nonvalvular atrial fibrillation. *Am J Med* 2000;109:45–51.

16. Feinberg WM, Kronmal RA, Newman AB, et al. Stroke risk in an elderly population with nonvalvular atrial fibrillation: the Cardiovascular Health Study. *J Gen Intern Med* 1999;14:56–59.

17. Yamaguchi T, for the Japanese Nonvalvular Atrial Fibrillation–Embolism Secondary Prevention Cooperative Study Group. Optimal intensity of warfarin therapy for secondary prevention of stroke in patients with nonvalvular atrial fibrillation. *Stroke* 2000;31:817–821.

18. Lechat P, Lardoux H, Mallet A, et al. Anticoagulant (fluindione)–aspirin combination in patients with high-risk atrial fibrillation. *Cerebrovasc Dis* 2001;12:245–252.

19. Gorter JW. Major bleeding during anticoagulation after cerebral ischemia: patterns and risk factors. Stroke Prevention in Reversible Ischemia Trial (SPIRIT) and European Atrial Fibrillation Trial (EAFT) study groups. *Neurology* 1999;53:1319–1327.

20. Wehinger C, Stollberger C, Langer T, et al. Evaluation of risk factors for stroke/embolism and of complications due to anticoagulant therapy in atrial fibrillation. *Stroke* 2001;32:2246–2252.

21. Atrial Fibrillation Investigators. Risk factors for stroke and efficacy of antithrombotic therapy in atrial fibrillation. *Arch Intern Med* 1994;154:1449–1457.

22. Evans A, Kalra L. Are the results of randomized controlled trials on anticoagulation in patients with atrial fibrillation generalizable to clinical practice? *Arch Intern Med* 2001;161:1443–1447.

23. Stroke Prevention in Atrial Fibrillation Investigators. Warfarin vs. aspirin for prevention of thromboembolism in atrial fibrillation. *Lancet* 1994;343:687–691.

24. Rosand J, Hylek EM, O'Donnell KC, et al. Warfarin-associated hemorrhage and cerebral amyloid angiopathy: a genetic and pathological study. *Neurology* 2000; 55:947–952.

25. Stroke Prevention in Atrial Fibrillation Investigators. Prospective identification of patients with nonvalvular atrial fibrillation at low-risk of stroke during treatment with aspirin. *JAMA* 1998;279:1273–1277.

26. Gage BF, Waterman AD, Shannon W, et al. Validation of clinical classification schemes for predicting stroke. Results from the national registry of atrial fibrillation. *JAMA* 2001;285:2864–2870.

27. Albers GW, Dalen JE, Laupacis A, et al. Antithrombotic therapy in atrial fibrillation. *Chest* 2001;119[Suppl]: 194S–206S.

28. Hart RG, Pearce LA, McBride R, et al. Factors associated with ischemic stroke during aspirin therapy in atrial fibrillation. *Stroke* 1999;30:1223–1229.

29. Stroke Prevention in Atrial Fibrillation Investigators Committee on Echocardiography. Transesophageal echocardiography correlates of thromboembolism in high-risk patients with nonvalvular atrial fibrillation. *Ann Intern Med* 1998;128:639–647.

30. Saxena R, Lewis S, Berge E, et al., for the International Stroke Trial Collaborative Group. Risk of early death and recurrent stroke and effect of heparin in 3169 patients with acute ischemic stroke and atrial fibrillation in the International Stroke Trial. *Stroke* 2001;32:2333–2337.

31. Lamassa M, Di Carlo AA, Pracucci G, et al. Characteristics, outcome, and care of stroke associated with atrial fibrillation in Europe. *Stroke* 2001;32:392–398.

32. Carlsson J, Miketic S, Flicker E, et al. Neurological events in patients with atrial fibrillation: outcome and preventive practices. *Z Kardiol* 2000;89:1090–1097.

33. Hart RG, Palacio S, Pearce LA. Atrial fibrillation, stroke, and acute antithrombotic therapy: analysis of randomized clinical trials. *Stroke* 2002;33:2722–2727.

34. Moroney JT, Bagiella E, Paik MC, et al. Risk factors for early recurrence after ischemic stroke. *Stroke* 1998;29:2118–2121.

35. International Stroke Trial Collaborative Group. The International Stroke Trial (IST): a randomized trial of aspirin, subcutaneous heparin, both, or neither among 19435 patients with acute ischemic stroke. *Lancet* 1997;349:1569–1581.

36. Berge E, Abdelnoor M, Nakstad PH, et al., for the HAEST Study Group (Heparin in Acute Embolic Stroke Trial). Low molecular-weight heparin vs. aspirin in patients with acute ischemic stroke and atrial fibrillation: a double blind randomized trial. *Lancet* 2000;355:1205–1210.

37. Publications Committee for the Trial of ORG 10172 in Acute Stroke Treatment (TOAST) Investigators. Low molecular weight heparinoid, ORG 10172 (danaparoid), and outcome after acute ischemic stroke. *JAMA* 1998; 279:1265–1272.

38. Bath PMW, Iddenden R, Bath FJ. Low-molecular-weight heparins and heparinoids in acute ischemic stroke. A meta-analysis of randomized controlled trials. *Stroke* 2000;31:1770–1778.

39. Bath PMW, Lindenstrom E, Boysen G, et al., for the TAIST Investigators. Tinzaparin in Acute Ischemic Stroke Trial (TAIST): a randomized, aspirin-controlled trial. *Lancet* 2001;358:702–710.

40. Hart RG, Bailey RD. An assessment of guidelines for prevention of ischemic stroke. *Neurology* 2002;59:977–982.

41. Mohr JP, Thompson JLP, Lazar RM, et al. A comparison of warfarin and aspirin for the prevention of recurrent ischemic stroke. *N Engl J Med* 2001;345: 1444–1451.

42. Jung DK, Devuyst G, Maeder P, et al. Atrial fibrillation with small subcortical infarcts. *J Neurol Neurosurg Psychiatry* 2001;70:344–349.

43. PROGRESS Collaborative Group. Randomised trial of perindopril-based blood-pressure-lowering regimen among 6105 individuals with previous stroke or transient ischaemic attack. *Lancet* 2001;358:1033–1041.

44. Gottdiener JS, Reda DJ, Williams DW, et al., for the VA Cooperative Study Group on Antihypertensive Agents. Effect of single-drug therapy on reduction of left atrial size in mild to moderate hypertension. *Circulation* 1998;98:140–148.

45. Dahlof B, Devereux RGB, Kjeldsen SE, et al. Cardiovascular morbidity and mortality in the Losartan Intervention for Endpoint Reduction in Hypertension (LIFE): a randomized trial against atenolol. *Lancet* 2002;359:995–1003.

46. Bell C, Kapral M, with the Canadian Task Force on Preventive Health Care. Use of ambulatory electrocardiography for the detection of paroxysmal atrial fibrillation in patients with stroke. *Can J Neurol Sci* 2000;27: 25–31.

Ischemic Stroke: Advances in Neurology, Vol. 92. Edited by
H.J.M. Barnett, Julien Bogousslavsky, and Heather Meldrum.
Lippincott Williams & Wilkins, Philadelphia © 2003.

31

Anticoagulants for Acute Ischemic Stroke

Eivind Berge and *Peter Sandercock

*Department of Internal Medicine, Ullevaal University Hospital, Oslo, Norway; *Department of Clinical Neurosciences, University of Edinburgh and Western General Hospital, Edinburgh, United Kingdom*

More than four-fifths of all strokes in Caucasians are ischemic strokes due to thromboembolic occlusion and cerebral infarction (1). The rationale for anticoagulant agents in acute ischemic stroke is therefore to suppress or halt any underlying thrombotic process, to reduce the volume of infarcted cerebral tissue, and to reduce the degree of neurologic deficit and consequent disability. Anticoagulants are also given to prevent stroke recurrence and to prevent or treat deep vein thrombosis and pulmonary embolism in patients who have had a stroke. However, anticoagulants can increase the risk of intracranial and extracranial hemorrhage, which might offset any benefits.

EVIDENCE FROM RANDOMIZED–CONTROLLED TRIALS AND SYSTEMATIC REVIEWS

A recent systematic review identified 21 randomized-controlled trials comparing anticoagulants with control among patients with acute ischemic stroke (2). The trials tested standard unfractionated heparin, low-molecular-weight heparin, heparinoid, direct thrombin inhibitors, and heparin given for just 24 h followed by oral anticoagulation. Most of the data came from trials in which unfractionated heparin was administered by subcutaneous injection in high dose (12,500 IU twice daily) or low dose (5,000 IU twice daily). In total, the trials included 23,427 patients with acute presumed ischemic stroke (2). The results are, however, dominated by the data from a single trial, the International Stroke Trial (IST), which included 19,435 patients (2,3). Most patients had a computed tomography scan to exclude intracranial hemorrhage before treatment was started, patients were generally randomized within 48 h of stroke onset, and treatment continued for about 2 weeks. A

systematic review of trials exclusively comparing low-molecular-weight heparins with control is also available (4). Since that review appeared, a further trial comparing low-molecular-weight heparin with control has been published (5). There are only a few trials directly comparing one anticoagulant agent with another or comparing different doses of the same agent (6–8).

Recurrent Ischemic Stroke During the Treatment Period

Immediate anticoagulation significantly reduced the relative odds of recurrent ischemic or unknown stroke (referred to as recurrent ischemic stroke for simplicity) within the first 2 weeks by 24% [95% confidence interval (CI) 12%–35%], from 3.6% in control subjects to 2.8% in treated patients, i.e., avoiding nine recurrences for every 1,000 patients treated. The effects of the different regimens tested were broadly consistent.

Symptomatic Intracranial Hemorrhage During the Treatment Period

Immediate anticoagulation significantly increased the relative odds of symptomatic intracranial hemorrhage by 152% (95% CI 92%–230%), from 0.5% in control subjects to 1.4% in treated patients, i.e., causing nine symptomatic intracranial hemorrhages for every 1,000 patients treated. Each of the regimens tested, when compared with control, appeared to increase the risk of symptomatic intracranial hemorrhage. The relative increase was consistent across the different regimens, although (because of small numbers) it was statistically significant only for unfractionated heparin. Indirect comparisons of different dosing regimens showed consistently higher bleeding risks with higher dose regimens. In the IST (3), patients allocated to subcutaneous unfractionated heparin were randomized to high dose (12,500 IU twice daily) or to low dose (5,000 IU twice daily). The proportions with symptomatic intracranial hemorrhage were 1.8% and 0.7%, respectively, a highly significant 11/1,000 excess with the higher dose ($2p$ < 0.00001). A systematic review of all trials directly comparing high- with low-dose anticoagulants in acute stroke supports the dose dependency of the bleeding risks (7,8).

Recurrent Stroke of Any Type During the Treatment Period

This combined endpoint encompasses both the benefits and the risks of anticoagulants and provides the best estimate of the effect of anticoagulants on recurrent events. Anticoagulation was not associated with a net reduction in the odds of this event (odds ratio 0.97; 95% CI 0.85–1.11) (Fig. 31-1).

Major Extracranial Hemorrhage During the Treatment Period

Hemorrhages into the gastrointestinal tract and elsewhere were reported in 0.4% of control subjects and 1.3% of treated patients, a significant threefold increase. With anticoagulants, for every 1,000 patients treated, nine had a major extracranial hemorrhage. The indirect comparisons of different agents show that the bleeding risks are higher with higher-dose regimens. In the IST, the risk of major extracranial bleeds was 2% among patients allocated high-dose unfractionated heparin and 0.6% among those allocated low-dose unfractionated heparin, a highly significant 14/1,000 excess with the higher dose ($2p$ < 0.00001) (3). A systematic review of all trials directly comparing high- with low-dose anticoagulants confirmed this dose dependency (7,8).

Deep Venous Thrombosis and Pulmonary Embolism During the Treatment Period

Data on the effects of anticoagulants on deep venous thrombosis were available only for 916 patients. There was heterogeneity of treatment effect between the trials, which makes it harder to interpret the overall estimate of treatment effect. Overall, symptomatic or asymptomatic deep venous thrombosis occurred in 43% of control subjects and 15% of treated patients, a highly significant 79% reduction in

relative odds with anticoagulants (95% CI 61%–85%). For every 1,000 patients treated, 280 avoided deep vein thrombosis. Fatal or nonfatal pulmonary embolism was not systematically studied in the trials. It was reported in only 0.9% of control subjects and 0.6% of treated patients, a significant 39% reduction in relative odds with anticoagulants (95% CI 17%–55%). For every 1,000 patients treated, 3 avoided pulmonary embolism. It is difficult to judge whether the reductions in deep venous thrombosis or pulmonary embolism are dose dependent from the indirect comparisons. In the IST, fatal or nonfatal pulmonary embolism occurred in 0.4% of those allocated high dose and 0.7% of those allocated low dose, a nonsignificant difference (3). A systematic review of all of the direct randomized comparisons confirmed the greater reduction in pulmonary embolism with higher doses, but the absolute benefit was very small (7,8).

If we allow for the likely underascertainment of pulmonary embolism and assume that the true rate in the control subjects was 3%, and then apply the same 39% proportional reduction (i.e., from 3% to 1.85%), for every 1,000 patients treated, about 12 avoid pulmonary embolism. However, even if the benefit is that large, it will still be substantially offset, as an extra nine patients will have a major extracranial hemorrhage associated with anticoagulants.

Death During the Treatment Period and at the End of Follow-Up

There was no significant effect on deaths during the treatment period; 8.7% of control subjects died compared with 8.5% of treated patients (95% CI 10% reduction in relative odds to 10% increase). By the end of the scheduled follow-up at 3 to 6 months, 20.6% of control subjects had died compared with 21.4% of treated patients, a nonsignificant 5% increase in the relative odds of death (95% CI 2% reduction to 12% increase).

Death or Dependency at the End of Follow-Up

The most important measure of outcome is the proportion of patients, at the end of follow-up, who are either alive but need help for everyday activities or who are dead. Overall, 60.1% of controls were dead or dependent compared with 59.7% of treated patients, a nonsignificant 1% relative odds reduction (95% CI 6% reduction to 5% increase in the odds of death).

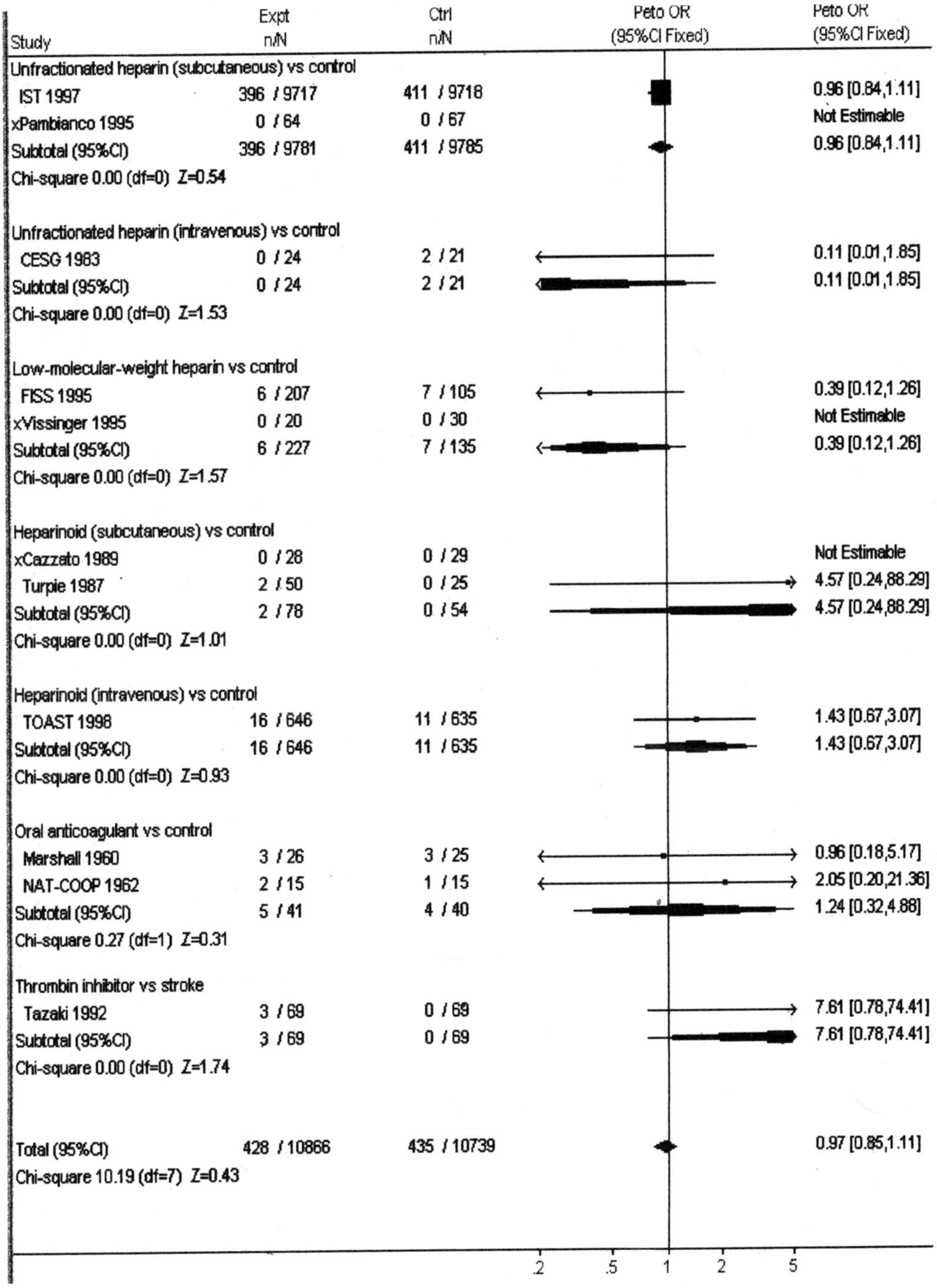

Study	Expt n/N	Ctrl n/N	Peto OR (95%CI Fixed)	Peto OR (95%CI Fixed)
Unfractionated heparin (subcutaneous) vs control				
IST 1997	396 / 9717	411 / 9718		0.96 [0.84,1.11]
xPambianco 1995	0 / 64	0 / 67		Not Estimable
Subtotal (95%CI)	396 / 9781	411 / 9785		0.96 [0.84,1.11]
Chi-square 0.00 (df=0) Z=0.54				
Unfractionated heparin (intravenous) vs control				
CESG 1983	0 / 24	2 / 21		0.11 [0.01,1.85]
Subtotal (95%CI)	0 / 24	2 / 21		0.11 [0.01,1.85]
Chi-square 0.00 (df=0) Z=1.53				
Low-molecular-weight heparin vs control				
FISS 1995	6 / 207	7 / 105		0.39 [0.12,1.26]
xVissinger 1995	0 / 20	0 / 30		Not Estimable
Subtotal (95%CI)	6 / 227	7 / 135		0.39 [0.12,1.26]
Chi-square 0.00 (df=0) Z=1.57				
Heparinoid (subcutaneous) vs control				
xCazzato 1989	0 / 28	0 / 29		Not Estimable
Turpie 1987	2 / 50	0 / 25		4.57 [0.24,88.29]
Subtotal (95%CI)	2 / 78	0 / 54		4.57 [0.24,88.29]
Chi-square 0.00 (df=0) Z=1.01				
Heparinoid (intravenous) vs control				
TOAST 1998	16 / 646	11 / 635		1.43 [0.67,3.07]
Subtotal (95%CI)	16 / 646	11 / 635		1.43 [0.67,3.07]
Chi-square 0.00 (df=0) Z=0.93				
Oral anticoagulant vs control				
Marshall 1960	3 / 26	3 / 25		0.96 [0.18,5.17]
NAT-COOP 1962	2 / 15	1 / 15		2.05 [0.20,21.36]
Subtotal (95%CI)	5 / 41	4 / 40		1.24 [0.32,4.88]
Chi-square 0.27 (df=1) Z=0.31				
Thrombin inhibitor vs stroke				
Tazaki 1992	3 / 69	0 / 69		7.61 [0.78,74.41]
Subtotal (95%CI)	3 / 69	0 / 69		7.61 [0.78,74.41]
Chi-square 0.00 (df=0) Z=1.74				
Total (95%CI)	428 / 10866	435 / 10739		0.97 [0.85,1.11]
Chi-square 10.19 (df=7) Z=0.43				

.2   .5   1   2   5

FIG. 31-1. Proportional effect of early anticoagulant therapy on the risk of any recurrent stroke (ischemic, hemorrhagic, or undetermined) during the treatment period. The estimate of treatment effect is expressed as an odds ratio (solid square) and its 95% confidnce interval (horizontal line). The size of the solid square is proportional to the amount of information available. An odds ratio of 1.0 corresponds to a treatment effect of zero, and odds ratio less than 1 suggests treatment is better than control, and an odds ratio greater than 1 suggests treatment is worse than control. The figures given to the right are relative odds ratios with 95% confidence intervals. With permission from Gubiz et al. (2).

EFFECTS OF ANTICOAGULANTS IN VARIOUS CATEGORIES OF PATIENTS

Suspected Cardioembolic Ischemic Stroke

Anticoagulants have often been advocated for the treatment of acute cardioembolic stroke, and in many centers in the United States, such patients are treated routinely with intravenous heparin (9). However, there is no evidence to support the use of anticoagulants in such circumstances. A subgroup analysis of more than 3,200 patients with acute ischemic stroke of suspected cardioembolic origin in all available randomized, controlled trials did not show net benefit from anticoagulants (2). The small Heparin in Acute Embolic Stroke Trial (HAEST) compared a low-molecular-weight heparin with aspirin in 449 patients with acute ischemic stroke and atrial fibrillation and did not show evidence of an advantage of low-molecular-weight heparin over aspirin (10).

"Progressing Hemispheric Stroke"

Likewise, many textbooks and reviews recommend immediate intravenous heparin for patients with "progressing stroke." However, there have not been any trials of intravenous heparin for "progressive stroke," and anticoagulants have not been shown to prevent neurologic deterioration better than aspirin (5,10,11).

"Basilar Thrombosis"

The IST included over 2,000 patients with posterior circulation infarcts, and there was no evidence that the effects of treatment in this subgroup were any different from those seen in the trial overall (3). However, it is likely that only a small proportion had occlusion of the basilar artery. A trial focused on patients with proven basilar occlusion might be justified, but trials that seek to recruit a type of patient only rarely encountered in clinical practice are notoriously difficult to do.

Carotid or Vertebral Artery Dissection

There is no evidence of benefit from the trials of anticoagulants in ischemic stroke in general and no randomized evidence at all in patients with ischemic stroke due to arterial dissection (12). Despite this, many clinicians are inclined to use anticoagulants for carotid or vertebral artery dissection.

Intracranial Venous Thrombosis

Two trials have evaluated heparin as a treatment for the whole spectrum of intracranial venous thrombosis (13,14), and a Cochrane systematic review of the randomized trials of anticoagulants is under way (15). Although the evidence is not strongly in favor of anticoagulants, they do appear safe in these patients.

USE OF ANTICOAGULANTS IN CLINICAL PRACTICE

Despite the lack of evidence from randomized-controlled trials, there are still occasions when clinicians may feel compelled to use anticoagulants in patients with acute ischemic stroke.

High Risk of Deep Venous Thrombosis

Guidelines vary in their recommendations about whether or not heparin should be used for deep venous thrombosis prophylaxis (16–20). Patients at high risk of deep venous thrombosis, for example, immobile patients with predisposing factors, may benefit from graded compression stockings or, alternatively, from low-dose heparin. However, there is no reliable evidence on the benefit of compression stockings or low-dose heparin in stroke patients or whether any benefit is additive to the effect of aspirin.

Non-Valvular Atrial Fibrillation

Patients with atrial fibrillation who have had a stroke or transient ischemic attack are likely to benefit from long-term oral anticoagulants as secondary prevention (21), but the best time to start anticoagulant therapy is not known. The early use of heparin in the acute phase has been discussed in Chapter 30. We recommend that all patients with acute ischemic stroke and atrial fibrillation be started on aspirin as soon as possible (10). Patients with minor ischemic strokes or transient ischemic attacks can be started on oral anticoagulants immediately, and aspirin should be stopped once the international normalized ratio is in the therapeutic range. Patients with large infarcts can be started on oral anticoagulants after 1 or 2 weeks, when the risk of hemorrhagic transformation of the infarct is lower.

Intracranial Venous Thrombosis

There is no firm evidence in favor of anticoagulants for intracranial thrombosis, although they appear to be safe (13,14). As described in Chapter 28, based on incomplete proof of efficacy, some neurologists recommend anticoagulation with heparin, especially if the patient is deteriorating, and some even suggest local thrombolysis if all else fails (14). In the collaborative European trial (14), after 3 weeks, patients allocated anticoagulants were put on oral anticoagulants for 3 months (analogous to the treatment of deep venous thrombosis in the leg), which seems sensible.

Management of Complications of Anticoagulant Treatment

The most life-threatening risks are intra- or extracranial hemorrhage. Management of severe hemorrhage consists of stopping any administration of anticoagulants, estimation of the clotting time, and reversal with intravenous protamine sulfate or vitamin K and clotting factor concentrates (with or without fresh frozen plasma), according to local protocols and preferably in consultation with the local hematology specialist (18). For reversal of low-molecular-weight heparin or heparinoids, consult the manufacturer's data sheet.

If an ischemic stroke occurs in a patient already receiving oral anticoagulants, the reason for the infarction must be sought. The cause is often an inadequate dose of anticoagulants (21), but infective endocarditis must be ruled out. Recurrent ischemic stroke despite an adequate international normalized ratio may necessitate the addition of low-dose aspirin, though this is likely to double the risk of intracranial hemorrhage (23,24).

IS THERE A FUTURE FOR ANTICOAGULANTS IN ACUTE ISCHEMIC STROKE?

Combination of Aspirin and Low-Dose Anticoagulant Treatment

As a part of a systematic review of anticoagulants versus antiplatelet agents for acute ischemic stroke, we sought to assess whether the addition of anticoagulants to antiplatelet agents offers any net advantage over antiplatelet agents alone (25). The data from this review suggested that the combination of low-dose unfractionated heparin and aspirin might be associated with net benefits over aspirin alone, and this might be worth testing in further large-scale, randomized-controlled trials.

Very Early Anticoagulation

A further trial is planned to randomize patients with nonlacunar ischemic stroke within 12 h of onset to full doses of intravenous unfractionated heparin or to aspirin 300 mg daily [Rapid Anticoagulation Prevents Ischaemic Damage (RAPID) Trial (26)]. Until the RAPID Trial is complete, there is no indication to use anticoagulants (either unfractionated heparin, low-molecular-weight heparin, or heparinoid, given either subcutaneously or intravenously) as routine treatment in patients with acute ischemic stroke in general or in particular etiologic subtypes.

REFERENCES

1. Warlow C, Dennis MS, van Gijn J, et al. *Stroke. A practical guide to management.* Oxford: Blackwell Science, 1996.
2. Gubitz G, Councell C, Sandercock P, et al. Anticoagulants for acute ischaemic stroke [Cochrane review]. In: *Cochrane library*, issue 4, 2002. Oxford: Update Software, 2002.
3. International Stroke Trial Collaborative Group. The International Stroke Trial (IST): a randomised trial of aspirin, subcutaneous heparin, both, or neither among 19435 patients with acute ischaemic stroke. *Lancet* 1997;349:1569–1581.
4. Bath PMW, Iddenden R, Bath FJ. Low-molecular-weight heparins and heparinoids in acute ischemic stroke. A meta-analysis of randomized controlled trials. *Stroke* 2000;31:1770–1778.
5. Bath PM, Lindenstrom E, Boysen G, et al. Tinzaparin in Acute Ischaemic Stroke (TAIST): a randomised aspirin-controlled trial. *Lancet* 2001;358:702–710.
6. Counsell C, Sandercock P. Low-molecular-weight heparins or heparinoids versus standard unfractionated heparin for acute ischaemic stroke [Cochrane review]. In: *Cochrane library*, issue 4, 2002. Oxford: Update Software, 2002.
7. Gubitz G, Sandercock P. Different doses of anticoagulant for acute ischaemic stroke [protocol for a Cochrane review]. In: *Cochrane library*, issue 4, 2002. Oxford: Update Software, 2002.
8. Gubitz G, Sandercock P, Counsell C. Immediate anticoagulant therapy for acute ischaemic stroke: a systematic review of seven randomised trials directly comparing different doses of the same anticoagulant. *Stroke* 2000; 31:308.
9. Moussouttas MM, Lichtman JH, Krumholtz HM, et al. The use of heparin anticoagulation in acute ischemic stroke among academic medical centres. *Stroke* 1999; 30:265.
10. Berge E, Abdelnoor M, Nakstad PH, et al. Low molecular-weight heparin versus aspirin in patients with acute ischaemic stroke and atrial fibrillation: a double-blind randomised study. *Lancet* 2000;355:1205–1210.
11. Publications Committee for the Trial of ORG 10172 in Acute Stroke Treatment (TOAST) investigators. Low molecular weight heparinoid, ORG 10172 (danaparoid), and outcome after acute ischemic stroke: a randomized controlled trial. *JAMA* 1998;279: 1265–1272.
12. Lyrer P, Erickson LP. Antithrombotic drugs for carotid artery dissection [Cochrane review]. In: *Cochrane library*, issue 4, 2002. Oxford: Update Software, 2002.
13. Einhaupl KM, Villringer A, Meister W, et al. Heparin

treatment in sinus venous thrombosis. *Lancet* 1991;338:597–600.

14. de Bruijn SF, Stam J. Randomized, placebo-controlled trial of anticoagulant treatment with low-molecular-weight heparin for cerebral sinus thrombosis. *Stroke* 1999;30:484–488.

15. Stam J, de Bruijn STFM, Deveber G. Anticoagulants for cerebral sinus thrombosis [protocol for a Cochrane review]. In: *Cochrane library*, issue 4, 2002. Oxford: Update Software, 2002.

16. Adams HP Jr, Brott TG, Crowell RM, et al. Guidelines for the management of patients with acute ischemic stroke. A statement for healthcare professionals from a special writing group of the Stroke Council, American Heart Association. *Stroke* 1994;25:1901–1914.

17. Albers GW, Amarenco P, Easton JD, et al. Antithrombotic and thrombolytic therapy for ischemic stroke. *Chest* 2001;119:300S–320S.

18. Scottish Intercollegiate Guidelines Network. *Antithrombotic therapy. A national clinical guideline.* Edinburgh: Scottish Intercollegiate Guidelines Network, Royal College of Physicians, 1999 (also available at *www.show.scot.nhs.uk/sign/clinical.htm*).

19. Scottish Intercollegiate Guidelines Network. *Prevention of venous thromboembolism. A national clinical guideline.* Edinburgh: Scottish Intercollegiate Guidelines Network, Royal College of Physicians, 2000 (also available at: *www.show.scot.nhs.uk/sign/clinical.htm*).

20. Royal College of Physicians of Edinburgh. Consensus Conference on Medical Management of Stroke. *J Neurol Neurosurg Psychiatry* 1999;66:128–129.

21. EAFT (European Atrial Fibrillation Trial) Study Group. Secondary prevention in non-rheumatic atrial fibrillation after transient ischaemic attack or minor stroke. *Lancet* 1993;342:1255–1262.

22. Bousser MG. Cerebral venous thrombosis: nothing, heparin, or local thrombolysis? *Stroke* 1999;30:481–483.

23. Turpie AG, Gent M, Laupacis A, et al. A comparison of aspirin with placebo in patients treated with warfarin after heart-valve replacement. *N Engl J Med* 1993;329:524–529.

24. Hart RG, Benavente O, Pearce LA. Increased risk of intracranial hemorrhage when aspirin is combined with warfarin: a meta-analysis and hypothesis. *Cerebrovasc Dis* 1999;9:215–217.

25. Berge E, Sandercock P. Anticoagulants versus antiplatelet agents for acute ischaemic stroke [Cochrane review]. In: *Cochrane library*, issue 4, 2002. Oxford: Update Software, 2002.

26. Chamorro A. Heparin in acute ischemic stroke: the case for a new clinical trial. *Cerebrovasc Dis* 1999;9[Suppl 3]:16–23.

Ischemic Stroke: Advances in Neurology, Vol. 92. Edited by
H.J.M. Barnett, Julien Bogousslavsky, and Heather Meldrum.
Lippincott Williams & Wilkins, Philadelphia © 2003.

32

Anticoagulants for Prevention of Ischemic Stroke: Current Concepts

J.P. Mohr

*Doris & Stanley Tananbaum Stroke Center, New York Presbyterian Hospital; Department of
Neurology, College of Physicians & Surgeons, Columbia University, New York, New York, U.S.A.*

The use of antithrombotics dates back to the early effort, said to have begun first in 1938, by the late, great Irving S. Wright, a Cornell–New York Hospital cardiologist. Judging from his *New York Times* obituary (he died at the age of 96), he was the first to use warfarin (the name itself an acronym for the Wisconsin Alumni Research Foundation, Incorporated), whose agriculture school investigations into rotten clover uncovered the compound that explained hemorrhages suffered by milk cows in Wisconsin. The interest and energy of Irving Wright widened the application for use of this compound in treatment to prevent ischemic stroke. Its use and definitions for stroke were some of the reasons for the initiation of a biannual series of January meetings called the Princeton Conference. The first such conference, held at the Nassau Inn (Wright was a Princeton graduate) in Princeton, NJ, U.S.A., in January 1954, entitled "Cerebral Vascular Diseases," was held under the "auspices" of the American Heart Association, with Irving Wright as chair and E. Hugh Luckey, M.D., a prominent New York Hospital internist, as editor. During this first session, early results of treatment of 57 patients with warfarin, 31 with valvular heart disease, and 29 in atrial fibrillation were presented by E. McDevitt, M.D., of Cornell. The second conference, held in 1956, was notable for having published a report, reprinted from a 1958 issue of the *Journal of Neurology,* featured a "Classification and Outline of Cerebrovascular Diseases," which also acknowledged among other entities the existence of a diagnosis termed "infarction of undetermined cause. At the third conference, in 1960, the subject of clinical diagnosis was defined in three stages of focal arterial disease, the last being "completed stroke." At the same conference, C.M. Fisher,

M.D., from the Massachusetts General Hospital's Neurology Service, presented results from anticoagulant therapy from the National Cooperative Study begun in 1958. Thus, well under way, and prior to large, current clinical trials, was the notion that antithrombotics, in this case warfarin, had a role in the treatment of ischemic stroke.

PREVENTION OF FIRST ISCHEMIC STROKE

There was a time when some serious investigators questioned the use of warfarin for any indication, given uncertainties of its safety and effectiveness (1,2). Some speculated that a clinical trial in the setting of nonvalvular atrial fibrillation was impractical because there would be few eligible patients, it would be too costly because of the need for pretreatment computed tomography scans, and it would not be likely to show any useful effect for warfarin (3). Since then, major clinical trials have shown a benefit for warfarin in the prevention of stroke in a wide variety of settings, among them following myocardial infarction (4); for those in atrial fibrillation, a reduction in rate of first stroke with warfarin has been superior when compared with aspirin and placebo (5), with any other physician-chosen therapy (6), and also with aspirin compared with placebo (7). Acceptably low complication rates for warfarin have been documented at international normalized ratio (INR) ranges showing a warfarin benefit (8).

The findings seem clear enough that treatment recommendations based on stratified risk factor analysis for patients with atrial fibrillation have even been formulated (9).

Many of the trials focused on the diagnosis of stroke, without strenuous effort to address questions of the stroke subtype, severity, or short- or long-term recurrence. As a result, the insights from these studies on secondary stroke prevention have necessarily been limited. Some of the larger studies have also been open label for the warfarin arm, which could have led to different clinical standards for reporting events for those in the different treatment groups (placebo, antiplatelet, or warfarin), depending on the bias of the clinician.

PREVENTION OF RECURRENT ISCHEMIC STROKE

Reported 5-year cumulative recurrence rates after prior cerebral ischemia range from 24% to 42%, with one-third of recurrences occurring within the first 30 days after the initial event. Therapeutic control of modifiable vascular risk factors is highly recommended but as yet has not shown a major effect on preventing recurrent stroke.

Early Versus Late Recurrence

Most of the interest in antithrombotics has been on prevention of late recurrence, say, over a period of 2 years or more. Part of the interest has been the assumption that sufficient time would be needed for the event rate to show itself, so that events in the first few hours or days, during hospitalization, might be difficult to study with any degree of success. In the Warfarin–Aspirin Recurrent Stroke Study (WARSS) (10), described in more detail below, special attention was paid to the recurrence rates within the first 30 days from enrollment to determine if a difference would be found separating warfarin from aspirin. The study group had a concern that recurrent events in the warfarin arm might be excessive during the period when warfarin effect on the INR was not yet "therapeutic" and thus might blunt any benefit found later. In the event, no differences were encountered, although the event rates (under 3% in the first month) were low.

Atrial Fibrillation

The results of primary prevention trials in a setting of atrial fibrillation make it widely assumed that not only those seeking prevention of first stroke (primary prevention) but also those already suffering a stroke with atrial fibrillation require dose-adjusted oral anticoagulation (target INR 2.5 ± 0.5). Although

warfarin has proved itself superior to a range of other therapies (6), including placebo (8), the recurrence rates even on warfarin are higher than those of first occurrence (5,11). The INR effects in secondary prevention trials show a similar-shaped curve to that for the primary prevention trials, flattening between INR 1.5 and 2.0 and remaining relatively stable for higher values to 3.0.

Issues of safety have not been as well established. Acceptably low hemorrhage rates have been reported for INRs of 2.0 to 3.0 in atrial fibrillation in some studies of prevention of first and recurrent stroke (12). Yet major hemorrhagic complications at an INR of 2.8 (treatment range 2.2 to 3.5) forced discontinuation of a recent trial, although the lower intensity range of 1.5 to 2.1 proved safe (13). These more recent experiences leave unsettled the actual safety of anticoagulants in the prevention of recurrent, as opposed to primary, ischemic stroke.

Noncardiogenic Stroke

As recently as 1989, a report from the World Health Organization expressed dissatisfaction with the lack of a proven medical therapy to prevent recurrent ischemic stroke (14). In the decade that followed, considerable effort was directed toward this problem, along several lines. Initially, concerns for safety with warfarin prompted work limited largely to antithrombotic agents of the platelet antiaggregant type.

Warfarin Versus Aspirin for Noncardiogenic Stroke

A recent double-blind study made a direct comparison of warfarin with aspirin for those for whom the therapy for the inferred ischemic stroke mechanism had yet not been settled. WARSS (10) took as its point of departure the goal of determining whether the 30% risk reduction in primary stroke prevention in the setting of atrial fibrillation could be approximated for noncardioembolic recurrent ischemic stroke. No precedent existed for such a finding except the supportive evidence that at least some instance of noncardioembolic stroke appeared on clinical grounds to suggest an embolic mechanism, even though none could be found, a category embraced by the general term "cryptogenic stroke" (15). A target of 30% rate reduction at least allowed for the calculation of sample size using the roughly 8%/year recurrence rate achieved in most trials with aspirin. The trial was, thus, never conceived as an equivalence trial. The patients in WARSS underwent a degree of laboratory workup reflecting current standards of care (Table 32-1).

The overall rates of stroke and death (372 of 2,206 patients, 16.9%) at 2 years (recorded at 761 days, 1 month beyond 2 years) approximated those of the original hypotheses used to calculate sample size and sufficed for prespecified analyses. By intent-to-treat analysis comparing the two treatment arms, there was no difference for the primary outcome of death or recurrent ischemic stroke [relative risk reduction (RRR) 1.13 for warfarin, 95% confidence interval (CI) 0.92–1.38, p = 0.25]. For patients treated with warfarin, 47 died and 149 experienced recurrent ischemic stroke, a total of 196 primary events among 1,103 (17.7%). For aspirin, 53 patients died and 123 experienced recurrent ischemic stroke, totaling 176 primary events among 1,103 patients (15.9%). Because over 30 patients (less than 1.5% of the total) ended their participation for a variety of uncontrollable reasons such as moving to another state, etc., a special computation was made to undertake an efficacy analysis for the remaining 2,164 patients. The findings of the trial were not changed.

Taken as a condensed summary, the overall findings failed to confirm a 30% superiority of warfarin over aspirin. The findings also failed to show a statistically significant difference between the two treatment arms. WARSS was not powered as an equivalence trial, and the results should be understood to have failed to confirm statistically significant differential therapeutic effects for the two treatments. A difference might exist, but the findings of the study do not allow a statement of difference or of equivalence. That said, even fewer data exist seeking differences for any clinically identifiable subtypes of ischemic stroke. The results leave unclear whether warfarin can be said to be justified for any but obvious cardioembolic strokes or whether each of the treatments appears justifiable for any of the stroke subtypes.

Some reviewers have considered that the investigators actually claimed WARSS to be an equivalence trial (16,17), so a comment appears useful here: The CI for the RR for warfarin versus aspirin (0.92–1.38) ruled out the 0.70 value that would have corresponded to such a benefit. Warfarin actually exhibited a 13% higher risk than aspirin. As WARSS remains the only adequately powered randomized clinical trial comparing these medications for recurrent stroke, this point estimate of the relative usefulness of these two medications is the best currently available. However, there is a 25% probability of observing a rate ratio as large as 1.13 in either direction when there is, in fact, no true difference between treatments. We thus could not rule out our original null hypothesis.

The generalizability of the results could be at issue. The percentages of ischemic stroke subtypes in the WARSS population varied somewhat from those of patients with stroke when adjusted for the removal of those ineligible: Absent from WARSS were patients with hemorrhage from any cause, those with inferred cardiogenic embolism (especially atrial fibrillation), and those too disabled by stroke or otherwise ineligible to participate in a clinical trial. The similarity of the recurrence rates among these subtypes is comparable with that found in the National Institute of Neurological and Communication Disorders and Stroke Data Bank (18) but somewhat different from those in other cohorts reported since then (19,20). When the data from WARSS for individual ischemic stroke subtypes were adjusted to match those of prior studies, the overall outcome was unchanged (Table 32-2).

Two other general findings are worth comment as well. First, several clinicians expressed concern that the time required for warfarin to take effect might bias the trial toward early recurrent events in the war-

TABLE 32-1. *Extent of workup for WARSS patients (n = 2,206)*

	No. of patients	%
CT	2,007	91.0
MRI	1,344	60.5
Duplex Doopler	1,691	76.7
Transcranial Doppler	596	27.0
Angiogram	845	38.3
CT or MRI	2,202	99.8
CT/MRI + any other test	2,056	93.2

CT, computed tomography; MRI, magnetic resonance imaging; WARSS, Warfarin–Aspirin Recurrent Stroke Study.

TABLE 32-2. *Hazard ratio for warfarin for overall results of WARSS versus three other observational studies adjusted for stroke subtype*

	Hazard ratio	95% CI	p
WARSS primary result	1.10	0.92–1.38	0.25
NOMASS weighting	1.11	0.90–1.36	0.33
Mayo weighting	1.08	0.88–1.32	0.47
SDB weighting	1.06	0.87–1.30	0.57

CI, confidence interval; NOMASS, Northern Manhattan Stroke Study; SDB, Stroke Data Bank; WARSS, Warfarin–Aspirin Recurrent Stroke Study.

farin arm, nullifying any beneficial effects later. To address this concern, a prespecified null hypothesis was explored for the slope of events for the first 30 days. In the event, there was no statistically significant difference between the two treatment groups for this period. A second concern related to safety and hemorrhage.

International Normalized Ratio Range, Complications, and Prevention of Recurrent Ischemic Stroke

Safety in WARSS at the 1.4 to 2.8 range was to prove adequate. To the surprise of many of the investigators, major hemorrhage rates proved comparable between the aspirin and warfarin groups, occurring in 68 patients, 38 of whom were randomized to the warfarin arm (3.44%) and 30 to the aspirin arm (2.71%). The differences were not statistically significant (RR for warfarin 1.28, 95% CI 0.80–2.07, $p = 0.304$), and the major adverse event rates were below the prespecified threshold for ending the trial early. By major hemorrhage was meant those with any intracranial or intraspinal hemorrhage, hemorrhage into the eye, or any hemorrhage in any other site leading to transfusion. Rates in WARSS for minor hemorrhage were significantly higher for warfarin than for aspirin, a finding replicated in other trials (Table 32-3).

At issue in any trial comparing warfarin with aspirin was a choice for the target INR. For WARSS, the range selected approximated that in the atrial fibrillation trials, where efficacy and safety had been demonstrated at ranges from 1.5 to 3.0. The range of 1.4 to 2.8 was selected also based in part on results from studies of the levels of prothrombin split product f1.2, indicating suppression of thrombosis could be achieved by values 1.4 and higher (21). The clinicians in the trial were prepared to accept this range as safe and presumably suitable for a test of efficacy. No data from clinical trials for safety of INR above 2.5 had been demonstrated at the time the trial was begun.

Complications with warfarin have been well documented in trials with no prior stroke (12,22,23), as well as in the stroke population, mainly elderly and at higher risk for hemorrhage (24,25). Few studies have addressed risks of serious hemorrhage in a setting of prior ischemic stroke. One such effort was the Stroke Prevention in Reversible Ischemia Trial (SPIRIT) (26). This study, begun after WARSS had started enrolling patients and having shared protocol details with WARSS, was an open-label warfarin comparison against lower-dose aspirin after transient ischemic attack and stroke, outcomes reviewed by a panel blinded as to therapy. No monitoring of INRs, institutional audits, or central laboratory performance of the INRs was part of the research plan. This study, undertaken with a planned INR range of 3.0 to 4.5 (actual reported INR mean of 3.5), was brought to an end after the first interim analysis. The complications of therapy were due almost entirely to hemorrhage, and these events mainly in the warfarin group (27). At the first interim analysis, 1,316 patients were reported to have been enrolled. Of them, 81 of 651 of the anticoagulated group had had events versus 36 of 665 in the aspirin group (hazard ratio 2.3, 95% CI 1.6–3.5). In this trial, the bleeding incidence, calculated from this small sample, was estimated to have been increased by a factor of 1.43 (95% CI 0.96–2.13) for each 0.5-U increase of the achieved INR. No reports from SPIRIT have appeared documenting the stability of the INRs in the treated patients over time or the percentages of patients above the upper or below the lower ranges of the planned INRs, so it cannot yet be inferred whether the serious hemorrhage rates were related to large fluctuations, to time well above the targeted range, or to any other variable apart from the reported mean. The study has undergone revision and

TABLE 32-3. *Aspirin versus warfarin safety in WARSS*

	Warfarin (n = 1,103)	Aspirin (n = 1,103)	Odds ratio (95% CI)	p
Death	47	53	0.88 (0.58–1.32)	0.61
from Hemorrhage	7	5	1.40 (0.42–5.13)	0.77
First hemorrhage				
Major	38	30	1.28 (0.78–2.10)	0.39
Minor	261	188	1.51 (1.22–1.87)	<0.001
All hemorrhages				
Major	44	30	1.48 (0.93–2.44)	0.10
Minor	413	259	1.61 (1.38–1.89)	<0.001

CI, confidence interval; WARSS, Warfarin–Aspirin Recurrent Stroke Study.

has restarted under a new name, ESPIRIT (European/Australian Stroke Prevention in Reversible Ischemia Trial) (28).

Apart from this open-label study, other efforts in nonstroke settings with higher INR ranges than those used in WARSS have also had mixed results where warfarin was compared with (29) or in combination with (30) aspirin. In these latter trials, the patient cohort has been mainly cardiac disease, not stroke.

Blinding of Therapy

Some investigators have expressed concerns that open-label studies allow a bias among treating physicians toward the treatment arm they already prefer, be it warfarin or platelet antiaggregants. For those patients receiving treatment deemed by a local investigator to be inferior, the threshold might be lower for reporting an outcome event that could allow the patient to end participation and be put on the alterative treatment deemed better by the investigator. A comparable concern would be for safety: For those physicians doubting the safety of warfarin, the first sign of a complication might suffice to withdraw the patient from the study. Finally, those on a warfarin program have a greater likelihood of being monitored more closely than those on, say, aspirin or another platelet antiaggregant. All of these concerns are obviated by a double-blind design, but only if the double-blind design works.

In WARSS, the existence of a true-aspirin/false-warfarin arm meant data accumulated for the false-INR values, those values created by the coordinating center to keep the physicians and patients blinded as to who was receiving what therapy. Inspection of the false-INR values for the aspirin arm allowed an estimate of whether the clinicians were using the INR value as a guide to their decisions as to outcome. The trial design for WARSS allowed tests of the effect on outcome from treatment biases of the participants. Analysis of the false-INR values for the aspirin arm (having no direct biologic effect on outcome) showed no indication that study physicians detected symptoms or signs suggesting stroke based on INR values reportedly higher or lower than the desired range. Further, the essentially identical mean and range of INR values used to treat the major subgroups of lacune, cryptogenic, and large-artery stroke provided no evidence that physicians selected target INR ranges based on bias toward treating certain clinically defined subgroups at different INR rates. In a Cox proportional hazards model for the log relative hazard, estimated Kaplan–Meier survival curves free of

primary events over a 2-year period were computed for those in the aspirin arm (false-INR values) and the warfarin arm. For those in the aspirin arm and on therapy, the estimated survival curves showed no variation and were essentially identical for those whose false INR was less than 1.4, in the range for WARSS (1.4–2.8), or greater than 2.8. No evidence was found indicating a relationship between outcome and false INRs. For the true-warfarin arm, however, a clear relationship was found between the INR value in the true-warfarin arm and outcomes, the event rates falling dramatically to a stable level for those patients whose INR was greater than 1.5.

Ischemic Stroke Subtypes and Differential Effects of Therapy in WARSS

Prior studies may have wisely shied away from attempts at characterizing the mechanism of the ischemic stroke. Such efforts have had a long history and a well-known degree of disagreement as to nomenclature and successful application of algorithms, having been described (31), refined (32), debated and contrasted with others (33), expanded (34), and, for at least some definitions, validated as clinically recognizable (35).

Accepting a minor degree of uncertainty in the exact application of diagnostic algorithms, the WARSS project classified recurrent ischemic strokes into three broad groups: lacunar, large artery, and cryptogenic. Given the debates that continue on the mechanism of infarction each of these is thought to represent, it was of interest to find the number and percentage of events in each of the three major infarct subtypes to be similar: For lacunar stroke, primary events occurred in 107 of 612 (17.5%) of patients on warfarin and in 95 of 625 (15.2%) of those on aspirin. For "cryptogenic" stroke, primary events occurred in 42 of 281 (14.9%) of patients on warfarin and in 48 of 295 (16.3%) of those on aspirin. For large-artery stroke, primary events occurred in 27 of 144 (18.7%) in patients on warfarin and in 18 of 115 (15.6%) of those on aspirin (Table 32-4).

Were no further efforts made to analyze the basis for the diagnosis in such cases, there would be ample basis for concluding that prior trials loosely diagnosing "stroke" or "ischemic stroke" should suffice to settle the essential homogeneity of the therapeutic effects between an anticoagulant and a platelet antiaggregant. However, in the analysis plan constructed by the investigators and reviewed with the National Institutes of Health-supported performance, safety, and monitoring board, a number of detailed subset

TABLE 32-4. *Outcome by baseline stroke subtype in WARSS*

| | | Probability of event at 2 yr | | | | |
	No.	Warfarin	Aspirin	Hazard ratio	95% CI	p
Cryptogenic	576	15.0	16.5	0.92[a]	0.61–1.39	0.68
Lacunar	1,237	17.1	15.2	1.15[a]	0.88–1.52	0.31
Large artery	259	18.8	15.7	1.22[a]	0.67–2.22	0.51
Other	63	36.7	21.2	1.99	0.77–5.15	0.15

CI, confidence interval; WARSS, Warfarin–Aspirin Recurrent Stroke Study.

analyses had been planned and were undertaken. The results were presented at the Joint International Stroke Meeting in San Antonio, Texas, U.S.A., in February 2002, in a special symposium devoted to WARSS. At that symposium, the general results from parallel studies conducted within the WARSS cohort were presented, showing no effect on recurrent stroke and no differential response to warfarin or aspirin for those showing an antiphospholipid profile considered sufficient for a diagnosis of the antiphospholipid syndrome or for those whose circulating values of the prothrombin split product F1.2 (formerly known as F1+2) were measured and/or for those with or without a cardiac patent foramen ovale.

Recalling the cryptogenic group as the only one showing the faintest hint of warfarin effect, but not statistically significant, exploratory analyses found a 30% risk reduction ($p = 0.02$) for those nonhypertensive individuals whose infarcts affected the cerebral convexity, the convexity plus a deep ipsilateral infarct, or whose infarct was "large and deep" (beyond the size bounds usually considered examples of lacunar infarction). For many clinicians, the cryptogenic subtype is suspected to contain many occult examples of embolism, even if no obvious source is found. This 30% risk reduction could mean such cases represent a link to the warfarin effects found at similar levels of risk reduction with warfarin. The data supporting this possibility come from a randomized, double-blind trial with prespecified subset analyses and, although they may not suffice for the most violent critics, could provide a link with a warfarin effect in atrial fibrillation to occult embolism without atrial fibrillation. Further studies would be useful, but support for yet another warfarin trial may be limited.

Similar subset analyses provided no comfort for those whose practice has been to consider warfarin the stronger of the two agents for large-artery disease and lacunes. In these settings, warfarin use, if anything, had a slightly higher rate of primary events.

The lacune group (1,237 patients) was of sufficient size that the lack of difference between the two treatment arms, even a clear numerical difference favoring aspirin, is likely to blunt further studies of this direct comparison. The large-artery stroke subgroup contained smaller numbers (259) but also showed no treatment differences by intent-to-treat analysis. Subset analyses showed a far higher recurrent rate for the warfarin arm in primary brainstem infarction. How these data impact on the ongoing trial comparing warfarin with aspirin (36), which seeks a 50% risk reduction favoring warfarin, can only be speculated.

Pursued below the first level of analysis, the WARSS findings suggest future trials should not be content merely to count "strokes" but would profit from a detailed data collection mechanism, from issues of diagnosis subtype to estimates of severity (37), only slowly emerging in more recent clinical trial designs. The field has gone beyond head counts and now needs information which bears on therapy directed at the cause. Infectious disease specialists wish to hear of the nature of the organism and its sensitivities to various antimicrobials as the expected point of departure in treating a fever of infectious origin. Until stroke specialists insist on the same, we will still be using the vascular equivalent of broad-spectrum antibiotics. We should follow this lead.

Combined Warfarin and Aspirin Therapy

Painful experience argues against the simple assumption that a decision between these two classes of drug can be avoided by their simple combination in the prevention of recurrent ischemic stroke. No trial has directly assessed this point, but "stroke" as an outcome in several trials suggests clinicians will be disappointed when they infer that the two agents can be managed safely if the INR is kept under 3.0.

A range of studies has pursued the possibility that a combination of aspirin and warfarin may achieve the best of both with the least complications. Sad to see, none of the efforts as yet appears either to show such benefits or to achieve them without worrisome hemorrhagic complications. Two sets of studies exist, the first after myocardial infarction. The original Coumadin Aspirin Reinfarction Study showed no superiority of fixed-dose warfarin (1 or 3 mg) plus aspirin (80 mg) compared with aspirin alone (160 mg). The recently completed Warfarin–Aspirin Reinfarction Study (WARIS-II) (38) achieved benefits for warfarin (INR 2.0 to 2.5) plus aspirin 75 versus aspirin 160 mg and for warfarin (INR 2.8 to 4.2) versus aspirin 160 mg, but the hope that hemorrhagic complications with the combination could be avoided given the adjustment of INR in the range of 2.0 to 2.5 was not realized: The hemorrhagic complication rates were comparable with those with the warfarin with high INR ranges. The CHAMP (Combination Hemotherapy and Mortality Prevention) Study (39) fits between these two extremes, testing warfarin (INR 1.5 to 2.5) plus aspirin 81 mg against aspirin 162 mg (no expected difference between 160 and 162 mg if none has been found for wider differences in dose). As in other studies, no benefits accrued for prevention of recurrent myocardial infarction, and the combination group had a far higher major bleeding rate of 1.28 versus 0.72 events/100 person-years ($p < 0.001$).

A recent study in a setting of atrial fibrillation has come to similar disappointing conclusions (40). This French 49-institution, placebo-controlled, double-blind, randomized trial included patients with atrial fibrillation over age 65 years who had had a prior "thromboembolic event" to fluindione plus placebo or fluindione plus aspirin at a targeted INR of 2.0 to 2.6. The primary endpoint was a combination of stroke (ischemic or hemorrhagic), myocardial infarction, systemic arterial emboli, or vascular death. The 157 patients were followed an average of a mere 0.84 year. The imbalance was great, with 10 nonfatal hemorrhagic complications in the combination group (13.1%) versus 1 in the anticoagulation-only group (1.2%) ($p = 0.003$).

The findings to date suffice to argue against safety, even given unsettled possible benefits from higher-dose combined therapies. The findings also argue that those inclined to use any combined therapy are unlikely, at best, to see enough patients in their practice to test any benefits or, at worst, to be aware of the risks from hemorrhagic complications amply documented in these studies. Assuming the findings are broadly representative for vascular disease in general, they may also damp enthusiasm for combined warfarin and aspirin therapy in other vascular beds, cerebrovascular in particular.

REFERENCES

1. Starkey I, Warlow C. The secondary prevention of stroke in patients with atrial fibrillation. *Arch Neurol* 1986;43:66–68.
2. Yatsu FM, Hart RG, Mohr JP, et al. Anticoagulation of embolic strokes of cardiac origin: an update. *Neurology* 1988;38:314–316.
3. Sandercock P, Warlow C, Bamford J, et al. Is a controlled trial of long-term oral anticoagulants in patients with stroke and non-rheumatic atrial fibrillation worthwhile? *Lancet* 1986;1:788–792.
4. Sixty Plus Reinfarction Study Research Group. A double-blind trial to assess long-term oral anticoagulant therapy in elderly patients after myocardial infarction. *Lancet* 1980;2:989–993.
5. Petersen P, Boysen G, Godtfredsen J, et al. Placebo-controlled, randomised trial of warfarin and aspirin for prevention of thromboembolic complications in chronic atrial fibrillation. The Copenhagen AFASAK Study. *Lancet* 1989;1:175–179.
6. Boston Area Anticoagulation Trial of Atrial Fibrillation Investigators. The effect of low-dose warfarin on the risk of stroke in patients with non-reheumatic atrial fibrillation. *N Engl J Med* 1990;323:1505–1511.
7. Stroke Prevention in Atrial Fibrillation Investigators. Warfarin versus aspirin for prevention of thromboembolism in atrial fibrillation: Stroke Prevention in Atrial Fibrillation III Study. *Lancet* 1996;348:633–639.
8. Ezekowitz MD, Bridgers SL, James KE, et al. Warfarin in the prevention of stroke associated with non-rheumatic atrial fibrillation. Veterans Affairs Stroke Prevention in Nonrheumatic Atrial Fibrillation. *N Engl J Med* 1992;327:1406–1412.
9. Goldstein LB, Adams R, Becker K, et al. Primary prevention of ischemic stroke: a statement for healthcare professionals from the Stroke Council of the American Heart Association. *Stroke* 2001;32:280–299.
10. Mohr JP, Thompson JL, Lazar RM, et al. A comparison of warfarin and aspirin for the prevention of recurrent ischemic stroke. *N Engl J Med* 2001;345:1444–1451.
11. EAFT Study Group. Secondary prevention in non-rheumatic atrial fibrillation after transient ischemic attack or minor stroke. *Lancet* 1993;342:1255–1262.
12. Gullov AL, Koefoed BG, Petersen P. Bleeding during warfarin and aspirin therapy in patients with atrial fibrillation: the AFASAK 2 Study. Atrial Fibrillation Aspirin and Anticoagulation. *Arch Intern Med* 1999;159:1322–1328.
13. Yamaguchi T. Optimal intensity of warfarin therapy for secondary prevention of stroke in patients with nonlvular atrial fibrillation: a multicenter, prospective, randomized trial. Japanese Nonvalvular Atrial Fibrillation–Embolism Secondary Prevention Cooperative Study Group. *Stroke* 2000;31:817–821.
14. World Health Organization Report 1989.
15. Mohr JP. Cryptogenic stroke [Editorial]. *N Engl J Med* 1988;318:1197–1198.
16. Lewis SC, Sandercock PAG. Warfarin or aspirin for recurrent ischemic stroke [Letter and reply]. *N Engl J Med* 2002;346:1169–1171.

17. Hankey GJ. Warfarin–Aspirin Recurrent Stroke Study (WARSS) trial: is warfarin really a reasonable therapeutic alternative to aspirin for preventing recurrent noncardioembolic ischemic stroke? *Stroke* 2002;33:1723–1726.

18. Hier DB, Foulkes MA, Swiontoniowski M, et al. Stroke recurrence within 2 years after ischemic infarction. *Stroke* 1991;22:155–161.

19. Sacco RL, Shi T, Zamanillo MC, et al. Predictors of mortality and recurrence after hospitalized cerebral infarction in an urban community: the Northern Manhattan Stroke Study. *Neurology* 1994;44:626–634.

20. Petty GW, Brown RD Jr, Whisnant JP, et al. Ischemic stroke subtypes: a population-based study of functional outcome, survival, and recurrence. *Stroke* 2000;3: 1062–1068.

21. Millenson MM, Bauer KA, Kistler JP, et al. Monitoring "mini-intensity" anticoagulation with warfarin: comparison of the prothrombin time using a sensitive thromboplastin with prothrombin fragment F1+2 levels. *Blood* 1992;79:2034–2038.

22. Yamaguchi T. Optimal intensity of warfarin therapy for secondary prevention of stroke in patients with nonvalvular atrial fibrillation: a multicenter, prospective, randomized trial. Japanese Nonvalvular Atrial Fibrillation–Embolism Secondary Prevention Cooperative Study Group. *Stroke* 2000;31:817–821.

23. Pengo V, Legnani C, Noventa F, et al. Oral anticoagulant therapy in patients with nonrheumatic atrial fibrillation and risk of bleeding. A Multicenter Inception Cohort Study. ISCOAT Study Group. Italian Study on Complications of Oral Anticoagulant Therapy. *Thromb Haemost* 2001;85:418–422.

24. Liu M, Counsell C, Sandercock P. Anticoagulants for preventing recurrence following ischaemic stroke or transient ischemic attack [Cochrane review]. In: *Cochrane library.* Oxford: Update Software, 2001:1.

25. Go AS, Hylek EM, Phillips KA, et al. Implications of stroke risk criteria on the anticoagulation decision in nonvalvular atrial fibrillation: the Anticoagulation and Risk Factors in Atrial Fibrillation (ATRIA) study. *Circulation* 2000;102:11–13.

26. Stroke Prevention in Reversible Ischemia Trial (SPIRIT) Study Group. A randomized trial of anticoagulants versus aspirin after cerebral ischemia of presumed arterial origin. *Ann Neurol* 1997;42:857–865.

27. Gorter JW. Major bleeding during anticoagulation after cerebral ischemia: patterns and risk factors. Stroke Prevention in Reversible Ischemia Trial (SPIRIT). European Atrial Fibrillation Trial (EAFT) Study Groups. *Neurology* 1999;53:1319–1327.

28. De Schryver EL. Design of ESPRIT: an international randomized trial for secondary prevention after non-disabling cerebral ischaemia of arterial origin. Euro-pean/Australian Stroke Prevention in Reversible Ischaemia Trial (ESPRIT) Group. *Cerebrovasc Dis* 2000;10:147–150.

29. Witte K, Thackray S, Clark AL, et al. Clinical trials update: IMPROVEMENT-HF, COPERNICUS, MUS-TIC, ASPECT-II, APRICOT and HEART. *Eur J Heart Fail* 2000;2:455–460.

30. Huynh T, ThÈroux P, Bogaty P, et al. Aspirin, warfarin, or the combination for secondary prevention of coronary events in patients with acute coronary syndromes and prior coronary artery bypass surgery. *Circulation* 2001;103:3069.

31. Mohr JP, Caplan LR, Melski JW, et al. The Harvard Cooperative Stroke Registry: a prospective registry. *Neurology* 1978;28:754–762.

32. Kunitz SC, Gross CR, Heyman A, et al. The pilot Stroke Data Bank: definition, design, and data. *Stroke* 1984;15: 740–746.

33. Tei H, Uchiyama S, Ohara K, et al. Deteriorating ischemic stroke in 4 clinical categories classified by the Oxfordshire Community Stroke Project. *Stroke* 2000; 31:2049–2054.

34. Gan R, Sacco RL, Kargman DE, et al. Testing the validity of the lacunar hypothesis: the Northern Manhattan Stroke Study experience. *Neurology* 1997;48: 1204–1211.

35. Madden KP, Karanjia PN, Adams HP Jr, et al. Accuracy of initial stroke subtype diagnosis in the TOAST Study. Trial of ORG 10172 in Acute Stroke Treatment. *Neurology* 1995;45:1975–1979.

36. Warfarin–Aspirin Symptomatic Intracranial Disease (WASID) Study Group. Prognosis of patients with symptomatic vertebral or basilar artery stenosis. *Stroke* 1998;29:1389–1392.

37. Sivenius J, Cunha L, Diener HC, et al. Antiplatelet treatment does not reduce the severity of subsequent stroke. European Stroke Prevention Study 2. *Neurology* 1999;53:825–829.

38. Hurlen M, Smith P, Arnesen H. Effects of warfarin, aspirin and the two combined, on mortality and thromboembolic morbidity after myocardial infarction. The WARIS-II (Warfarin–Aspirin Reinfarction Study) design. *Scand Cardiovasc J* 2000;34:168–171.

39. Fiore LD, Ezekowitz MD, Brophy MT, et al. Department of Veterans Affairs Cooperative Studies Program Clinical Trial comparing combined warfarin and aspirin with aspirin alone in survivors of acute myocardial infarction: primary results of the CHAMP Study. *Circulation* 2002;105:557–563.

40. Lechat P, Lardoux H, Mallet A, et al. Anticoagulant (fluindione)–aspirin combination in patients with high-risk atrial fibrillation. A randomized trial. *Cerebrovasc Dis* 2001;12:245–252.

Ischemic Stroke: Advances in Neurology, Vol. 92. Edited by
H.J.M. Barnett, Julien Bogousslavsky, and Heather Meldrum.
Lippincott Williams & Wilkins, Philadelphia © 2003.

33

Antithrombotic Therapy for Atherosclerotic Intracranial Arterial Stenosis

Marc I. Chimowitz

Department of Neurology, Emory University and Stroke Program, Department of Neurology Emory University Hospital, Atlanta, Georgia, U.S.A.

Atherosclerotic stenosis of the major intracranial arteries (carotid siphon, middle cerebral artery, vertebral artery, basilar artery) is an important cause of stroke, accounting for approximately 5% to 10% of ischemic strokes in the U.S.A. or at least 40,000 strokes annually (1). The importance of intracranial atherosclerosis as a cause of stroke is underscored when one considers that two other common causes of stroke, nonvalvular atrial fibrillation and extracranial carotid stenosis, account for approximately 70,000 and 85,000 strokes, respectively, in the U.S.A. each year (2,3). Blacks, Asians, and Hispanics appear to be at particularly high risk of stroke from intracranial arterial stenosis (4,5), possibly because of the high incidence of hypertension in these patients.

Previous studies, only one of which was prospective (6), suggest that the annual risk of stroke in patients with intracranial stenosis is 3% to 15% (Table 33-1) (6–10). Retrospective studies have suggested that patients with basilar or intracranial vertebral artery stenosis (11) (Fig. 33-1), severe intracra-

nial stenosis (greater than 80%) (7), or intracranial atherosclerosis with ischemic events while on antithrombotic therapy may be at highest risk of stroke (12). Treatment of patients with intracranial arterial stenosis has traditionally consisted of antithrombotic therapy (antiplatelet therapy or anticoagulation) and management of vascular risk factors. More recently, angioplasty with or without stenting

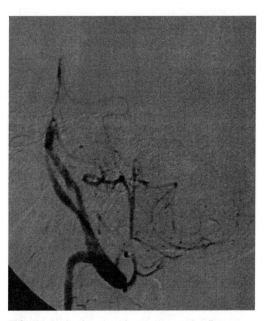

FIG. 33-1. Angiogram shows severe basilar artery stenosis in a patient presenting with a pontine infarct. Therapeutic options include anticoagulation, antiplatelet therapy, and angioplasty/stenting, but there are no data from randomized, controlled studies to indicate the optimal therapy.

TABLE 33-1. *Risk of stroke in patients with stenosis of the major intracranial arteries*

Intracranial artery	Annual risk of stroke
Carotid siphon	4%–12% in any territory, 8% in same territory (6,8,10)
Middle cerebral artery	10% in any territory, 8% in same territory (6,8,10)
Vertebral artery	4%–13% in any territory, 3%–8% in same territory (7,9,11)
Basilar artery	3%–15% in any territory, 2.5%–11% in same territory (7,9,11)

has emerged as a potential therapeutic option, but data on the efficacy and safety of this procedure for intracranial stenosis are rudimentary (13). This chapter will focus on antithrombotic therapy for intracranial arterial stenosis.

ANTITHROMBOTIC THERAPY FOR SYMPTOMATIC INTRACRANIAL STENOSIS

Despite the importance of intracranial stenosis as a cause of ischemic stroke, there have been no prospective trials comparing different antithrombotic agents in patients with this disease. Antiplatelet agents (aspirin, ticlopidine, clopidogrel, combination aspirin and extended-release dipyridamole) are frequently used in this setting based on studies that have shown a benefit of these agents for lowering the risk of stroke in patients with noncardioembolic transient ischemic attack (TIA) or minor stroke (14). However, the efficacy of antiplatelet agents has not been established specifically in patients with symptomatic intracranial large-artery disease. Only one of these agents (aspirin 1,300 mg/day) has been evaluated in a population of patients with intracranial arterial stenosis. In the Extracranial/Intracranial (EC/IC) Bypass Trial, there was no significant benefit of surgical bypass over aspirin in patients with symptomatic stenosis of the intracranial carotid or middle cerebral artery (6). However, the absence of a placebo arm in that study does not permit the conclusion that aspirin is specifically efficacious for the treatment of intracranial stenosis. In fact, the relatively high rate of stroke in patients with carotid siphon or middle cerebral artery stenosis who were treated with aspirin (1,300 mg/day) in the medical arm of the EC/IC Bypass Study (7.7%–9.5%/patient-year) suggests the need for more efficacious therapies for this disease (6,10).

Ticlopidine, another antiplatelet agent, was shown to be slightly more effective than aspirin for secondary stroke prevention in patients with noncardioembolic TIA or minor stroke (15). However, the efficacy of ticlopidine in patients with symptomatic intracranial stenosis has not been established either. A *post hoc* analysis of the Ticlopidine–Aspirin Stroke Study (TASS) suggests that ticlopidine may be more effective in blacks than in whites (16). As blacks are at higher risk of intracranial large-artery stenosis, it might be inferred that ticlopidine is effective therapy for this disease. However, blacks are also at higher risk of intracranial small-vessel disease, for which ticlopidine may be effective. If cerebral angiography had been performed routinely in TASS, clarification of the role of ticlopidine in patients with intracranial

large-artery stenosis might have been possible. However, angiography was performed in only approximately half the patients in this study, most of whom had carotid territory symptoms. Of note is that in the subgroup of patients with extracranial carotid stenosis greater than 70%, ticlopidine was significantly less effective than aspirin for preventing stroke (17). This finding raises a question about the efficacy of ticlopidine for the treatment of intracranial large-artery stenosis. Moreover, the association of neutropenia and thrombotic thrombocytopenic purpura with ticlopidine has raised concerns about the safety profile of this agent.

Clopidogrel, a safer congener of ticlopidine, has been compared with aspirin (325 mg/day) in the Clopidogrel Versus Aspirin in Patients at Risk of Ischemic Events (CAPRIE) Trial (18). Although clopidogrel was slightly more effective than aspirin in preventing stroke, myocardial infarction, or vascular death in patients presenting with myocardial infarction, stroke, or peripheral vascular disease, clopidogrel was not significantly more effective than aspirin in the stroke cohort alone. Moreover, the CAPRIE Trial did not provide data on the relative efficacy of clopidogrel versus aspirin in patients with stroke caused by intracranial arterial stenosis. Although the combination of extended-release dipyridamole and low-dose aspirin (50 mg daily) was significantly more effective than either agent alone for preventing stroke in patients presenting with TIA or stroke in the European Stroke Prevention Study (ESPS) II Trial (19), this study also did not address the efficacy of combined extended-release dipyridamole and aspirin in patients with intracranial arterial stenosis.

Combination antiplatelet therapy has become the preferred antithrombotic treatment for some vascular disorders. Randomized studies have shown that combining aspirin with ticlopidine or clopidogrel is more effective than aspirin alone or warfarin for preventing myocardial infarction following coronary artery angioplasty with stenting (20). Additionally, a recent study showed that clopidogrel in addition to aspirin was significantly ($p < 0.001$) more effective than aspirin alone for preventing the composite endpoint of death from cardiovascular causes, nonfatal myocardial infarction, or stroke in patients with acute coronary syndromes followed for a mean of 9 months (21). However, there were significantly more ($p = 0.001$) patients with major bleeding in the combination treatment group. There are no data on the safety and efficacy of combined aspirin and clopidogrel in patients presenting with TIA or stroke, though studies addressing this are ongoing.

Warfarin is frequently used for the treatment of intracranial stenosis based on the results of nonrandomized, retrospective studies of patients with symptoms suggestive of vertebrobasilar disease (22,23). In a retrospective, nonangiographic study of patients with vertebrobasilar symptoms, Whisnant et al. (23) found that patients treated with anticoagulation had a lower risk of stroke in the first 6 months of treatment compared with untreated patients; however, the rates of stroke beyond 6 months were similar in both groups.

There has been only one study comparing warfarin directly with aspirin in patients with intracranial arterial stenosis; however, this was a retrospective, nonrandomized study (7). Eligibility criteria for the study were (a) angiographically proven 50% to 99% stenosis of one of the major intracranial arteries, (b) a TIA or stroke in the distribution of the stenotic artery, and (c) therapy with aspirin or warfarin (based on local physician preference). The most common dose of aspirin was 325 mg/day, and the dose of warfarin was typically adjusted to maintain prothrombin times in the range of 1.2 to 1.6 times control values. The study was performed prior to the widespread application of the international normalized ratio (INR). Primary endpoints in this study were ischemic stroke in any vascular territory, myocardial infarction, or sudden death. Hemorrhages were classified as major (fatal hemorrhage, any intracranial hemorrhage, bleeding requiring hospitalization, bleeding requiring transfusion) or minor (any other bleeding complication).

Of the 151 patients in the study, 88 patients (58%) were treated with warfarin and 63 patients (42%) were treated with aspirin. There were no significant differences in the frequency of risk factors for stroke between the two groups. Major ischemic events (ischemic stroke, myocardial infarction, or sudden death) occurred in 26 patients on aspirin during 143 patient-years of follow-up and in 14 patients on warfarin during 166 patient-years of follow-up ($p < 0.01$, log rank test). Hemorrhagic complications occurred in 13 patients on warfarin (3 major, 10 minor) during 166 patient-years of follow-up and in 2 patients on aspirin (both minor) during 143 patient-years of follow-up ($p < 0.01$, log rank test) (7). Cox proportional hazards analysis showed that the relative risk of stroke, myocardial infarction, or sudden death in patients treated with warfarin was 0.45 [95% confidence interval (CI) 0.23–0.86] compared with patients treated with aspirin. The major effect of warfarin was to prevent stroke.

Patients with moderate intracranial stenosis (50%–69%) had a lower risk of stroke in the same vascular territory than patients with a severe intracranial stenosis (70%–99%). Of 62 patients with 50%–69% intracranial stenosis, 5 patients (6%) had a stroke in the same territory as the stenotic artery during a median follow-up of 20 months [4 of 28 (14%) on aspirin, 1 of 34 (3%) on warfarin]. In comparison, of 89 patients with 70%–99% intracranial stenosis, 9 patients (10%) had a stroke in the same territory as the stenotic artery during a median follow-up of 14 months [5 of 35 (14%) on aspirin, 4 of 54 (7%) on warfarin]. Patients with stenosis of the vertebral or basilar arteries had a higher rate of stroke in the same vascular territory than patients with carotid siphon or middle cerebral artery stenosis (basilar artery 11%/year, vertebral artery 8%/year, carotid siphon 2%/year, middle cerebral artery 3%/year) (11).

Whereas this study suggests that warfarin may be more efficacious than aspirin 325 mg/day for the treatment of symptomatic intracranial arterial stenosis, the retrospective, nonrandomized, unblinded study design does not provide definitive evidence regarding the use of warfarin versus aspirin in this setting. Moreover, the results of a recent randomized, double-blind trial [WARSS (Warfarin–Aspirin Recurrent Stroke Study)] of 2,206 patients with noncardioembolic stroke treated with warfarin (INR 1.4–2.8) or aspirin (325 mg/day) suggest further caution in concluding that warfarin is more effective than aspirin for intracranial arterial stenosis (24). In WARSS, the rates of the primary endpoint (recurrent stroke or death) were 17.8%/2 years in the warfarin group versus 16%/2 years in the aspirin group ($p = 0.25$) (24). As only a small percent of patients in WARSS had documented intracranial arterial stenosis, the results of WARSS do not clarify whether warfarin or aspirin is more effective for this disease. However, the fact that warfarin was not superior to aspirin in any of the major subgroups of stroke patients enrolled in WARSS (those with lacunar or cryptogenic stroke) should raise the question as to whether warfarin is superior to aspirin for intracranial arterial stenosis.

A definite recommendation regarding the comparative efficacy and safety of warfarin versus aspirin for intracranial stenosis must await the results of an ongoing study: the Warfarin–Aspirin Symptomatic Intracranial Disease (WASID) Trial (25). This is a National Institutes of Health-funded, randomized, double-blind clinical trial in which 806 patients with TIA or minor stroke caused by angiographically proven stenosis (50%–99%) of a major intracranial artery will be randomized to warfarin (INR 2–3) or aspirin (1,300 mg/day). This study will (a) determine whether warfarin or aspirin is more effective for preventing stroke and vascular death in these patients and (b) identify subgroups of patients with rates of ischemic stroke in the territory of the stenotic intracranial artery that are sufficiently high to justify a subsequent trial comparing intracranial angioplasty/stenting with medical therapy in these patients.

Until the results of WASID are known, how should patients with intracranial arterial stenosis be treated? If possible, patients should be offered the opportunity to participate in ongoing clinical trials such as WASID that evaluate medical therapies (see *http://www.sph.emory.edu/WASID* for a list of WASID sites). If this is not feasible, vascular risk management and individual physician choice of antithrombotic therapy should be the cornerstone of treatment. Currently, there are insufficient data to determine whether warfarin or antiplatelet therapy is superior or which antiplatelet agent is most effective for intracranial arterial stenosis (26).

ACKNOWLEDGMENT

The author is a recipient of a grant from the National Institutes of Health/National Institute of Neurological and Communication Disorders and Stroke (RO1-NS36643-01A1) to fund the WASID Trial.

REFERENCES

1. American Heart Association. *Heart and stroke facts: 1996 statistical supplement.* American Heart Association, 1995.
2. Executive Committee for the Asymptomatic Carotid Atherosclerosis Study. Endarterectomy for asymptomatic carotid artery stenosis. *JAMA* 1995;273:1421–1428.
3. Stroke Prevention in Atrial Fibrillation Study Group. Preliminary report of the Stroke Prevention in Atrial Fibrillation Study. *N Engl J Med* 1990;322:863–868.
4. Gorelick PB. Distribution of atherosclerotic cerebrovascular lesions. Effects of age, race, and sex. *Stroke* 1993;24[Suppl]:I16–I19.
5. Sacco RL, Kargman D, Gu Q, et al. Race–ethnicity and determinants of intracranial atherosclerotic cerebral infarction. The Northern Manhattan Stroke Study. *Stroke* 1995;26:14–20.
6. EC/IC Bypass Study Group. Failure of extracranial-intracranial arterial bypass to reduce the risk of ischemic stroke. Results of an international randomized trial. *N Engl J Med* 1985;313:1191–1200.
7. Chimowitz MI, Kokkinos J, Strong J, et al. The Warfarin–Aspirin Symptomatic Intracranial Disease Study. *Neurology* 1995;45:1488–1493.
8. Wechsler LR, Kistler JP, Davis KR, et al. The prognosis of carotid siphon stenosis. *Stroke* 1986;17:714–718.
9. Moufarrij NA, Little JR, Furlan AJ, et al. Basilar and distal vertebral artery stenosis: long term follow-up. *Stroke* 1986;17:938–942.
10. Bogousslavsky J, Barnett HJM, Fox AJ, et al., for the EC/IC Bypass Study Group. Atherosclerotic disease of the middle cerebral artery. *Stroke* 1986;17:1112–1120.
11. Warfarin–Aspirin Symptomatic Intracranial Disease (WASID) Study Group. Prognosis of patients with symptomatic vertebral or basilar artery stenosis. *Stroke* 1998;29:1389–1392.
12. Thijs VN, Albers GW. Symptomatic intracranial atherosclerosis: outcome of patients who fail antithrombotic therapy. *Neurology* 2000;55:490–497.
13. Chimowitz MI. Angioplasty or stenting is not appropriate as first-line treatment of intracranial stenosis. *Arch Neurol* 2001;58:1690–1692.
14. Antiplatelet Trialists' Collaboration. Secondary prevention of vascular disease by prolonged antiplatelet treatment. *Br Med J* 1988;296:320–331.
15. Hass WK, Easton JD, Adams HP Jr, et al. A randomized trial comparing ticlopidine hydrochloride with aspirin for the prevention of stroke in high risk patients. *N Engl J Med* 1989;321:501–507.
16. Weisberg LA, for the Ticlopidine–Aspirin Stroke Study Group. The efficacy and safety of ticlopidine in non-whites: analysis of a patient subgroup from the Ticlopidine–Aspirin Stroke Study. *Neurology* 1993;43:27–31.
17. Grotta JC, Norris JW, Kamm B, for the TASS Baseline and Angiographic Data Subgroup. Prevention of stroke with ticlopidine: who benefits most? *Neurology* 1992;42:111–115.
18. CAPRIE Steering Committee. A randomised, blinded, trial of clopidogrel versus aspirin in patients at risk of ischaemic events (CAPRIE). *Lancet* 1996;348:1329–1339.
19. Diener HC, Cunha L, Forbes C, et al. European Stroke Prevention Study 2. Dipyridamole and acetylsalicylic acid in the secondary prevention of stroke. *J Neurol Sci* 1996;143:1–13.
20. CURE Study Investigators. The Clopidogrel in Unstable Angina to Prevent Recurrent Events (CURE) Trial programme: rationale, design, and baseline characteristics including a meta-analysis of the effects of thienopyridines in vascular disease. *Eur Heart J* 2000;21:2033–2041.
21. Clopidogrel in Unstable Angina to Prevent Recurrent Events Trial investigators. Effects of clopidogrel in addition to aspirin inpatients with acute coronary syndromes without ST-segment elevation. *N Engl J Med* 2001;345:494–502.
22. Millikan CH, Siekert RG, Shick RM. Studies in cerebrovascular disease: III. The use of anticoagulant drugs in the treatment of insufficiency or thrombosis within the basilar arterial system. *Mayo Clin Proc* 1955;30:116–126.
23. Whisnant JP, Cartlidge NEF, Elveback LR. Carotid and vertebral–basilar transient ischemic attacks: effect of anticoagulants, hypertension, and cardiac disorders on survival and stroke occurrence—a population study. *Ann Neurol* 1978;3:107–115.
24. Mohr JP, Thompson JLP, Lazar RM, et al., for the Warfarin–Aspirin Recurrent Stroke Study Group. A comparison of warfarin and aspirin for the prevention of recurrent ischemic stroke. *N Engl J Med* 2001;345:1444–1451.
25. Major ongoing stroke trials. Warfarin versus aspirin for intracranial disease. *Stroke* 1999;30:2256–2261.
26. Benesch C, Chimowitz MI, for the WASID investigators. Best treatment for intracranial arterial stenosis? 50 years of uncertainty. *Neurology* 2000;55:465–466.

Ischemic Stroke: Advances in Neurology, Vol. 92. Edited by
H.J.M. Barnett, Julien Bogousslavsky, and Heather Meldrum.
Lippincott Williams & Wilkins, Philadelphia © 2003.

34

Antithrombotic Therapy in Small Subcortical Strokes (Lacunar Infarcts)

Oscar Benavente

*Department of Medicine, Division of Neurology, University of Texas Health Science Center,
San Antonio, Texas, U.S.A.*

Ischemic stroke is a syndrome with multiple etiologies and diverse pathogenic mechanisms. Therefore, adequate prevention of stroke recurrence should be targeted to the underlying mechanism responsible for the first stroke subtype, assuming that subsequent strokes are likely to be the same type as the first one.

In the past, clinical trials for secondary stroke prevention testing antithrombotic agents included a wide variety of stroke subtypes and drew a single conclusion regarding the efficacy of the intervention (1). Unfortunately, this approach led to inconclusive results about specific therapies for specific stroke subtypes. Stroke research has evolved; over the last decade, we have learned that different subtypes of stroke respond differently to specific interventions for secondary stroke prevention (i.e., cardioembolic stroke, carotid artery stenosis) (2–4). Despite this progress, it is still unclear which is the best strategy to prevent stroke recurrence in patients who suffer a small subcortical stroke (S3), commonly referred to

as a lacunar infarct, an important type of stroke. S3s comprise more than 25% of brain infarcts (5–13) (Table 34-1) and are particularly frequent in Hispanic Americans and African Americans (14), occur at a younger age than other types of ischemic strokes (15), and are the most common cause of vascular dementia (16,17).

Classic lacunar syndromes are commonly accompanied by a small, deep infarction, and each syndrome typically is associated with specific locations (18). These lesions are located deep in the cerebral hemispheres or brainstem, their size ranges from 3 to 15 mm in diameter, and most are caused by occlusion of a single small deep penetrating artery (20–22). Although relatively small in volume, S3s can cause functionally devastating neurologic deficits because of their location.

Are S3s simply small strokes, or do they respond to a specific type of cerebrovascular disease? Whereas any etiology of brain ischemia (e.g., cardiogenic

TABLE 34-1. *Frequency of patients with small subcortical stroke (S3) in case series*

Study	No. of patients with ischemic stroke	% of S3
Rothrock et al. (11)	500	27
Mohr et al. (12)	579	23
Yip et al. (10)	676	29
Bamford et al. (9)	515	21
Chamorro et al. (5)	1,273	26
Boon et al. (8)	755	27
Kolominsky-Rabas et al. (6)	583	26
Wolfe et al. (7)	862	33
Bogousslavsky et al. (13)	778	19
Aggregate	6,521	26

Criteria for S3 differed between studies.

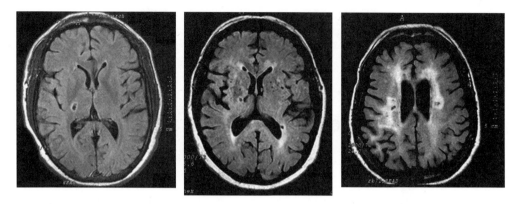

FIG. 34-1. Spectrum of white matter disease observed in participants of the Secondary Prevention of Small Subcortical Stroke (SPS3) pilot study. The number of small subcortical strokes (S3s) correlates with the extent of white matter abnormality (29).

embolism or carotid stenosis) can occasionally cause S3 (23–26), most S3s result from intrinsic diseases of the small penetrating arteries. Two pathologic types of small artery disease are responsible for most S3s: (a) lipohyalinosis, characterized by segmental disorganization of the vessel wall with replacement by fibrin and collagen deposits, and (b) microatheroma, where a small atheromatous plaque occludes the origin of the affected vessel, which tends to result in larger lesions. The latter is believed to be responsible for larger subcortical infarcts, whereas lipohyalinosis tends to affect smaller arteries leading to smaller subcortical infarcts (22,27). The presence of multiple S3s and associated extensive white matter abnormalities by magnetic resonance imaging supports the presence of cerebral small-artery disease (28–30) (Fig. 34-1). In short, the majority of S3s represent manifestations of intracranial small artery disease.

Risk factors for S3 (advancing age, hypertension, and diabetes) are similar to those of atherothrombotic stroke. Perhaps, the exception is hyperlipidemia, which does not to appear to be a risk factor for S3 (26). About 70% of patients with S3 in recent studies have a history of hypertension (31–34). Hypertension appears to play a key role in the development of widespread cerebral small-artery disease. Autopsy-based studies show an association between hypertension and the presence of multiple S3s (35,36).

STROKE RECURRENCE IN PATIENTS WITH SMALL SUBCORTICAL STROKE

While initial S3s often cause relatively mild neurologic disability and carry a low fatality rate (15,37), multiple or recurrent S3s give rise to more severe clinical manifestations including lacunar state (*état lacunaire*) and vascular dementia. From longitudinal studies, the rate of recurrent stroke among patients with S3 ranged from 4% to 11% (4,9,15,34,38–41) (Table 34-2) comparable with and perhaps slightly higher than other common types of cerebral ischemia. Most (about 60%) recurrent strokes in S3 patients are

TABLE 34-2. *Recurrent ischemic stroke in patients with small subcortical stroke (S3)*

Study	No. of patients with S3	Recurrent stroke
Bamford et al. (9)	102	11
Sacco et al. (34)	78	10
Clavier et al. (38)	172	4
Boiten and Lodder (15)	103	5
Samuelson et al. (54)	81	7
Miyao et al. (39)	190	9
Salgado et al. (41)	145	7
Petty et al. (40)	72	7
WARSS[a] (4)	1,237	8
Aggregate	2,180	8

WARSS, Warfarin–Aspirin Recurrent Stroke Study.
[a]Outcome stroke or death, patients assigned to aspirin or warfarin.

also S3s, supporting a distinctive pathomechanism. In the Secondary Prevention of Small Subcortical Stroke (SPS3) pilot study, patients with symptomatic recent S3, assigned to antiplatelet therapy plus strict control of hypertension, had an early recurrent stroke rate higher than previously reported, particularly among Hispanic Americans: 22%/year [95% confidence interval (CI) 11–42) (42). The presence of white matter abnormalities appears to predict a higher rate of recurrent stroke in S3 patients (39). White matter abnormalities on neuroimaging studies of S3 patients may be an indicator of the severity and extent of small-artery disease; therefore, white matter abnormalities may be an independent risk factor for stroke recurrence and cognitive decline in S3 patients as well as ethnicity.

SMALL SUBCORTICAL STROKE AND RISK OF VASCULAR DEMENTIA

Vascular dementia is the second most common cause of dementia after Alzheimer's disease, accounting for about 15% of all cases of dementia, with another 10% considered "mixed' cases of Alzheimer's disease and vascular dementia (43). Patients with S3 are at risk of developing vascular dementia. S3 is the most common stroke subtype that predisposes to vascular dementia (16,17,43). In two prospective studies, 11% and 23% of patients with first-ever S3 developed vascular dementia over the following 3 years (44,45). The estimated rate of clinically diagnosed vascular dementia in S3 patients has been reported as 3%/year to 5%/year (39,44). The incidence of vascular dementia was related to the rate of stroke recurrence: Demented patients had a significantly higher rate of stroke recurrence than patients who did not develop dementia (56% versus 17%). Conversely, S3s (most asymptomatic) are increased in vascular dementia (46–48), in which they are typically multiple and bilateral (45). It seems reasonable to hypothesize that interventions that reduce stroke recurrence may also prevent cognitive decline from vascular dementia in S3 patients.

ANTIPLATELET THERAPY IN SMALL SUBCORTICAL STROKES

Despite the fact that most S3s are due to disease of the small cerebral arteries, it is highly probable that the final common pathway in S3s and atherothrombotic stroke involves platelet aggregation and thrombus formation. Therefore, it is sensible to speculate that antithrombotic agents that are proven to be beneficial in atherothrombotic strokes would be effective in preventing stroke recurrence and vascular dementia following S3.

Whereas S3 represents more than 25% of all ischemic strokes, there have been no stroke prevention trials focusing on this important stroke subtype. Therefore, all the data concerning safety and efficacy of antiplatelet therapy in S3 patients derive from subgroup analyses of clinical trials where all ischemic strokes were studied together. Only five randomized clinical trials for secondary stroke prevention reported the outcomes in subgroups of participants with S3 as their index event separately (4,49–52).

In the French AICLA aspirin trial, a total of 603 patients with ischemic cerebral events were included in this double-blind study to determine whether high-dose aspirin or aspirin plus dipyridamole would reduce stroke recurrence over a 3-year period compared with placebo. Ninety-seven patients with S3 as a qualifying event were enrolled. Recurrent stroke was reduced by 69% ($p = 0.03$) among those with S3 given aspirin with or without dipyridamole versus 31% (p = NS) for those with nonlacunar ischemic stroke. This yielded an absolute stroke reduction among S3 patients of 18% over 3 years (26% placebo versus 8% treatment) (95% CI 2–34) (51).

The Canadian–American Ticlopidine Study (ticlopidine versus placebo) enrolled 26% of the participants with S3 as the qualifying event (n = 275). The overall risk reduction of composite outcome (stroke, myocardial infarction, and vascular death) was 30% (95% CI 8–48) in favor of ticlopidine. The relative risk reduction for the endpoint of stroke and stroke death among S3 patients assigned to ticlopidine was 50%/year (from 10%/year to 5%/year) with a wide CI (95% CI 0.76 –76). For nonlacunar stroke type, the reduction for similar endpoint was only 23%; however, the differences did not achieve statistical significance (52).

The Cilostazol Stroke Prevention Study, conducted in Japan, randomized more than 1,000 S3 patients (75% of the total number of patients) to cilostazol or placebo within 6 months of the index event. All S3s were confirmed at study entry by neuroimaging studies; the primary outcome was stroke recurrence. The overall risk reduction was 42% in favor of cilostazol. S3 patients had a slightly superior benefit with a risk reduction of 43% (95% CI 3–67), favoring active treatment (49).

A fourth trial, the Chinese Acute Stroke Trial (CAST), randomized more than 6,000 patients with lacunar stroke as the index event to aspirin or placebo and considered stroke recurrence or death at 30 days of entry. The event rate during this short period of time was 2.6% in those assigned to aspirin versus

2.9% in the placebo group, representing a 10% relative risk reduction (95% CI −0.5–1.1). Although this trial cannot be considered strictly a secondary stroke prevention owing to the short follow-up, the results support the effect of antiplatelet agents in patients with S3 (50).

Recently, the Warfarin–Aspirin Recurrent Stroke Study (WARSS) randomized 2,206 patients with non-cardioembolic stroke to aspirin or oral anticoagulant with a mean follow-up of 2 years; 1,237 of the enrolled patients had a lacunar infarct as an index event. The outcome of stroke or death in patients with S3 was 8%/year on aspirin and 9%/year in the warfarin group; this trend in favor of aspirin did not reach statistical significance ($p = 0.31$). This study has the largest sample size of S3 patients with a long-term follow-up. Unfortunately, this trial was underpowered to definitively detect a differential efficacy for aspirin over warfarin in this stroke subtype (4). According to WARSS, existing data favor use of antiplatelet agents instead of warfarin for secondary prevention in S3 patients.

Based on the available evidence, it seems reasonable to speculate that antithrombotic agents have similar or superior effect to prevent stroke recurrence in patients with S3 when compared with other stroke subtypes. However, all the studies to date have been underpowered to determine the efficacy of the intervention, and in addition, the index event was not strictly defined or documented by neuroimaging test, except in one (49). This has the potential problem of studying patients without a homogeneous mechanism (i.e., small-artery disease). Methodologic weaknesses limit the validity and ability to generalize the results of these studies.

There is a need for further research in this area, with randomized clinical trials focusing on populations with S3, to develop risk stratifications and better define the risk/benefit of the use of antiplatelet agents. Intracranial small-artery disease remains understudied relative to its importance as a cause of neurologic disability. The SPS3 Phase III National Institutes of Health/National Institute of Neurological and Communication Disorders and Stroke-funded trial will enroll 2,500 with recent symptomatic S3 documented by magnetic resonance imaging. Patients will be randomized in a factorial design to two interventions: (a) antiplatelet therapy: (i) aspirin 325 mg/day or (ii) aspirin plus clopidogrel 75 mg/day; and (b) systolic targets of blood pressure control: (i) "intensive" less than 130 mm Hg or (ii) "usual" 130 to 149 mm Hg. Follow-up will be for 3 years, and the outcomes are recurrent stroke, cognitive decline (vascular dementia), and vascular death. With use of intensive clinical and magnetic resonance imaging

evaluation at study entry, subgroups of S3 patients with different natural histories and different responses to antiplatelet therapy and blood pressure control will be sought. The study will start enrolling patients in early 2003.

At present, there is no definitive answer as to what is the best strategy for stroke prevention in patients with index S3. The evidence favors the use of antiplatelet agents over oral anticoagulants for stroke prevention (4). Aspirin, in doses between 75 and 325 mg/day, remains the standard initial antiplatelet agent for patients with S3. The combination of aspirin plus dipyridamole or clopidogrel may be acceptable options for secondary stroke prevention in this stroke subtype. In patients intolerant to aspirin, clopidogrel should be used as initial therapy. Adding clopidogrel to aspirin for secondary stroke prevention may produce additional benefits, but there is no evidence yet to support the use of this therapy. Until the results of clinical trials are available, the recommendations based on other stroke subtypes seem sensible (1,53).

ACKNOWLEDGMENT

I gratefully acknowledge Dr. Robert G. Hart for his advice and criticism in reviewing the manuscript. This work was supported in part by National Institutes of Health/National Institute of Neurological and Communication Disorders and Stroke grant R01 NS 38529.

REFERENCES

1. Antithrombotic Trialists' Collaboration. Collaborative meta-analysis of randomised trials of antiplatelet therapy for prevention of death, myocardial infarction, and stroke in high risk patients. *Br Med J* 2002;324:71–86.
2. Barnett HJM, Taylor DW, Eliasziw M. Benefit of carotid endarterectomy in symptomatic patients with moderate and severe stenosis. *N Engl J Med* 1998;339: 1415–1425.
3. SPAF I. Warfarin verus aspirin for the prevention of thromboembolism in atrial fibrillation: results of the Stroke Prevention in Atrial Fibrillation II Study. *Lancet* 1994;343:687–691.
4. Mohr JP, Thompson JLP, Lazar RM, et al. A comparison of warfarin and aspirin for the prevention of recurrent ischemic stroke. *N Engl J Med* 2001;345:1444–1451.
5. Chamorro A, Sacco R, Mohr JP, et al. Clinical-computed tomographic correlations of lacunar infarction in the Stroke Data Bank. *Stroke* 1991;22:175–181.
6. Kolominsky-Rabas PL, Weber M, Gefeller O, et al. Epidemiology of ischemic stroke subtypes according to TOAST criteria. Incidence, recurrence, and long-term survival in ischemic stroke subtypes: a population-based study. *Stroke* 2001;32:2735–2740.
7. Wolfe CDA, Rudd AG, Howard R, et al. Incidence and case fatality rates of stroke subtypes in a multiethnic

population: the South London Stroke Register. *J Neurol Neurosurg Psychiatry* 2002;72:211–216.
8. Boon A, Lodder J, Heuts-van Raak L, et al. Silent brain infarcts in 755 consecutive patients with a first-ever supratentorial ischemic stroke. *Stroke* 1994;25: 2384–2390.
9. Bamford JM, Sandercock P, Jones L, et al. The natural history of lacunar infarction: the Oxfordshire Community Stroke Project. *Stroke* 1987;18:545–551.
10. Yip PK, Jeng JS, Lee TK, et al. Subtypes of ischemic stroke. A hospital-based stroke registry in Taiwan (SCAN-IV). *Stroke* 1997;28:2507–2512.
11. Rothrock JF, Lyden PD, Brody ML. Analysis of ischemic stroke in an urban southern California population. *Arch Intern Med* 1993;153:619–624.
12. Mohr JP, Caplan LR, Melski JW, et al. The Harvard Cooperative Stroke Registry: a prospective registry. *Neurology* 1978;28:754–762.
13. Bogousslavsky J, Van Melle G, Regli F. The Lausanne Stroke Registry: analysis of 1,000 consecutive patients with first stroke. For the Lausanne Stroke Registry Group. *Stroke* 1988;19:1083–1092.
14. Hartmann A, Rundek T, Mast H, et al. Mortality and causes of death after first ischemic stroke. The Northern Manhattan Stroke Study. *Neurology* 2001;57: 2000–2005.
15. Boiten J, Lodder J. Prognosis for survival, handicap and recurrence of stroke in lacunar and superficial stroke. *Cerebrovasc Dis* 1993;3:221–226.
16. Ross G, Petrovitch H, White L, et al. Characterization of risk factors for vascular dementia: the Honolulu–Asia Aging Study. *Neurology* 1999;53:337–343.
17. Tatemichi TK, Desmond D, Paik M, et al. Clinical determinants of dementia related to stroke. *Ann Neurol* 1993;33:568–575.
18. Schoneville W, Tuhrim S, Singer M, et al. Diffusion-weighted MRI in acute lacunar syndromes: a clinical–radiological correlation study. *Stroke* 1999;30: 2066–2069.
19. Lindgren A, Staaf G, Geiger B, et al. Clinical lacunar syndromes as predictors of lacunar infarcts. A comparison of acute clinical lacunar syndromes and findings on diffusion-weighted MRI. *Acta Neurol Scand* 2000; 101:128–134.
20. Fisher CM. Lacunar strokes and infarcts: a review. *Neurology* 1982;32:871–876.
21. Fisher CM. Lacunes: small, deep cerebral infarcts. *Neurology* 1965;15:774–784.
22. Fisher CM. Thalamic pure sensory stroke: a pathologic study. *Neurology* 1978;35:126–128.
23. Boiten J, Luyckx GJ, Kessels F, et al. Risk factors for lacunes. *Neurology* 1996;47:1109.
24. Inzitari D, Eliasziw M, Sharp B, et al. Risk factors and outcome of patients with carotid stenosis presenting with lacunar stroke. *Neurology* 2000;54: 660–666.
25. Wong KS, Gao S, Chan YL, et al. Mechanisms of acute cerebral infarction in patients with middle cerebral artery stenosis: a diffusion-weighted imaging and microemboli monitoring study. *Ann Neurol* 2002;52: 74–81.
26. You R, McNeil JJ, O'Malley HM, et al. Risk factors for lacunar infarction syndromes. *Neurology* 1995;45: 1483–1487.
27. Caplan L. Intracranial branch atheromatous disease: a neglected, understudied, and underused concept. *Neurology* 1989;39:1246–1250.
28. Boiten J, Lodder J, Kessels F. Two clinically distinct lacunar infarct entities? *Stroke* 1993;24:652–656.
29. Benavente O, Palacio S, Kesava P, et al. White matter abnormalities in lacunar stroke patients. *Stroke* 2001; 32:28(abst).
30. Benavente O, Eliasziw M, Streifler J, et al. Prognosis of lacunar stroke patients in association with leukoaraiosis. *Stroke* 2001;32:366(abst).
31. Lammie AG, Brannan F. Nonhypertensive cerebral small-vessel disease. *Stroke* 1997;28:2222–2229.
32. Lodder J, Bamford JM. Are hypertension or cardiac embolism likely causes of lacunar infarction? *Stroke* 1990;21:375–381.
33. Mast H, Thompson AJ, Lee SH, et al. Hypertension and diabetes mellitus as determinants of multiple lacunar infarcts. *Stroke* 1995;26:30–33.
34. Sacco SE, Whisnant JP, Broderick JP, et al. Epidemiological characteristics of lacunar infarcts in a population. *Stroke* 1991;22:1236–1241.
35. Dozono K, Ishii N, Nishihara Y, et al. An autopsy study of the incidence of lacunes in relation to age, hypertension, and arteriosclerosis. *Stroke* 1991;22:993–996.
36. Tuszynski MH, Petito CK, Levy DE. Risk factors and clinical manifestations of pathologically verified lacunar infarctions. *Stroke* 1989;20:990–999.
37. Brainini M, Seiser A, Czvitkovits B, et al. Stroke subtype is an age-independent predictor of first-year survival. *Neuroepidemiology* 1992;11:190–195.
38. Clavier I, Hommell M, Besson G, et al. Long-term prognosis of symptomatic lacunar infarcts. *Stroke* 1994; 25:2005–2009.
39. Miyao S, Takano A, Teramoto J, et al. Leukoaraiosis in relation to prognosis for patients with lacunar infarction. *Stroke* 1992;23:1434–1438.
40. Petty GW, Brown RDJ, Whisnant JP, et al. Ischemic stroke subtypes: a population-based study of functional outcome, survival, and recurrence. *Stroke* 2000;31: 1062–1068.
41. Salgado AV, Ferro JM, Gouveia-Oliveira A. Long-term prognosis of first-ever lacunar stroke. *Stroke* 1996;27: 661–666.
42. Benavente O, Hart RG, Palacio S, et al. Stroke recurrence, cognitive impairment and white matter abnormalities are frequent in Hispanic Americans with lacunar stroke. *Cerebrovasc Dis* 2002;13[Suppl 3]:1–100.
43. Snowdon DA, Greiner LH, Mortimer JA. Brain infarction and the clinical expression of Alzheimer disease. The Nun Study. *JAMA* 1997;277:813–817.
44. Samuelsson M, Soderfelt B, Olsson GB. Functional outcome in patients with lacunar infarction. *Stroke* 1996; 27:842–846.
45. Loeb C, Gandolfo C, Bino G. Intellectual impairment and cerebral lesions in multiple cerebral infarcts. A clinical-computed tomography study. *Stroke* 1988;19: 816–820.
46. Esiri MM, Wilcock GK, Morris JH. Neuropathological assessment of the lesions of significance in vascular dementia. *J Neurol Neurosurg Psychiatry* 1997;63: 749–753.
47. Erkinjuntti T, Haltia M, Palo J, et al. Accuracy of the clinical diagnosis of vascular dementia: a prospective

and post-mortem neuropathological study. *J Neurol Neurosurg Psychiatry* 1988;51:1037–1044.

48. Meyer JS, McClintic KL, Rogers RL. Aetiological considerations and risk factors for multi-infarct dementia. *J Neurol Neurosurg Psychiatry* 1988;51:1489–1497.

49. Gotoh F, Tohgi H, Hirai S, et al. Cilostazol Stroke Prevention Study: a placebo-controlled double-blind trial for secondary prevention of cerebral infarction. *J Stroke Cerebrovasc Dis* 2000;9:147–157.

50. Chinese Acute Stroke Trial. CAST: randomised placebo-controlled trial of early aspirin use in 20,000 patients with acute ischaemic stroke. *Lancet* 1997;349:1641–1649.

51. Bousser MG, Eschwege E, Haguenau M, et al. "AICLA" controlled trial of aspirin and dipyridamole in the secondary prevention of athero-thrombotic cerebral ischemia. *Stroke* 1983;14:5–14.

52. Gent M, Blakeley JA, Easton D. The Canadian American Ticlopidine Study (CATS) in thromboembolic stroke. *Lancet* 1989;1:1215–1220.

53. Albers GW, Amarenco P, Easton D, et al. Antithrombotic and thrombolytic therapy for ischemic stroke. *Chest* 2001;119[Suppl]:300–320.

54. Samuelson M, Lindell D, Norrving B. Presumed pathogenetic mechanisms of recurrent stroke after lacunar infarction. *Cerebrovasc Dis* 1996;6:128–136.

On page 281, in the last paragraph:
The first sentence should begin : We will now address key issues... (address was misspelled).
The third sentence should read: Investigators must decisde which primary hypothesis and outcome endpoints are mos important (endpoints was misspelled.)

Ischemic Stroke: Advances in Neurology, Vol. 92. Edited by
H.J.M. Barnett, Julien Bogousslavsky, and Heather Meldrum.
Lippincott Williams & Wilkins, Philadelphia © 2003.

35

North American Perspective of Antiplatelet Agents

Philip B. Gorelick

Department of Neurosciences, Rush Medical College, Chicago, Illinois, U.S.A.

Aspirin has been commercially available for more than 100 years, and its forerunner, salicylic acid, has been used to treat fever and ease pain since ancient times (1). In the 1700s, a clergyman, Edward Stone, hypothesized that the bark of the willow might cure fever. He pulverized the bark, brewed a tea, and showed that it did reduce fever. About 70 years later, salicin, or salicylic acid, was identified as the active ingredient of the willow; however, it was found to be bitter and irritating to the stomach. In the mid to late 1800s, chemists in Europe tried to synthesize a less toxic form of the agent. In 1898, Felix Hoffmann was credited for synthesizing a pure and stable form of an acetate derivative, acetylsalicylic acid, which was later referred to as aspirin ("a" to denote acetyl and "spirin" to denote the meadowsweet, **Spiraea ulmaria,** the origin of the salicylic acid) (1).

In the 1950s, Lawrence Craven reported the use of aspirin to prevent coronary and cerebral thrombosis (2,3). Craven was aware that surgical patients (e.g., dental extraction, tonsillectomy procedures) who took aspirin might experience hemorrhage after surgery as thrombus formation was impaired. Craven's observation became the precursor of large-scale, multicenter clinical trials of aspirin and other antiplatelet agents for prevention of cerebral ischemia. Interestingly, it was not until the early 1970s that John Vane determined the mechanism of aspirin therapy: suppression of the biosynthesis of prostaglandins (PGs) (1,4,5). In addition to aspirin, we now have other antiplatelet agents and combination antiplatelet therapy to choose from for stroke prevention. In this chapter, we will discuss the mechanism, safety, efficacy, and cost of the antiplatelet agents available for ischemic stroke prevention.

Limitations of the randomized controlled trial (RCT) and meta-analysis (systemic review), data sources that we use to assist in making clinical decisions, are reviewed elsewhere (6–13).

MECHANISM OF ACTION FOR ANTIPLATELET AGENTS

Antiplatelet agents are drugs that (a) inhibit a measurable property of platelets such as adhesion, retention, or aggregation; (b) inhibit platelet-induced thrombus formation; and (c) prolong survival of radioactively labeled platelets in clinical or experimental conditions in which platelet survival may be decreased (14–17). Aspirin, the thienopyridines (ticlopidine and clopidogrel), dipyridamole, and the platelet glycoprotein IIb/IIIa receptor inhibitors all have unique mechanisms of action for platelet inhibition (14–25). The mechanisms of action of commonly used antiplatelet agents are listed in Table 35-1.

EFFICACY OF ANTIPLATELET AGENTS

We will now addess key issues about the use of aspirin and other antiplatelet agents in stroke prevention. This information is derived largely from RCTs that study efficacy (26). Investigators must decide which primary hypothesis and outcome endpints are most important. Albers (27) has reviewed the most relevant outcomes to stroke/transient ischemic attack (TIA) patients. The composite endpoint of stroke, myocardial infarction, and vascular death represents an important outcome cluster in patients with atherosclerosis and is frequently used in recurrent stroke prevention RCTs. However, stroke/TIA patients gen-

Chapter 35: *North American Perspective of Antiplatelet Agents* by Philip B. Gorelick, pages 281-288
The second European Stroke Prevention Study is abbreviated as both ESPS-2 and ESPS-II; both refer to the same
study. The correct abbreviation is ESPS-2.

TABLE 35-1. *Mechanisms of action of antiplatelet agents for stroke prevention*

Agent	Mechanism of action
1. Aspirin	1. Selectively acetylates the hydroxyl group of a serine residue at position 529 within the polypeptide chain of platelet prostaglandin G/H_1 to cause irreversible loss of cyclooxygenase activity, which results in decreased conversion of arachidonate to prostaglandin G_2 and consequently the synthesis products of prostaglandin G_2, prostaglandin H_2 and thromboxane A_2 (the latter induces irreversible platelet aggregation) (14–17).
2. Ticlopidine and clopidogrel[a]	2. Believed to inhibit the binding of adenosine 5-diphosphate (ADP) to its platelet receptor (glycoprotein IIb/IIIa, low-affinity type 2 purinergic receptor) with direct inhibition of fibrinogen binding to this receptor. Drugs of this class of agents may interfere with von Willebrand factor binding to platelet receptors, may improve enhanced erythrocyte aggregability, and have a decreased effect with higher plasma fibrinogen concentrations (18–22).
3. Dipyridamole immediate release (DIR) and dipyridamole extended	3. Suggested mechanisms of action include: (a) inhibition of platelet phosphodiesterase enzyme, which leads to an increase in intraplatelet cyclic AMP and resultant release (DER)[b] potentiation of the platelet-inhibitory actions of prostacyclin; (b) direct release of eicosanoid (e.g., prostacyclin) by vascular endothelium; and (c) inhibition of cellular uptake and metabolism of adenosine (platelet-inhibiting and vasodilating compound) (16, 17, 23).
4. Platelet glycoprotein IIb/IIIa	4. The platelet-membrane glycoprotein receptors are a family of integrin and nonintegrin receptors that are involved in platelet adhesion or aggregation (24, 25). Drugs that inhibit glycoprotein IIb/IIIa receptors inhibit platelet aggregation by preventing binding of fibrinogen to the receptors.

[a]The structures of ticlopidine and clopidogrel are similar; however, clopidogrel has the addition of a carboxymethyl side chain.

[b]DIR has variable absorption kinetics (23), whereas DER, the reformulated, slow-release, higher-dose preparation, has higher and more consistent circulating concentrations of dipyridamole (Fitzgerald GA, Thrombosis and Vascular Biology Newsletter, Spring 2001).

erally have a high risk of stroke recurrence during the ensuing several years and a lower risk of myocardial infarction and vascular death. Thus, the composite endpoint may have disadvantages as chance variations in the incidence of myocardial infarction or death could detract from the benefit of therapy for recurrent stroke prevention. For this reason, some experts advocate recurrent stroke as the primary outcome endpoint in prevention studies for patients with stroke or TIA.

Aspirin Dose

The proper aspirin dose for recurrent stroke prevention has been a longstanding controversy. Advo-

cates of higher doses of aspirin (e.g., 2, 3, or 4 325-mg tablets/day) have argued that there is greater efficacy for recurrent stroke prevention at these higher doses and cite superior platelet inhibition as a rationale for higher-dose aspirin use (28). Lower-dose aspirin enthusiasts cite single trials and meta-analyses that claim a lack of dose–response effect for efficacy of aspirin in recurrent stroke prevention and gastrotoxicity data (indigestion, nausea, heartburn, vomiting, and possibly gastrointestinal bleeding) to advocate for lower-dose aspirin use (29). Based on the cumulative evidence, the U.S. Food and Drug Administration now recommends an aspirin dose of 50 to 325 mg/day for stroke prevention in patients who have a history of symptomatic cerebrovascular disease (30). There is a paucity of data, however, that directly compare the efficacy and safety of high, medium, and low doses of aspirin in recurrent stroke prevention (31,32).

Aspirin and Prevention of a First Stroke

The weight of the data suggests that aspirin is not beneficial in stroke prevention unless one is at high risk of stroke (e.g., history of prior stroke or TIA) (33–46). Several observational studies of self-selected regular users of aspirin in low-risk persons suggest increases in the incidence of stroke (37–40,46). However, in the Nurses' Health Study cohort, women who took 1 to 6 aspirins/week had a reduced risk of large-artery infarction, whereas those who used 15 or more aspirins/week had an increased risk of subarachnoid hemorrhage, especially among older or hypertensive women (43).

The Physicians' Health Study, an RCT, showed a slightly increased risk of stroke among those taking aspirin (325 mg every other day), primarily in the subgroup with hemorrhagic stroke (34), and a British RCT of doctors showed that disabling strokes were somewhat more common among those allocated to aspirin therapy (500 mg/day) (33). The Hypertension Optimal Treatment study, another RCT, showed no increase in the incidence of stroke in those with vascular risk factors who received aspirin 75 mg/day (41). In the Primary Prevention Project (42), there was a trend for fewer strokes in the aspirin (100 mg/day) treatment arm.

In a meta-analysis, Hart et al. (44) hypothesize that the effect of aspirin therapy for stroke prevention of persons with major risk factors for vascular disease may be intermediate between those with manifest vascular disease, where there is a decrease in stroke risk with aspirin therapy, and those with low risk, where there might be a small increase in risk due to aspirin-associated intracra-nial hemorrhage. Controversies regarding aspirin use for the prevention of a first stroke will be resolved by additional well-designed RCTs (45,46).

Aspirin Therapy in the Early Phase of Acute Ischemic Stroke

Meta-analysis of combined data from the International Stroke Trial (IST) and Chinese Acute Stroke Trial (CAST) of 40,000 individual patients who received aspirin versus control (placebo) therapy for acute ischemic stroke has been reported (47–49). The main findings are listed in Table 35-2. Overall, early aspirin therapy was of benefit for a wide range of patients mainly to reduce the risk of early stroke recurrence. The aspirin dose in IST was 300 mg/day for 2 weeks and in CAST 160 mg/day for 4 weeks.

Aspirin Therapy for Recurrent Ischemic Stroke Prevention

Major aspirin trials for recurrent ischemic stroke prevention have reported administration of aspirin doses as low as 30 mg/day and as high as 1,300 or 1,500 mg/day. As aspirin became the gold standard therapy for recurrent stroke prevention, placebo comparator studies gave way to aspirin versus aspirin at different doses or aspirin versus other antiplatelet agents. Several major recurrent stroke prevention RCTs show that aspirin is effective for reducing death/recurrent stroke risk or combined endpoints (e.g., nonfatal stroke, nonfatal myocardial infarction, vascular death) (50–53). However, in the U.K. Transient Ischemic Attack Study, the signal was less clear as the trend for reduction in major stroke, myocardial infarction, and vascular death was noted only after the results for the 300- and 1,200-mg aspirin dose groups were combined

TABLE 35-2. *Main findings from a metaanalysis of the international stroke trial and Chinese acute stroke trial (47–49)*

Outcome[a]	↓ or ↑ per 1,000 with aspirin	2 *p*-value
1. Recurrent ischemic stroke	↓ by 7	<0.000001
2. Death without further stroke	↓ by 4	0.05
3. Hemorrhagic stroke or hemorrhagic transformation	↑ by 2	0.07
4. Stroke/death in hospital	↓ by 9	0.001

[a]There was no significant heterogeneity of the proportional benefit of aspirin in subgroup-specific analyses.

(51). The Antiplatelet Trialists' Collaboration summarized data for approximately 10,000 patients with stroke or TIA and reported a 3-year benefit of about 40 of 1,000 ($2p < 0.00001$) for reduction of vascular events (nonfatal myocardial infarctions, nonfatal strokes, or vascular deaths) and found, among a wider range of patients at high risk of occlusive vascular disease after some years of aspirin therapy (75–325 mg/day) or some other antiplatelet regimen, worthwhile protection against myocardial infarction, stroke, and death (54). Comparisons of other antiplatelet agents versus aspirin or placebo are discussed in subsequent sections of this chapter.

Stroke Recurrence While on Aspirin

In clinical practice, it is not uncommon to encounter ischemic stroke or TIA patients who have ischemic stroke recurrence while being treated with aspirin. These cases have been referred to as "aspirin failures." Explanations for ischemic stroke recurrence in these patients have included noncompliance, inadequate aspirin dose, resistance to aspirin effect, irrelevance of the biological effect of aspirin in relation to the specific pathogenetic mechanism of cerebral ischemia, and other mechanisms (55–58). Helgason et al. (55,56) have shown incomplete platelet inhibition in some ischemic stroke patients on 325 mg of aspirin/day. With aspirin dose escalation, most develop complete inhibition of platelet aggregation, though there may be individual variability. Bornstein et al. (58) found a trend toward a higher frequency of aspirin failure in patients taking lower doses of aspirin (less than 500 mg/day) and statistically significant findings for aspirin failure among hyperlipidemic individuals and those with ischemic heart disease. Higher doses of aspirin may be needed to block platelet activation when there are hemodynamic (shear) forces (57). These studies suggest individual variation in aspirin response and the need for correlative studies of platelet function and clinical outcome in ischemic stroke patients (59).

Aspirin and Carotid Endarterectomy

In the ASA and Carotid Endarterectomy (ACE) trial, the risk of stroke, myocardial infarction, and death within 30 days and 3 months of endarterectomy was lower for patients taking 81 or 325 mg of acetylsalicylic acid/day than those taking 650 or 1,300 mg/day (60,61). At 3 months, the risk was lowest for the 325-mg aspirin treatment group.

Aspirin in Atrial Fibrillation

RCTs suggest that (a) adjusted-dose warfarin reduces the risk of stroke in atrial fibrillation by about 60% compared with placebo; (b) aspirin reduces the risk by about 20% compared with placebo; and (c) warfarin reduces the risk by about 40% compared with aspirin (62–64). Atrial fibrillation patients may be identified who have a low risk of stroke (about 1%/year) and who may be suitable candidates for aspirin therapy (325 mg/day) and those who have much higher risks of stroke (about 8%/year) and who may be suitable candidates for warfarin. Those atrial fibrillation patients at low risk of stroke may be those *without* a history of hypertension, recent congestive heart failure, left ventricular fractional shortening of ≤25%, previous thromboembolism, systolic blood pressure higher than 160 mm Hg, or women older than 75 years of age (62).

Aspirin and Hemorrhagic Stroke Frequency in Recurrent Stroke Prevention Studies

The risk of hemorrhagic stroke in patients on aspirin for recurrent stroke prevention is generally low (65–67). However, this could vary by race–ethnic group, whereby the risk may be higher for some groups (e.g., Asians) (68,69). He et al. (70), in a meta-analysis of collaborative trials, reported a reduction of myocardial infarction by 137 of 10,000, a reduction of ischemic stroke by 39 of 10,000, but an increase of hemorrhagic stroke by 12 of 10,000 with aspirin use. Whereas there may be a modest dose–response effect for aspirin use (more than 1,225 mg/week) on intracerebral hemorrhage risk in a city hospital setting (71), there are data to suggest that this may not be the case in the clinical trial setting (65).

Aspirin and Angiotensin-Converting Enzyme (ACE-I) Inhibitor Antagonism

Angiotensin-converting enzyme (ACE-I) inhibitors are a popular class of antihypertensives and may be used frequently in conjunction with aspirin for cardiovascular disease and stroke prevention. They prevent the breakdown of bradykinin, which promotes the synthesis of the vasodilating PGs, PGE_2 and PGI_2, and relaxation of smooth muscle. An antagonistic interaction is believed to be mediated by aspirin inhibition of PG synthesis, which is likely to be dose dependent. That is, the synthesis of PGI_2 and thromboxane A_2 is affected at higher (e.g., 300 mg/day or higher) but not lower doses of aspirin administration (72–74).

Beyond Aspirin: Other Antiplatelet Agents and Combinations

From aggregate analysis of recurrent stroke prevention studies, it is estimated that the relative risk reduction of aspirin over placebo for the combined endpoint stroke, myocardial infarction, or vascular death is 13% (75), and the risk of stroke alone is reduced by 15% (76). Thus, there is room for improvement as about five of six strokes could occur on aspirin therapy (77). Can we improve the outcomes with other antiplatelet agents?

Ticlopidine, Clopidogrel, and Aspirin plus Extended-Release Dipyridamole or Immediate-Release Dipyridamole

Each of these therapies has been shown to further reduce stroke risk over aspirin alone (78). The exception, the combination of aspirin plus immediate-release dipyridamole, was tested against a placebo rather than aspirin therapy or did not show convincing evidence for stroke reduction in individual studies (79).

Ticlopidine

In the Canadian–American Ticlopidine Study (CATS), patients with major ischemic stroke were randomly allocated to treatment with ticlopidine (250 mg b.i.d./day) or placebo (80). By intent-to-treat analysis, the risk of the composite endpoint stroke, myocardial infarction, or vascular death was reduced by 23.3% ($p = 0.020$). In the Ticlopidine–Aspirin Stroke Study (TASS), patients with minor stroke or TIA received ticlopidine (250 mg b.i.d./day) or aspirin (650 mg b.i.d./day) (81). By intent-to-treat analysis, the risk of nonfatal stroke

or death was reduced by 12% ($p = 0.048$) at 3 years.

In a TASS *post hoc* analysis, it was determined that nonwhites had about 10% fewer adverse events and a more favorable risk reduction profile than whites (82). Presently, we are carrying out a recurrent stroke prevention RCT, the African American Antiplatelet Stroke Prevention Study (AAASPS), of ticlopidine (250 mg b.i.d./day) versus aspirin (325 mg b.i.d./day) in African Americans with noncardioembolic ischemic stroke (83). As of October 2001, the target enrollment of 1,800 subjects had been completed. Each will be followed for up to 2 years. The primary outcome endpoint is recurrent stroke, myocardial infarction, and vascular death.

Clopidogrel

In the Clopidogrel Versus Aspirin in Patients at Risk of Ischemic Events (CAPRIE) Study, 19,185 patients were enrolled, of whom over 6,000 entered from each of the following three groups: recent ischemic stroke, recent myocardial infarction, and symptomatic peripheral arterial disease (84). Patients were randomly allocated to clopidogrel 75 mg/day or aspirin 325 mg/day and followed on average for about 1.9 years. There was a marginal reduction of 8.7% (95% confidence interval 0.3, 16.5%, $p = 0.043$) favoring clopidogrel over aspirin for the outcome cluster ischemic stroke, myocardial infarction, and vascular death. Additional analysis showed that the largest benefit occurred in the peripheral arterial disease group where over 75% of the therapeutic advantage of clopidogrel over aspirin was observed (85). The study, however, was not statistically powered to analyze the data from the three separate entry subgroups for the primary outcome.

Aspirin plus Extended- or Immediate-Release Dipyridamole

Use of immediate-release dipyridamole (150–300 mg/day) poses several disadvantages: (a) variable absorption kinetics (23); (b) three or four times daily dosing schedule that is likely to reduce compliance (77); and (c) coupling of the agent with possible gastrotoxic doses of aspirin (900 mg/day or higher) to show efficacy (77). Furthermore, the efficacy of immediate-release dipyridamole in combination with aspirin for stroke prevention has been questioned.

Wilterdink and Easton (79) and Easton (29) provide expert reviews of the key issues regarding the efficacy and safety of dipyridamole. One concern has been the adequacy of the statistical power of the early aspirin plus immediate-release dipyridamole studies. Relatively small numbers of study subjects were enrolled in these RCTs that pitted aspirin plus immediate-release dipyridamole against an active comparator agent such as aspirin. One of the stronger clinical signals in favor of this combination therapy for stroke prevention came from the first European Stroke Prevention Study (ESPS-I); however, this was a placebo comparator study and did not include an aspirin-only arm (86).

In the ESPS-II, an RCT of 6,602 ischemic stroke or TIA patients, study subjects were allocated randomly to receive aspirin 25 mg plus the newly formulated extended-release dipyridamole 200 mg b.i.d., aspirin 25 mg b.i.d., extended-release dipyridamole 200 mg b.i.d., or placebo (87). The main finding of the ESPS-2 was a 23.1% reduction for stroke in favor of the combination therapy over aspirin alone.

Critics have charged that the ESPS-2 aspirin comparator dose of 50 mg/day was too low; a placebo arm should not have been included; dropout rates were high and there were unexpected imbalances in compliance rates among treatment groups; one site had over 400 fictitious patients that had to be withdrawn from the statistical analysis; and the predominant effect was to reduce nonfatal stroke, yet there was little effect on death (88).

Rationale for low-dose aspirin administration in ESPS-2 was to minimize side effects and maintain an appropriate dose ratio with extended-release dipyridamole to maximize inhibition of thrombus formation. Furthermore, the investigators believed that the benefit of aspirin had not been conclusively proven in 1989 when the trial was initiated (51) and, exclusion of patients from the site with fictitious data did not alter the main study findings. Finally, mortality may not have been reduced substantially as in the first several years after ischemic stroke, nonfatal ischemic stroke may be the key outcome endpoint, and mortality from other causes may be substantially less frequent (27). The Food and Drug Administration carried out a comprehensive review of the study data and sites, found the results to be substantial, and approved aspirin (25 mg) plus extended-release dipyridamole (200 mg) twice-daily dosing for stroke prevention in patients with TIA or ischemic stroke in late 1999.

Indirect Comparisons of Aspirin and Other Antiplatelet Agents

A recent consensus statement on antithrombotic therapy from the American College of Chest Physicians provides indirect comparisons of aspirin versus clopidogrel, aspirin versus ticlopidine, and aspirin versus aspirin plus extended-release dipyridamole for the outcome endpoint stroke and the composite outcome endpoint stroke, myocardial infarction, and vascular or sudden death (78). The absolute risk reduction of the other antiplatelet agents over aspirin and the number needed to treat are listed in Table 35-3 (89). One must be cautious in the interpretation of these data as they do not represent direct head-to-head comparison of the

TABLE 35-3. *Indirect comparison of absolute risk reduction (ARR) and number-needed-to-treat (NNT) for aspirin versus clopidogrel (CAPRIE), aspirin versus ticlopidine (TASS), and aspirin versus aspirin plus extended-release dipyridamole in patients with cerebrovascular disease according to the ACCP (78, 89)[a]*

Study	Recurrent stroke prevention (%)		Recurrent stroke, myocardial infarction, vascular (sudden)[b] death (%)	
	ARR	NNT	ARR	NNT
CAPRIE (84)	0.8 (p = 0.28)	125	1 (p = 0.26)	100
TASS (81)	2.5 (p = 0.02)	40	2.3 (p = 0.20)	43
ESPS-2 (87)	3.0 (p = 0.006)	33	3.6 (p = 0.01)	28

ACCP, American College of Chest Physicians; ESPS, European Stroke Prevention Study.
[a]Within each respective study, the ARR favors the nonaspirin agent over aspirin at 2 years.
[b]Sudden death was reported in ESPS-II.

nonaspirin antiplatelet agents, doses of aspirin in the various studies differ (e.g., CAPRIE 325 mg/day, TASS 1,300 mg/day, ESPS-2 50 mg/day), study designs are disparate, and confidence intervals for the point estimates overlap. Furthermore, the individual RCTs may not have been statistically powered to study recurrent stroke or the composite endpoint recurrent stroke, myocardial infarction, or vascular (sudden) death.

SAFETY OF ANTIPLATELET AGENTS

The details of the safety profile for commercially available antiplatelet agents with indications for recurrent stroke prevention are listed in the individual RCT study publications (50–53,80–82, 84,87) and recently reviewed by Diener and Ringleb (90). The main side effects of aspirin are dyspepsia and gastrointestinal bleeding. Gastrointestinal side effects may be driven by aspirin dose. The main side effects of ticlopidine are diarrhea, gastrointestinal symptoms of various types, rash, neutropenia, and thrombocytopenia. Because of the hematologic side effects, a complete blood count with differential and platelet count must be obtained at baseline and every 2 weeks during the 3 months after initiation of ticlopidine therapy. Thrombotic thrombocytopenia purpura is estimated to occur in 1 of 2,000 to 4,000 ticlopidine users. Rapid recognition and treatment of thrombotic thrombocytopenia purpura are needed as the condition may be fatal. Aplastic anemia also may occur with ticlopidine.

The main side effects of clopidogrel are rash, diarrhea, and various gastrointestinal symptoms. Clopidogrel is not associated with neutropenia and infrequently may be associated with thrombotic thrombocytopenia purpura (91). Overall, clopidogrel is about as safe as aspirin but has a side effect profile that is more favorable than ticlopidine. The main side effects of aspirin plus extended-release dipyridamole are headache, various gastrointestinal symptoms, and dizziness. Analysis of cardiac events in patients with coronary heart disease or myocardial infarction at entry into ESPS-2 showed that dipyridamole administration did not result in a higher number of cardiac events such as angina pectoris, myocardial infarction, or death from all causes (92). Headache after aspirin plus extended-release dipyridamole administration usually occurs within the first 10 to 14 days of treatment and is self-limited (93).

COST

Aspirin is a commonly used agent, is available as an over-the-counter drug, and is inexpensive. Whereas ticlopidine, clopidogrel, and aspirin plus extended-release dipyridamole may provide added recurrent stroke prevention over aspirin, these agents are more expensive than aspirin. In the U.S.A., the cost of these newer agents varies based on region and the availability of generic agents. Ticlopidine is available as a generic agent; however, clopidogrel and extended-release dipyridamole are not. Immediate-release dipyridamole is available as a generic agent; however, immediate-release dipyridamole has variable absorption kinetics (23) as well as other disadvantages (see Aspirin plus Extended- or Immediate-Release Dipyridamole). Cost-effectiveness analyses, which have inherent limitations, suggest that in high-risk patients, ticlopidine therapy is cost-effective over aspirin to prevent stroke (94) as is aspirin plus extended-release dipyridamole over aspirin and clopidogrel over aspirin (except in extreme scenarios or possibly otherwise) (95,96).

CONCLUSION

Aspirin is a widely available, easy-to-use, and inexpensive agent for recurrent stroke prevention. According to the AACP guidelines, aspirin is an option for initial therapy in a dose range of 50 to 325 mg/day. For patients who cannot afford antiplatelet agents beyond aspirin or who cannot tolerate the other agents, aspirin is the main antiplatelet agent for recurrent stroke prevention. Many physicians in the United States are prescribing aspirin plus extended-release dipyridamole or clopidogrel as initial therapy for recurrent stroke prevention in accordance with the American College of Chest Physicians recommendations. Aspirin plus extended-release dipyridamole is the first Food and Drug Administration-approved combination antiplatelet agent for recurrent stroke prevention, offers enhanced stroke prevention over low doses of aspirin alone (78), and is cost-effective (95). Clopidogrel is marginally better than aspirin alone but may be substantially better than aspirin in high-risk persons such as those with peripheral arterial disease (85) or multiple cardiovascular risk factors when clopidogrel is used in combination with aspirin (the safety and efficacy of this combination therapy is being tested in the MATCH Study) (90). As combination antiplatelet therapy has become popular in North America, a three-arm clinical trial comparing aspirin, aspirin plus extended-release dipyridamole, and aspirin plus clopidogrel would be useful to determine evidence-based treatment guidelines for these agents in recurrent stroke prevention. Furthermore, more information is needed on the biology of "aspirin failure" and on the use of ticlopidine in high-risk populations such as African Americans (83).

New and innovative antithrombotic strategies are needed for recurrent stroke prevention (97). Further testing of combination antiplatelet therapies is necessary to overcome the modest efficacy of, for example, aspirin (98). Disappointment with the glycoprotein IIb/IIIa oral inhibitors, which have been associated with excessive mortality (99), and the failure of warfarin to out perform aspirin in a head-to-head recurrent stroke prevention comparison (100) leaves the research pipeline somewhat depleted at this time and emphasizes the need to carefully study the use of the available antiplatelet agents in combination or possibly with other novel or standard antithrombotics. A soon-to-be-released statement from the Antithrombotic Trialists' Collaboration will provide additional insights about aspirin dose and combination therapy.

ACKNOWLEDGMENT

This work was supported in part by National Institutes of Health/National Institute of Neurological and Communication Disorders and Stroke subcontract R01 NS33430.

REFERENCES

1. Weisman SM, Rabe CS. Aspirin: new tricks for an old drug. *Primary Care Rep* 1998;4:239–246.
2. Craven LL. Prevention of coronary and cerebral thrombosis. *Mississippi Valley Med J* 1956;78: 213–215.
3. Fields WS, Lemak NA. *A history of stroke. Its recognition and treatment.* New York: Oxford University Press, 1989:115–121.
4. Vane JR. Inhibition of prostanglandin synthesis as a mechanism of action for aspirin-like drugs. *Nat (New Biol)* 1971;231:232–235.
5. Moncada S, Vane JR. Arachidonic acid metabolites and the interactions between platelets and blood-vessel walls. *N Engl J Med* 1979;300:1142–1147.
6. Gorelick PB. Are more subjects better in a randomized controlled trial? In: Fisher M, Bogousslavsky J, eds. *Current review of cerebrovascular disease.* 3rd ed. Boston: Butterworth Heinemann, 1999: 220–221.
7. Begg C, Cho M, Eastwood S, et al. Improving the quality of reporting randomized controlled trials. The CONSORT statement. *JAMA* 1996;276: 637–639.
8. Charlton BG. Fundamental deficiencies in the mega-trial methodology. *Curr Trials Cardiovasc Med* 2001; 2:2–7.
9. Petitti DB. *Meta-analysis, decision analysis and cost-effectiveness analysis. Methods for quantitative synthesis in medicine.* New York: Oxford University Press, 1994:3–243.
10. Cappelleri JC, Ioannidis JPA, Schmid CH, et al. Large trials vs. meta-analysis of smaller trials. How do their results compare? *JAMA* 1996;276:1332–1338.
11. Colditz GA, Burdick E, Mosteller F. Heterogeneity in meta-analysis of data from epidemiologic studies: a commentary. *Am J Epidemiol* 1995;4:371–382.
12. Counsell C, Warlow C, Sandercock P, et al. (Cochrane Collaboration Stroke Review Group Editorial Board). Meeting the need for systematic reviews in stroke care. *Stroke* 1995;26:498–502.
13. Hankey GJ. Policy and practice in the prevention of stroke: between the ideal and the affordable. In: Norris J, Hachinski V, eds. *Stroke prevention.* New York: Oxford University Press, 2001:313–334.
14. Patrono C. Aspirin as an antiplatelet drug. *N Engl J Med* 1994;330:1287–1294.
15. Moncada S, Vane JR. Arachidonic acid metabolites and the interaction between platelets and blood-vessel walls. *N Engl J Med* 1979;300:1142–1147.
16. Fuster V, Chesebro JH. Antithrombotic therapy: role of platelet-inhibitor drugs. II. Pharmacologic effects of platelet-inhibitor drug (second of three parts). *Mayo Clin Proc* 1981;56:185–195.
17. Weiss HJ. Properties of platelets. *N Engl J Med* 1978; 298:1344–1348.
18. Teitelbaum P. Pharmacodynamics and pharmacokinetics of ticlopidine. In: Haas WK, Easton JD, eds. *Ticlopidine, platelets, and vascular disease.* New York: Springer-Verlag, 1993:27–40.
19. Herbert JM, Frehl D, Vallee E, et al. Clopidogrel, a novel antiplatelet and antithrombotic agent. *Cardiovasc Drug Rev* 1993;11:180–198.
20. Sharis PJ, Cannon CP, Lascalzo J. The antiplatelet effects of ticlopidine and clopidogrel. *Ann Intern Med* 1998;129:394–405.
21. Tanahashi N, Fukuuchi Y, Tomita M, et al. Ticlopidine improves the enhanced erythrocyte aggregability in patients with cerebral infarction. *Stroke* 1993;24: 1083–1086.
22. Tohgi H, Takahashi H, Kashiwaya M, et al. Effect of plasma fibrinogen concentration on the inhibition of platelet aggregation after ticlopidine compared with aspirin. *Stroke* 1994;25:2017–2021.
23. Fitzgerald GA. Dipyridamole. *N Engl J Med* 1987; 316:1247–1256.
24. Lefkovits J, Plow EF, Topol EJ. Platelet glycoprotein IIb/IIIa receptors in cardiovascular medicine. *N Engl J Med* 1995;332:1553–1559.
25. Vorcheimer DA, Badimon JJ, Fuster V. Platelet glycoprotein IIb/IIIa receptor antagonists in cardiovascular disease. *JAMA* 1999;281:1407–1414.
26. Feasby TE. The appropriateness and effectiveness of stroke prevention. In: Norris J, Hachinski V, eds.

On page 288, the following should be inserted:

Addendum: After the submission of this chapter, new information about aspirin and other antiplatelet efficacy and dose was published. See the following reference: Antithrombotic Trialists' Collaboration. Collaborative meta-analys of randomised trials of antiplatelet therapy for prevention of death, myocardial infarction, and stroke in high risk patients. *BMJ* 2002; 324:71-86.

Stroke prevention. New York: Oxford University Press, 2001:295–312.

27. Albers GW. Choice of endpoints in antiplatelet trials. Which outcomes are most relevant to stroke patients? *Neurology* 2000;54:1022–1028.

28. Dyken ML, Barnett HJM, Easton JD, et al. Low-dose aspirin and stroke: "It ain't necessarily so." *Stroke* 1992;23:1395–1399.

29. Easton JD. Antiplatelet therapy. In: Norris J, Hachinski V, eds. *Stroke prevention.* New York: Oxford University Press, 2001:195–209.

30. Food and Drug Administration, Department of Health and Human Services. Internal analgesic, antipyretic, and antirheumatic drug products for over-the-counter human use; final rule for professional labeling of aspirin, buffered aspirin, and aspirin in combination with antacid drug products. *Fed Reg* 1998;63: 56802–56819.

31. Barnett HJM, Eliasziw M, Meldrum HE. Drugs and surgery in the prevention of ischemic stroke. *N Engl J Med* 1995;332:238–248.

32. Barnett HJM, Kaste M, Meldrum H, et al. Aspirin dose in stroke prevention. Beautiful hypotheses slain by ugly facts. *Stroke* 1996;27:588–592.

33. Peto R, Gray R, Collins R, et al. Randomized trial of prophylactic daily aspirin in British male doctors. *Br Med J* 1988;296:313–316.

34. Steering Committee of the Physicians' Study Research Group. Final report on the aspirin component of the ongoing Physicians' Health Study. *N Engl J Med* 1989;321:129–135.

35. Fuster V, Cohen M, Halperin J. Aspirin in the prevention of coronary disease. *N Engl J Med* 1989;321: 183–185.

36. Young FE, Nightingale SL, Temple RA. The preliminary report of the findings of the aspirin component of the ongoing Physicians' Health Study. The FDA perspective on aspirin for the primary prevention of myocardial infarction. *JAMA* 1988;259: 3158–3160.

37. Pagnani-Hill, Chao A, Ross R, et al. Aspirin use and chronic diseases: a cohort study of the elderly. *Br Med J* 1989;299:1247–1250.

38. Kronmal RA, Hart RG, Manolio TA, et al. Aspirin use and incident stroke in the Cardiovascular Health Study. *Stroke* 1998;29:887–894.

39. Voko Z, Koudstaal PJ, Botts ML, et al. Aspirin use and risk of stroke in the elderly: the Rotterdam Study. *Neuroepidemiology* 2001;20:40–44.

40. Manson JE, Stamfer MJ, Colditz GA, et al. A prospective study of aspirin use and primary prevention of cardiovascular disease in women. *JAMA* 1991;266: 521–527.

41. Hannson L, Zanchetti A, Carruthers SG, et al. Effects of intensive blood-pressure lowering and low-dose aspirin in patients with hypertension: principal results of the Hypertension Optimal Treatment (HOT) randomised trial. *Lancet* 1998;351: 1755–1762.

42. Collaborative Group of the Primary Prevention Project (PPP). Low-dose aspirin and vitamin E in people at cardiovascular risk: a randomised trial in general practice. *Lancet* 2001;357:89–95.

43. Iso H, Hennekens CH, Stampfer MJ, et al. Prospective study of aspirin use and risk of stroke in women. *Stroke* 1999;30:1764–1771.

44. Hart RG, Halperin JL, McBride R, et al. Aspirin for the primary prevention of stroke and other major vascular events. Arch *Neurol* 2000;57:326–332.

45. Buring JE, Bogousslavsky J, Dyken M. Aspirin and stroke. *Stroke* 1998;29:885–886.

46. Barnett HJM, Eliasziw M. Aspirin benefit remains elusive in primary stroke prevention. Arch *Neurol* 2000;57:306–308.

47. International Stroke Trial Collaborative Group. The International Stroke Trial (IST): a randomized trial of aspirin, subcutaneous heparin, both or neither among 19,435 patients with acute ischemic stroke. *Lancet* 1997;349:1569–1581.

48. CAST (Chinese Acute Stroke Trial) Collaborative Group. CAST: a randomized placebo-controlled trial of early aspirin use in 20,000 patients with acute ischemic stroke. *Lancet* 1997;349: 1641–1649.

49. Chen ZM, Sandercock P, Pan HL, et al. Indications for early aspirin use in acute ischemic stroke. A combined analysis of 40,000 randomized patients from the Chinese Acute Stroke Trial and the International Stroke Trial. *Stroke* 2000;31:1240–1249.

50. Canadian Cooperative Study Group. A randomized trial of aspirin and sulfinpyrazone in threatened stroke. *N Engl J Med* 1978;299:53–59.

51. UK-TIA Study Group. The United Kingdom Transient Ischemic Attack (UK-TIA) Aspirin Trial: final results. *J Neurol Neurosurg Psychiatry* 1991;54: 1044–1054.

52. Dutch TIA Trial Study Group. A comparison of two doses of aspirin (30mg vs. 283mg a day) in patients after a transient ischemic attack or minor ischemic stroke. *N Engl J Med* 1991;325:1261–1266.

53. SALT Collaborative Group. Swedish Aspirin Low-Dose Trial (SALT) of 75mg aspirin as secondary prophylaxis after cerebrovascular ischemic events. *Lancet* 1991;338:1345–1349.

54. Antiplatelet Trialists' Collaboration. Collaborative overview of randomised trials of antiplatelet therapy—I: prevention of death, myocardial infarction, and stroke by prolonged antiplatelet therapy in various categories of patients. *Br Med J* 1994;308: 81–106.

55. Helgason CM, Tortorice KL, Winkler SR, et al. Aspirin response and failure in cerebral infarction. *Stroke* 1993;24:345–350.

56. Helgason CM, Hoff JA, Kondos GT, et al. Platelet aggregation in patients with atrial fibrillation taking aspirin or warfarin. *Stroke* 1993;24:1458–1461.

57. Ratnatunga CP, Edmondson SF, Rees GM, et al. High-dose aspirin inhibits shear-induced platelet reaction involving thrombin generation. *Circulation* 1992;85: 1077–1082.

58. Bornstein NM, Karepov VG, Aronovich BD, et al. Failure of aspirin treatment after stroke. *Stroke* 1994; 25:275–277.

59. Kawasaki T, Ozeki Y, Igawa T, et al. Increased platelet sensitivity to collagen in individuals resistant to low-dose aspirin. *Stroke* 2000;31:591–595.

60. Taylor DW, Barnett HJM, Haynes RB, et al. Low-dose and high-dose acetylsalicylic acid for patients under-

going carotid endarterectomy: a randomized controlled trial. *Lancet* 1999;353:2179–2184.

61. Gorelick PB. Carotid endarterectomy. Where do we draw the line? *Stroke* 1999;30:1745–1750.

62. SPAF III Writing Committee for the Stroke Prevention in Atrial Fibrillation Investigators. Patients with nonvalvular atrial fibrillation at low risk of stroke during treatment with aspirin. Stroke Prevention in Atrial Fibrillation III Study. *JAMA* 1998;279:1273–1277.

63. Hart RG, Pearce LS, McBride R, et al. Factors associated with ischemic stroke during aspirin therapy in atrial fibrillation. Analysis of 2012 participants in the SPAFI–III clinical trials. *Stroke* 1999;30:1223–1229.

64. Hart RG, Halperin JL. Atrial fibrillation and thromboembolism: a decade of progress in stroke prevention. *Ann Intern Med* 1999;131:668–695.

65. Mayo NE, Levy AR, Goldberg MS. Aspirin and hemorrhagic stroke [Letter]. *Stroke* 1991;22:1213–1214.

66. Petty GW, Brown RD, Whisnant JP, et al. Frequency of major complications of aspirin, warfarin and intravenous heparin for secondary stroke prevention. A population-based study. *Ann Intern Med* 1999;130:14–22.

67. Stroke Prevention in Reversible Ischemia Trial (SPIRIT) Study Group. A randomized trial of anticoagulants versus aspirin after cerebral ischemia of presumed arterial origin. *Ann Neurol* 1997;42:857–865.

68. Wong KS, Mo KV, Lam WWM, et al. Aspirin-associated intracerebral hemorrhage. Clinical and radiologic features. *Neurology* 2000;54:2298–2301.

69. Tokuda Y, Kato J. Letter. *JAMA* 1999;282:732.

70. He J, Whelton PK, Vu B, et al. Aspirin and risk of hemorrhagic stroke: a meta-analysis of randomized controlled trials. *JAMA* 1998;280:1930–1935.

71. Thrift AG, McNeil J, Forbes A, et al. Risk of primary intracerebral hemorrhage associated with aspirin and nonsteroidal anti-inflammatory drugs: case-control study. *Br Med J* 1999;318:759–764.

72. Guazzi MD, Campodonico J, Celeste F, et al. Antihypertensive efficacy of angiotensin converting enzyme inhibition and aspirin counteraction. *Clin Pharmacol Ther* 1998;63:79–86.

73. Nawarskas JJ, Spinler SA. Update on the interaction between aspirin and angiotensin-converting enzyme inhibitors. *Pharmacotherapy* 2000;20:698–710.

74. Teerlink JR, Massie BM. The interaction of ACE inhibitors and aspirin in heart failure: torn between two lovers. *Am Heart J* 1999;138:193–197.

75. Algra A, van Gijn J. Aspirin at any dose above 30mg offers only modest protection after cerebral ischemia. *J Neurol Neurosurg Psychiatry* 1996;60:197–199.

76. Johnson ES, Lanes SF, Wentworth CE, et al. A meta-regression analysis of the dose–response effect of aspirin on stroke. *Arch Intern Med* 1999;159:1248–1253.

77. Gorelick PB. Aspirin plus extended-release dipyridamole: a new combination antiplatelet agent for secondary stroke prevention. *National Stroke Association Stroke Clinical Updates* 2000;10:1–4.

78. Albers GW, Amarenco P, Easton JD, et al. Antithrombotic and thrombolytic therapy for ischemic stroke. *Chest* 2001;119:300S–320S.

79. Wilterdink JL, Easton JD. Dipyridamole plus aspirin in cerebrovascular disease. *Arch Neurol* 1999;56:1087–1092.

80. Gent M, Blakely JA, Easton JD, et al. The Canadian American Ticlopidine Study (CATS) in thromboembolic stroke. *Lancet* 1989;1:1215–1220.

81. Hass WK, Easton JD, Adams HP Jr, et al. A randomized trial comparing ticlopidine hydrochloride with aspirin for the prevention of stroke in high-risk patients. *N Engl J Med* 1989;321:501–507.

82. Weisberg LA, for the Ticlopidine Aspirin Stroke Study Group. The efficacy and safety of ticlopidine and aspirin in non-whites: analysis of a patient subgroup from the Ticlopidine Aspirin Stroke Study. *Neurology* 1993;43:27–31.

83. Gorelick PB, Leurgans S, Richardson D, et al., for the AAASPS Investigators. African American Antiplatelet Stroke Prevention Study: clinical trial design. *J Stroke Cerebrovasc Dis* 1998;7:426–434.

84. CAPRIE Steering Committee. A randomized, blinded, trial of clopidogrel versus aspirin in patients at risk of ischemic events (CAPRIE). *Lancet* 1996;348:1329–1339.

85. Gorelick PB, Born GVR, D'Agostino RB, et al. Therapeutic benefit. Aspirin revisited in light of the introduction of clopidogrel. *Stroke* 1999;30:1716–1721.

86. ESPS Group. European Stroke Prevention Study. *Stroke* 1990;21:1122–1130.

87. Diener HC, Cunha L, Forbes C, et al. European Stroke Prevention Study 2. Dipyridamole and acetylsalicylic acid in the secondary prevention of stroke. *J Neurol Sci* 1996;143:1–13.

88. Bornstein NM. Acetylsalicylic acid (aspirin). In: Norris J, Hachinski V, eds. *Stroke prevention.* New York: Oxford University Press, 2001:177–194.

89. Albers GW, Easton JD, Sacco RL, et al. Antithrombotic and thrombolytic therapy for ischemic stroke. *Chest* 1998;114:683S–698S.

90. Diener H-C, Ringleb P. Antithrombotic secondary prevention after stroke. *Curr Treat Options Neurol* 2001;3:451–462.

91. Bennett CL, Connors JM, Carwile JM, et al. Thrombotic thrombocytopenia purpura associated with clopidogrel. *N Engl J Med* 2000;342:1773–1777.

92. Diener H-C, Darius H, Bertrand-Hardy JM, et al. Cardiac safety in the European Stroke Prevention Study 2 (ESPS-2). *Int J Clin Pract* 2001;55:162–163.

93. Theis JGW, Deichsel G, Marshall S. Rapid development of tolerance to dipyridamole- associated headaches. *Br J Clin Pharmacol* 1999;48:750–755.

94. Oster G, Huse DM, Lacey MJ, et al. Cost-effectiveness of ticlopidine in preventing stroke in high risk patients. *Stroke* 1994;25:1149–1156.

95. Sarasin FP, Gaspoz J-M, Bounameaux H. Cost-effectiveness of new antiplatelet regimens used as secondary prevention of stroke or transient ischemic attack. *Arch Intern Med* 2000;160:2773–2778.

96. Shah H, Gondek K. Aspirin plus extended-release dipyridamole or clopidogrel compared with aspirin

monotherapy for the prevention of recurrent ischemic stroke: a cost-effectiveness analysis. *Clin Ther* 2000; 22:362–370.

97. Gotoh F, Tohgi H, Hirai S, et al. Cilostazol stroke prevention study: a placebo-controlled double-blind trial for secondary prevention of cerebral infarction. *J Stroke Cerebrovasc Dis* 2000;9:147–157.

98. Hankey GJ, Sudlow CLM, Dunbabin DW. Thienopyridines or aspirin to prevent stroke and other serious vascular events in patients at high risk of vascular disease? A systematic review of the evidence from randomized trials. *Stroke* 2000;31:1779–1784.

99. Wilterdink JL, Easton JD. Stroke prevention in 2001. In: Bogousslavsky J, ed. *Drug therapy for stroke prevention.* New York: Taylor and Francis, 2001:1–13.

100. Mohr JP, Thompson JLP, Lazar RM, et al. A comparison of warfarin and aspirin for the prevention of recurrent ischemic stroke. *N Engl J Med* 2001;345:1444–1451.

Ischemic Stroke: Advances in Neurology, Vol. 92. Edited by
H.J.M. Barnett, Julien Bogousslavsky, and Heather Meldrum.
Lippincott Williams & Wilkins, Philadelphia © 2003.

36

Antiplatelet Agents

European Perspective

Juhani Sivenius and *Markku Kaste

Department of Neurology, University of Kuopio; Department of Neurology, Kuopio University
Hospital; Kuopio, Finland; *Department of Neurology, University of Helsinki; Department of
Neurology, Helsinki University Central Hospital, Helsinki, Finland

NEED FOR SECONDARY PREVENTION OF STROKE

Stroke is the second most common cause of death worldwide (1), and the loss of quality-adjusted life-years caused by stroke is more substantial than for any other disease (2). It imposes an enormous economic and human burden (3). Each year about 1.5 million people suffer a new stroke in the United States and Europe (4). Ischemic stroke is by far the most frequent subtype of acute stroke, with more than 80% of all stroke patients suffering from focal ischemia (5). Patients with a recent ischemic stroke or transient ischemic attack (TIA) are at high risk for further cerebrovascular or vascular events and vascular death. The recurrence risk after a TIA or ischemic stroke ranges from 5% to 20% per year (6). Numerous trials and meta-analyses have left little doubt that antiplatelet therapy reduces stroke risk in patients with prior stroke or TIA. Our aim is to review the European practice of antiplatelet therapy in stroke prevention, given that the therapy varies enormously and that there are no scientific data on European practice.

AVAILABLE AGENTS FOR SECONDARY PREVENTION

Use of platelet inhibition as an antithrombotic strategy emerged from biochemical studies, which revealed the pivotal role of platelets in thrombus formation. Clinical studies of antiplatelet therapy for stroke prevention have focused primarily on acetylsalicylic acid (ASA, aspirin) and secondarily on ticlo-pidine, dipyridamole (DP), and clopidogrel. The antithrombotic action of ASA is related to its ability to irreversibly inhibit cyclooxygenase, thereby suppressing production of thromboxane A_2 in platelets, which induces platelet aggregation and vasoconstriction in response to various stimuli such as thrombin (7). DP inhibits phosphodiesterases in platelets and thereby elevates cyclic adenosine monophosphate (cAMP), which results in vasodilation, platelet anti-aggregation, and inhibition of thromboxane A_2 (8). Ticlopidine (9) and clopidogrel (10) selectively inhibit adenosine diphosphate (ADP)-induced platelet binding to fibrinogen by affecting ADP-dependent activation of glycoprotein IIb/IIIa complex on platelet surface.

Acetylsalicylic Acid

ASA is the best-studied medical therapy in stroke prevention and the most commonly prescribed agent for secondary stroke prevention. Meta-analysis of the Antithrombotic Trialists' Collaboration showed that antiplatelet therapy among those with previous stroke or TIA was followed by odds reduction of 22% (SE 4) in the risk of having nonfatal stroke, nonfatal myocardial infarction, or vascular death per 1,000 patients treated (11). Aspirin is highly cost effective and generally well tolerated. Nonetheless, its clinical benefits in stroke prevention are less than ideal, mainly because of its relatively small magnitude of effect. Of the 10 controlled studies available comparing aspirin and placebo in the secondary prevention of ischemic stroke, only three trials were large enough to have appropriate power to answer the question of whether aspirin is effective [United Kingdom Transient Ischaemic Attack (UK-TIA) Study (12), Swedish Aspirin Low-dose Trial (SALT) (13), and European Stroke Prevention Study 2 (ESPS2) (14)]. In these three trials, aspirin reduced the relative risk of the combined endpoint of stroke, myocardial infarction, and death from vascular causes by 13% (15). The absolute risk reduction was 3%. This relatively unsatisfactory result explains why other antiplatelet drugs such as ticlopidine and clopidogrel were developed and investigated. The general opinion in Europe is that small doses of aspirin (30 to 250 mg) are as effective as larger doses but have much fewer side effects. This opinion is supported by the study of Tijssen (16), who performed a meta-analysis that included more than 9,000 patients from 10 studies. The studies were categorized according to dose ranges (1,000–1,300 mg, 300 mg, 50–75 mg). There was no relationship between the dose of ASA and risk reduction, which varied from 9% (300 mg) to 14% (50–75 mg), overall 13%. The same result was achieved in an independent meta-analysis by Algra et al. (17). However, the Antithrombotic Trialists' Collaboration came to the conclusion that the effects of doses lower than 75 mg daily were less certain (11).

Ticlopidine

There are two large North American studies in patients with cerebrovascular disease: the Ticlopidine-Aspirin Stroke Study (TASS) (18) and the Canadian-American Ticlopidine Study (CATS) (19). TASS was a randomized study comparing ticlopidine (250 mg twice daily) with aspirin (650 mg twice daily) in 3,069 patients with TIA and minor stroke who were followed for an average of 3.3 years. Intention-to-treat analysis gave a relative risk reduction of 12% for the combined endpoint of nonfatal stroke or death from all causes. CATS was a randomized, double blind, placebo-controlled trial to prevent stroke recurrence (ticlopidine 250 mg twice daily) involving 1,072 patients with a substantial completed stroke. Follow-up lasted an average of 2 years. Intention-to-treat analysis gave a relative risk reduction of 23.3% ($p = 0.02$) for the combined endpoints (nonfatal stroke, nonfatal myocardial infarction, and vascular death). The treatment was effective in both men and women. Adverse events associated with ticlopidine included severe neutropenia, skin rash, and diarrhea. All of these side effects were reversible after treatment was withdrawn. A complete blood cell count with differential and platelet count should be per-

formed before starting treatment and every 2 weeks during the first 3 months of ticlopidine therapy.

Clopidogrel

The efficacy of the ticlopidine derivative clopidogrel was studied in the Clopidogrel versus Aspirin in Patients at Risk of Ischemic Events (CAPRIE) Study (20), which was one of the largest randomized trials of secondary prevention of stroke, myocardial infarction, and vascular death. In the CAPRIE Study, clopidogrel 75 mg and aspirin 325 mg daily were compared in patients with recent ischemic stroke, recent myocardial infarction, or symptomatic peripheral arterial disease. Patients were treated and followed for a minimum of 1 year and a maximum of 3 years with a mean follow-up of 1.9 years (Table 36-1).

There were more than 6,300 patients in each of the three clinical subgroups, for a total of 19,185 patients. The primary endpoint of the study was the risk of the combined outcome of ischemic stroke, myocardial infarction, or vascular death. There were 1,960 validated first events included in the primary outcome cluster on which an intention-to-treat analysis showed an absolute risk reduction of 0.5% and a relative risk reduction of 8.7% ($p = 0.043$) in favor of clopidogrel. There were no significant differences in adverse events, and there was no increased risk of neutropenia in the clopidogrel group in contrast to the ticlopidine groups of CATS and TASS. The investigators concluded that the overall safety profile of clopidogrel is at least as good as that of medium-dose aspirin.

Clopidogrel is an effective alternative for secondary prevention of stroke. It is especially suitable for those who cannot tolerate aspirin. Because it was more effective than ASA in the CAPRIE Study, it also could be used primarily instead of ASA in high-risk patients, as well as for patients who have ischemic symptoms despite use of ASA or combination therapy with ASA and DP.

Combined Use of Acetylsalicylic Acid and Dipyridamole

The benefits of DP in combination with ASA were first shown in the European Stroke Prevention Study 1 (ESPS1) (21). In that double blind study of 2,500 patients with prior stroke or TIA, treatment with a combination of immediate-release DP (75 mg three times daily) plus ASA (330 mg three times daily) was compared with placebo. The 2-year relative risk reduction of fatal and nonfatal strokes was 38% ($p < 0.0001$) and that of stroke and all-cause mortality was

TABLE 36-1. *CAPRIE Study: primary and secondary endpoints, intention-to-treat analysis (20)*

Outcome event	Treatment group	First outcome events	Event rate/yr	Relative risk reduction (95% CI)	*p* Value
Ischemic stroke, MI, or	Clopidogrel	939	5.32%	8.7%	0.043
vascular death	ASA	1,021	5.83%	(0.3%, 16.5%)	
Vascular death	Clopidogrel	350	1.9%	7.6%	0.29
	ASA	378	2.06%	(−6.9%, 20.1%)	
Any stroke, MI, or death	Clopidogrel	1,133	6.43%	7.0%	0.081
from any cause	ASA	1,207	6.9%	(−0.9%, 14.2%)	
Death from any cause	Clopidogrel	560	3.05%	2.2%	0.71
	ASA	571	3.11%	(−9.9%, 12.9%)	

ASA, acetylsalicylic acid; CI, confidence interval; MI, myocardial infarction.

33.5%. The results of ESPS1 demonstrate the value of combined antiplatelet therapy in the secondary prevention of stroke; however, the study design did not include a treatment arm provided with ASA alone.

ESPS2 (14) was designed to clarify the efficacy of combined ASA and slow-release DP with low-dose ASA alone, the efficacy of low-dose ASA alone, and placebo in a 2×2 factorial design. ASA was given at a dose of 25 mg two times a day and slow-release DP at a dose of 200 mg two times a day. The trial included 6,602 patients with prior TIA (23.7%) or ischemic stroke (76.3%). Patients were followed for 2 years. The relative risk reduction was 37% for the combination therapy in the prevention of stroke, 18% ($p = 0.013$) for ASA alone, and 16% ($p = 0.039$) for DP alone in comparison with placebo (Table 36-2). Combined ASA+DP was 23% more effective than ASA alone in stroke prevention ($p = 0.006$). Combined ASA+DP compared with ASA alone was associated with a 12% relative risk reduction in the primary outcome of stroke and death from any cause (Fig. 36-1). Thus, the preventive benefit of combination therapy in ESPS2 was of a similar magnitude to that observed in ESPS1. ESPS2 showed the superiority of ASA+DP over ASA alone.

The results of ESPS2 also show that adding DP to a small dose of ASA does not influence the tolerability compared with any of the study drugs given alone. The patients tolerated all of the treatment alternatives, and there were few severe adverse events. There were two to three times more bleeding events (including mild bleeds) in the patients who used ASA either alone or combined with DP. A bleeding complication was the cause for termination about four times more frequently in the ASA groups (1.2%) than in the placebo group (0.3%). Headache was significantly more common (8%) in the patients who used DP, whereas it occurred in about 2% in the other groups. This difference disappeared within the first 3 months.

It can be calculated from the results of ESPS2 that ASA prevents stroke in 29 of 1,000 treated patients, whereas ASA+DP prevents stroke in 58 of 1,000 treated patients. It also can be calculated (22) that one must treat 35 patients with ASA in order to prevent one stroke but only 17 patients with ASA+DP.

The Antithrombotic Trialists' Collaboration stated that the results of ESPS2 suggested a worthwhile further reduction in stroke but that it also is plausible that these findings (which were not supported by other studies) arose largely or wholly by chance (11). Another possible explanation for the better result in ESPS2 than in the previous studies could be the new, slow-release formulation of DP (11).

There has been critical commentary about the ESPS2 study design, for example, use of a placebo when the efficacy of ASA was proven, use of low-dose aspirin, and one study site that enrolled fictitious patients. Additional study of ASA and DP is ongoing in the European/Australian Stroke Prevention in Reversible Ischaemia Trials (ESPRIT), in which the combination of aspirin plus DP is being compared to aspirin alone in TIA and stroke patients (23).

DISCUSSION

Several platelet inhibitors (aspirin, ticlopidine, clopidogrel, and the combination of ASA with slow-release DP) have proven effective in patients with various causes of TIA/ischemic stroke (11,14,18,19,20). Recommendations about the choice of antiplatelet drugs in patients with TIA or stroke have been published but are not unanimous. The recommendations of the European Stroke Initiative (EUSI) (24) have been approved by the European Stroke Council (ESC), the European Neurological Society (ENS), and the European Federation of Neurological Societies (EFNS) and reflect a European consensus for

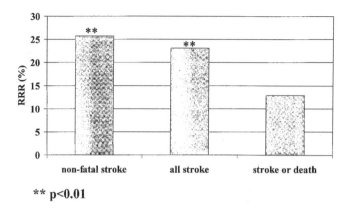

** p<0.01

FIG. 36-1. In the European Stroke Prevention Study 2, combined sustained release dipyridamole 200 mg and acetylsalicylic acid (ASA) 25 mg twice daily produced a significant 23% relative risk reduction of fatal and nonfatal stroke, a significant 25.7% reduction in nonfatal stroke, and a nonsignificant 12.9% reduction in stroke or death from any cause compared with ASA alone (14).

TABLE 36-2. *Effect of individual treatments on stroke endpoint, combined endpoint of stroke or death, and death*

	Stroke			Stroke or death			Death		
	No. of events/ patients (%)	Relative risk reduction (%)	p Value	No. of events/ patients (%)	Relative risk reduction (%)	p Value	No. of events/ patients (%)	Relative risk reduction (%)	p Value
ASA-DP vs. placebo	157/1,650 (9.5)			286/1,650 (17.3)			185/1,650 (11.2)		
		37.0	<0.001		24.4	<0.001		8.5	0.32
	250/1,649 (15.2)			378/1,649 (22.9)			202/1,649 (12.2)		
ASA-DP vs. ASA	157/1,650 (9.5)			286/1,650 (17.3)			185/1,650 (11.2)		
		23.1	0.006		12.6	0.056		−2.8	0.78
	206/1,649 (12.5)			330/1,649 (20.0)			182/1,649 (11.0)		
ASA-DP vs. DP	157/1,650 (9.5)			286/1,649 (17.3)			185/1,650 (11.2)		
		24.7	0.002		10.1	0.073		1.8	0.82
	−211/1,654 (12.8)			321/1,654 (19.4)			188/1,654 (11.4)		
ASA vs. placebo	206/1,649 (12.5)			330/1,649 (20.0)			182/1,649 (11.0)		
		18.1	0.013		13.2	0.017		10.9	0.20
	250/1,649 (15.2)			378/1,649 (22.9)			202/1,649 (12.2)		
DP vs. placebo	211/1,654 (12.8)			321/1,654 (19.4)			188/1,654 (11.4)		
		16.3	0.04		15.4	0.015		7.2	0.45
	250/1,649 (15.2)			378/1,649 (22.9)			202/1,649 (12.2)		

ASA, acetylsalicylic acid; DP, dipyridamole. ASA-D; combination of acetylsalicylic acid and dipyridamole. Pairwise comparison with survival analysis. Results of ESPS2 (14).

stroke prevention. These recommendations state that ASA should be given as a first choice, or the combination of ASA and DP, where available. (Table 36-3). Clopidogrel also may be prescribed as a first choice, when ASA is not tolerated, and in high-risk patients or patients with ischemic events taking ASA. Patients who do not tolerate ASA or clopidogrel may be treated with DP alone. Clopidogrel should be given instead of ticlopidine when thienopyridines are prescribed. However, patients who already have been treated with ticlopidine for a long time should continue taking it

There is a paucity of data regarding how these recommendations translate into clinical practice and which factors affect the choice of antiplatelet drugs in patients with a recent ischemic cerebrovascular event. In a study from the Vienna Stroke Register (25), the most important factor influencing the use of clopidogrel was aspirin administration before an index event. The investigators found a high interhospital variability in the use of the combination of ASA with slow-release DP. The relation between ASA and clopidogrel use also varied significantly between departments. Thus, for clopidogrel and ASA+DP, the most prominent factor influencing their use or nonuse was divergent interpretation of the available evidence. Other main factors were the higher cost (clopidogrel) or individual experience and side effects (ASA+DP).

In secondary prevention of stroke, there now are alternatives to the less expensive but less effective ASA. The combination of ASA with DP is somewhat more expensive, and clopidogrel is even more expensive. Both the ASA-DP combination and clopidogrel are more effective than ASA (26,27). Among TIA or stroke patients, the number needed to treat to prevent one stroke with aspirin was 100. The number is 62 using clopidogrel and 53 using the combination of ASA and slow-release DP (28). Adding DP to ASA or substituting clopidogrel for ASA is more expensive than ASA alone in stroke prevention, but more cost effective in high-risk patients if they can be identified (28).

There is a common trend to use combinations of drugs with different functional mechanisms to improve outcomes in many diseases. The use of combination therapies is a generally accepted view in hypertension, diabetes, and malignancies. It makes sense to use two or more therapies if they are additive and have no harmful interaction. In epilepsy, one drug is prescribed and used up to the highest recommended dose or until side effects occur. If seizures continue, a second drug is added. This may not be an appropriate strategy in stroke prevention. When a TIA or minor stroke has occurred, the next event might be a transient occlusion of the trunk of middle cerebral artery (MCA), but it also could be a permanent occlusion of the MCA. Thus, in stroke patients, it may be difficult to justify the use of a less effective therapy, although it may be a less expensive alternative (e.g., ASA). Table 36-4 compares the three most effective therapies over ASA alone that have been evaluated in controlled studies. It is evident that the combination of ASA with DP is more effective than low-dose ASA, and both ticlopidine and clopidogrel are more effective than ASA alone. It appears that in the long run, ASA combined with DP is more effective and less costly compared with aspirin alone (29).

Other combinations of drugs probably will become available in the future. An attractive approach may be to combine aspirin with clopidogrel. It is reasonable to expect that this combination is superior to aspirin only, because each component of the combination works by a different mechanism of action. However, without a randomized trial, we cannot be certain that the combination is effective and safe. A clinical trial to study these agents, the Management of Atherothrombosis with Clopidogrel in High-Risk Patients

---

TABLE 36-3. *EUSI recommendations (31)*

1. Low- or medium-dose ASA (50–325 mg) can be be given as first-choice agent to reduce stroke recurrence (level I). Where available, the combination of ASA (25 mg) and dipyridamole (200 mg) twice daily may be given (level I).
2. Clopidogrel is slightly more effective than aspirin for prevention of atherothrombotic events (level I). It may be prescribed as first choice, when aspirin is not tolerated or efficacious, and in special situations, such as high-risk patients or a previous event on aspirin (level III).
3. Patients starting treatment with thienopyridine derivatives should receive clopidogrel instead of ticlopidine because it has fewer side effects (level I). Patients who already have been treated with ticlopidine for a long time should be maintained on this regimen because the most severe side effects (neutropenia and rash) appear at the beginning of treatment.
4. Patients who do not tolerate either ASA or clopidogrel may be treated with dipyridamole retard, 2 × 200 mg daily (level I).

ASA, acetylsalicylic acid; EUSI, European Stroke Initiative.

TABLE 36-4. *Relative risk reduction (%) with each study medication compared with aspirin therapy in three major controlled studies, intention-to-treat analysis*

Endpoint	TASS (18)	CAPRIE (20)	ESPS2 (14)
Stroke	21	8	23
Stroke or death	12	NA	13
Stroke, MI, vascular death[b]	NA	7	21
Vascular death	−4	2	−2

MI, myocardial infarction.
Daily treatment: Ticlodipine Aspirin Stroke Study (TASS): ticlopidine 500 mg vs. aspirin 1,300 mg; Clopidoprel versus Aspirin in Patients at Risk of Ischemic Events (CAPRIE): clopidogrel 75 mg vs. aspirin 325 mg; European Stroke Prevention Study 2 (ESPS2): aspirin 50 mg + dipyridamole 400 mg vs. aspirin 50 mg.
[a]Clinical subgroup "ischemic stroke" in CAPRIE study.
[b]Combined endpoint "vascular events" in ESPS2 study.

Trial (MATCH), was launched 1 year ago. The patients in that study had a recent TIA or ischemic stroke and at least one additional risk factor such as diabetes or prior atherothrombotic event. They will be randomized to either clopidogrel 75 mg plus ASA 325 mg/day or clopidogrel 75 mg/day alone. The results will be available in about 2 years. In the meantime, the combination of clopidogrel and ASA may be appropriate for patients with a history of recent cardiac ischemia who appear to be at a low risk of hemorrhagic complications or if they have suffered a stroke while undergoing another antiplatelet therapy (30).

CONCLUSIONS

There are a number of recommendations for optimal therapy to prevent recurrent stroke in patients with TIA or ischemic stroke. The recommendations made by the EUSI (Table 36-3) reflect the European perspective and has been approved by the ESC, ENS, and EFNS (24). According to EUSI recommendations, the first choice is ASA (50–325 mg) or the combination of ASA (25 mg) and slow-release DP (200 mg) twice daily in countries where this is available. Clopidogrel (75 mg) may be prescribed as a first choice or when aspirin is not tolerated or is not efficacious (31).

There are no studies suggesting procedures to follow if the effective therapies of combined aspirin and DP or clopidogrel fail, and the patient has suffered a new TIA or ischemic stroke while undergoing these therapies. Certainly, one must be assured that all the investigational studies to reveal the cause of recurrent ischemic event have been performed; if indicated, some of these studies must be repeated. If there is any reason to suspect a cardiac cause for ischemic attacks, then anticoagulant therapy should be started. The indication for carotid surgery in case of major stenotic lesion should be reconsidered if surgery was postponed. One option would be to try a combination treatment with aspirin, DP, and clopidogrel. Naturally, the effectiveness and safety of this combination has never been evaluated, but such a combination theoretically is attractive.

Antiplatelet therapy should be started immediately when the diagnosis of TIA or ischemic stroke has been made. Because the risk of a new event is greatest in the early phase after the index event, the urgency of sending a patient for investigations is strongly emphasized. There are no studies about the duration of antiplatelet therapy. Most reasonable would be to continue as long as the risk is present. Because the most common reason for ischemic cerebrovascular disease is atherosclerosis, it is presumed that treatment should continue for the rest of the patient's life if there are no contraindications for it. This is the main reason for developing drugs and doses of drugs that can be tolerated by patients and that do not lose their effectiveness over the years.

REFERENCES

1. Murray CJ, Lopez AD. Mortality by cause for eight regions of the world: global burden of disease study. *Lancet* 1997;349:1269–1276.
2. The World Bank. *World development report 1993: investing in health.* New York: Oxford University Press, 1993
3. Kaste M, Fogelholm R, Rissanen A. Economic burden of stroke and the evaluation of new therapies. *Public Health* 1998;112:103–112.
4. Sandercock PAG, van del Belt AGM, Lindley RI, et al. Antithrombotic therapy in acute ischaemic stroke: an overview of the completed randomized trials. *J Neurol Neurosurg Psychiatry* 1993;56:17–25.
5. Bonita R. Epidemiology of stroke. *Lancet* 1992;339:342–344.
6. Wilterdink JL, Easton JD. Vascular event rates in patients with atherosclerotic cerebrovascular disease. *Arch Neurol* 1992;49:857–863.
7. Patrono C. Aspirin as an antiplatelet drug. *N Engl J Med* 1994;18:1287–1294.

8. Müller TH, Su CA, Weisenberg H, et al. Dipyridamole alone or combined with low dose acetylsalicylic acid inhibits platelet aggregation in human whole blood ex vivo. *Br J Clin Pharmacol* 1990;30:179–186.

9. Kent RA. Ticlopidine. *Lancet* 1991;337:459–460.

10. Herber J, Frehel D, Vallee E, et al. Clopidogrel, a novel antiplatelet and antithrombotic agent. *Cardiovasc Drug Rev* 1993;11:180–198.

11. Antithrombotic Trialists' Collaboration. Collaborative meta-analysis of randomised trials of antiplatelet therapy for prevention of death, myocardial infarction, and stroke in high risk patients. *BMJ* 2002;324:71–86.

12. UK-TIA Study Group. United Kingdom Transient Ischaemic Attack (UK-TIA) aspirin trial: interim results. *BMJ* 1988;296:316–320.

13. The Salt Collaborative Group. Swedish Aspirin Low-dose Trial (SALT) of 75 mg aspirin as secondary prophylaxis after cerebrovascular ischaemic events. *Lancet* 1991;338:1345–1349.

14. Diener HC, Cunha L, Forbes C, et al. European Stroke Prevention Study 2. DP and acetylsalicylic acid in the secondary prevention of stroke. *J Neurol Sci* 1996;143: 1–13.

15. Diener H-C. Stroke prevention. Antiplatelet and thrombolytic therapy. In *Neurologic clinics: stroke, vol. 19.* Philadelphia: WB Saunders Company, 2000:343–355.

16. Tijssen JG. Low-dose and high-dose acetylsalicylic acid, with and without dipyridamole: a review of clinical trial results. *Neurology* 1998;51[3 Suppl 3]: S15–S16.

17. Algra A, van Gijn J. ASA at any dose above 30 mg offers only modest protection after cerebral ischemia. *J Neurol Neurosurg Psychiatry* 1996;60:197–199.

18. Hass WK, Easton JD, Adams HP Jr, et al. A randomized trial comparing ticlopidine hydrochloride with aspirin for the prevention of stroke in high-risk patients. Ticlopidine Aspirin Stroke Study Group. *N Engl J Med* 1989; 321:501–507.

19. Gent M, Blakely JA, Easton JD, et al. The Canadian American Ticlopidine Study (CATS) in thromboembolic stroke. *Lancet* 1989;1:1215–1220.

20. CAPRIE Steering Committee. A randomized, blinded, trial of clopidogrel versus aspirin in patients at risk of ischemic events (CAPRIE). *Lancet* 1996;348: 1329–1339.

21. ESPS Group. The European Stroke Prevention Study. Preliminary results. *Lancet* 1987;2:1351–1345.

22. Cook RJ, Sackett DL. The number needed to treat: a clinically useful measure of treatment effect. *BMJ* 1995; 310:452–454.

23. De Schryver EL. Design of ESPRIT: an international randomized trial for secondary prevention after non-disabling cerebral ischaemia of arterial origin. European/Australian Stroke Prevention in Reversible Ischaemia Trials (ESPRIT) group. *Cerebrovasc Dis* 2000;10: 147–150.

24. Hacke W, Kaste M, Olsen TS, et al., for the EUSI Executive Committee. European Stroke Initiative recommendations for stroke management. *Cerebrovasc Dis* 2000;10:335–351.

25. Lalouschek W, Land W, Mullner M, on behalf of the Vienna Stroke Study Group. Current strategies of secondary prevention after a cerebrovascular event. *Stroke* 2001;32:2860–2866.

26. Wilterdink JL, Easton JD. Dipyridamole plus aspirin in cerebrovascular disease. *Arch Neurol* 1999;56: 1087–1092.

27. Hankey GJ, Sudlow CLM, Dunbabin DW. Thienopyridines or aspirin to prevent stroke and other serious vascular events in patients at high risk of vascular events. A systematic review of the evidence from randomized trials. *Stroke* 2000;31:1779–1784.

28. Hankey GJ, Warlow CP. Treatment and secondary prevention of stroke: evidence, costs, and effects on individuals and populations. *Lancet* 1999;354:1457–1463.

29. Sarasin FP, Gaspoz J-M, Bounameux H. Cost-effectiveness of new antiplatelet regimens used as secondary prevention of stroke or transient ischemic attack. *Arch Intern Med* 2000;160:2773–2778.

30. Albers GW, Amarenco P. Combination therapy with clopidogrel and aspirin. Can the cure results be extrapolated to cerebrovascular patients? *Stroke* 2001;32: 2948–2949.

31. Bogousslavsky J, Kaste M, Olsen TS, et al., for the EUSI Executive Committee. Risk factors and stroke prevention. *Cerebrovasc Dis* 2000;10[Suppl 3]:12–21.

Ischemic Stroke: Advances in Neurology, Vol. 92. Edited by
H.J.M. Barnett, Julien Bogousslavsky, and Heather Meldrum.
Lippincott Williams & Wilkins, Philadelphia © 2003.

37

Commentary on Antiplatelet Agents

Saran Jonas

Department of Neurology, New York University Medical Center, New York, New York, U.S.A.

The results of the randomized trials of antiplatelet agents are reviewed from the viewpoint of a stroke neurologist. Where results for an agent are available from only a single trial, the statistical analyses of the investigators are presented. Some agents have undergone several trials. Such results have been combined by Anne Zeleniuch-Jacquotte, M.D., Department of Environmental Medicine, New York University School of Medicine (1), and are given as an effect of treatment on the composite endpoint of stroke and death (S+D), new nonfatal stroke of any type or death from any cause, and are presented as odds ratios (ORs). OR for S+D = $[(S+D)_t/(N_t - (S+D)_t)]/[(S+D)_c/(N_c - (S+D)_c)]$, where t is treatment and c is control. The complement of S+D is survival free of new stroke. OR < 1.0 indicates that treatment gives a better outcome than control management; OR > 1.0 indicates the converse.

RESULTS OF TRIALS

Aspirin Versus Placebo in Various Populations

Aspirin [acetylsalicylic acid (ASA)] has been demonstrated ($p < 0.05$ or better) to reduce S+D in three groups of people: (a) patients with recent stroke or transient ischemic attack (TIA) (OR: 0.83); (b) patients who entered into study during acute ischemic stroke (OR: 0.90); and (c) people with nonvalvular atrial fibrillation (NVAF) (OR: 0.79; Table 37-1).

In contrast, in studies of people without such previous conditions (total N of these studies = 29,570), ASA was not shown to have a statistically confirmed beneficial effect on S+D [OR 0.97, 95% confidence interval (CI) 0.87–1.08, $p > 0.05$, NS].

Effect of Aspirin Versus Placebo in Women

Jonas and Zeleniuch-Jacquotte (2) previously analyzed by sex the S+D outcomes of aspirin trials among patients treated after stroke or TIA. The ORs were identical for 3,691 men (0.82) and 1,596 women (0.82), although the results were statistically significant only for men ($p = 0.01$). Considering differences in sample size and event rate, we concluded that the results were compatible with the view that aspirin was equally effective in women as in men.

Optimal Dose of Aspirin

In the analyses, results were combined without regard to daily dose of aspirin, which ranged from 50

TABLE 37-1. *Effect on S+D odds ratios of aspirin versus placebo in various populations*

Population (no. of trials)	Total no. of participants	Odds ratio	95% Confidence interval	p Value
Previous stroke or TIA (11)	9,468	0.83	0.75–0.92	<0.001
Acute ischemic stroke (3)	31,132	0.90	0.83–0.98	<0.05
Nonvalvular atrial fibrillation (3)	2,574	0.79	0.65–0.97	<0.05
Without the above factors (3)	29,750	0.97	0.87–1.08	NS

S+D, composite endpoint of stroke and death; TIA, transient ischemic attack.

For previous stroke or TIA: ten trials (see "The Aspirin Papers" of the Antiplatelet Trialists' Collaboration (12): AITIA, Reuther, Canadian Cooperative, Toulouse-TIA, AICLA, Danish Cooperative, Britton, Danish Low Dose, UK TIA, and SALT; the eleventh trial: ESPS2 (13). Acute ischemic stroke trials: CAST, IST, and MAST-I (see the CAST paper (14). Nonvalvular atrial fibrillation trials: SPAF, AFASAK, EAFT (see "The Aspirin Papers,"). "Without the above factors": UK doctors; US physicians (see "The Aspirin Papers"); Meade et al. (15).

TABLE 37-2. *Direct comparisons between ASA doses: effect on S+D odds ratios in patients with previous stroke or transient ischemic attack*

Cohort	S+D (higher/ lower dose)	Total no. of participants (higher/lower dose)	Odds ratio (higher/lower dose)	95% Confidence interval	p Value
UK TIA: ASA 1,200 vs. 300 mg/d	193/191	815/806	1.00	0.79–1.26	NS
Dutch TIA: ASA 283 vs. 30 mg/d	260/250	1,576/1,555	1.03	0.85–1.25	NS

ASA, acetylsalicylic acid; S+D, composite endpoint of stroke and death.

mg [European Stroke Prevention Study 2 (ESPS2)] to 1,500 mg (Swedish Cooperative Study) (Table 37-2). The justification for combining results without regard to dose derives from the UK TIA Trial (3) and the Dutch TIA Trial (4). The UK Trial showed that 1,200 mg of aspirin was no better than 300 mg daily; in the Dutch trial, aspirin 283 mg offered no benefit over 30 mg. These results are compatible with the interpretation that high or moderate doses of aspirin are no more efficacious than low doses.

Dipyridamole or Ticlopidine Versus Placebo

By indirect comparison with placebo, the S+D ORs for dipyridamole (DP), aspirin, and ticlopidine are similar (0.83–0.84). The results for ticlopidine did not reach statistical significance (Table 37-3).

Dipyridamole or Ticlopidine Versus Aspirin

By direct comparison, DP and aspirin are equal, and ticlopidine is superior to aspirin (OR: 0.81; 95% CI: 0.69–0.95; Table 37-4).

Clopidogrel Versus Aspirin

Clopidogrel 75 mg was compared to aspirin 325 mg daily in the Clopidogrel versus Aspirin in Patients at Risk of Ischaemic Events (CAPRIE) Trial (5). For the 6,431 patients admitted after ischemic stroke, Barnett and Eliasziw (6) found a relative risk reduction of 8.0% for subsequent ischemic stroke, favoring clopidogrel ($p = 0.31$, NS). For the entire cohort (19,185 patients, of whom 12,754 had been admitted because of MI or peripheral arterial disease), Rupprecht et al. (6) determined relative risk reduction of 5.2% for subsequent ischemic stroke, but this was not significant (95% CI: −7.9% to 16.7%). [The published data do not permit S+D analysis for the 6,431 ischemic stroke patients, and the sponsors have refused to release these data (6).]

Aspirin Versus Anticoagulation

Aspirin reduced S+D occurrence in patients treated because of NVAF (OR vs. placebo 0.79; $p < 0.05$; Table 37-1). In their review of the five primary prevention studies of warfarin in NVAF (aspirin also was used in three of these studies), Ezekowitz and Levine (7) commented, "All trials....were terminated early because of the benefit demonstrated with warfarin." Against placebo, the stroke risk was reduced by 68% with warfarin and by 36% with aspirin.

Mohr et al. (8) reported the Warfarin-Aspirin Recurrent Stroke Study (WARSS) results of aspirin 325 mg daily versus warfarin [international normalized ratio (INR) 1.4–2.8] in patients with noncar-

TABLE 37-3. *Effect on S+D odds ratios of various agents versus placebo in patients with previous stroke or transient ischemic attack*

Agent (no. of trials)	Total no. of participants	Odds ratio	95% Confidence interval	p Value
Aspirin (11)	9,468	0.83	0.75–0.92	<0.001
Dipyridamole (2)	3,472	0.83	0.71–0.98	<0.05
Ticlopidine (5)	1,206	0.84	0.64–1.10	NS

S+D, composite endpoint of stroke and death.
Aspirin trials: see Table 37.1. Dipyridamole: ESPS2 (see Table 37.1) and Stoke ("The Aspirin Papers," see Table 37.1). The five ticlopidine trials are CATS, Ross Russell, McKenna-III, Tokyo, and Ciufetti (see "The Aspirin Papers").

TABLE 37-4. *Direct comparison of various agents with ASA: effect on S+D odds ratios in patients with previous stroke or transient ischemic attack*

Agents (no. of trials)	Total no. of participants	Odds ratio	95% Confidence interval	p Value
Ticlopidine (2)	3,409	0.81	0.69–0.95	<0.05
Dipyridamole (1)	3,303	0.96	0.82–1.14	NS

ASA, acetylsalicylic acid; S+D, composite endpoint of stroke and death.
Ticlopidine: TASS and Japanese B; data are from "The Aspirin Papers" (see Table 37.1). Dipyridamole: ESPS2 (see Table 37.1).

dioembolic ischemic stroke. The primary endpoint was recurrent ischemic stroke or death from any cause. The authors calculated the hazard ratio for this combined endpoint was 1.13 (close to OR of 1.14) favoring aspirin; the difference was not statistically significant (95% CI: 0.92–1.38; $p = 0.25$). The results indicate that aspirin is as effective as warfarin in ischemic stroke of noncardioembolic origin.

One of the three acute stroke studies (International Stroke Trial [IST] (9); N = 19,435) had subcutaneous heparin (5,000 or 12,500 international units twice daily), aspirin (300 mg daily), and placebo arms. For S+D in the first 2 weeks after acute ischemic stroke, aspirin was not inferior to heparin (OR for heparin vs. aspirin: 1.08).

The Heparin in Acute Embolic Stroke Trial (HAEST) (10) compared the low-molecular-weight heparin dalteparin with aspirin 160 mg/d in 449 atrial fibrillation patients with acute ischemic stroke. The 14-day outcomes for S+D showed an OR of 0.73 favoring aspirin, but the difference was not statistically significant.

Aspirin Plus Anticoagulation

The IST data allow comparison of the effect on early stroke recurrence of aspirin + heparin versus aspirin alone (N = 9,719). For intracranial hemorrhage or recurrent ischemic stroke, there was no significant difference after 2 weeks of treatment (OR for aspirin + heparin vs. aspirin alone: 0.99).

The report of Meade et al. (see legend to Table 37-1) gives the S+D outcomes of prophylactic regimens in primary prevention in men at high risk for vascular events. At mean follow-up of 6.7 years, the fatal strokes + nonfatal strokes + nonstroke deaths were 12 + 17 + 91 in 1,277 subjects taking warfarin (mean INR 1.47) + aspirin (75 mg daily), and 1 + 25 + 109 in 1,272 subjects taking placebo. OR was 0.87, but the difference was not statistically significant.

Aspirin Plus Dipyridamole

For ASA+DP versus placebo, the OR for S+D was 0.68 ($p < 0.0001$; Table 37-5). ASA+DP showed a favorable OR of 0.89 against aspirin alone, but the p

TABLE 37-5. *Effect on S+D odds ratios of ASA in combination with DP in patients with previous stroke or transient ischemic attack*

Agents (no. of trials)	Total no. of participants	Odds ratio	95% Confidence interval	p Value
ASA + DP vs. placebo (5)	6,577	0.68	0.60–0.77	<0.0001
ASA + DP vs. ASA (5)	5,056	0.89	0.77–1.03	NS

ASA, acetylsalicylic acid; DP, dipyridamole; S+D, composite endpoint of stroke and death.
ASA + DP vs. placebo: ESPS2 (see Table 37.1), plus ESPS1, AICLA, Toulouse-TIA, and Toulouse-II (from "The Aspirin Papers"). ASA + DP vs. ASA: ESPS2; plus AICLA, Toulouse-TIA, ACCSG, and Capildeo (from "The Aspirin Papers"). The odds ratio (OR) for ASA + DP vs. placebo of 0.68 is composed of OR of 0.71 for ESPS2 (3,299 patients; the treatment was Aggrenox: aspirin 25 mg combined with slow-release DP 200 mg; one such tablet was given twice daily), and OR of 0.65 for the other four studies (ASA + conventional DP 150–255 mg/d). These results imply that conventional DP in doses no greater than 225 mg daily is as effective as DP 400 mg daily in slow-release form. However, the apparent uniformity of benefit is not seen in trials against ASA. OR for ASA + DP vs. ASA in ESPS2 (N = 3,299 patients; total of 616 S+D) is 0.84. The combined OR for the other four studies (N = 1,757; total of 283 S+D) is 0.98. In three of these four studies, conventional DP was given in daily doses of 150–300 mg (for the unpublished 183-patient Capildeo study—reference: "The Aspirin Papers"—DP dose is not stated). These data imply that conventional DP in doses of 150–300 mg daily is *not* as effective as slow-release DP 400 mg daily. If this is so, is Aggrenox superior because of the slow-release formulation or the higher dose? The study of Chevolet et al. (16) suggests that the formulation is not relevant in the steady state. In humans, similar plasma dipyridamole levels and inhibitory effects on platelet adenosine uptake were obtained with conventional DP 100 mg four times daily and slow-release DP 200 mg twice daily.

value of this result was not statistically significant, and the 95% confidence interval was 0.77 to 1.03. (For further discussion of these results, see legend to Table 37-5.)

OVERVIEW OF ANTIPLATELET AGENTS, WITH COST CONSIDERATIONS

Tables 37-6A and 37-6B summarize the costs of the various antiplatelet agents and their S+D ORs in patients with previous ischemic stroke or TIA. The results of the studies directly comparing aspirin with DP or with clopidogrel show no statistically significant difference in S+D outcome and therefore no justification for the use of expensive DP or very expensive clopidogrel (available only as proprietary Plavix) rather than aspirin, which is inexpensive. The only candidates warranting consideration for use in place of aspirin monotherapy are ticlopidine and ASA+DP.

Ticlopidine is statistically superior to aspirin by direct comparison (OR: 0.81; $p < 0.05$). Based on published clinical trial results, ticlopidine should be the first choice for secondary stroke prevention in noncardiac situations where financial and logistical factors permit. However, according to the manufacturer's entry on Ticlid (proprietary ticlopidine) in the *Physicians' Desk Reference* (11): "Because TICLID is associated with a risk of life-threatening blood dyscrasias including thrombotic thrombocytopenic purpura (TTP) and neutropenia/agranulocytosis (see BOXED WARNINGS and WARNINGS) TICLID should be reserved for patients who are intolerant or allergic to aspirin therapy or who have failed aspirin therapy." The boxed warning estimates the incidence of neutropenia as 2.4%, agranulocytosis 0.08%, and TTP one per 2,000 to 4,000.

ASA+DP has an OR of 0.89 on *direct* comparison with aspirin monotherapy, but this apparent superiority fails to reach statistical significance (95% CI: 0.77–1.03; Table 37-3). However, by *indirect* comparison of each regimen against placebo, ASA+DP seems almost twice as effective as aspirin alone in reducing S+D (OR of 0.68 for ASA+DP vs. 0.83 for ASA alone). Both ORs have strong p values. One might consider that the combination would have shown a statistically verified benefit over aspirin if the total N in the studies of ASA+DP versus aspirin had been somewhat larger.

Because there are no recognized dangerous consequences unique to DP, the only disadvantage to the combination is cost (Table 37-6B: $13.15–$26.20 for 30 days with generic DP; the 30-day cost is $82.95 with proprietary Aggrenox). The wager is the increased expense against the chance that ASA+DP actually is better than aspirin alone.

TABLE 37-6A. *Regimens, their lowest costs, and their effect (compared with placebo) on S+D odds ratios*

Agents and daily doses	30-Day cost	Odds ratio: regimen vs. placebo (*p* value)
ASA	$1.00	0.83 (<0.001)
DP	$12.15–$25.20	0.83 (<0.05)
Ticlopidine 500 mg	$84.69	0.84 (NS)
ASA + DP	$13.15–$26.20	0.68 (<0.0001)

TABLE 37-6B. *Regimens, their lowest costs, and their effect (compared with aspirin) on S+D odds ratios*

Agents and daily doses	30-Day cost	Odds ratio: regimen vs. ASA (*p* value)
ASA	$1.00	1.00
DP 400 mg	$25.20	0.96 (NS)
Clopidogrel (Plavix) 75 mg (no generic form)	$90.65	0.96 (NS)
ASA + DP	$13.15–$26.20	0.89 (NS)
Ticlopidine 500 mg	$84.69	0.81 (<0.05)

ASA, acetylsalicylic acid; DP, dipyridamole; S+D, composite endpoint of stroke and death.
Drug costs were obtained from *www.drugstore.com* on December 26, 2001.
From various *drugstore.com* prices, the 30-day ASA cost is approximated as $1.00. The only trial of DP vs. ASA is ESPS2: DP 400 mg daily in a slow-release form, which is not available commercially. For conventional DP 50 mg, the best *drugstore.com* price is $25.20 for 400 mg daily. For the ESPS1 dose of DP 225 mg daily + ASA, the 30-day cost would be $12.15 + $1.00 = $13.15. For the ESPS2 dose of DP 400 mg + ASA, the 30-day cost would be $25.20 + $1.00 = $26.20. (The proprietary preparation used in ESPS2 was Aggrenox: cost for 30 days would be $82.95.)

OVERVIEW OF ASPIRIN AND ANTICOAGULANTS

Aspirin given during acute ischemic stroke reduces S+D during the first 2 weeks as effectively as unfractionated heparin. Adding heparin to aspirin offers no demonstrable advantage.

Aspirin is as good as warfarin in preventing death or recurrence of ischemic stroke when given during long-term follow-up after an initial ischemic stroke. The combination of warfarin with aspirin for long-term primary prophylaxis is not demonstrably superior to treatment with aspirin alone.

Limited data show no suggestion of inferiority of aspirin to low-molecular-weight heparin in preventing death or new stroke in the first 2 weeks after stroke from NVAF.

Aspirin is significantly better than placebo for primary stroke prevention during long-term use in NVAF but is not as effective as warfarin. Warfarin is the long-term treatment of choice in patients with NVAF.

REFERENCES

1. Jonas S, Zeleniuch-Jacquotte A. Effect of antiplatelet agents on survival free of new stroke: a meta-analysis. *Stroke Clinical Updates (National Stroke Association)* 1998;VIII:1–4 [corrections and correspondence in *Stroke Clinical Updates (National Stroke Association)* 1998;VIII:1–6].
2. Jonas S, Zeleniuch-Jacquotte A. Effect of aspirin on risk of stroke or death in women who have suffered cerebral ischemia. *Cerebrovasc Dis* 1994:4:157–162.
3. UK-TIA Study Group. The United Kingdom Transient Ischaemic Attack (UK-TIA) Aspirin Trial: final results. *J Neurol Neurosurg Psychiatry* 1991;54:1044–1054.
4. The Dutch TIA Trial Study Group. A comparison of two doses of aspirin (30 mg vs. 283 mg a day) in patients after a transient ischemic attack or minor ischemic stroke. *N Engl J Med* 1991;325:1261–1266.
5. CAPRIE Steering Committee. A randomized, blinded, trial of clopidogrel versus aspirin in patients at risk of ischaemic events (CAPRIE). *Lancet* 1996;348:1329–1339.
6. Rupprecht HJ, on behalf of the CAPRIE Investigators. Consistency of the benefit of clopidogrel across a range of vascular-related endpoints: results from CAPRIE. *Eur Heart J* 1998;19:52(abst P484).
7. Ezekowitz MD, Levine JA. Preventing stroke in patients with atrial fibrillation. *JAMA* 1999;281:1830–1835.
8. Mohr JP, Thompson JLP, Lazar RM, et al., for the Warfarin-Aspirin Recurrent Stroke Study Group. A comparison of warfarin and aspirin for the prevention of recurrent ischemic stroke. *N Engl J Med* 2001;345:1444–1451.
9. International Stroke Collaborative Group. The International stroke Trial (IST): a randomised trial of aspirin, subcutaneous heparin, both, or neither among 19 435 patients with acute ischaemic stroke. *Lancet* 1997;349:1569–1581.
10. Berge E, Abdelnoor M, Nakstad PH, et al. Low molecular-weight heparin versus aspirin in patients with acute ischemic stroke and atrial fibrillation: a double-blind randomized study. *Lancet* 2000;355:1205–1210.
11. *Physicians' desk reference,* 55th ed. Montvale, NJ: Medical Economics Company, 2001:2786–2789.
12. Antiplatelet Trialists' Collaboration. Collaborative overview of randomised trials of antiplatelet therapy—I: prevention of death, myocardial infarction, and stroke by prolonged antiplatelet therapy in various categories of patients. *BMJ* 1994;308:81–106.
13. The ESPS2 Group. European Stroke Prevention Study 2. *J Neurol Sci* 1997;151:S1–S77.
14. CAST (Chinese Acute Stroke Trial) Collaborative Group. CAST: randomised placebo-controlled trial of early aspirin use in 20000 patients with acute ischaemic stroke. *Lancet* 1997;349:1641–1649.
15. The Medical Research Council's General Practice Research Framework. Thrombosis prevention trial: randomised trial of low-intensity oral anticoagulation with warfarin and low-dose aspirin in the primary prevention of ischemic heart disease in men at increased risk. *Lancet* 1998;351:233–241.
16. Chevolet CL, Van de Velde V, Weisenberger H, et al. Bioequivalence of two dipyridamole preparations and inhibitory effect on the platelet adenosine uptake in Man. *Arch Int Pharmacodyn* 1981;253:321–322.

Ischemic Stroke: Advances in Neurology, Vol. 92. Edited by
H.J.M. Barnett, Julien Bogousslavsky, and Heather Meldrum.
Lippincott Williams & Wilkins, Philadelphia © 2003.

38

Treatment of Symptomatic Arteriosclerotic Carotid Artery Disease

H.J.M. Barnett, Heather Meldrum, M. Eliasziw, and *G.G. Ferguson

*The John P. Robarts Research Institute, London, Ontario, Canada; and *Department of Clinical Neurological Sciences, University of Western Ontario, London, Ontario, Canada*

Stroke-free survival after carotid endarterectomy (CE) exceeds that of similar patients given only best medical therapy. This chapter examines the evidence determining which symptomatic patients benefit most, have modest benefit, or are harmed by CE. Recommendations are based upon data from the North American Symptomatic Carotid Endarterectomy Trial (NASCET) and the Aspirin and Carotid Endarterectomy (ACE) Trial (1–3). Additional information has come from the publications of the European Carotid Surgery Trial (ECST) (4). Earlier trials and observational case series are no longer relevant to decision making.

NORTH AMERICAN SYMPTOMATIC CAROTID ENDARTERECTOMY TRIAL AND ASPIRIN AND CAROTID ENDARTERECTOMY TRIAL DESIGNS AND RESULTS

NASCET randomized 2,885 patients who had recent focal retinal or hemisphere symptoms, within the territory of supply of a carotid artery, proven by conventional angiography to have an arteriosclerotic stenosis ≥30%. Half of the patients were randomized to best medical care plus CE and the other half to best medical care alone. Patients who had evidence of vital organ failure, reasonable likelihood of a cardioembolic stroke, or cancer likely to cause death within 5 years were excluded. The protocol required proof of surgical expertise with a perioperative rate of stroke or death ≤6% (1).

The ACE Trial, which was conducted in parallel to NASCET by the same stroke neurologists and surgeons, had no medical arm. It evaluated the optimum dose of aspirin for the perioperative period and provided 90-day postoperative data on 2,469 patients: 1,214 had asymptomatic disease and 1,255 had symptoms related to severe stenosis (3).

NASCET found clear benefit from CE for patients with severe (≥70%) stenosis (1). As shown in Table 38-1, the surgical patients had a 2-year absolute risk reduction (ARR) in stroke of 15.9% compared to the medical patients. To prevent one stroke in 2 years requires that only six patients receive CE, provided the perioperative rate is at or near the 5.8% achieved in NASCET (5). Patients with moderate disease (50%–69%) benefitted but to a lesser extent (2). With a surgical complication rate of 6.9%, the number needed to treat (NNT) at 2 years was 19, with an ARR of 5.3% (Table 38-1). With less than 50%, stenosis benefit was not found.

The ECST had several features at variance to NASCET: if the trialists thought they knew that a patient should or should not receive CE, they were not entered; the degree of stenosis was measured by a formula that suggested a stenosis greater than that obtained with the NASCET formula (NASCET's denominator for measurement was the width of the artery in the upper part of its cervical course; ECST's denominator was the diameter of what was thought to be the normal width of the diseased bulb); surgeons' skills were not vetted prior to patient entry; and data sufficient to determine stroke by cause were not recorded (4). Despite these differences, after remeasuring the ECST angiograms by the NASCET method, the results for patients with severe stenosis were similar (5). For ECST patients with ≥70% stenosis, ARR was 12.9%, and NNT was 8 (Table 38-1). The perioperative complication rate of stroke and death was 5.6%. The

TABLE 38-1. *Two-year risk of ipsilateral stroke and number needed to treat by carotid endarterectomy in symptomatic patients*

	No. of patients in specified trial	Medical risk (%) at 2 yr	Surgical risk (%) at 2 yr	Absolute risk reduction (%)	Relative risk reduction (%)	Needed to treat[a]	Perioperative stroke and death rate (%)
Symptomatic 70%–99%							
NASCET	659	24.5	8.6	15.9	65	6	5.8
ECST[b]	501	19.9	7.0	12.9	65	8	5.6
Symptomatic 50%–69%							
NASCET	858	14.6	9.3	5.3	36	19	6.9
ECST	684	9.7	11.1	−1.4	−14	—	9.8

ECST, European Carotid Surgery Trial; NASCET, North American Symptomatic Carotid Endarterectomy Trial.
[a]Needed to treat indicates number of patients needed to treat by endarterectomy to prevent one additional ipsilateral stroke in 2 years after the procedure compared to medical therapy alone.
[b]Additional data supplied by Dr. P. Rothwell.
From Barnett HJM, Eliasziw M, Meldrum HE. The prevention of ischemic stroke. *BMJ* 1999;318:1539–1543, with permission.

684 ECST patients with a moderate (50%–69%) degree of stenosis had a perioperative rate of 9.8%. Benefit was not achieved; ARR was −1.4%.

PATIENTS AT HIGHER OPERATIVE RISK

Multivariate analyses were done on 26 baseline and intraoperative variables, and a higher perioperative risk was detected in some NASCET patients (Fig. 38-1) (6). Two variables were unexpected. First, a worse outlook for the left-sided lesions (6.7% compared with 3.0%). This also was observed in the ACE Trial, with a perioperative stroke and death rate of 6.6% for left-sided procedures compared to 4.2% for right-sided procedures ($p = 0.005$) (3). A retrospective study of 1,280 endarterectomies over a 3-year period identified an increased risk from left-sided CE [odds ratio: 1.72; 95% confidence interval (CI): 1.07–2.76] (7).

Second, an unexpected reduction in perioperative complications in NASCET patients with prior coronary artery bypass grafting (CABG) compared to those without CABG was observed (1.0% vs. 6.0%). Similarly, the ACE Trial detected that patients with a history of coronary artery disease without CABG had a perioperative stroke and death risk of 5.9% compared with 3.4% for patients with prior CABG ($p = 0.16$). Post-CABG patients are known to survive satisfactorily with major surgery, possibly due to extra vigilance. Improved cardiac function and lifestyle changes may offer further protection from cardiac complications causing perioperative death.

COMPLICATIONS OF CAROTID ENDARTERECTOMY

Stroke and Death

Balancing risk between medical and surgical treatment is at the core of decision making for CE. Table 38-2 shows the perioperative outcome events in the NASCET and symptomatic ACE patients submitted to CE. The risk of any stroke or death and risk of disabling stroke or death were similar between NASCET (6.5, 2.0) and ACE (5.9, 2.2) (8). The low rate of fatal and nonfatal myocardial infarction (MI) in both trials reflects the exclusion of patients with recent MI, recent heart failure, and unstable angina.

At the Operative Site

The complications from NASCET and ACE combined are listed in Table 38-3. The three deaths from wound hematoma are reminders of the need to practice total control of bleeders and to ensure scrupulous arterial suturing. At times, a highly degenerative arteriosclerotic lesion may be encountered and a patch may be desirable.

Cranial nerve injuries are reported in larger numbers than in some reported case series, but none were permanent. Like mild wound hematomas, they reflect the meticulous attention of the study coordinators who reported any type of complication, no matter how trivial.

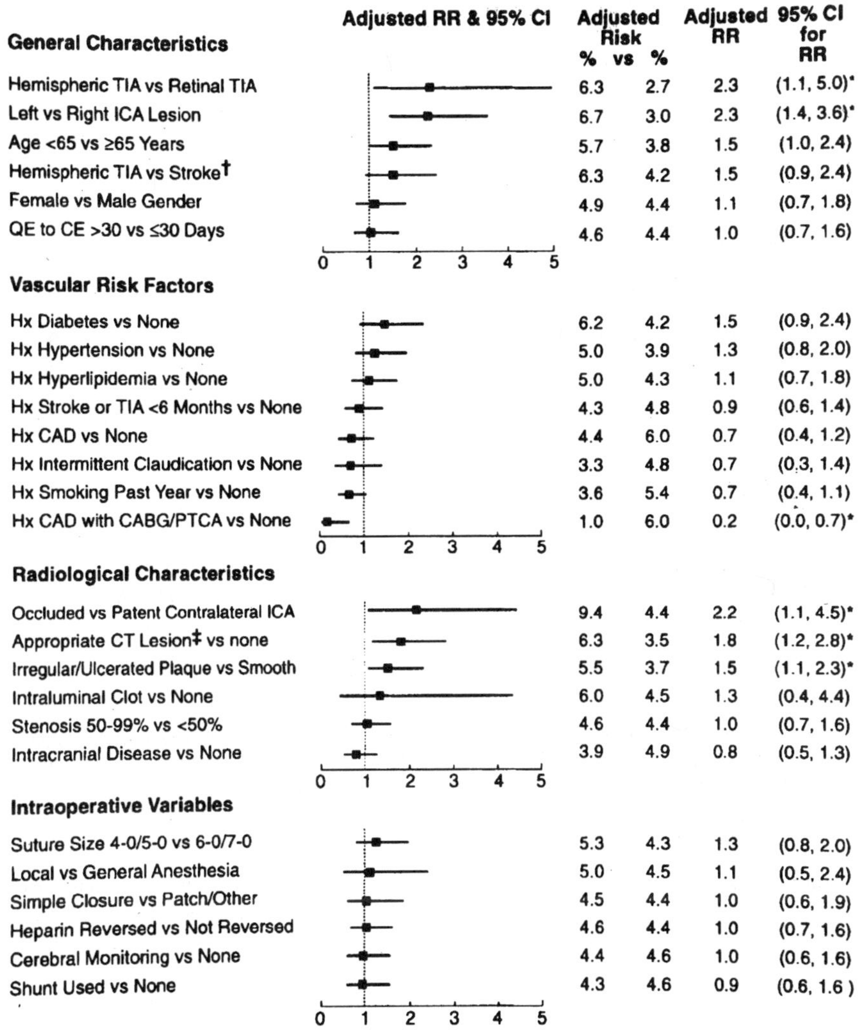

General Characteristics

Adjusted RR & 95% CI | **Adjusted Risk % vs %** | **Adjusted RR** | **95% CI for RR**

General Characteristics	Adjusted Risk % vs %	Adjusted RR	95% CI for RR
Hemispheric TIA vs Retinal TIA	6.3 2.7	2.3	(1.1, 5.0)*
Left vs Right ICA Lesion	6.7 3.0	2.3	(1.4, 3.6)*
Age <65 vs ≥65 Years	5.7 3.8	1.5	(1.0, 2.4)
Hemispheric TIA vs Stroke†	6.3 4.2	1.5	(0.9, 2.4)
Female vs Male Gender	4.9 4.4	1.1	(0.7, 1.8)
QE to CE >30 vs ≤30 Days	4.6 4.4	1.0	(0.7, 1.6)

Vascular Risk Factors

Vascular Risk Factors	Adjusted Risk % vs %	Adjusted RR	95% CI for RR
Hx Diabetes vs None	6.2 4.2	1.5	(0.9, 2.4)
Hx Hypertension vs None	5.0 3.9	1.3	(0.8, 2.0)
Hx Hyperlipidemia vs None	5.0 4.3	1.1	(0.7, 1.8)
Hx Stroke or TIA <6 Months vs None	4.3 4.8	0.9	(0.6, 1.4)
Hx CAD vs None	4.4 6.0	0.7	(0.4, 1.2)
Hx Intermittent Claudication vs None	3.3 4.8	0.7	(0.3, 1.4)
Hx Smoking Past Year vs None	3.6 5.4	0.7	(0.4, 1.1)
Hx CAD with CABG/PTCA vs None	1.0 6.0	0.2	(0.0, 0.7)*

Radiological Characteristics

Radiological Characteristics	Adjusted Risk % vs %	Adjusted RR	95% CI for RR
Occluded vs Patent Contralateral ICA	9.4 4.4	2.2	(1.1, 4.5)*
Appropriate CT Lesion‡ vs none	6.3 3.5	1.8	(1.2, 2.8)*
Irregular/Ulcerated Plaque vs Smooth	5.5 3.7	1.5	(1.1, 2.3)*
Intraluminal Clot vs None	6.0 4.5	1.3	(0.4, 4.4)
Stenosis 50-99% vs <50%	4.6 4.4	1.0	(0.7, 1.6)
Intracranial Disease vs None	3.9 4.9	0.8	(0.5, 1.3)

Intraoperative Variables

Intraoperative Variables	Adjusted Risk % vs %	Adjusted RR	95% CI for RR
Suture Size 4-0/5-0 vs 6-0/7-0	5.3 4.3	1.3	(0.8, 2.0)
Local vs General Anesthesia	5.0 4.5	1.1	(0.5, 2.4)
Simple Closure vs Patch/Other	4.5 4.4	1.0	(0.6, 1.9)
Heparin Reversed vs Not Reversed	4.6 4.4	1.0	(0.7, 1.6)
Cerebral Monitoring vs None	4.4 4.6	1.0	(0.6, 1.6)
Shunt Used vs None	4.3 4.6	0.9	(0.6, 1.6)

FIG. 38-1. Multivariate analysis of 26 baseline and intraoperative variables for 30-day perioperative risk of stroke and death. Within each category, the results have been ordered by decreasing adjusted relative risks (RR). Unexpected were results in left-sided lesions and prior coronary artery interventions. *Statistically significant at $p <$ 0.05. †Hemispheric transient ischemic attack versus hemispheric stroke as the qualifying event (QE). ‡Ipsilateral ischemic lesion on entry computed tomographic scan. Hx, history; ICA, internal carotid artery; PTCA, percutaneous transluminal coronary angioplasty. (From Ferguson GG, Eliasziw M, Barr HWK, et al., for the North American Symptomatic Carotid Endarterectomy Trial (NASCET) Collaborators. The North American Symptomatic Carotid Endarterectomy Trial. Surgical results in 1415 patients. *Stroke* 1999;30:1751–1758, with permission.)

TABLE 38-2. *Perioperative (30-day) outcome events (percentage of group)*

Outcome event	NASCET symptomatic (N = 1,415)	ACE symptomatic (N = 1,255)	NASCET and ACE symptomatic (N = 2,670)
Any stroke or death	6.5	5.9	6.2
Disabling stroke or death	2.0	2.2	2.1
Any stroke or death or MI	7.3	6.4	6.9
Nonfatal MI	0.9	0.9	0.9
Fatal MI	0.1	0.1	0.1

ACE, Aspirin and Carotid Endarterectomy Trial; ECST, European Carotid Surgery Trial; MI, myocardial infarction; NASCET, North American Symptomatic Carotid Endarterectomy Trial.

From Barnett HJM, Meldrum HE, Eliasziw M, for the North American Symptomatic Carotid Endarterectomy Trial (NASCET) Collaborators. The appropriate use of carotid endarterectomy. *CMAJ* 2002;166(9):1169–1179, with permission.

TABLE 38-3. *Perioperative (30-day) complications from endarterectomy (percentage of group)*

Complication	NASCET and ACE symptomatic (N = 2,670)	
	Mild or moderate[a]	Severe[b]
Surgical		
Wound hematoma	6.6	0.3[c]
Wound infection	1.2	0
Other wound complication	0.3	0
Cranial nerve injury	6.8	0
Medical		
Arrhythmia	1.6	0
Congestive heart failure	0.9	0
Angina pectoris	1.2	0
Hypertension	1.1	0
Hypotension	2.9	0
Respiratory disorder	1.6	0.1[d]
Confusion	0.9	0

ACE, Aspirin and Carotid Endarterectomy Trial; NASCET, North American Symptomatic Carotid Endarterectomy Trial.
[a]Mild or moderate: Transient complication that did not result in permanent disability.
[b]Severe: Complication that resulted in permanent functional disability or death.
[c]Three of seven fatal.
[d]Fatal.
Adapted from Barnett HJM, Meldrum HE, Eliasziw M, for the North American Symptomatic Carotid Endarterectomy Trial (NASCET) Collaborators. The appropriate use of carotid endarterectomy. *CMAJ* 2002;166(9):1169–1179, with permission.

Medical Complications in the Thirty-Day Period

Intraoperative hypertension and more commonly intraoperative hypotension occurred, but all responded to immediate therapy (Table 38-3). Postoperative respiratory complications were infrequent, although there was one death. Pulmonary embolism was absent, probably due to early mobilization.

COMPLICATIONS AND USE OF CONVENTIONAL ANGIOGRAPHY

The trials required conventional angiography and, when complicated by a disabling stroke, the patient was not eligible for entry. Among 2,885 NASCET patients, 20 nondisabling strokes occurred within 24 hours of angiography (0.7%). From a systematic review of the literature, five of six strokes complicating angiography were reported as transient or nondisabling (9); thus, four disabling strokes can be estimated as the total in the NASCET centers following angiography, a 0.1% disabling stroke rate (10).

A previous study examined the incidence of stroke due to angiography in 360 patients from an academic center and 209 from a community hospital. All of the 659 patients had >50% carotid stenosis. No difference was found between the institutions in the performance of angiography. In total only one disabling stroke (0.2) and two nondisabling strokes (0.3%) occurred, yielding a combined rate of 0.5% (11). This report showed that both academic and nonacademic institutions could achieve an acceptably low angiographic complication rate (11).

The harm done by misidentification of patients for CE by noninvasive studies is hard to quantify. Patients are exposed to the risks of CE because of overreading the degree of stenosis. Despite advances in noninvasive imaging methods, overreading persists and mostly occurs around the 50% angiographic threshold of stenosis (12–14). The patient then faces a 2% risk of disabling stroke from CE, 20 times the risk of 0.1% from angiography. Carotid near occlusion, commonly misread by noninvasive methods because of reduced blood flow, was observed in 7.6% of NASCET angiograms (15).

Misreading occurs in approximately 15% of images. There is serious expense involved in caring for patients with disabling stroke after unwarranted CE or by strokes occurring when denied appropriate CE because of unsatisfactory imaging. Most patients should have conventional angiography performed by an expert neuroradiologist before CE (11–13,16).

SUBGROUPS WITH MOST, LEAST, AND NO BENEFIT FROM CAROTID ENDARTERECTOMY

The NASCET and ACE Trials gathered data on 4,119 symptomatic patients, of whom 2,670 received CE and 1,449 (all in NASCET) had medical care alone. Because of the scrupulousness of the prospective data gathering and the large number of patients, it was appropriate to examine a number of subgroups seeking patients most likely to benefit from CE and to identify conditions that modify or negate benefit. The following observations are important because the endarterectomy trials that tested against best medical care will not be repeated.

Influence of Degree of Stenosis on Benefit from Carotid Endarterectomy

The NASCET and ECST Trials indicate that patients treated medically with severe degrees of stenosis (70%–94%) are at highest risk (2,4). After endarterectomy, risk difference was highest in severe patients. Compared to severe patients, medically treated patients with moderate stenosis had a lower risk of stroke and death, but the risk from CE was slightly higher. For these reasons, although benefit was achieved from CE, it was less than with severe disease. Below 50% stenosis no benefit was found. The special category of the near occlusions is covered separately.

Influence of Age on Benefit from Carotid Endarterectomy

Patients (n = 409) 75 years or older in NASCET were at high risk. At 2 years, with ≥70% stenosis, the risk of ipsilateral stroke and death with medical therapy was 36.5%; at 50% to 69% stenosis, the risk was 24.3% (17). Surgical risk was not greater than in the younger patients; benefit was higher with an ARR of 28.9% and a 2-year NNT of 3. With 50% to 69% stenosis, ARR was 17.3%, giving an NNT of 6. Healthy symptomatic elderly patients without threatening heart disease, vital organ failure, or mortality-threatening cancer are ideal candidates for CE.

Influence of Gender on Benefit from Carotid Endarterectomy

Between NASCET and ACE, 1,208 women and 2,825 men were randomized to the trials. There was a moderate increase in perioperative risk in women (7.6%) compared to men (5.9%) (18). Risk reduction at 5 years with ≥70% stenosis was only slightly and not significantly different: 15.1% for women and 17.3% for men. NNT for women at 5 years was 7 and for men was 6. The benefit for women with 50% to 69% stenosis was only present when they had a high-risk profile. In the highest-risk category (seven risk factors) the benefit for men was 15.4% and for women was 8.9%. Lower-risk profiles gave no or negative benefit for women. The seven risk factors that emerged from multivariate analyses of a full profile of potential risks were hemisphere, not retinal presentation; history of diabetes mellitus; previous stroke; age 70 years or older; stroke not TIA as the presenting event; >180 mm Hg systolic or >100 mm Hg diastolic pressures; and history or electrocardiographic evidence of MI.

Women with severe stenosis and women with a higher-risk profile in the moderate category should be considered for CE.

Highest-Risk Time Period After the First Ischemic Event in Patients with Carotid Stenosis

Most calculations of risk of stroke in clinical trial populations have been calculated forward from the time of entry into the study and have used the event closest to this time to begin the evaluations of risk. NASCET put into its database earlier historical information about ischemic events. These "index events" often were months before the "entry event". The risk was recalculated for patients entering NASCET from the time of the index events.

At 90 days after an index event of hemisphere TIA, the risk of ipsilateral stroke was 20.1% (n = 603); after an index event of hemisphere stroke, the risk was 2.3% (n = 526) (19). Half of these stroke events occurred in the first 7 days after the index event. By contrast, using the events immediately prior to entry instead of the index events to calculate risk of ipsilateral stroke in these two groups of patients yielded figures of 5.5% and 4.8%, respectively.

The occurrence of the first hemispheric TIA must be regarded as an urgent signal threatening serious consequences. Trials evaluating surgical and medical therapy after index events are clearly indicated. Patients will need to go directly from emergency rooms to be screened for trial entry.

Benefit of Carotid Endarterectomy for Patients Presenting Solely with Transient Monocular Blindness

In NASCET 496 patients had experienced only recent (6 months) transient monocular blindness.

Medically treated they were shown to be a group with only half the risk experienced by patients presenting with hemisphere TIA (20). A risk profile was developed by multivariate analyses that included age 75 years or older, male sex, distant history of hemisphere TIA or stroke, history of intermittent claudication, stenosis 80% to 94%, and absence of collaterals. As a rule, patients with severe stenosis had multiple risk factors. The 3-year medical risk of ipsilateral stroke varied markedly with two, three, or more than three risk factors from 1.8% to 12.3% to 24.2%, respectively. Favoring CE, the ARR benefit ranged from negative 2.2% to 4.9% to 14.3%.

In conclusion, patients with transient molecular blindness alone and with a low-risk profile should not receive endarterectomy. Patients should be considered for CE if they have a high-risk profile even with moderate stenosis.

Value of Carotid Endarterectomy with Intracranial Stenosis

Traditionally tandem intracranial arteriosclerotic disease was thought to negate the value of CE. NASCET discouraged randomization of patients with the most severe intracranial lesions but one third (n = 956) of the randomized patients had tandem lesions. In medically treated patients compared to patients without the lesion, relative risk of stroke varied with the degree of extracranial stenosis from 1.3 (95% CI: 0.9–1.9) with <50% stenosis to 1.8 (95% CI: 1.1–3.2) with ≥85% stenosis (21). The risk of stroke from CE was not increased in the presence of intracranial arteriosclerotic disease. The 3-year risk of ipsilateral stroke between medically and surgically treated patients by degree of stenosis is listed in Table 38-4.

Increased risk with medical treatment alone and lack of increased risk with CE yielded an ARR favoring CE as the degree of extracranial stenosis increased. To prevent one ipsilateral stroke in 3 years, NNT decreased as the degree of stenosis increased and reached a low of three for patients with ≥85% extracranial stenosis. Rather than being a contraindication to CE, this group of patients receives increased benefit from CE.

Cause of Stroke in Patients with Carotid Artery Stenosis

Not all strokes that occur in patients who have stenosed carotid arteries arise from this lesion. In NASCET 1,039 strokes occurred at an average follow-up of 5 years: 17 intracerebral hemorrhages, one subarachnoid hemorrhage, and 1,021 ischemic strokes. Of the latter, 698 were judged to be of large-artery origin, 211 lacunar, and 112 cardioembolic (22). The cardioembolic number was a lower figure than might have occurred had the protocol not excluded patients likely to be at risk of a cardioembolic stroke based on cardiac history and findings. The likelihood of the occurrence of a non–large-artery stroke increased with decreasing degrees of stenosis. In patients with <70% stenosis, one third of subsequent strokes were not of large-artery origin. This figure was 20% in patients with ≥70% stenosis.

Close attention must be given to the heart, aorta, and small vessels in all patients with threatened stroke, including those with obvious carotid lesions. The occurrence of strokes not affected by CE (cardioembolic) or less benefited (lacunar) is of greater importance when dealing with subjects with asymptomatic carotid stenosis.

TABLE 38-4. *Number of patients with and without intracranial artery disease needed to undergo carotid endarterectomy to prevent one ipsilateral stroke in three years, according to degree of internal carotid artery stenosis*

Degree of ICA stenosis	Ipsilateral IAD	
	Absent	Present
50%–69%	26	12
70%–84%	7	5
85%–99%	6	3

IAD, intracranial artery disease; ICA, internal carotid artery.
Adapted from Kappelle LJ, Eliasziw M, Fox AJ, et al., for the North American Symptomatic Carotid Endarterectomy Trial (NASCET) Group. Importance of intracranial atherosclerotic disease in patients with symptomatic stenosis of the internal carotid artery. *Stroke* 1999;30:282–286.

Lacunar Stroke in Patients with Carotid Stenosis

Commonly, large-artery disease coexists with small-vessel disease. Not knowing whether patients with lacunar strokes would benefit from CE, they were entered into NASCET with the combination of extracranial disease and recognizable clinicoradiologic features of lacunar stroke. Of 1,158 patients with hemisphere strokes entered into NASCET, 493 (43%) had evidence of disease in both large and small arteries (23). With medical therapy alone, the patients in this category had a lower risk of large-artery stroke and a higher risk of lacunar stroke than patients presenting without lacunar disease.

The lacunar strokes were described as "probable" when they fulfilled the full diagnostic criteria used in NASCET. In the nonlacunar group with ≥50% carotid stenosis, CE at 3 years reduced the medically derived stroke risk from 24.9% to 9.7% (ARR 15.2%) (Fig. 38-2). With a "probable" lacunar stroke at entry the subsequent risk of stroke was reduced from 25.5% to 16.5%, an ARR of 9.0%.

Symptomatic patients presenting with evidence of disease in the neck and in the small vessels can be recommended for CE, but the benefit will not be as great as without lacunar disease.

Leukoaraiosis in the Presence of Carotid Stenosis

The white matter changes, called leukoaraiosis, that came to light in the computed tomography (CT) and later the magnetic resonance imaging (MRI) era were common in NASCET patients. A total of 493 of 2,618 patients with CT scans at entry had restricted (n = 354) or widespread (n = 139) leukoaraiosis (24). Treated medically the 3-year stroke risks were 20.2%, 27.3%, and 37.2% for patients without, with restricted, and with widespread leukoaraiosis, respectively. The perioperative risk was proportional to the severity of the white matter change, rising from 5.3% with none to 13.9% with widespread evidence of leukoaraiosis. Despite the high operative risk, CE reduced the absolute risk of stroke at 3 years.

Patients with leukoaraiosis who have symptoms and are candidates for CE should be advised to undergo the procedure, but they should be told to expect less benefit than patients without this condition.

Carotid Endarterectomy When One Carotid Artery is Occluded and the Opposite is Severely or Moderately Stenosed and Symptomatic

This uncommon condition is known to carry a poor prognosis. The prospect of a second occlusion makes

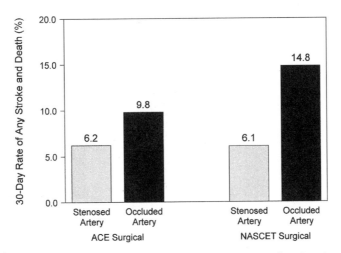

FIG. 38-2. Risk of ipsilateral stroke at 3 years by presenting stroke category and treatment group for patients with 50% to 99% internal carotid artery stenosis. The numbers of patients represented in each bar, from left to right, are 172, 160, 57, 69, 41, and 38. For probable lacunes, the absolute relative risk of stroke was reduced by 9.0% with carotid endarterectomy compared with 15.2% reduction in the absence of lacunar stroke at entry. Med, medically treated; Surg, surgically treated. (From Inzitari D, Eliasziw M, Sharpe BL, et al., for the North American Symptomatic Carotid Endarterectomy Trial (NASCET) Group. Risk factors and outcome of patients with carotid artery stenosis presenting with lacunar stroke. *Neurology* 2000;54:660–666, with permission.)

it imperative that salvage of the stenosed artery be considered. NASCET had 61 patients with this combination. More commonly the artery opposite to the symptoms was moderately stenosed (n = 559); the artery was only severely narrowed in 57. The perioperative rate of stroke and death was high at 14.8% when the opposite artery was occluded but was not above the usual perioperative rate (6.1%) if the opposite artery had any degree of stenosis short of occlusion (25). Similar ACE patients (n = 82) had a perioperative risk of 9.8% (Fig. 38-3) (26). These perioperative rates are formidable but contrast favorably to the medically treated risk at 2 years of stroke ipsilateral to the symptomatic artery of 69.4%. The ARR favoring CE in NASCET was 45.1% when the symptomatic artery was the site of severe stenosis.

Although the risk is higher, benefit from CE has been established with this combination.

Carotid Endarterectomy in the Presence of Extremely Severe Stenosis

In a small number of patients with symptoms related to arteries that are most severely stenosed, the flow is reduced to the point where the internal carotid artery is narrowed. The narrowing may be so great that the amount of contrast in the angiogram is reduced to a thin thread. This condition is called near occlusion. The narrowing is accompanied by evidence of intracranial collateral circulation, dilution of the contrast in the intracranial carotid artery and its major branches from collateral circulation, and delayed passage of contrast up the internal compared with the external carotid artery. Near occlusions were present in 7.6% of NASCET patients. The surgical risk was not above usual but the medical risk was lower, resulting in an ARR of 7.9%. A small number of patients (n = 13) had only a string or thread of contrast. They probably do not require CE. In NASCET, the outlook was good; only a few patients went on to have ipsilateral stroke. It appears that when patients reach this degree of narrowing and have not experienced a disabling stroke, collateral supply is adequate to maintain them free of stroke (NASCET unpublished data 2002).

The conclusion is that patients with near occlusion, probably not those reduced to a thread, will benefit but to a lesser degree than patients with severe stenosis short of occlusion. The outlook treated medically is about the same as in patients with only moderate symptomatic stenosis.

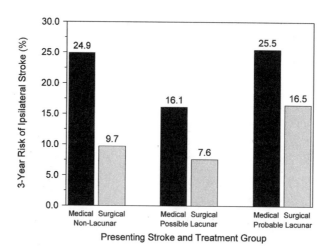

FIG. 38-3. Thirty-day perioperative stroke and death in patients with contralateral occlusion compared with the rate in patients with only contralateral stenosis. Data are from surgically treated patients with symptomatic stenosis in the Aspirin and Carotid Endarterectomy (ACE) Trial or the North American Symptomatic Carotid Endarterectomy Trial (NASCET). The numbers of patients represented in the bars are, from left to right, 1,210, 82, 1354, and 61. (Modified from Inzitari D, Eliasziw M, Gates P, et al., for the North American Symptomatic Carotid Endarterectomy Trial (NASCET) Group. The causes and risk of stroke in subjects with an asymptomatic internal carotid artery. *N Engl J Med* 2000;342:1693–1700.)

Collateral Circulation and Carotid Endarterectomy

Approximately half of patients with severe symptomatic carotid stenosis have angiographic evidence of collateral circulation compensating for the reduced blood flow caused by arterial narrowing. Substantial amounts of filling through anterior and posterior communicating arteries and retrograde through ophthalmic arteries are encountered. Evidence of the efficacy of these channels in improving cerebral blood flow in patients with severe stenosis in NASCET was shown by comparing the 2-year risk of hemisphere stroke of 27.8% when collaterals were absent to 11.3% when collaterals were present (27). Without collaterals the 2-year risk after CE was 8.4%, with collaterals 5.4%. ARR favoring CE was 19.4% without collaterals but only 5.4% when they were present, a paradox explained by the exceptionally high medical risk without collaterals.

Although the surgical risk is increased, the risk difference strongly commends the use of CE.

Impact of Intraluminal Thrombi

Conventional angiography may disclose thrombi beyond severe stenosis in the carotid artery. NASCET patients with ≥85% stenosis had a 5.5% chance of having a thrombus seen within the artery (28). For medically treated patients, this lesion carried a 30-day risk that was triple that seen without its presence. Surgical risk from CE doubled when thrombus was visible. However, followed for 1 year, the risk of stroke was 25.3% with medical therapy but decreased to 16.0% after CE. Endarterectomy is recommended despite increased risk. A period of antithrombotic therapy for a few weeks before endarterectomy may reduce the risk of CE, but the evidence is sparse and anecdotal (29).

Aspirin Dose Perioperatively

In 2,804 patients randomized preoperatively to take either 81, 325, 650, or 1,300 mg of aspirin, stroke, death, or MI occurred less frequently in the combined low-dose arm compared to the combined high-dose arm (3). Although not reaching statistical significance the optimum of the two low doses was 325 mg. These results should not be extrapolated to decisions about optimum dose for long-term stroke prophylaxis.

CONCLUSION

All patients with symptoms related to *severe carotid stenosis* fare better with CE than with medical care alone. In the absence of life-threatening disease they should receive CE. Some symptomatic patients face an excessive risk of stroke when treated medically compared to those without these conditions, and because the risk of CE is not more than 6.0%, they benefit most (Table 38-5). Other patients with *severe carotid stenosis* are at high medical and high perioperative risk but will benefit from CE.

Many, but not all, patients with *moderate stenosis* benefit from CE. For most patients, the benefit is small compared to patients with severe stenosis. Some patients may be harmed.

A reduced risk of stroke with medical treatment occurs in patients who have carotid stenosis and present with lacunar stroke or in patients with near occlusion of the symptomatic carotid artery. The operative risk is at usual levels (6%), but the benefit is only muted.

Precautions Necessary to Apply the Trial Conclusions

Surgical expertise must be at least that in the NASCET and ACE trials. The perioperative compli-

TABLE 38-5. *Patients with most, muted, and no benefit from carotid endarterectomy*

With severe stenosis (≥70%)		With moderate stenosis (50%–69%)
Benefit: most	Benefit: muted	No benefit

Medical risk: high
Surgical risk: usual (6%)
  1. Elderly (≥75 yr)
  2. Tandem intracranial lesion
  3. No collaterals
  4. Hemisphere, not retinal, symptoms
	Medical risk: high
	Surgical risk: high (>6%)
	  1. Contralateral carotid occlusion
	  2. Widespread leukoaraiosis
	  3. Intraluminal thrombus
		Medical risk: low
		Surgical risk: usual (6%)
		  1. Transient monocular blindness only, with few risk factors
		  2. Females with few risk factors

cation rates of stroke in any territory and death should not exceed 6%. Disabling stroke should not exceed 2%.

The conclusions from randomized trials came from patients submitted to CE after the important factor of the degree of stenosis was measured by conventional angiography. The stroke rate from this procedure must be carried out in a facility with no more than 0.1% risk of disabling stroke. The substitution of other noninvasive varieties of imaging is leading to inappropriate endarterectomies because the correlation between invasive testing and noninvasive methods remains inexact.

Patients with organ failure, heart disease likely to be mortal or to cause stroke, and patients with cancer with a fatal outlook should be treated medically. Those who would perform angioplasty/stenting in these sick patients are working with only anecdotal and conflicting data. Ideally, such patients should be entered into a clinical trial to evaluate the efficacy of angioplasty/stenting.

All patients who are potential candidates for CE should receive scrupulous medical management. The manageable risks of increased blood pressure, high blood sugar or cholesterol, cigarette smoking, and impaired cardiac function need lifetime care. Antithrombotic medication, with aspirin as first choice, is recommended.

REFERENCES

1. North American Symptomatic Carotid Endarterectomy Trial Collaborators. Beneficial effect of carotid endarterectomy in symptomatic patients with high-grade stenosis. *N Engl J Med* 1991;325:445–453.
2. Barnett HJM, Taylor DW, Eliasziw M, et al., for the North American Symptomatic Carotid Endarterectomy Trial Collaborators. Benefit of carotid endarterectomy in symptomatic patients with moderate and severe stenosis. *N Engl J Med* 1998;339:1415–1425.
3. Taylor DW, Barnett HJM, Haynes RB, et al., for the ASA and Carotid Endarterectomy (ACE) Trial Collaborators. Low-dose and high-dose acetylsalicylic acid for patients undergoing carotid endarterectomy: a randomized controlled trial. *Lancet* 1999;353:2179–2184.
4. European Carotid Surgery Trialists' Group. Randomised trial of endarterectomy for recently symptomatic carotid stenosis: final results of the MRC European Carotid Surgery Trial (ECST). *Lancet* 1998;351:1379–1387.
5. Barnett HJM, Eliasziw M, Meldrum HE. The prevention of ischemic stroke. *BMJ* 1999;318:1539–1543.
6. Ferguson GG, Eliasziw M, Barr HWK, et al., for the North American Symptomatic Carotid Endarterectomy Trial (NASCET) Collaborators. The North American Symptomatic Carotid Endarterectomy Trial. Surgical results in 1415 patients. *Stroke* 1999;30:1751–1758.
7. Kucey DS, Bowyer B, Iron K, et al., for the University of Toronto Carotid Study Group. Determinants of outcome after carotid endarterectomy. *J Vasc Surg* 1998;28:1051–1058.
8. Barnett HJM, Meldrum HE, Eliasziw M, for the North American Symptomatic Carotid Endarterectomy Trial (NASCET) Collaborators. The appropriate use of carotid endarterectomy. *CMAJ* 2002; 166(9):1169–1179.
9. Hankey GJ, Warlow CP, Molyneux AJ. Complications of cerebral angiography for patients with mild carotid territory ischaemia being considered for carotid endarterectomy. *J Neurol Neurosurg Psychiatry* 1990;53:542–548.
10. Eliasziw M, Rankin RN, Fox AJ, et al., for the North American Symptomatic Carotid Endarterectomy Trial (NASCET) Group. Accuracy and prognostic consequences of ultrasonography in identifying severe carotid artery stenosis. *Stroke* 1995;26:1747–1752.
11. Johnston DCC, Chapman KM, Goldstein LB. Low rate of complications of cerebral angiography in routine clinical practice. *Neurology* 2001;57:2012–2014.
12. Johnston DCC, Goldstein LB. Clinical carotid endarterectomy decision making. Noninvasive vascular imaging versus angiography. *Neurology* 2001;56:1009–1015.
13. Norris JW, Rothwell PM. Noninvasive carotid imaging to select patients for endarterectomy. Is it really safer than conventional angiography? *Neurology* 2001;56:990–991.
14. Eliasziw M, Smith RF, Singh N, et al., for the North American Symptomatic Carotid Endarterectomy Trial (NASCET) Group. Further comments on the measurement of carotid stenosis from angiograms. *Stroke* 1994;25:2445–2449.
15. Morgenstern LB, Fox AJ, Sharpe BL, et al., for the North American Symptomatic Carotid Endarterectomy Trial (NASCET) Group. The risks and benefits of carotid endarterectomy in patients with near occlusion in the carotid artery. *Neurology* 1997;48:911–915.
16. Qureshi AI, Suri MFK, Ali Z, et al. Role of conventional angiography in evaluation of patients with carotid artery stenosis demonstrated by doppler ultrasound in general practice. *Stroke* 2001;32:2287–2291.
17. Alamowitch S, Eliasziw M, Algra A, et al., for the North American Symptomatic Carotid Endarterectomy Trial (NASCET) Group. Risk, causes and prevention of ischemic stroke in elderly patients with symptomatic internal carotid artery stenosis. *Lancet* 2001;357:1154–1160.
18. Alamowitch S, Eliasziw M, Taylor DW, et al., for the North American Symptomatic Carotid Endarterectomy Trial (NASCET), and the ASA and Carotid Endarterectomy (ACE) Trial Collaborators. The risk and benefit of endarterectomy in women with symptomatic internal carotid artery disease. *(in press).*
19. Eliasziw M, Kennedy J, Hill MD, et al., for the North American Symptomatic Carotid Endarterectomy Trial (NASCET) Group. Acute neurovascular syndromes: differential prognosis after acute cerebral ischemia in patients with internal carotid artery stenosis. *(in press).*
20. Benavente O, Eliasziw M, Streifler JY, et al., for the North American Symptomatic Carotid Endarterectomy Trial (NASCET) Collaborators. Prognosis after tran-

sient monocular blindness associated with carotid artery stenosis. *N Engl J Med* 2001;345:1084–1090.

21. Kappelle LJ, Eliasziw M, Fox AJ, et al., for the North American Symptomatic Carotid Endarterectomy Trial (NASCET) Group. Importance of intracranial atherosclerotic disease in patients with symptomatic stenosis of the internal carotid artery. *Stroke* 1999;30:282–286.

22. Barnett HJM, Gunton RW, Eliasziw M, et al., for the North American Symptomatic Carotid Endarterectomy Trial (NASCET) Group. The causes and severity of ischemic stroke in patients with internal carotid artery stenosis. *JAMA* 2000;283:1429–1436.

23. Inzitari D, Eliasziw M, Sharpe BL, et al., for the North American Symptomatic Carotid Endarterectomy Trial (NASCET) Group. Risk factors and outcome of patients with carotid artery stenosis presenting with lacunar stroke. *Neurology* 2000;54:660–666.

24. Streifler JY, Eliasziw M, Benavente OR, et al., for the North American Symptomatic Carotid Endarterectomy Trial Group. Prognostic importance of leukoaraiosis in patients with symptomatic internal carotid artery stenosis. *Stroke* 2002; 33(6):1651–1655.

25. Gasecki AP, Eliasziw M, Ferguson GG, et al., for the North American Symptomatic Carotid Endarterectomy

Trial (NASCET) Group. Long-term prognosis and effect of endarterectomy in patients with symptomatic severe carotid stenosis and contralateral carotid stenosis or occlusion: results from NASCET. *J Neurosurg* 1995; 83:778–782.

26. Inzitari D, Eliasziw M, Gates P, et al., for the North American Symptomatic Carotid Endarterectomy Trial (NASCET) Group. The causes and risk of stroke in subjects with an asymptomatic internal carotid artery. *N Engl J Med* 2000;342:1693–1700.

27. Henderson RD, Eliasziw M, Fox AJ, et al., for the North American Symptomatic Carotid Endarterectomy Trial (NASCET) Group. Angiographically-defined collateral circulation and the risk of stroke in patients with severe carotid artery stenosis. *Stroke* 2000;31:128–132.

28. Villarreal J, Silva J, Eliasziw M, et al., for the North American Symptomatic Carotid Endarterectomy Trial (NASCET) Group. Prognosis of patients with intraluminal thrombus in the internal carotid artery. *Stroke* 1998;29:276.

29. Pelz DM, Buchan A, Fox AJ, et al. Intraluminal thrombus of the internal carotid arteries: angiographic demonstration of resolution with anticoagulant therapy alone. *Radiology* 1986;160:369–373.

Ischemic Stroke: Advances in Neurology, Vol. 92. Edited by
H.J.M. Barnett, Julien Bogousslavsky, and Heather Meldrum.
Lippincott Williams & Wilkins, Philadelphia © 2003.

39

Treatment of Asymptomatic Arteriosclerotic Carotid Artery Disease

H.J.M. Barnett, Heather Meldrum, *D.J. Thomas, and M. Eliasziw

*The John P. Robarts Research Institute, London, Ontario, Canada; and
*Department of Clinical Neurology, Institute of Neurology; Department of Neurology,
St. Mary's Hospital, London, United Kingdom*

A major question facing the medical community is whether there is a group of subjects with asymptomatic arteriosclerotic carotid arterial narrowing who will benefit from carotid endarterectomy (CE). This chapter addresses the available evidence from case series and randomized trials.

PREVALENCE OF THE DISEASE

Community Surveys

Community surveys have used ultrasound to study the prevalence of asymptomatic carotid artery disease in the general population (1–5). After age 50 years, important degrees of atheroma become common. In 5,201 subjects aged 65 years or older, moderate (50%–74%) stenosis occurred in 5.3% of men and 4.0% of women, and severe (75%–99%) stenosis in 2.3% of men and 1.1% of women (4). The severity of stenosis became equal by gender over age 70 years in 1,348 subjects (5). Two million North Americans are estimated to have asymptomatic stenosis of an internal carotid artery (6).

Vascular Laboratory Referrals

Subjects with bruits of the internal carotid artery are commonly referred for ultrasound to identify carotid stenosing lesions. Asymptomatic bruits have been estimated to occur in subjects 45 years or older in 4.4% to 12.5% of the population in the United States (7,8). Several caveats apply: bruits decline and disappear as the stenosis becomes sufficiently severe to reduce flow; all neck bruits are not due to internal carotid artery stenosis; and transmitted aortic valve

murmurs must be excluded. In 336 individuals with bruits in the upper neck, 61% had >35% carotid stenosis, 11% with the bruit confined to the supraclavicular region (9). The Framingham Study with 5,148 subjects, after 8 years of follow-up, reported carotid bruit audible in 66 men and 105 women without symptoms (10). The incidence doubled from 3.5% at 44 to 54 years to 7.0% at 65 to 79 years.

A vascular laboratory investigated 2,380 subjects for a variety of reasons other than vascular symptoms or signs: as part of a general checkup or because of light-headedness, headache, neck pain, faintness, or falls (11). Among these subjects, 526 had asymptomatic stenosis. The prevalence increased with age. At 75 to 84 years, there was >50% carotid stenosis in 6.1% of women and 6.9% of men.

Racial Differences

Racial differences influence the localization of atheroma. A study of 1,006 carotid artery ultrasound examinations involved 151 Caucasians, 515 Hispanics, 173 African-Americans, and 167 Asians. Stenosis ≥60% was found in 21.5% of Caucasians, 10.1 % of Hispanics, 8.7% of African-Americans, and 10.5% of Asians (12).

NATURAL HISTORY FROM LONGITUDINAL OBSERVATIONAL STUDIES

Longitudinal prospective observational studies have been conducted in several series involving hundreds of subjects proven by imaging to have asymptomatic carotid artery stenosis. These studies did not

TABLE 39-1. *Annual risks of ipsilateral stroke and of stroke and vascular death*

Author	No. of patients	Annual ipsilateral stroke risk by degree of stenosis	Annual risk of stroke and vascular death
Mackey et al. 1997 (13)	357	2.8 (≥80%)	8.5 (≥80%)
			2.4 (<80%)
		1.4 (≥50%)	5.5 (≥50%)
Hennerici et al. 1987 (14)	339	3.4 (≥80%)	
		1.2 (≥50%)	7.1 (>50%)
Chambers and Norris 1986 (15)	113	2.8 (75%–100%)	12.6 (>75%)
Bogousslavsky et al. 1986 (16)	38	2.0 (≥90%)	6.6 (>90%)
Meissner et al. 1987 (17)	292	1.3 (assumed >50%)[a]	9.3 (assumed >50%)[a]
Autret et al. 1987 (18)	228	1.1 (50%–99%)	6.7 (>50%)

[a]Abnormal ocular pneumoplethysmography.

contain identical subjects because they came to the vascular laboratories for various reasons. A few were community surveys, such as older individuals urged to submit to screening and follow-up.

Incidence of Stroke

Six studies were selected because they included the largest number of subjects followed without surgical intervention over periods ranging from 2.5 to 4.0 years with repeated noninvasive examinations (Table 39-1) (13–18). Mean subject age ranged from 60 to 69 years, and subjects had ≥50% stenosis. The risk of outcomes by stenotic degree indicates the importance of increasing stenosis. The annual risk of ipsilateral stroke was as low as 1.1% and exceeded 3.0% only with ≥80% stenosis.

Incidence of Vascular and Nonvascular Death

Vascular deaths are more common in subjects with the highest degrees of stenosis. In one study, the annual rate was 0.4% in subjects with <50% stenosis and 3% with ≥80% stenosis (13). The annual risk of combined outcome of any stroke and vascular death shows that at least a three-fold increase of these events over ipsilateral stroke can be expected (Table 39-1). Nonvascular deaths occur at an annual rate of 2.0% (13–15).

Incidence of Occlusion and Risk of Stroke

More occlusions occurred with severe than moderate stenosis. Table 39-2 indicates that the annual risk of occlusion ranged from 6.3% to 12.2%, the latter in subjects with ≥80% stenosis. The figure of 7.9% in the small series of subjects with ≥90% stenosis was lower than expected compared to the other studies with lesser degrees of stenosis. The risk of having a stroke with an occluded artery was highest at 25.0% in the study that followed patients with >90% stenosis (16). In the other studies, the risk ranged from 11.8% to 14.8%.

Incidence of Nonfatal Myocardial Infarction

Two studies have reported nonfatal myocardial infarction (MI) separately. In one study, the annual rate of nonfatal MI was 1.2% with <80% stenosis and 3.3% at ≥80% (13). In 113 patients with ≥75% stenosis, the incidence of any MI was 7.5% annually (15). The incidence increases with the severity of the stenosis (Fig. 39-1).

In summary, the observational studies demonstrated in subjects with asymptomatic carotid stenosis that vascular death and fatal and nonfatal MI are more common occurrences than ischemic stroke. Risk of stroke, carotid occlusion, and MI increase with the degree of stenosis.

TABLE 39-2. *Annual risks of occlusion and stroke*

Author	Annual risk of occlusion	Risk of stroke with occlusion
Mackey et al. 1997 (13)	12.2 (≥80%)	14.8%
Hennerici et al. 1987 (14)	7.1 (>50%)	12.2%
Chambers and Norris 1986 (15)	6.3 (>75%)	11.8%
Bogousslavsky et al. 1986 (16)	7.9 (>90%)	25.0%

Data not available for Meissner et al. and Autret et al.

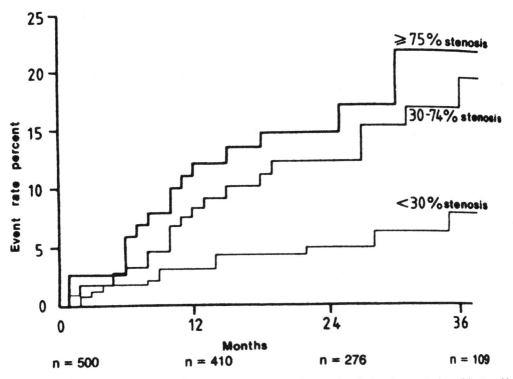

FIG. 39-1. Kaplan-Meier event-free survival curves demonstrating cardiac ischemic events in subjects with increasing severity of stenosis detected at ultrasound examination at time of entry into study. (From Chambers BR, Norris JW. Outcome in patients with asymptomatic neck bruits. *N Engl J Med* 1986;315:860–865, with permission.)

TRENDS IN NUMBERS OF CAROTID ENDARTERECTOMIES PERFORMED IN ASYMPTOMATIC SUBJECTS

Publication of the North American Symptomatic Carotid Endarterectomy Trial (NASCET) and the Asymptomatic Carotid Atherosclerosis Study (ACAS) was followed by a doubling of the annual performance of CE (19) (R. Pokras, *personal communication, 1999*). Many surveys do not distinguish between patients with and without symptoms but attribute the increase to the Clinical Alert from ACAS (20–22).

A 1981 sampling of Medicare patients identified 1,302 patients who underwent endarterectomy of whom one fourth were asymptomatic (23). Subsequent Medicare surveys indicated that CE was performed in asymptomatic subjects 30% to 75% of the time (24,25). Fifty-four percent of 2,804 individuals who underwent endarterectomy between 1994 and 1997 in 50 academic centers in North America had no symptoms (26).

Marked variations exist between Canada, the United States, and Europe regarding the acceptance and application of endarterectomy for asymptomatic subjects. Skepticism in Europe has led to the conduct of a multicenter observational study seeking to identify subjects at highest risk (27). Another large European study, the Asymptomatic Carotid Surgery Trial (ACST), is continuing with nearly 3,000 subjects to determine the efficacy of CE (28). Of 270 stroke neurologists surveyed, neurologists from Florida (65%) and Indiana (35%) were more likely than Canadian neurologists (11%) to refer subjects for CE sometimes or often (29). Medicolegal concerns were a reason for referring patients in the Florida sample (27%) and were much less for Canadian neurologists (3%). Of 185 stroke neurologists surveyed, CE was recommended by 48% of North American neurologists and 28% of European neurologists (30).

Without distinguishing between symptomatic and asymptomatic subjects, Tu et al. (31) reported on endarterectomy in California, New York, and Ontario, Canada. Between 1984 and 1989, the numbers in all three regions declined. The rates reversed from 1989 to 1995, with the number of endarterectomies highest in California and lowest in Ontario.

RESULTS FROM RANDOMIZED TRIALS

Between 1984 and 1995, five randomized trials testing medical care against CE for asymptomatic subjects were published (32–36).

The first trial published randomized 29 subjects and followed 28 nonrandomized individuals with asymptomatic cervical bruits and abnormal ocular pneumoplethysmography (32). With a mean 32 months of follow-up, the results for the combined randomized and nonrandomized groups were not encouraging, with five strokes or deaths in the medical group and seven in the surgical group.

The second study randomized 406 individuals with <90% stenosis (33). There are several design flaws in this study. Too many patients in the medical arm crossed over to receive CE, eventually 334 of the 406 randomized subjects. Therapeutic decisions cannot be made from such a flawed protocol.

The third study randomized 71 subjects and followed 87 nonrandomized eligible subjects with 50% to 99% stenosis (34). The use of aspirin was discouraged in the surgical arm but was prescribed in medical subjects. The study was stopped prematurely at 30 months because of eight MIs in the surgical arm and none in the medical arm. There were three strokes in the surgical group and none in the medical group. There were too few ischemic events to reach any conclusion. Of note is the preponderance of MI and stroke in the randomized surgical arm that received no aspirin.

The Veterans Affairs (VA) Study randomized 444 men with ≥50% angiographic stenosis (35). The surgical and medical groups had 211 and 233 subjects, respectively. The outcome events were transient ischemic attack, stroke, and death. Baseline characteristics were similar to those in ACAS (36), except for the absence of women in the VA trial and a doubling in current smokers in the veterans group (50% vs. 25%). In the surgical group, eight declined CE and eight had bilateral CE. Calculating perioperative morbidity and mortality from 203 subjects, four deaths (2%) and five strokes (2.5%) yielded a combined rate of 4.5%. Four nonfatal MI events occurred (2.0%). Including angiography, the risk of stroke and death in the perioperative period was 4.8%. The 30-day rate of stroke in the medical group was 0.5%, and there was one death from suicide. With follow-up to 96 months (mean 47.9 months), statistically significant benefit was observed only when transient ischemic attacks were included among the outcome events. The 4-year risk of ipsilateral stroke (including 30-day perioperative

deaths) was 9.9% and 6.6% for medically and surgically treated patients, respectively. The difference was not statistically significant, and the 2-year number needed to treat is calculated to be approximately 61 subjects. When stroke and death were the outcome events, the results were identical in both arms of the trial.

ACAS followed 1,659 randomized subjects with ≥60% stenosis measured by Doppler ultrasound (36). Angiography was required for subjects randomized to CE. Of the 825 subjects in the surgical arm, 741 had conventional angiography. While still asymptomatic, 45 subjects crossed over from the medical arm to the surgical arm.

Outcome events were ipsilateral stroke, any perioperative stroke or death, any stroke, or death. The severity of disabling stroke (category 2–5 on the Glasgow Coma Scale) was analyzed. Ipsilateral stroke, any perioperative stroke. or death occurred in 52 subjects at 2.7 years of average follow-up in the medical group and in 33 in the surgical group. Benefit was shown for CE compared to best medical therapy. The relative risk reduction was 53%; however, the absolute risk reduction of ipsilateral stroke out to 5 years was 5.9% (medical risk 11% − surgical risk 5.1%). The annualized absolute risk reduction was 1.2%. A differential benefit in any of the deciles of stenosis could not be determined.

Because of the small numbers of outcome events of disabling ipsilateral stroke at a median 2.7 years of follow-up (medical N = 24, surgical N = 21), no benefit from CE could be identified. In the 1,091 men, perioperative events occurred in 1.7% (n = 9) and in the 568 women 3.6% (n = 10). Women were not shown to benefit from CE, but there were too few outcome events for definitive analysis.

In the perioperative period, only 19 subjects had a stroke in any territory or died (2.3%), including four strokes and one fatal stroke resulting from angiography. Because 101 surgical subjects did not undergo CE, the actual perioperative rate of any stroke or death was 2.7% (adding the 1.5% risk of CE and the 1.2% risk of angiography). Among the 724 subjects who underwent endarterectomy, 10 nonfatal strokes and one fatal MI (1.5%) were recorded in the 30-day perioperative period. During the comparable 30-day period, the medical subjects experienced a 0.4% rate of stroke or death.

Despite the statistically significant results from ACAS, sufficient doubt about the clinical importance allowed continuation of another large randomized trial of asymptomatic subjects. The ACST, which has a design similar to ACAS, seeks 3,200 subjects (28).

ACST plans to analyze by degrees of stenosis. It will identify strokes by side and cause: large artery, lacunar, cardioembolic. It will conduct analyses involving gender differential and disabling compared to nondisabling strokes.

ANCILLARY INFORMATION FROM OTHER RANDOMIZED TRIALS

Asymptomatic Carotid Artery in the North American Symptomatic Carotid Endarterectomy Trial and European Carotid Surgery Trial

Investigators reported on the outlook for 1,820 patients in NASCET with contralateral asymptomatic stenosis (Fig. 39-2) (37). At 5 years among 216 patients with ≥60% asymptomatic stenosis, the highest risk of ipsilateral stroke (18.5%) was found with 75% to 94% stenosis. The annualized risk in this group was 3.7%. In patients with 60% to 74% stenosis and those with nearly occluded arteries the annualized risk was lower at 2.9%. At 5 years, among 1,604 patients with <60% asymptomatic stenosis the annualized risk of first stroke was only 1.6%. Of the 1,820 patients, 86 developed an ICA occlusion. The 5-year risk of stroke in the territory of the occluded artery was 9.4%, an annualized stroke risk of 1.9%. The cause of stroke was identified. At 5 years with 60% to 99% stenosis the risk of first ipsilateral stroke

attributable to the large-artery lesion was 9.9%, cardioembolic cause 2.1%, and lacunar stroke 6%.

The European Carotid Surgery Trial (ECST) Investigators identified 970 patients with 30% to 99% asymptomatic stenosis of the contralateral artery (38). Of these, 127 had 70% to 99% stenosis and 55 patients had a symptomless contralateral occluded artery. The annual risk of stroke with 70% to 99% stenosis was 1.9% and dropped to less than half this figure for patients with lesser degrees of stenosis. After occlusion the 3-year risk was 3.7%, slightly more than 1% per year. The causes of stroke were not identified.

Asymptomatic Subjects in the Aspirin and Carotid Endarterectomy Trial

The Aspirin and Carotid Endarterectomy (ACE) Trial randomized patients to study the optimum aspirin dose prior to CE (26). Most of the surgeons were NASCET participants and participants whose skill was vetted by strict criteria. Among the 2,804 patients in ACE, 1,214 totally asymptomatic subjects underwent CE. Follow-up was 90 days; long-term risk could not be evaluated. The perioperative 30-day complication rate of any stroke and death was 4.4%. In the presence of a contralateral occlusion (N = 154), the rate was 12.3%.

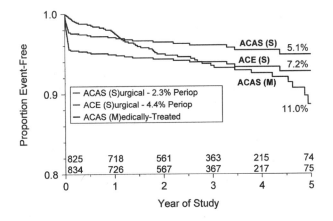

FIG. 39-2. Bar graphs showing the 5-year risk of ipsilateral stroke by degrees of stenosis in the North American Symptomatic Carotid Endarterectomy Trial's "asymptomatic other side." The numbers on top of the bars show the 5-year risk of ipsilateral stroke in each category of stenosis. The number of patients at risk in each group is shown below the horizontal axis. The annualized ipsilateral stroke risk was highest (3.7%) in the 75%–94% group, and intermediate (2.9%) with 60%–74% stenosis and with near occlusion (95%–99%). In aggregating patients below 60%, the annualized risk was 1.6%. Despite lack of visible disease, almost 1% of these patients had a stroke each year, presumably from heart, aorta, or small-vessel disease. (From Inzitari D, Eliasziw M, Gates P, et al. The causes and risk of stroke in patients with asymptomatic internal-carotid-artery stenosis. *N Engl J Med* 2000;342:1693–1700, with permission.)

APPLICATION OF DATA FROM THE TRIALS AND STUDIES

Risk of Stroke

In general, the risk of ipsilateral stroke is low and only reaches levels that exceed the optimum operative risk in subjects with highest degrees of stenosis. If the cause of stroke is taken into consideration, surgical benefit becomes even less achievable.

Areas of Uncertainty about Efficacy of Carotid Endarterectomy

Prevention of disabling stroke has been incompletely studied. The ACAS data were inconclusive. In the Mackey natural history study, only six strokes (14%) were disabling. In the ACE trial, with no medical group, postoperative strokes were disabling in 17% of 149 strokes in asymptomatic subjects.

Data are accumulating about the perioperative complication rate favoring men. In the ACAS and ACE asymptomatic subjects, the combined complication rates were 3.1% for men and 4.6% for women (39).

The data from large observational studies point to increasing risk with increasing degrees of stenosis (13–15). The randomized trials lacked a sufficient number of events to confirm or deny this hypothesis. It seems likely that the increasing risk of stroke with increasing severity of stenosis found in symptomatic patients eventually will be confirmed in asymptomatic subjects.

Number Needed to Treat

The concept of estimating numbers needed to treat to prevent stroke within a given time period is helpful in evaluating the effectiveness of CE. There is a striking difference between the number calculated for symptomatic patients and asymptomatic subjects. Six symptomatic patients with 70% to 99% stenosis need to be treated to prevent one stroke within 2 years and only three in the elderly (≥75 years). This contrasts sharply with the 67 calculated for asymptomatic subjects. If the assumption is correct that the causes of stroke in subjects in ACAS and the asymptomatic side of NASCET are reasonably similar, a calculation has been made that to prevent one large-artery stroke, 111 asymptomatic subjects need to be submitted to CE (37).

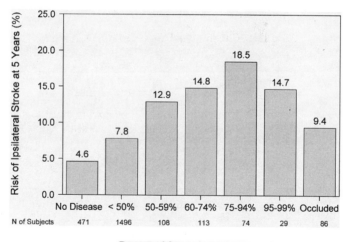

FIG. 39-3. The medical and surgical 5-year Kaplan-Meier curves of freedom from ipsilateral stroke, perioperative stroke, and death indicate a 5.9% difference favoring endarterectomy at 5 years in the Asymptomatic Carotid Atherosclerosis Study. Between years 4 and 5, a series of stroke of unknown cause occurred in the medical arm. The number of patients available for analysis at each year of follow-up appears along the horizontal axis. At year 5 the numbers were very small. Superimposed is the projected outcome of 1,214 asymptomatic individuals from the Aspirin and Carotid Endarterectomy Trial based on the 4.4% stroke and death rate at 30 days, extrapolating the outcomes to 5 years. Using the projected 7.2% rate at 5 years, the difference between treatment groups is 3.8%, only 0.8% benefit per year. The surgical benefit is too small to justify the procedure in these 1,214 subjects. (From Barnett HJM, Meldrum HE, Eliasziw M. The appropriate use of carotid endarterectomy. *CMAJ* 2002;166:1169–1179.)

TABLE 39-3. *Thirty-day stroke and death operative risk*

Author or study	Year	No. of patients	No. of events	Type of study	30-Day stroke, death
ACAS (26)	1995	724	11	Randomized trial	1.5%
Hertzer et al. (40)	1997	1,174	19	Single institution	1.6%
Cebul et al. (41)	1998	322	8	Medicare	2.5%
Goldstein et al. (42)	1998	463	13	Multi-institutional	2.8%
Karp et al. (24)	1998	1,002	32	Medicare	3.2%
Bratzler et al. (43)	1996	350	13	Medicare	3.7%
Kucey et al. (44)	1998	305	12	Multi-institutional	4.0%
VA, Hobson et al. (35)	1993	203	9	Randomized trial	4.5%
Kresowik et al. (25)	2001	7,604	342	Medicare	4.5%
ACE Trial (36)	1999	1,214	70	Multi-institutional	4.4%
Wong et al. (45)	1997	117	6	Multi-institutional	5.2%
Hartmann et al. (46)	1999	54	3	Single institution	5.6%
Total		**13,532**	**538**		**4.0%**

ACAS, Asymptomatic Carotid Atherosclerosis Study; ACE, Aspirin and Carotid Endarterectomy; VA, Veterans Affairs Cooperative Study Group.

Are Surgeons Meeting the Necessary Perioperative Complication Rates?

The challenge facing surgeons has been to approximate the 1.5% perioperative stroke and death rate reported in ACAS. Expert surgeons in the ACE Trial achieved an acceptable perioperative complication rate of 6.4% in 1,292 symptomatic patients. The same surgeons had a 4.4% perioperative complication rate in 1,214 asymptomatic subjects. Projected out to 5 years, stroke-free survival was not achieved (Fig. 39-3).

Table 39-3 lists the variability in achieving the necessary perioperative rate of ≤3% in asymptomatic subjects. Of ten case series and two randomized trials only four reports (2,683 subjects) achieved a perioperative complication rate at or below 3.0% (36,40–42). The other eight studies (10,849 subjects) were well above the critical threshold with an average of 4.5% (24–26,35,43–46).

Endarterectomy Concomitant with Major Vascular Surgery

Based on the assumption that strokes in subjects with asymptomatic carotid stenosis submitted to major vascular surgery were related to the carotid lesion, it became popular to perform CE concomitantly with these procedures. Eventually, it was noted that this combination of procedures resulted in aggregating the perioperative risks of the two (47). Stroke was as likely to be on the opposite side of the carotid lesion (15,48). It emerged that the common source of stroke complicating coronary artery bypass grafting was not hemodynamic but was thromboembolism from the disease in the aorta into which the bypass was inserted. In a Medicare survey, when 236 patients had both CE and coronary artery bypass grafting, the perioperative rate of stroke and death was a prohibitive 17.4% (25). CE combined with major vascular surgery should be avoided.

Acceptance of Carotid Endarterectomy

The extraordinary increase in the number of CEs performed in the last decade implies that many practitioners in the United States favor CE for asymptomatic subjects. Individual surgical commentary endorses the benefit as a carte blanche in these subjects (49). Despite this endorsement a number of warnings have appeared. Describing the ACAS results, Lanska and Kryscio (50) state that "the application of an early stopping rule is open to question; the demonstrated statistically significant results are of small magnitude and no consensus exists concerning their clinical importance and generalizability . . . population screening for asymptomatic carotid stenosis is unwarranted." Another critique concludes that "although surgery effectively prevents ipsilateral stroke, the stroke risk and absolute reduction are small; surgery does not prevent stroke and death overall...the cost of surgery relative to the cost of stroke for the population at risk is large" (51).

A consensus panel of the American Heart Association concluded: "For patients with a surgical risk <3% and life expectancy of at least 5 years: Proven indications: Ipsilateral CE is acceptable for stenotic lesions (≥60% diameter reduction of distal outflow tract) with or without ulceration and with or without antiplatelet therapy, irrespective of contralateral artery status, ranging from no disease to occlusion [Grade A recommendation]" (52). The consensus panel of the National Stroke Association reiterated the need for a perioperative complication rate of <3% (53).

A unique paradox has emerged with respect to CE in asymptomatic subjects. Population screening to identify subjects with the appropriate lesions is not recommended. Nevertheless, entrepreneurs are flooding mailboxes and websites with advertisements promising longer stroke-free life to those who come to church basements and community halls to be screened by ultrasound for "dangerous lesions."

There is no disagreement that only some skilled surgeons can achieve the requisite low morbidity and mortality rate of ACAS (54). The vexed but pertinent question for the referring physician or the patient who is referred for CE is the availability of information about the skill of the surgeon who will perform the endarterectomy (55). Surgical audits are being invited (56). Audits must be carried out by impartial individuals and preferably by experts in neurologic examination who will not overlook minor strokes. A report of 2,000 physicians sampled from the master file of the American Medical Association showed that knowledge of local surgical skills are largely unknown (42). Of 1,006 responses, only 19% knew the perioperative mortality rate for CE in their institutions.

RECOMMENDATIONS FOR MANAGEMENT OF PATIENTS WITH ASYMPTOMATIC CAROTID STENOSIS

1. The large majority of asymptomatic individuals should be treated with rigorous medical therapy alone. Management of hypertension, diabetes mellitus, hypercholesterolemia, and cigarette smoking is mandatory. Other less common risks must be managed. Both patient and physician must regard risk factor management as a lifetime commitment.

2. Antiplatelet therapy is recommended. The authors strongly favor aspirin.

3. Patients should be familiar with symptoms of focal hemisphere and retinal origin and should be urged to report them immediately. Physicians should be acquainted with symptoms that cannot be attributed to a carotid lesion (e.g., vertigo,

dizziness, blackouts, drop attacks, amnestic events, episodes of confusion, isolated episodes of diplopia).

4. Occasionally, on empirical grounds, subjects with the highest degrees of stenosis (≥80%) may be considered for endarterectomy. The surgeon should be capable of performing endarterectomy with a ≤3% stroke and death perioperative rate, validated by independent audit.

5. Subjects with contralateral occlusion and an ipsilateral asymptomatic stenosis should be treated medically to avoid the excessive morbidity and mortality of endarterectomy that accompany this combination.

6. Subjects with asymptomatic carotid lesions proceeding to other major vascular surgical procedures are not candidates for endarterectomy.

7. Population screening is not warranted. Routine auscultation for bruits cannot be recommended.

8. For practitioners in Europe, participation in the ACST should be considered until patient entry is closed.

REFERENCES

1. Ramsey DE, Miles RD, Lambeth A, et al. Prevalence of extracranial carotid artery disease: A survey of an asymptomatic population with noninvasive techniques. *J Vasc Surg* 1987;5:584–588.
2. Colgan MP, Strode GR, Sommer JD, et al. Prevalence of asymptomatic carotid disease: results of duplex scanning in 348 unselected volunteers. *J Vasc Surg* 1988;8: 674–678.
3. Ricci S, Flaminio OF, Celani MG, et al. Prevalence of internal carotid-artery stenosis in subjects older than 49 years: a population study. *Cerebrovasc Dis* 1991;1: 16–19.
4. O'Leary DH, Polak JF, Kronmal RA, et al., on behalf of the CHS Collaborative Research Group. Distribution and correlates of sonographically detected carotid artery disease in the cardiovascular health study. *Stroke* 1992;23:1752–1760.
5. Prati P, Vanuzzo D, Casaroli M, et al. Prevalence and determinants of carotid atherosclerosis in a general population. *Stroke* 1992;23:1705–1711.
6. Barnett HJM, Eliasziw M, Meldrum HE, et al. Do the facts and figures warrant a 10-fold increase in the performance of carotid endarterectomy on asymptomatic patients? *Neurology* 1996;46:603–608.
7. Wiebers DO, Whisnant JP, Sandok BA, et al. Prospective comparison of a cohort with asymptomatic carotid bruit and a population-based cohort without carotid bruit. *Stroke* 1990;21:984–988.
8. Heyman A, Wilkinson WE, Heyden S, et al. Risk of stroke in asymptomatic persons with cervical arterial bruits. *N Engl J Med* 1980;302:838–841.
9. Chambers BR, Norris JW. Clinical significance of asymptomatic neck bruits. *Neurology* 1985;35: 742–745.

10. Wolf PA, Kannel WB, Sorlie P, et al. Asymptomatic carotid bruit and risk of stroke. *JAMA* 1981;245:1441–1445.

11. Josse MO, Touboul PJ, Mas JL, et al. Prevalence of asymptomatic internal carotid artery stenosis. *Neuroepidemiology* 1987;6:150–152.

12. Wang MY, Mimran R. Mohit A, et al. Carotid stenosis in a multiethnic population. *J Stroke Cerebrovasc Dis* 2000;9:64–69.

13. Mackey AE, Abrahamowicz M, Langlois Y, et al., and the Asymptomatic Cervical Bruit Study Group. Outcome of asymptomatic patients with carotid disease. *Neurology* 1997;48:896–903.

14. Hennerici M, Hülsbömer HB, Hefter H, et al. Natural history of asymptomatic extracranial arterial disease. *Brain* 1987;100:777–791.

15. Chambers BR, Norris JW. Outcome in patients with asymptomatic neck bruits. *N Engl J Med* 1986;315:860–865.

16. Bogousslavsky J, Despland PA, Regli F. Asymptomatic tight stenosis of the internal carotid artery: long-term prognosis. *Neurology* 1986;36:861–863.

17. Meissner I, Wiebers DO, Whisnant JP, et al. The natural history of asymptomatic carotid artery occlusive lesions. *JAMA* 1987;258:2704–2707.

18. Autret A, Saudeau D, Bertrand PH, et al. Stroke risk in patients with carotid stenosis. *Lancet* 1987;1:888–890.

19. Pokras R, Dyken ML. Dramatic changes in the performance of endarterectomy for diseases of the extracranial arteries of the head. *Stroke* 1988;19:1289–1290.

20. NINDS clinical advisory. Carotid endarterectomy for patients with asymptomatic internal carotid stenosis. September 28, 1994.

21. Huber TS, Wheeler KG, Cuddeback JK, et al. Effect of the asymptomatic carotid atherosclerosis study on carotid endarterectomy in Florida. *Stroke* 1998;29:1099–1105.

22. Morasch MD, Parker MA, Feinglass J, et al. Carotid endarterectomy: Characterization of recent increases in procedure rates. *J Vasc Surg* 2000;31:901–909.

23. Winslow CM, Solomon DH, Chassin MR, et al. The appropriateness of carotid endarterectomy. *N Engl J Med* 1988;318:721–727.

24. Karp HR, Flander D, Shipp CC, et al. Carotid endarterectomy among Medicare beneficiaries. *Stroke* 1998;29:46–52.

25. Kresowik TF, Bratzler D, Karp HR, et al. Multistate utilization, processes, and outcomes of carotid endarterectomy. *J Vasc Surg* 2001;33:227–235.

26. Taylor DW, Barnett HJM, Haynes RB, et al., for the ASA and Carotid Endarterectomy (ACE) Trial Collaborators. Low-dose and high-dose acetylsalicylic acid for patients undergoing carotid endarterectomy: a randomized controlled trial. *Lancet* 1999;353:2179–2184.

27. Nicolaides AN. Asymptomatic carotid stenosis and risk of stroke. Identification of a high risk group (ACSRS). A natural history study. *Int Angiol* 1995;14:21–23.

28. Halliday AW, for the steering committee and for the collaborators. The Asymptomatic Carotid Surgery Trial (ACST) rationale and design. *Eur J Vasc Surg* 1994;8:703–710.

29. Chaturvedi S, Meinke JL, St. Pierre E, et al. Attitudes of Canadian and U.S. neurologists regarding carotid endarterectomy for asymptomatic stenosis. *Can J Neurol Sci* 2000;27:116–119.

30. Masuhr F, Busch M, Einhaupl KM. Differences in medical and surgical therapy for stroke prevention between leading experts in North America and Western Europe. *Stroke* 1998;29:339–345.

31. Tu JV, Hannan EL, Anderson GM, et al. The fall and rise of carotid endarterectomy in the United States and Canada. *N Engl J Med* 1998;339:1441–1447.

32. Clagett GP, Youkey JR, Brigham RA, et al. Asymptomatic cervical bruit and abnormal ocular pneumoplethysmography: a prospective study comparing two approaches to management. *Surgery* 1984;96:823–830.

33. CASANOVA Study Group. Carotid surgery versus medical therapy in asymptomatic carotid stenosis. *Stroke* 1991;22:1229–1235.

34. Mayo Asymptomatic Carotid Endarterectomy Study Group. Results of a randomized controlled trial of carotid endarterectomy for asymptomatic carotid stenosis. *Mayo Clin Proc* 1992;67:513–518.

35. Hobson RW, Weiss DG, Fields WS, et al., and the Veterans Affairs Cooperative Study Group. Efficacy of carotid endarterectomy for asymptomatic carotid stenosis. *N Engl J Med* 1993;328:221–227.

36. Executive Committee for the Asymptomatic Carotid Atherosclerosis Study. Endarterectomy for asymptomatic carotid artery stenosis. *JAMA* 1995;273:1421–1428.

37. Inzitari D, Eliasziw M, Gates P, et al. The causes and risk of stroke in patients with asymptomatic internal-carotid-artery stenosis. *N Engl J Med* 2000;342:1693–1700.

38. The European Carotid Surgery Trialists Collaborative Group. Risk of stroke in the distribution of an asymptomatic carotid artery. *Lancet* 1995;345:209–212.

39. Alamowitch S, Eliasziw M, Taylor DW, et al., for the North American Symptomatic Carotid Endarterectomy Trial (NASCET) and the ASA and Carotid Endarterectomy (ACE) Trial Collaborators. The risk and benefit of endarterectomy in women with symptomatic internal carotid artery disease. *(in press)*.

40. Hertzer NR, O'Hara PJ, Mascha EJ, et al. Early outcome assessment for 2228 consecutive carotid endarterectomy procedures: the Cleveland Clinic experience from 1989 to 1995. *J Vasc Surg* 1997;26(1):1–10.

41. Cebul RD, Snow JR, Pine R, et al. Indications, outcomes, and provider volumes for carotid endarterectomy. *JAMA* 1998;279:1282–1287.

42. Goldstein LB, Samsa GP, Matchar DB, et al. Multicenter review of preoperative risk factors for endarterectomy for asymptomatic carotid artery stenosis. *Stroke* 1998;29:750–753.

43. Bratzler DW, Oehlert WH, Murray CK, et al. Carotid endarterectomy in Oklahoma Medicare beneficiaries: patient characteristics and outcomes. *J Okla St Med Assoc* 1996;89:423–429.

44. Kucey DS, Bowyer B, Iron K, et al. Determinants of outcome after carotid endarterectomy. *J Vasc Surg* 1998;23:1051–1058.

45. Wong J, Findlay J, Suarez-Almazor M. Regional performance of carotid endarterectomy. Appropriateness, outcomes and risk factors for complications. *Stroke* 1997;228:891–898.

46. Hartmann A, Hupp T, Koch H, et al. Prospective study on the complication rate of carotid surgery. *Cerebrovasc Dis* 1999;9:152–156.

47. Robertson JT, Fraser JC. Evaluation of carotid

endarterectomy with and without coronary artery bypass surgery. In: Moossy J, Reinmuth OM, eds. *Cerebrovascular diseases.* New York: Raven Press, 1981: 261.

48. Ropper AH, Wechsler LR, Wilson LS. Carotid bruit and the risk of stroke in elective surgery. *N Engl J Med* 1982;307:1388–1390.

49. Loftus CM, Hopkins LN. Paradoxical indications for carotid artery reconstruction. *Neurosurgery* 1995;36: 99–100.

50. Lanska DJ, Kryscio RJ. Endarterectomy for asymptomatic internal carotid artery stenosis. *Neurology* 1997; 48:1481–1490.

51. Frey JL. Asymptomatic carotid stenosis: surgery's the answer, but that's not the question. *Ann Neurol* 1996;39: 405–406.

52. Biller J, Feinberg WM, Castaldo JE, et al. Guidelines for carotid endarterectomy: a statement for healthcare professionals from a special writing group of the Stroke Council, American Heart Association. *Stroke* 1998;29: 554–562.

53. Gorelick PB, Sacco RL, Smith DB, et al. Prevention of a first stroke: a review of guidelines and a multidisciplinary consensus statement from the National Stroke Association. *JAMA* 1999;281:1112–1120.

54. Ruby ST, Robinson D, Lynch JT, et al. Outcome analysis of carotid endarterectomy in Connecticut: the impact of volume and specialty. *Ann Vasc Surg* 1996;10:22–26.

55. Barnett HJM, Broderick JP. Carotid endarterectomy, another wake-up call. *Neurology* 2000;55:746–747.

56. Goldstein LB, Moore WS, Robertson JT, et al. Complication rates for carotid endarterectomy. A call to action. *Stroke* 1997;28:889–890.

57. Barnett HJM, Meldrum HE, Eliasziw M. The appropriate use of carotid endarterectomy. *CMAJ* 2002;166: 1169–1179.

Ischemic Stroke: Advances in Neurology, Vol. 92. Edited by
H.J.M. Barnett, Julien Bogousslavsky, and Heather Meldrum.
Lippincott Williams & Wilkins, Philadelphia © 2003.

40

Extracranial to Intracranial Bypass

Catharina J.M. Klijn and J. van Gijn

*Department of Neurology, University Medical Center Utrecht
and the Rudolf Magnus Institute for Neuroscience, Utrecht, The Netherlands*

Extracranial to intracranial (EC/IC) bypass surgery in the treatment of ischemic stroke is based on the notion that ischemic stroke in some patients is caused by failure of blood flow to the brain rather than by embolism (1). In such "hemodynamically compromised" patients, augmentation of blood flow to the symptomatic hemisphere by EC/IC bypass theoretically might be beneficial. This involves mainly patients with transient or at most moderately disabling symptoms of cerebral ischemia associated with ipsilateral occlusion of the internal carotid artery (ICA) (1,2), who have a risk of recurrent stroke of 5% to 6% per year (3). In these patients, treatment options such as carotid endarterectomy or angioplasty are not feasible.

This theory was put to the test in the International EC/IC Bypass Study. This randomized trial addressed the question whether a bypass between the superficial temporal artery (STA) and a cortical branch of the middle cerebral artery (MCA) could prevent ischemic stroke in patients with symptomatic ICA occlusion, intracranial ICA stenosis, or MCA stenosis or occlusion better than medical treatment alone (4). In 1985, after inclusion of 1,377 patients (960 with symptomatic ICA occlusion and 417 with intracranial ICA stenosis or MCA stenosis or occlusion) over a period of 8 years, the study showed that the operation was not effective despite good operative results (5). Subgroup analysis failed to show any trends toward a benefit of the operation in any of the prespecified subgroups, such as patients with ongoing symptoms after demonstration of ICA occlusion or patients with frequent transient ischemic attacks (≥6) and poor collateral blood supply (5,6). As a result, the operation has been largely abandoned throughout the world (7). Proponents of the hemodynamic theory, however, noted that the EC/IC Bypass Study did not restrict inclusion of patients to those who were at high risk for recurrent stroke, that is, those in whom compromised blood flow to the hemisphere ipsilateral to the occluded carotid artery had been demonstrated (8–12). If such patients at high risk can be identified, the role of the EC/IC bypass operation for prevention of recurrent ischemic stroke in patients with symptomatic carotid artery occlusion should be reappraised.

In this chapter, we will not discuss other indications for the operation, such as surgical treatment of large cerebral aneurysms.

WHICH PATIENTS ARE MOST AT RISK?

Symptoms occurring in patients with occlusion of the carotid artery may vary widely in frequency, severity, and duration. Symptoms may involve the eye and the brain. In patients with an occlusion of the carotid artery who never had any symptoms, collateral pathways probably are sufficient because in these patients the risk of recurrent ischemic stroke is low (approximately 1%–2% per year) (13,14). The same applies to patients who had symptoms only before the occlusion of the carotid artery was found but not thereafter (12,15). One might speculate that in these patients, symptoms arose as a result of thromboembolism before the carotid artery became occluded and that collateral pathways could adequately sustain blood flow to the brain once the occlusion had occurred. Furthermore, patients with only retinal symptoms and not symptoms of cerebral ischemia are at relatively low risk for stroke; none of 16 of such patients in one study (16) and none of 24 in another study (12) had an ischemic stroke during follow-up of more than 2 years.

In patients with ongoing symptoms of cerebral ischemia (e.g., after documentation of carotid occlusion) there are indicators of hemodynamic compromise that may further distinguish high-risk patients from those at relatively low risk for recurrent ischemic stroke. Typical features from the history that may suggest hemodynamic compromise, such as limb shaking or precipitation of symptoms by rising or exercise, are associated with a relatively high risk of recurrent cerebral ischemic events (hazard ratio: 5.0; 95% confidence interval: 1.4–17.2; $p = 0.01$) (12). However, such symptoms occur in only a minority of patients (about 14%–20%) (12,17). The presence of leptomeningeal pathways on angiography was associated with a worse outcome in one study (12) but not in another study (16). The number of collateral pathways was inversely related to the risk of ischemic stroke in a single study (18). Several studies using a variety of techniques have shown that decreased hemodynamic reserve is associated with a relatively high risk of stroke, probably on the order of 9% to 18% per year (15,16,18–21). However, other studies did not find such an association (12,22–24). Some of these studies can be criticized because the study population was not homogeneous in that asymptomatic patients were included (18–20,22,23), patients with intracranial carotid artery or MCA lesions or extracranial carotid artery stenosis (15,21–24) were included, or some patients were censored due to surgical intervention (12,22). Nevertheless, accumulating evidence leads to the tentative conclusion that high-risk patients can be distinguished from those at relatively low risk by a number of methods that provide information on the hemodynamic status of the hemisphere at risk.

At this time, the preferred method for measurement of the hemodynamic status of the hemisphere at risk probably is positron emission tomography (PET) with measurement of the oxygen extraction fraction, but this technique involves the use of unstable radioactive tracers and is not widely available. Hemodynamic compromise also can be measured by other techniques, such as transcranial Doppler ultrasonography (TCD), stable xenon (Xe) or Xe 133 inhalation techniques, or iodine (I 123)-labeled IMP single photon emission computed tomography before and after vasodilatory stimuli such as breath holding, carbogen inhalation, or acetazolamide. Correlations between different hemodynamic measures, such as oxygen extraction fraction by PET and TCD CO_2 reactivity (25), or changes in regional blood flow velocity and volumetric flow after acetazolamide (26), have been disappointingly low. It remains unclear whether the different techniques identify the same patients at high risk and which technique most accurately predicts the

occurrence of a future stroke. Noninvasive magnetic resonance (MR) techniques, such as MR perfusion, diffusion, and spectroscopy, may provide new prognostic indicators in the near future (27).

EXTRACRANIAL TO INTRACRANIAL BYPASS

The EC/IC Bypass Study clearly showed that the STA-MCA bypass did not prevent recurrent stroke better than medical treatment alone in patients with symptomatic carotid artery occlusion in general (5). Currently, it is unknown whether the EC/IC bypass confers benefit in a subgroup of patients at high risk for recurrent stroke because there is clinical or technical evidence for a hemodynamically compromised hemisphere on the side of the carotid artery occlusion. Many studies have reported improvement of cerebral hemodynamic measurements after STA-MCA bypass operation (28–31), but no comparisons with similar patients who were not operated on are available. Others found that improvement of hemodynamic measures did not occur after operation (32) or did not occur consistently (33,34). Improvement of hemodynamic measures has been shown especially in patients in whom such measures were most disturbed before operation (35–37). A caveat is that improvement of cerebral blood flow shortly after STA-MCA bypass surgery may not last over time (36,38) and that cerebral hemodynamic measures may improve spontaneously (20,22,39).

If STA-MCA bypass surgery is considered in the subgroup of patients with carotid artery occlusion who are at high risk for recurrent ischemic stroke, it should be kept in mind that the number of complications of surgery in this subgroup may be higher than that reported in the EC/IC Bypass Study. One study reported a complication rate of STA-MCA bypass surgery close to 12% in patients who were considered neurologically unstable (40). Patients who on theoretical grounds have the most to gain by EC/IC bypass surgery also may carry the highest perioperative risk.

Over the last years, a new technique for the EC/IC bypass operation has been developed, the so-called *high-flow EC/IC bypass* (41,42). This bypass connects the STA (or external carotid artery) not with a small artery at the brain convexity but with the intracranial distal part of the ICA or the proximal part of the MCA, by means of a venous (or arterial) transplant. The intracranial anastomosis is made with the Excimer laser, which allows construction of an anastomosis with one of the large arteries proximal in the vascular tree without the need to temporarily clamp

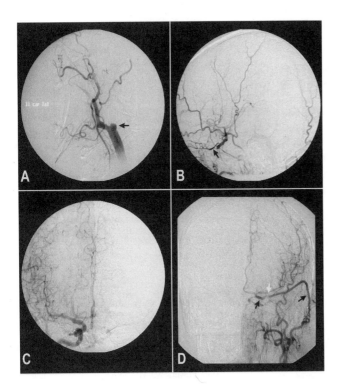

FIG. 40-1. Angiogram of a 76-year-old man who was referred because of recurrent attacks of expressive dysphasia, right-sided weakness and numbness, and transient monocular blindness of the left eye that occurred one to six times per day and mostly after he rose from a sitting or lying position. Selective catheterization of the left common carotid artery showed **(A)** occlusion of the internal carotid arrow (*arrow*) and **(B)** filling of the left middle cerebral artery (MCA) via the ophthalmic artery *(arrow)*. **(C)** Selective catheterization of the right common carotid artery showed filling of the left anterior but not the left MCA. **(D)** Angiography 1 month postoperatively demonstrated the patent bypass (*black arrows*) and clip artifact (*white arrow*). (Adapted from Klijn CJ, Kappelle LJ, van der Grond J, et al. A new type of extracranial/intracranial bypass for recurrent haemodynamic transient ischaemic attacks. *Cerebrovasc Dis* 1998;8: 184–187, with permission.)

the recipient arteries. An example of this type of bypass is given in Figure 40-1. The amount of flow that can be obtained through this bypass is higher than that reported for the conventional STA-MCA bypass (43). The hemodynamic effect of the high-flow EC/IC bypass on the blood flow to the hemisphere at risk may be larger than that of the STA-MCA bypass, but direct comparisons of such measures in patients with symptomatic carotid artery occlusion are not yet available. Preliminary results have shown that the Excimer laser-assisted EC/IC bypass operation is a potentially promising procedure for revascularization of the brain in patients with symptomatic carotid artery occlusion at high risk for recurrent stroke, but it carries a substantial risk in these patients (44).

OTHER TREATMENT OPTIONS

While further evidence on the efficacy of EC/IC bypass surgery in certain subgroups of patients is awaited, patients in the mean time will present with recurrent symptoms of cerebral ischemia attributable to an occluded carotid artery and expect us to advise them on the best available treatment. Before giving a brief overview of treatment options, we should acknowledge that for the greater part of these options there is no evidence from controlled studies, and most of the decisions are based on pathophysiological plausibility, admittedly a shaky basis.

All patients should be treated with an antithrombotic agent, which probably should be aspirin in most cases. If patients have ongoing transient ischemic attacks despite taking aspirin, oral anticoagulation may be prescribed instead (3), particularly in the presence of a possible source of cardiac embolism. All vascular risk factors (such as hyperlipidemia, diabetes mellitus, smoking, and being overweight) should be actively assessed and rigorously treated, as in all stroke patients. The treatment of hypertension should be performed prudently because aggressive treatment may induce cerebral ischemic symptoms in patients with symptomatic carotid artery occlusion (45). In our experience and that of other investigators (46), temporary tapering of antihypertensive drugs (unless contraindicated because of cardiac disease) may result in cessation of symptoms in some patients. To avoid episodes of hypotension induced by the patient rising from a sitting or supine position, we recommend (bed) rest during critical periods, especially in patients who report rising as a precipitating factor of symptoms.

Patients with symptomatic carotid artery occlusion who have a severe (70%–99%) stenosis of the contralateral asymptomatic ICA may be advised to undergo endarterectomy of this stenosis. This operation usually is not recommended for patients with an incomplete anterior circle of Willis in whom the contralateral ICA cannot contribute to the blood supply of the hemisphere on the side of the carotid occlusion. Serious concomitant disease that increases a patient's risk of operation may be a reason to refrain from contralateral carotid endarterectomy.

In patients with a severe stenosis of an external carotid artery ipsilateral to a symptomatic ICA occlusion (a rare finding in our experience), endarterectomy of the external carotid artery should be considered if patients are not at particularly high risk of surgery because of concomitant disease.

CONCLUDING REMARKS

An EC/IC bypass operation may benefit patients with symptomatic carotid artery occlusion who are at high risk for recurrent ischemic stroke, but presently there is insufficient evidence to support this. Such evidence can only be obtained by a new randomized controlled trial. The characteristics of the patients who should be included in such a trial are subject to debate. Probably only patients who had symptoms of the brain (and not those with only symptoms of the eye) should be included, and preferably only when such symptoms continued after the occlusion of the carotid artery was documented. Several methods probably can be used to assess the hemodynamic status of the hemisphere at risk. A new trial that uses a high oxygen extraction fraction by PET as the inclusion criterion for hemodynamic compromise is expected to start in the near future (H.P. Adams Jr., *personal communication*, 2002) (11).

ACKNOWLEDGMENT

C.J.M. Klijn was supported by the Netherlands Heart Foundation (94.085).

REFERENCES

1. Klijn CJM, Kappelle LJ, Tulleken CAF, et al. Symptomatic carotid artery occlusion. A reappraisal of hemodynamic factors. *Stroke* 1997;28:2084–2093.
2. Derdeyn CP, Grubb RL Jr, Powers WJ. Cerebral hemodynamic impairment. Methods of measurement and association with stroke risk. *Neurology* 1999;53:251–259.
3. Klijn CJM, Kappelle LJ, Algra A, et al. Outcome in patients with symptomatic occlusion of the internal carotid artery or intracranial arterial lesions: a meta-analysis of the role of baseline characteristics and type of antithrombotic treatment. *Cerebrovasc Dis* 2001;12:228–234.
4. The EC/IC Bypass Study group. The international cooperative study of extracranial/intracranial arterial anastomosis (EC/IC bypass study): methodology and entry characteristics. *Stroke* 1985;16:397–406.
5. The EC/IC Bypass Study Group. Failure of extracranial-intracranial arterial bypass to reduce the risk of ischemic stroke. Results of an international randomized trial. *N Engl J Med* 1985;313:1191–1200.
6. Barnett HJM, Sackett D, Haynes B, et al. Are the results of the extracranial-intracranial bypass trial generalizable? *N Engl J Med* 1987;316:820–824.
7. Caplan LR, Piepgras DG, Quest DO, et al. EC-IC bypass 10 years later: is it valuable? *Surg Neurol* 1996;46:416–423.
8. Ausman JI, Diaz FG. Critique of the extracranial-intracranial bypass study. *Surg Neurol* 1986;26:218–221.
9. Day AL, Rhoton AL, Little JR. The extracranial-intracranial bypass study. *Surg Neurol* 1986;26:222–226.
10. Sundt TM Jr. Was the international randomized trial of extracranial-intracranial arterial bypass representative of the population at risk? *N Engl J Med* 1987;316:814–816.
11. Adams HPJ, Powers WJ, Grubb RL Jr, et al. Preview of a new trial of extracranial-to-intracranial anastomosis. The Carotid Occlusion Surgery Study. *Neurosurg Clin N Am* 2001;36:613–624.
12. Klijn CJM, Kappelle LJ, van Huffelen AC, et al. Recurrent ischemia in symptomatic carotid occlusion: prognostic value of hemodynamic factors. *Neurology* 2000;56:1806–1812.
13. Powers WJ, Derdeyn CP, Fritsch SM, et al. Benign prognosis of never-symptomatic carotid occlusion. *Neurology* 2000;54:878–882.
14. Vernieri F, Pasqualetti P, Passarelli F, et al. Outcome of carotid artery occlusion is predicted by cerebrovascular reactivity. *Stroke* 1999;30:593–598.
15. Yamauchi H, Fukuyama H, Nagahama Y, et al. Significance of increased oxygen extraction fraction in five-year prognosis of major cerebral arterial occlusive diseases. *J Nucl Med* 1999;40:1992–1998.
16. Grubb RL Jr, Derdeyn CP, Fritsch SM, et al. Importance of hemodynamic factors in the prognosis of symptomatic carotid occlusion. *JAMA* 1998;280:1055–1060.
17. Klijn CJM, van Buren PA, Kappelle LJ, et al. Outcome in patients with symptomatic occlusion of the internal carotid artery. *Eur J Vasc Endovasc Surg* 2000;19:579–586.
18. Vernieri F, Pasqualetti P, Matteis M, et al. Effect of collateral blood flow and cerebral vasomotor reactivity on the outcome of carotid artery occlusion. *Stroke* 2001;32:1552–1558.
19. Kleiser B, Widder B. Course of carotid artery occlusions with impaired cerebrovascular reactivity. *Stroke* 1992;23:171–174.
20. Widder B, Kleiser B, Krapf H. Course of cerebrovascular reactivity in patients with carotid artery occlusions. *Stroke* 1994;25:1963–1967.

21. Webster MW, Makaroun MS, Steed DL, et al. Compromised cerebral blood flow reactivity is a predictor of stroke in patients with symptomatic carotid artery occlusive disease. *J Vasc Surg* 1995;21:338–345.

22. Yokota C, Hasegawa Y, Minematsu K, et al. Effect of acetazolamide reactivity and long-term outcome in patients with major cerebral artery occlusive diseases. *Stroke* 1998;29:640–644.

23. Hasegawa Y, Yamaguchi T, Tsuchiya T, et al. Sequential change of hemodynamic reserve in patients with major cerebral artery occlusion or severe stenosis. *Neuroradiology* 1992;34:15–21.

24. Powers WJ, Tempel LW, Grubb RL Jr. Influence of cerebral hemodynamics on stroke risk: one-year follow-up of 30 medically treated patients. *Ann Neurol* 1989;25: 325–330.

25. Sugimori H, Ibayashi S, Fujii K, et al. Can transcranial Doppler really detect reduced cerebral perfusion states? *Stroke* 1995;26:2053–2060.

26. Demolis P, Tran Dinh YR, Giudicelli J-F. Relationships between cerebral regional blood flow velocities and volumetric blood flows and their respective reactivities to acetazolamide. *Stroke* 1999;27:1835–1839.

27. Klijn CJM, Kappelle LJ, van der Grond J, et al. Magnetic resonance techniques for the identification of patients with symptomatic carotid artery occlusion at high risk of cerebral ischemic events. *Stroke* 2000;31: 3001–3007.

28. Iwama T, Hashimoto N, Hayashida K. Cerebral hemodynamic parameters for patients with neurological improvements after extracranial-intracranial arterial bypass surgery: evaluation using positron emission tomography. *Neurosurgery* 2001;48:504–512.

29. Takagi Y, Hashimoto N, Iwama T, et al. Improvement of oxygen metabolic reserve after extracranial-intracranial bypass surgery in patients with severe haemodynamic insufficiency. *Acta Neurochir (Wien)* 1997;139:52–56.

30. Karnik R, Valentin A, Ammerer H, et al. Evaluation of vasomotor reactivity by transcranial Doppler and acetazolamide test before and after extracranial-intracranial bypass in patients with internal carotid artery occlusion. *Stroke* 1992;23:812–817.

31. Yamashita T, Kashiwagi S, Nakano S, et al. The effect of EC-IC bypass surgery on resting cerebral blood flow and cerebrovascular reserve capacity studies with stable Xe-CT and acetazolamide test. *Neuroradiology* 1991; 33:217–222.

32. De Weerd AW, Veering MM, Mosmans PCM, et al. Effect of the extra-intracranial (STA-MCA) arterial anastomosis on EEG and cerebral blood flow. A controlled study on patients with unilateral cerebral ischemia. *Stroke* 1982;13:674–679.

33. Vorstrup S, Lassen NA, Henriksen L, et al. CBF before and after extra-intracranial bypass surgery in patients with ischemic cerebrovascular disease studied with ^{133}Xe inhalation tomography. *Stroke* 1985;16:616–626.

34. Ishikawa T, Yasui N, Suzuki N, et al. STA-MCA bypass surgery for internal carotid artery occlusion. Comparative follow-up study. *Neurol Med Chir (Tokyo)* 1992;32: 5–9.

35. Laurent JP, Lawner PM, O'Connor M. Reversal of intracerebral steal by STA-MCA anastomosis. *J Neurosurg* 1982;57:629–632.

36. Yonekura M, Austin G, Hayward W. Long-term evaluation of cerebral blood flow, transient ischemic attacks, and stroke after STA-MCA anastomosis. *Surg Neurol* 1982;18:123–130.

37. Powers WJ, Martin WRW, Herscovitch P, et al. Extracranial-intracranial bypass surgery: hemodynamic and metabolic effects. *Neurology* 1984;34:1168–1174.

38. Tanahashi N, Stirling Meyer J, Rogers RL, et al. Long term assessment of cerebral perfusion following STA-MCA by-pass in patients. *Stroke* 1985;16:85–91.

39. Derdeyn CP, Videen TO, Fritsch SM, et al. Compensatory mechanisms for chronic cerebral hypoperfusion in patients with carotid occlusion. *Stroke* 1999;30: 1019–1024.

40. Sundt TM Jr, Whisnant JP, Fode NC, et al. Results, complications, and follow-up of 415 bypass operations for occlusive disease of the carotid system. *Mayo Clin Proc* 1985;60:230–240.

41. Tulleken CAF, Verdaasdonk RM, Mansvelt Beck RJ, et al. The modified excimer laser-assisted high-flow bypass operation. *Surg Neurol* 1996;46:424–429.

42. Tulleken CAF, van der Zwan A, Verdaasdonk RM, et al. High-flow excimer laser-assisted extra-intracranial and intra-intracranial bypass. *Oper Tech Neurosurg* 1999;2: 142–148.

43. van der Zwan A, Tulleken CAF, Hillen B. Flow quantification of the non-occlusive excimer laser-assisted EC-IC bypass. *Acta Neurochir (Wien)* 2001;143: 647–654.

43a. Klijn CJ, Kappelle LJ, van der Grond J, et al. A new type of extracranial/intracranial bypass for recurrent haemodynamic transient ischaemic attacks. *Cerebrovasc Dis* 1998;8:184–187.

44. Klijn CJM, Kappelle LJ, van der Zwan A, et al. Excimer laser-assisted high-flow EC/IC bypass in patients with symptomatic carotid artery occlusion at high risk of recurrent cerebral ischemia: safety and long-term outcome. *Stroke* 2002;33(10):2451–2458.

45. Hankey GJ, Gubbay SS. Focal cerebral ischaemia and infarction due to antihypertensive therapy. *Med J Aust* 1987;146:412–414.

46. Leira EC, Ajax T, Adams HP. Limb-shaking carotid transient ischemic attacks successfully treated with modification of the antihypertensive regimen. *Arch Neurol* 1997;7:904–905.

Ischemic Stroke: Advances in Neurology, Vol. 92. Edited by
H.J.M. Barnett, Julien Bogousslavsky, and Heather Meldrum.
Lippincott Williams & Wilkins, Philadelphia © 2003.

41

Angioplasty and Stenting

Martin M. Brown

Institute of Neurology, University College London; Acute Brain Injury Service,
The National Hospital for Neurology and Neurosurgery, London, United Kingdom

Carotid endarterectomy is the major surgical treatment for prevention of stroke from carotid artery atherosclerosis. The application of carotid surgery for stroke prevention is supported by more than 50 years of experience and several large randomized trials that have established the benefit of surgery in patients with severe, recently symptomatic carotid stenosis. However, recent advances in endovascular interventional techniques are threatening the preeminence of this surgery for this indication. This should be no surprise, given that angioplasty and stenting now are widely used in the coronary and lower limb vessels, with an acceptably low complication rate similar to more invasive surgery at these sites. The pathology of atherosclerosis in different arteries is similar, yet there has been resistance to angioplasty and stenting for stroke prevention because of anxiety about the risks of cerebral embolism. Despite this, angioplasty and stenting have been increasingly used to treat carotid and vertebral artery stenosis, and recently the early results of a large multicenter randomized trial of carotid surgery versus carotid endovascular treatment have been reported (1). These new and emerging data are reviewed in this chapter. Technology is advancing rapidly, and experience of carotid stenting has improved; self-expanding stents designed for use in the carotid artery have been developed; and new devices to protect against cerebral embolism during stenting are being introduced. The time is ripe for further randomized trials of carotid stenting compared to carotid surgery.

ADVANTAGES AND DISADVANTAGES OF ENDOVASCULAR TREATMENT

The main advantage of endovascular treatment (angioplasty or stenting) is the avoidance of an incision in the neck. The incision, dissection, and retraction needed to reach the carotid artery to perform an endarterectomy may injure cranial nerves. The neck wound can become infected, and hematomas may cause discomfort, require surgical evacuation, and occasionally threaten life by causing tracheal compression. The surgical incision also injures cutaneous nerves, resulting in numbness around the scar, which occasionally may extend up to the face. Some patients are troubled by keloid formation. All of these disadvantages of surgery are avoided by endovascular treatment, although insertion of the catheter in the groin also may lead to hematoma formation with local complications and the occasional need for surgical evacuation. It is important to note that the complications of the incision associated with surgery rarely lead to long-lasting complaints or permanent disability. Moreover, the angiographic puncture may injure the femoral artery with occasional aneurysm formation or peripheral embolism. Endovascular procedures are accompanied by the general risks of angiography, including contrast reactions and radiation exposure. Surgery is associated with risks myocardial infarction, deep vein thrombosis, and pulmonary embolism, which appear to be very rare after angioplasty or stenting. However, surgery is being increasingly performed under local anesthesia, which may avoid some of these risks. However, where general anesthesia is used, the systemic effects of the anesthetic and muscle relaxants, the discomfort of intubation, and pneumonia are additional complications that weigh against surgery because angioplasty and stenting currently almost always are performed under local anesthesia.

One potential advantage of surgery is that the surgeon is able to protect the brain by clamping the distal internal carotid artery before carrying out the endarterectomy procedure. In contrast, until recently, angioplasty and stenting had to be carried out without protection, risking embolism during dilation of the stenosis. Both experimental studies in the laboratory and monitoring using transcranial Doppler during carotid angioplasty have confirmed that embolism is very frequent during balloon dilation and stenting (2–4). However, the recent development of protection devices removes this objection to endovascular techniques so long as they can be deployed safely. Perhaps the most important advantage of surgery is that it is tried and tested, with large numbers of vascular surgeons and neurosurgeons trained in the procedure. In contrast, there are few interventionists with experience of more than a handful of cases of angioplasty or stenting in the carotid artery.

There are a number of other complications of angioplasty and stenting (Table 41-1). Inadvertent subintimal insertion of the guidewire or catheter may result in arterial dissection, which may lead to vessel occlusion or chronic pseudoaneurysm formation. Balloon dilation may result in hemorrhage into the plaque or thrombosis secondary to plaque fracture, with the resulting acute closure and occlusion of the artery or embolic stroke. Stents are partly designed to avoid this

TABLE 41-1. *Complications of angioplasty and stenting*

Acute complications
Mechanical
   Intimal dissection
   Arterial spasm
   Plaque rupture
   Vessel rupture
   Balloon rupture
   Carotid sinus stimulation
      Bradycardia and asystole
      Hypotension
   Pseudoaneurysm formation
Neurologic
   Hemodynamic ischemia
   Cerebral embolism
   Vessel occlusion
Angiographic
   Groin hematoma
   Puncture-site pain
   Contrast reactions
   Hemorrhage from anticoagulation
   Femoral artery thromboembolism
Delayed complications
   Cerebral embolism
   Vessel occlusion
   Cerebral hemorrhage
   Hyperfusion syndrome
   Restenosis
   Stent collapse

complication, but often because of the size of the catheter, they cannot be deployed across a severe stenosis without first using an expandable balloon catheter to dilate the stenosis sufficiently to insert the stent. Once a stent is deployed, the struts should prevent a free intimal flap and maintain laminal flow across the stenosis. However, plaque debris may be extruded through the struts in the stent as the stent expands, and the stent itself may provide a site for thrombosis until it becomes covered in endothelium.

Rarer complications of endovascular treatment include hemodynamic ischemia during occlusion of the artery from balloon inflation or hypotension secondary to stimulation of the carotid sinus, which leads to bradycardia and occasionally brief periods of asystole. Hypotension due to dilation of the carotid bulb may be troublesome for 48 hours after the procedure. Bradycardia nowadays is minimized by pretreatment with atropine. Successful stenting occasionally may precipitate the hyperperfusion syndrome, similar to that seen after carotid endarterectomy (5). Some of the early cases of carotid stenting were complicated by the late occurrence of stent collapse, possibly as a result of pressure on the neck. New designs of stents have been developed to avoid this kind of complication.

These potential complications of endovascular treatment indicate that it is essential to establish the safety of endovascular treatment in comparison with surgery before the new techniques become widely used in preference to surgery. Moreover, the long-term efficacy of carotid angioplasty and stenting in preventing stroke has not been established. Restenosis certainly is more common after endovascular techniques than after surgery, and long-term follow-up is required to establish how often this leads to recurrent stroke.

CASE SERIES

Series of patients treated by balloon angioplasty for carotid stenosis first appeared 20 years ago, and only very small numbers of patients were treated (6). However, increasingly large series of patients treated by carotid angioplasty or stenting have been reported from individual centers (7). In 2001, the two largest series reported a total of 472 and 528 patients, with a rate of stroke or death within 30 days of treatment of 4.2% and 7.4%, respectively (8,9). In general, all the individual case series of angioplasty and stenting reported stroke and death rates around the time of the procedure consistent with the results of carotid surgery reported in the North American Symptomatic Carotid Endarterectomy Trial (NASCET) and the European Carotid Surgery Trial (ECST) (10,11). The exponential growth in carotid stenting is shown by the global carotid stenting survey, which in March 2001 reported that a total of 6,327 patients had been treated with a 30-day stroke and death rate of 6.2% (Michael H. Wholey, *personal communication*).

The results from case series are encouraging, but caution is required because the patients included in the series often are highly selected. For example, 40% of the cases included in the global registry, and many of the series, were asymptomatic and many had restenosis after carotid endarterectomy. Treatment of these patients is safer than treating recently symptomatic atheromatous stenosis. Few papers adequately describe the degree of stenosis treated. In addition, series with poor results are unlikely to be reported. All these factors may lead case series to underestimate the risks of treatment. On the other hand, in many of these series a substantial proportion of the symptomatic patients were said to have contraindications to surgery, which may have increased their surgical risks above average. In some series, the completeness of follow-up after discharge from hospital is uncertain.

RANDOMIZED TRIALS

The potential hazards of carotid stenting were emphasized by the first two randomized trials reported. Both were stopped early because of an excess of treatment-related strokes in the stented patients. The first trial of carotid stenting was stopped after only 23 patients had been randomized at a single center in Leicester, England, because five of seven patients treated by stenting had a stroke at the time of the procedure (12). In contrast, there were no strokes in the ten surgical patients. The second stopped trial, the Wallstent Study, was stopped after 219 patients had been randomized because the rate of stroke or death within 30 days of treatment in the stenting group was 12.1% compared to 4.5% in the surgical group ($p = 0.049$) (13).

It is likely that these disappointing results reflect poor technique at inexperienced centers and possibly poor stent design. The results argue strongly against the indiscriminate introduction of stenting and emphasize the importance of training and supervision of interventionists with little experience with carotid artery angioplasty or stenting. In contrast, another small randomized trial of carotid stenting versus carotid endarterectomy performed in a single community hospital was carried out on a total of 104 randomized patients without a single patient in either group sustaining a stroke (14).

None of these trials are large enough to provide convincing data. The Carotid and Vertebral Artery Transluminal Angioplasty Study (CAVATAS) is the only published randomized study to complete randomization with an adequate sample size (1). Five hundred sixty patients were randomized in CAVATAS from nine countries and 24 centers, the majority in the United Kingdom, but there also were centers in Australia, Canada, the United States, and other countries in Europe. The trial had two separate arms including patients with carotid stenosis unsuitable for surgery and patients with vertebral artery stenosis, who were both randomized between endovascular treatment and medical care alone. However, only small numbers of patients were randomized in these two groups, and the main published analysis was restricted to the third arm of the trial in which patients were randomized with carotid stenosis suitable for surgery between endovascular treatment (251 patients) and carotid endarterectomy (253 patients). Randomization started in 1992 and was completed in 1997. Centers were required to have a designated vascular surgeon or neurosurgeon with expertise in carotid endarterectomy, but they were not required to have a radiologist with expertise in carotid angioplasty. However, all the radiologists were required to have obtained training in neuroradiology and the techniques of angioplasty at other sites. CAVATAS is unique in conducting a randomized trial at the early stage of the introduction of the new procedure. The trial incorporates results from the learning curve and the development of new technology for carotid angioplasty and stenting techniques. The topic of the learning curve is discussed in more detail later.

The inclusion criteria for CAVATAS required patients to have stenosis of the carotid artery that investigators believed needed treatment and was suitable for both carotid endarterectomy and endovascular treatment. Patients were excluded if they were thought to be unsuitable for surgery or endovascular treatment, if they had thrombus in the carotid artery, or if they had severe intracranial carotid artery stenosis. The trial was designed to compare two policies: referral to surgery and referral for endovascular treatment. Hence, centers could randomize patients after noninvasive investigations if they routinely referred patients for treatment without performing angiography. Nevertheless, most centers performed conventional angiography or high-quality magnetic resonance angiography before the patients were randomized between carotid surgery and carotid endovascular treatment.

Almost all the patients randomized in CAVATAS were symptomatic, with only 4% of patients randomized without any relevant symptoms (Table 41-2). The majority had amaurosis fugax (25%) or transient ischemic attack (TIA; 38%); the remainder of symptomatic patients having an hemisphere stroke. The majority of patients had severe carotid stenosis on the treated side (mean stenosis 86% using the common carotid method or 75% using the NASCET method). There was a high percentage of vascular risk factors in the randomized patients, and contralateral carotid occlusion was twice as common in CAVATAS (8%) than in ECST (3%) or NASCET (4%). In the surgical patients, general anesthesia was used in 93% of cases and local anesthesia in 7%. Perioperative shunts and patches were used in 64% and 63% of the operations, respectively. CAVATAS started before the invention of arterial stents, and all patients in the first 2 years of the study underwent percutaneous transluminal angioplasty with balloon catheters. From 1994 onward, stenting was allowed within the protocol but stents usually were used as a secondary procedure after an unsatisfactory balloon dilation. The majority of patients allocated endovascular treatment received balloon angioplasty alone, but 55 (22%) of the patients in the endovascular arm were treated by stenting. All the patients were given aspirin or an alternative antiplatelet agent, and patients treated by endovascular techniques also were anticoagulated with heparin at the time of the procedure and for a minimum of 24 hours afterward. Best medical management, including antiplatelet therapy, was prescribed throughout follow-up in both groups.

The number of strokes in any arterial territory lasting more than 7 days and death from any cause occurring within 30 days after the first treatment analyzed by intention to treat were identical in the two groups (Table 41-3). The rate of disabling stroke or death within 30 days of treatment was 5.9% in patients randomized to surgery and 6.0% in patients randomized to endovascular treatment. The rate of any stroke lasting more than 7 days or death within 30 days of treatment was 9.9% in patients randomized to surgery and 10% in patients randomized to

TABLE 41-2. *Baseline characteristics of patients with carotid stenosis randomized in CAVATAS*

	Endovascular treatment (n = 251)	Surgical treatment (n = 253)
Demographics		
Female	30	30
Mean age (yr)	67	67
Symptoms leading to randomization		
Amaurosis fugax	24	25
Transient ischemic attack	37	39
Retinal infarct	2	1
Hemisphere stroke	25	26
Symptoms >6 mo before randomization	8	6
Never symptomatic	4	3
Vascular risk factors at randomization		
Hypertension	53	58
Mean SBP (mmHg)	152	152
Mean DBP (mmHg)	84	84
Ischemic heart disease	39	37
Previous history of myocardial infarction	19	17
Peripheral vascular disease	24	20
Diabetes	14	13
Current cigarette smoking	28	27
Exsmoker	50	50
Cholesterol >6.5 mmol/L	34	32
Atrial fibrillation	5	5
Other cardiac embolic source	1	2
Angiographic characteristics		
Mean percentage ipsilateral carotid stenosis (CC method)	87	86
Contralateral carotid artery occlusion	10	8

Figures are percentage numbers in each group, except where stated.
CAVATAS, Carotid and Vertebral Artery Transluminal Angioplasty Study; DBP, diastolic blood pressure; SBP, systolic blood pressure.

TABLE 41-3. *Outcome events within 30 days of treatment in patients with carotid stenosis randomized in CAVATAS, analyzed by intention to treat*

	Endovascular arm (n = 251)	Surgery arm (n = 253)	p Value
Major outcome events			
Death	2.8	1.6	NS
Disabling stroke	3.6	4.3	NS
Nondisabling stroke	3.6	4.0	NS
Death or disabling stroke	6.4	5.9	NS
Death or any stroke	10.0	9.9	NS
Other outcome events			
Cranial nerve palsy	0	8.7	<0.0001
Hematoma (requiring surgery or prolonging hospital stay)	1.2	6.7	<0.0015
Myocardial infarction (nonfatal)	0	1.2	NS
Pulmonary embolus	0	0.8[a]	NS

CAVATAS, Carotid and Vertebral Artery Transluminal Angioplasty Study.
Figures are percentage of patients. Only strokes lasting >7 days in any territory were included.
[a]One fatal, included above.

endoluminal treatment. CAVATAS counted only strokes lasting more than 7 days in order to match the criterion used in ECST and to avoid bias from potential underreporting of TIA or minor stroke in surgical patients operated under general anesthesia and returned to high-dependency intensive care or surgical wards. It was reasoned that minor neurologic events more likely would be detected after endovascular treatment because the procedure was done under local anesthesia and patients often were returned to a neurologic ward.

Analysis of the minor risks of treatment confirmed that endovascular treatment was safer than surgery in terms of minor morbidity. Cranial or peripheral nerve palsy was reported in 9% of surgical patients but never after endovascular treatment ($p < 0.0001$). Major groin or neck hematoma that prolonged hospi-

tal stay or required transfusion occurred significantly less often after endovascular treatment than after surgery (1% vs. 7%; $p < 0.00015$). Endovascular treatment also was safer than surgery with regard to myocardial infarction (three in surgical patients, none in endovascular patients) and pulmonary embolus (two in surgical patients and none in endovascular patients).

One important finding from CAVATAS was that about one third of the strokes, counted within 30 days of treatment, were delayed in onset for up to 3 weeks after the day of treatment in both the surgical and endovascular groups. Intracerebral hemorrhage, presumably resulting from the hyperperfusion syndrome, accounted for two cases of delayed stroke in the surgical group and three in the endovascular group (Fig. 41-1).

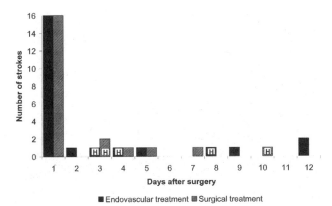

FIG. 41–1. Timing of strokes that occurred within 2 weeks of treatment in the Carotid and Vertebral Artery Transluminal Angioplasty Study (CAVATAS) and lasted more than 7 days. Day 1, day of treatment; H, cerebral hemorrhage.

Survival analysis over 3 years of follow-up showed that both surgery and endovascular treatment were equally effective at preventing ipsilateral stroke (Fig. 41-2). Ninety-six surviving patients at the time of the main analysis had more than 3 years of follow-up, and the event rate in these patients remained very low. At 3 years of follow-up, the rate of death or disabling stroke in any territory, including treatment related events, was 14.3% in the endovascular group and 14.2% in the surgical groups. Survival analysis with adjustment for age, sex, and trial center showed no difference between the two groups with a hazard ratio for any disabling stroke or death (endovascular treatment/surgery) of 1.03 (95% confidence interval: 0.64–1.64; $p = 0.9$).

CAVATAS confirmed that endovascular treatment could be performed successfully in the majority of patients considered suitable for treatment, with an 89% technical success rate. Interestingly, the rate of angiographic stroke, including those related to guidewire insertion, before balloon inflation (or stent deployment if this was done without balloon angioplasty) in the endovascular arm was 1.2%. These strokes were included in the 30-day complication rate of 10%.

The rate of stenosis at 1-year follow-up was measured in CAVATAS patients using ultrasound at the centers where available. Severe (70%–99%) contralateral stenosis was significantly more common 1 year after endovascular treatment than after surgery (14.5% vs. 4.0%; $p < 0.001$). However, this did not result in a significant number of recurrent strokes, and there was no association between severe stenosis at 1 year and the few strokes that were recorded during follow-up. However, it is worth noting that follow-up in these patients was limited and the longer-term outcome in these patients with restenosis or residual stenosis because of poor initial technique remains uncertain. CAVATAS is continuing follow-up with the aim of determining whether endovascular treatment can be regarded as effective beyond 2 or 3 years after treatment.

There has been particular interest in analysis of the subgroup of patients treated by stenting in CAVATAS, given the radiologic view that the results are superior using stenting compared to balloon angioplasty alone. Subgroup analysis certainly suggests that the early outcomes were superior in the patients treated by primary stenting. Only one (2%) of the 55 stented patients had a stroke when the stent was deployed. However, two (4%) ischemic strokes and two (4%) cerebral hemorrhages occurred between 2 and 11 days after stenting. Hence, stenting appeared safer at the time of deployment but was associated with a similar number of delayed strokes. There were no strokes at all in stented patients during follow-up. However, the rate of restenosis to more than 50% after stenting was only slightly less than after balloon angioplasty alone (42% vs. 52%), although carotid occlusion at 1-year follow-up was less common (2% vs. 5%).

One can conclude from CAVATAS that endovascular treatment and carotid endarterectomy appear to have very similar major risks and long-term benefits. However, the confidence intervals surrounding the comparison of the two treatments in terms of the hazard ratio were wide. This implies that a significant difference between the two procedures in risks and long-term benefits has not been excluded by CAVATAS, although the results are clearly encouraging for further studies. CAVATAS certainly confirmed the advantage of endovascular treatment in

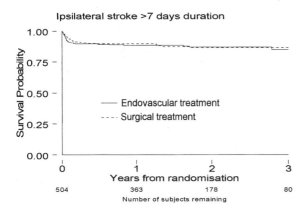

FIG. 41–2. Survival analysis showing number of patients in the Carotid and Vertebral Artery Transluminal Angioplasty Study (CAVATAS) free of ipsilateral stroke lasting more than 7 days.

terms of avoiding the minor complications of carotid endarterectomy. However, the rate of stroke at the time of the procedure was relatively high at 10% in both arms.

There are several possible explanations for the higher rate of procedural stroke in CAVATAS than in other randomized trials of carotid surgery. First, the result might merely be due to chance given the wide confidence intervals. Many of the surgeons operating in CAVATAS also treated patients in ECST, and the 9.9% rate of operative stroke in CAVATAS is not significantly different than the 7.5% rate of stroke in ECST (11). Furthermore, the difference is unlikely to be due to variation in surgical skills because there was no evidence on subgroup analysis of any significant difference between centers. Moreover, the rates of cranial neuropathy, wound hematoma, and myocardial infarction were very similar to those recorded in NASCET (15). Therefore, it is likely that the surgeons and anesthetists in the two trials had similar skills and similar techniques. The most likely explanation for the higher morbidity rate in both groups is the inclusion of patients at higher than average risk from treatment. Case mix is one of the major risk factors in carotid surgery and it is possible that the availability of endovascular treatment in the trial centers may have encouraged the inclusion of less fit patients for surgery in CAVATAS. In accordance with this explanation, there was substantially more patients with vascular risk factors, particular ischemic heart disease assigned to surgery in CAVATAS than in ECST. Patients included in NASCET were also highly selected, whereas there were a few exclusion criteria in CAVATAS. The similarity of the outcome events in the two arms of CAVATAS argues for the high rate of procedural stroke being caused by the characteristics of the patients. One contribution to the high rate of perioperative stroke may have been the number of delayed strokes counted within thirty days after treatment. However, NASCET also reported that 30% of surgical outcome events were delayed between the second and twenty eighth post operative days (15).

The fact that a substantial proportion of patients had severe stenosis on ultrasound at 1-year follow-up after angioplasty or stenting is a concern. Most of these patients had restenosis, but a proportion was related to persistent residual stenosis after inadequate dilation. Improved techniques may reduce this proportion in the future. However, the fact that there were very few strokes during follow-up in the angioplasty group even though the atheromatous plaque was not removed and given the incidence of restenosis is intriguing. This may reflect the fact that injury to the arterial wall by balloon dilation and stent insertion stimulates smooth muscle proliferation and neointimal endothelialization of the plaque. Restenosis reflects the excessive healing process and not recurrence of atheromatous plaque. It appears likely that this process prevents embolization, which is the main cause of stroke associated with carotid atherosclerosis. There is some evidence that when symptoms occur in association with restenosis after angioplasty, they result from hemodynamic ischemia and not emboli (16). Restenosis after endovascular treatment may be found to be clinically unimportant, although clearly longer-term follow-up is required before this conclusion can be justified.

A number of studies have shown that carotid angioplasty and stenting are associated with a substantially greater incidence of microembolism detected by transcranial Doppler ultrasound than carotid endarterectomy (2–4). CAVATAS has demonstrated that this does not translate into a major difference in the risk of symptomatic stroke, but there still is concern that microembolism might result in subclinical brain damage. However, extensive neuropsychological tests in two large subgroups of patients in CAVATAS at two centers did not show any significant differences in the neuropsychologic sequela of endovascular treatment and surgery at 6 months after treatment, which provides reassurance with respect to the safety of treatment in patients without symptomatic stroke (17,18).

CAVATAS also incorporated quality of life and economics evaluation (19). There was little difference in the quality of life after the two procedures, but the differences that were detected favored endovascular treatment. The economics evaluation demonstrated the substantial cost advantage of endovascular treatment, which was approximately half the cost of surgical treatment. This primarily reflected a shorter length of hospital stay after endovascular treatment. The procedural costs (operating room or radiology) were very similar. However, given that stents were only used in a proportion of patients, the difference between the two procedures may disappear if stents and protection devices are routinely used or if the length of surgical stay is reduced substantially in the future.

THE LEARNING CURVE

The interventional technique used to treat carotid stenosis has developed considerably over the last 10 years. Initially, simple inflatable silastic balloon catheters were used. The technique and safety improved with the introduction of long guiding catheters and sheaths, narrower guidewires, and lower profile balloons. In early series of balloon angioplasty, the initial dilation of the carotid artery was often less than complete, although in many cases this was followed by remodeling, which resulted in improvement of the initial results over time (20). Over the last 5 years, there has been increased use of primary stenting rather than simple balloon angioplasty. Initially, stents mounted over a balloon designed for use at other sites were used, but now several manufacturers produce self-expanding stents designed for use in the carotid artery. There is no doubt that on average the technique of stenting used today produces superior anatomic results. This improvement of technology might be expected to improve the safety of endovascular treatment. Surprisingly there is little evidence to support this hypothesis. In CAVATAS, the rate of stroke associated with endovascular treatment did not change over the 6 years of the study. However, this may be misleading because new inexperienced centers joined the trial toward the end of recruitment. One would expect there to be a learning curve with increasing experience, and this is what was found in CAVATAS when the results were analyzed by individual center experience. This showed that the average rate of stroke in the first 30 patients treated in any center was 11.1% but fell to 4.0% once an individual center had treated more than 50 patients (Table 41-4). The global carotid stent registry also reports lower morbidity rates at centers performing a larger number of procedures. In one of the largest series from the group with the largest experience of carotid stenting in North America, the incidence of minor stroke declined from 6.8% to 5.8%, then to 5.3% and then 4% over the 4 years from 1994 onward (9). In the last 2 years, there were

TABLE 41-4. *Improvement in 30-day rate of stroke and death with increasing experience in CAVATAS centers*

Patient no.	Endovascular treatment	Surgical treatment
1–30	11.1	10.8
31–50	7.5	10.0
51–100	4.0	6.4

CAVATAS, Carotid and Vertebral Artery Transluminal Angioplasty Study.
Data from all arms of the trial have been combined. The figures in the first row are the risks in the first 30 patients treated at any one center, averaged for all the CAVATAS centers combined. The second and third rows show the subsequent risk in the centers that randomized >30 patients.

no major strokes or neurologic deaths. However, it is not clear to what extent the improvement in results comes from increased experience, meticulous technique, better technology, or careful selection of patients.

PROTECTION DEVICES

The fact that an inexperienced investigator appears to have a high complication rate is a marked disincentive to the development of carotid stenting. However, the introduction of protection devices for use during carotid stenting is a major recent advance that can be expected to improve the safety of carotid stenting and allow the procedure to be used more widely, with the reassurance that if things go wrong the patient is protected against major embolism. A number of protection devices have been developed. These include filters and occlusion balloons on guidewires, which can be placed distal to the carotid stenosis before stent insertion and deployed to catch any embolic material released during stenting. Initial experience confirms that they catch embolic debris, and recent case series suggest that the use of protection devices at the time of stenting reduces the risks of immediate complications (9,21,22). One particularly elegant protection system has been developed by Parodi et al. (21). This system involves inserting an antiembolism system proximal to the stenosis. The antiembolism system includes two balloons that are deployed to simultaneously occlude the common carotid and external carotid arteries. The guiding catheter is externally connected to the contralateral femoral vein with an interposed blood filter. This results in reversal of the direction of blood flow in the internal carotid artery, which allows angioplasty and stent insertion to be performed safely so that any debris is washed away from the brain. However, it is possible that the use of a protection device will increase the hazards in some patients, for example, if the device leads to a significant reduction in cerebral blood flow or there is difficulty removing the device. The preliminary experience suggests that these are uncommon complications. Clearly, the use of protection devices, with the exception of the Parodi device, will not prevent stroke while crossing the stenosis to deploy the filter or occlusion balloon, and none of the devices will prevent delayed stroke after removal of the device.

VERTEBRAL ARTERY ANGIOPLASTY AND STENTING

There are little data on vertebral artery angioplasty and stenting. This reflects two facts. First, only about

24% of strokes occur in the vertebrobasilar territory and only about 23% of these have significant vertebral artery stenosis (21a,21b). Hence, only about 5% of stroke and TIA patients are likely to have vertebral artery stenosis. Second, patients are rarely investigated by angiography for vertebrobasilar stroke or TIA, and noninvasive investigations do not visualize the common site of vertebral artery atherosclerosis, which is at the origin of the vertebral artery. However, a number of a case series have suggested that vertebral artery stenosis can be easily treated by angioplasty and stenting, with a very low complication rate of less than 5% (23–28). Initial experience suggested that elastic recoil and restenosis were very common after balloon angioplasty alone for vertebral artery origin stenosis. Recent experience suggests that much better results are obtained with vertebral artery stenting (28). In one series, 50 patients treated with vertebral stenting had no procedure-related complications and only a 10% incidence of restenosis at 6 months (22). CAVATAS included patients with vertebral artery stenosis randomized between endovascular treatment and medical treatment, but only 16 patients were randomized in this group, and the results have not yet been reported.

THE FUTURE OF CAROTID STENTING

The relative high rate of procedural stroke in both surgical and endovascular groups in CAVATAS, and in the other two of carotid stenting trials that were stopped, has caused concern and argues strongly against using the results to promote the general introduction of carotid stenting as an alternative to surgery. However, there is some evidence that carotid stenting is safer than balloon angioplasty, and there is every hope that use of protection devices will reduce the risk of embolism at the time of the procedure. Endovascular treatment has advantages for the patient, mainly the atraumatic nature of the procedure, the lack of the incision in the neck, and the brief hospital admission. Further randomized trials of carotid stenting are justified and are needed to provide more convincing data on safety and efficacy. There currently is great enthusiasm among many interventional radiologists and cardiologists for the introduction of carotid stenting, but equally a number of vascular surgeons are vehemently opposed to the procedure on the grounds of its potential hazards. Large clinical trials are required to resolve this controversy and to prevent the indiscriminate introduction of carotid stenting without adequate evidence. A number of randomized clinical trials of carotid stenting started recruiting centers in 2001. These include the Stent-protected Percutaneous Angioplasty versus Carotid Endarterectomy (SPACE) Study in Germany, the Endarterectomy Versus Angioplasty in Patients with Severe Symptomatic Carotid Stenosis Study (EVA-3S) in France, the Carotid Revascularization Endarterectomy versus Stenting Trial (CREST) in the United States, and the International Carotid Stenting Study (ICSS), also known as CAVATAS-2, which is the follow-up study to CAVATAS. Undoubtedly, these trials will provide important and invaluable information about the risks and benefits of carotid stenting in comparison with carotid endarterectomy.

PROTOCOL FOR THE INTERNATIONAL CAROTID STENTING STUDY

The ICSS protocol has stringent requirements for center enrollment to ensure the safety of participants. Centers require a neurologist or physician with an interest in cerebrovascular diseases, a vascular surgeon or neurosurgeon with expertise in carotid endarterectomy, and a radiologist with training in carotid angiography and the techniques of angioplasty and stenting. Surgeons are required to have performed at least 50 carotid endarterectomies with an annual rate of more than 10 cases. The interventionalists are required to have performed at least 50 stenting procedures, 10 of which must have been in the carotid artery, using modern techniques. All investigators are required to produce an audit of their recent results and the data are submitted to a credentialing committee. Radiologists are required to attend approved courses on carotid stenting and have had their technique approved by an experienced carotid stenting expert. Centers are only approved once the credentialing committee is satisfied with the experience and skills of the center's surgeons and interventionalists.

To allow inexperienced centers to join, ICSS has developed the concept of probationary centers. These centers may join the study on a probationary basis if they fulfill all the other requirements for centers but do not have audited data on ten recent carotid stenting procedures. These centers are allowed to randomize patients within ICSS between carotid surgery and stenting, but if the patient is randomized to stenting, the stenting must be performed under the supervision and proctoring of an experienced carotid interventionalist. The probationary centers only become fully enrolled when the proctor is satisfied with the centers' skills and results. The trial results from probationary centers will be analyzed separately from the fully enrolled centers. This has the advantage of providing randomized data about the learning curve in carotid stenting while ensuring the safety of participants because of the proctoring arrangements.

The patients included in ICSS are required to have severe, recently symptomatic, atherosclerotic extracranial, internal, or bifurcation carotid artery stenosis. Patients must be fit and suitable for both surgical and endovascular intervention and able to give informed consent. Because of concerns about the long-term implications of implanted metal and the desire to include only atherosclerotic disease, patients are required to be older than 40 years, but there is no upper age limit. Exclusion criterion include major stroke with no useful functional recovery, stenosis unsuitable for stenting (e.g., because of tortuous anatomy or proximal stenosis, visible thrombus, or pseudoocclusion with a string sign); stenosis not suitable for surgery (e.g., high stenosis, rigid neck, medically not fit for surgery); and life expectancy less than 2 years.

Randomization is by telephone call or fax to the randomization center at the Clinical Trials Unit in Oxford, which allows 24-hour randomization from anywhere in the world. Randomization is stratified within each center and deploys a computerized program to minimize the main risk factors and balance them between the arms of the trial. Randomization is stratified over time to balance for any improvements or change in technology over the course of the trial.

The trial requires that stenting or surgery be performed as soon as possible after randomization. All patients will receive best medical care. Protection devices and stents used in the trial are required to be CE marked and approved by the steering committee, but otherwise radiologists are not restricted to the use of any one device. Local and general anesthesia may be used for patients randomized to carotid endarterectomy. The primary outcome measure is long-term survival free of disabling stroke; secondary outcomes include any stroke or death, TIA, long-term survival free of ipsilateral stroke, quality of life and economics measures, myocardial infarction, cranial nerve palsy and hematoma within 30 days of treatment, and stenosis to more than 70% or occlusion on ultrasound at follow-up.

ICSS plans a sample size of 2,000 patients. This has been calculated on the basis of an equivalence between the two procedures. Sample size calculations under these circumstances are difficult because one must estimate the difference between the two procedures with regard to risks or benefits that would influence the clinicians' choice between the two treatments. The sample size of 2,000 will give 95% confidence intervals of ±2 percentage points for dis-

abling stroke and death within 30 days of treatment and ±3 percentage points for disabling stroke during follow-up.

More than 40 centers throughout the world, including Europe, Australia, and North America, have expressed a firm interest in joining ICSS. The trial has set up a web page where further information about progress can be obtained. The current address is *www.ion.ucl.ac.uk/cavatas_icss/*

REFERENCES

1. CAVATAS Investigators. Endovascular versus surgical treatment in patients with carotid stenosis in the Carotid and Vertebral Artery Transluminal Angioplasty Study (CAVATAS): a randomised trial. *Lancet* 2001;357: 1729–1737.
2. Ohki T, Marin ML, Lyon RT, et al. Ex vivo human carotid artery bifurcation stenting: correlation of lesion characteristics with embolic potential. *J Vasc Surg* 1998;27:463–471.
3. Crawley F, Clifton A, Buckenham T, et al. Comparison of hemodynamic cerebral ischemia and microembolic signals detected during carotid endarterectomy and carotid angioplasty. *Stroke* 1997;28:2460–2464.
4. Orlandi G, Fanucchi S, Fioretti C, et al. Characteristics of cerebral microembolism during carotid stenting and angioplasty alone. *Arch Neurol* 2001;58:1410–1413.
5. McCabe DJH, Brown MM, Clifton A. Fatal reperfusion hemorrhage after carotid stenting. *Stroke* 1999;30: 2483–2486.
6. Brown MM. Balloon angioplasty. *Neurol Res* 1992; 14[Suppl]:159–173.
7. Brown MM. Carotid angioplasty and stenting: are they therapeutic alternatives? *Cerebrovasc Dis* 2001;11: 112–118.
8. Wholey MH, Tan WA, Toursarkissian B, et al. Management of neurological complications of carotid artery stenting. *J Endovasc Ther*2001;8:341–353.
9. Roubin GS, New G, Iyer SS, et al. Immediate and late clinical outcomes of carotid artery stenting in patients with symptomatic and asymptomatic carotid artery stenosis: a 5-year prospective analysis. *Circulation* 2001;103:532–537.
10. Barnett HJM, Taylor DW, Eliasziw M, et al. Benefit of carotid endarterectomy in patients with symptomatic moderate or severe stenosis. *N Engl J Med* 1998;339: 1415–1425.
11. European Surgery Trialists' Collaborative Group. Randomised trial of endarterectomy for recently symptomatic carotid stenosis: final results of the MRC European Carotid Surgery Trial (ECST). *Lancet* 1998;351: 1379–1387.
12. Naylor AR, Bolia A, Abbott RJ, et al. Randomized study of carotid angioplasty and stenting versus carotid endarterectomy: a stopped trial. *J Vasc Surg* 1998;28: 326–334.
13. Alberts MJ. Results of a multicentre prospective randomized trial of carotid artery stenting vs. carotid endarterectomy. *Stroke* 2001:32:325(abst).
14. Brooks WH, McClure RR, Jones MR, et al. Carotid

angioplasty and stenting versus carotid endarterectomy: randomized trial in a community hospital. *J Am Coll Cardiol* 2001;38:1589–1595.

15. Ferguson GG, Eliasziw M, Barr HW, et al. The North American Symptomatic Carotid Endarterectomy Trial: surgical results in 1415 patients. *Stroke* 1999;30: 1751–1758.

16. Crawley F, Clifton A, Taylor RS, et al. Symptomatic restenosis after carotid percutaneous transluminal angioplasty. *Lancet* 1998,352:708–709.

17. Crawley F, Stygall J, Lunn S, et al. Comparison of microembolism detected by transcranial Doppler and neuropsychological sequela of carotid surgery and percutaneous transluminal angioplasty. *Stroke* 2000;31: 1329–1334.

18. Sivaguru A, Gaines PA, Beard J, et al. Neuropsychological outcome after carotid angioplasty: a randomised control trial. *J Neurol Neurosurg Psychiatry* 1999;66: 262(abst).

19. Davies A, Brown MM, Buxton M, et al. The cost effectiveness of carotid angioplasty and stenting compared to surgery for the treatment of carotid stenosis. An economic evaluation based on the Carotid and Vertebral Transluminal Angioplasty Study (CAVATAS). *(Submitted for publication)*.

20. Crawley F, Clifton A, Markus H, et al. Delayed improvement in carotid artery diameter after carotid angioplasty. *Stroke* 1997;28:574–579.

21. Parodi JC, La Mura R, Ferreira LM, et al. Initial evaluation of carotid angioplasty and stenting with three different cerebral protection devices. *J Vasc Surg* 2000;32: 1127–1136.

21a. Bamford J, Sandercock P, Dennis M, et al. Classification and natural history of clinically identifieable subtypes of cerebral infarction *Lancet* 1991;337: 1521–1526.

21b. Crawley F, Clifton A, Brown MM. Treatable lesions demonstrated on vertebral angiography for posterior circulation ischaemic events. *Br J Radiol* 1998;71: 1266–1270.

22. Reimers B, Corvaja N, Moshiri S, et al. Cerebral protection with filter devices during carotid artery stenting. *Circulation* 2001;104:12–15.

23. Chastain HD, Campbell MS, Iyer S, et al. Extracranial vertebral artery stent placement: in-hospital and follow-up results. *J Neurosurg* 1999; 9:547–552.

24. Malek AM, Higashida RT, Phatouros CC, et al. Treatment of posterior circulation ischemia with extracranial percutaneous balloon angioplasty and stent placement. *Stroke* 1999;30:2073–2085.

25. Piotin M, Spelle L, Martin JB, et al. Percutaneous transluminal angioplasty and stenting of the proximal vertebral artery for symptomatic stenosis. *Am J Neuroradiol* 2000;21:727–731.

26. Jenkins JS, White CJ, Ramee SR, et al. Vertebral artery stenting. *Catheter Cardiovasc Interv* 2001;54:1–5.

27. Mukherjee D, Roffi M, Kapadia SR, et al. Percutaneous intervention for symptomatic vertebral artery stenosis using coronary stents. *J Invasive Cardiol* 2001;13: 363–366.

28. Cloud G, Crawley F, Clifton A, et al. Vertebral artery origin angioplasty and primary stenting: safety and restenosis rates in a prospective series. *J Neurol Neurosurg Psychiatr* in press.

Ischemic Stroke: Advances in Neurology, Vol. 92. Edited by
H.J.M. Barnett, Julien Bogousslavsky, and Heather Meldrum.
Lippincott Williams & Wilkins, Philadelphia © 2003.

42

Choice and Timing of Specific Stroke Treatment

Geoffrey A. Donnan, Henry Ma, *Stefan Schwarz, *Dimitrios Georgiadis,
and *Werner Hacke

National Stroke Research Institute, Austin & Repatriation Medical Centre, Heidelberg West,
Victoria, Australia; and *Department of Neurology, University of Heidelberg, Heidelberg, Germany

The range of treatments available for acute ischemic stroke has expanded considerably in recent years. The effectiveness of their application may be responsible in part for differing case fatality rates seen in different parts of the world (1). Given this increase in the range of management strategies for stroke, the choice and timing of their administration warrant discussion. The broad categories range from evidence-based strategies such as the use of thrombolysis, aspirin, and management in stroke care units (SCUs), to general measures such as swallowing competence and deep venous thrombosis (DVT) prophylaxis. Specific surgical interventions, including craniectomy, may be considered, as well as early secondary prevention strategies (Table 42-1).

TABLE 42-1. *Categories of treatment for acute ischemic stroke*

1. Acute evidence-based strategies
   - Thrombolysis
   - Aspirin
   - Stroke care units
2. General measures
   - Airway management
   - Swallowing management
   - Chest
   - Blood pressure
   - Glucose levels
   - Deep venous thrombosis prophylaxis
3. Specific surgical intervention
   - Posterior fossa
   - Anterior fossa
4. Early secondary prevention
   - Antiplatelet agents
   - Anticoagulation
   - Carotid endarterectomy
   - Blood pressure lowering

In general, the timing of various therapeutic interventions is limited to the evolution of the ischemic process. There is a great deal of emerging evidence that may suggest that the duration of the ischemic penumbra varies considerably from patient to patient (2). This may depend upon factors such as the underlying mechanism of ischemia and the rate of recanalization. There is evidence that the ischemic penumbra may persist for up to 48 hours after stroke onset, but in some cases, it may be as short as 3 hours or less (3,4). Regardless of this, it may be that the survival of the bulk of ischemic tissue is dependent upon early energy failure and ionic imbalances, whereas smaller volumes are dependent upon neurotoxic and inflammatory processes and even less on apoptosis (Fig. 42-1) (5). If this is the case, it may provide a ready explanation as to why thrombolysis, the most potent form of therapy, has so far been shown only to be effective within 3 hours of stroke onset (6). The concept of "time is brain" is generally a good one, regardless of the intervention planned.

The choice and timing of acute stroke treatments will depend upon the time that patients present. Clearly, thrombolysis is no longer applicable for patients who present beyond the critical 3-hour time window for this therapy, but other therapies (see later) may be. In this chapter, we give an overview of the choice of application of specific treatments with an emphasis on early intervention. Other aspects will be discussed in greater detail in subsequent chapters. Because the therapeutic approach is so strongly time based, management and therapies can be discussed in the prehospital phase, emergency room, and then SCU.

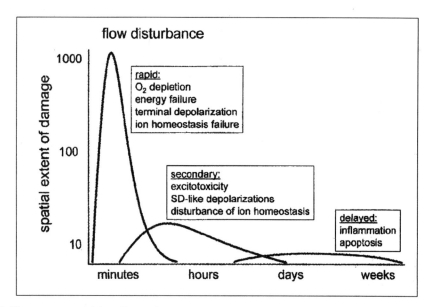

FIG. 42-1. Time sequence of the effects of various mechanisms of ischemic damage after stroke onset. (From Heiss et al. (5), with permission.)

PREHOSPITAL

Clinical Recognition of Stroke

This is one of the major problems of prehospital stroke management. Given that those persons making the calls to ambulance services (usually victims or relatives) may fail to adequately recognize stroke as the problem, the initial emergency call may not be accurate. In aphasic or otherwise unresponsive patients, an eyewitness history of the stroke onset should be obtained with particular respect to the exact time symptoms began. Even upon the arrival of an emergency team, the skill of paramedical groups in diagnosing neurologic disorders often is well below their skill in other areas such as cardiovascular or respiratory disease. This problem is being overcome to a certain degree by the development of a number of simple neurologic scoring systems for stroke that can be applied by ambulance officers at the site of the event. For example, the Los Angeles Prehospital Stroke Screen (LAPSS) has been found to have reasonable validity and may be a useful screening tool for focal neurologic events (7). Similar scoring systems have been developed elsewhere (8). Fortunately, ongoing refinement of these scoring systems is likely because the need for early diagnosis increases with the increasing choice of therapies.

First Aid

The earliest intervention is first aid provided by those who may be present at onset of stroke, such as

family members or, shortly after, ambulance personnel. During transport, the safety of the airway, breathing, and circulation have to be monitored. If available, a bedside test for serum glucose levels should be performed to exclude hyperglycemic or hypoglycemic states, which may mimic the clinical picture of acute stroke. An intravenous line may be introduced. Although there is no empirical evidence for the benefit of this practice, most guidelines recommend the routine administration of supplemental oxygen via a nasal catheter (2–3 L/min) (9). Arterial hypertension should be left untreated unless the values are extremely high (above 220/120 mm Hg). If very high blood pressure levels need to be treated, great care must be taken not to lower the blood pressure too rapidly or too extensively because a sudden drop in blood pressure in acute stroke may cause additional secondary ischemic damage. In patients with ischemic stroke, intubation and artificial ventilation are not necessarily required. However, rapid intubation is obligatory in comatose patients at risk of aspiration or respiratory insufficiency.

Potential Therapies

Currently, there are no specific therapies that can be administered by ambulance personnel to treat acute ischemic stroke. Obviously, one of the great hopes is that forms of neuroprotection will be useful at this time, so that therapeutic windows can be widened for other interventions such as thrombolysis, which may be given once an image has been obtained to exclude cerebral hemorrhage. Disappointingly, trials to date have not shown neuroprotectants to be effective in this setting, although the number of trials where therapy has been admitted before hospital arrival is small (10). In some instances, it may be reasonable to administer aspirin if the clinical event is clearly ischemic in nature (11,12), although most ambulance teams in the majority of countries are not yet sufficiently trained to make this decision.

Prehospital Barriers to Rapid Transfer to the Emergency Room

A number of studies have been performed to address this issue (13,14). Perhaps somewhat surprisingly, one of the most constant findings is that contacting the local doctor produces significant delays. Other factors include lack of the use of ambulance service, nighttime onset, lesser severity, and onset at home.

EMERGENCY ROOM

Recognition

As for the prehospital assessment, recognition in the emergency room that stroke is the problem is paramount, although the assessment is somewhat more sophisticated. The questions that need to be answered immediately are as follows:

1. Is it a stroke?
2. Where is the lesion?
3. What is the likely underlying pathogenic mechanism?

It has been demonstrated by a number of authors that the sensitivity, specificity, and accuracy for early stroke diagnosis using clinical criteria only are low (15,16). However, this can be improved considerably with the assistance of neuroimaging, particularly computed tomography (CT) to identify cerebral hemorrhage (6) and magnetic resonance imaging (MRI) using diffusion-weighted imaging (DWI) to identify the site of infarction (17). Infarct topography then may give some indication as to the likely underlying mechanism (18). Although clinical scores may give some clue as to the likelihood of underlying cerebral hemorrhage (19), this is not particularly reliable and urgent neuroimaging is the most appropriate course.

Investigations

The minimum set of investigations is listed in Table 42-2. These investigations should be performed as

TABLE 42-2. *Investigations for acute ischemic stroke*

Minimum set
- Computed tomography (noncontrast)
- Electrocardiography
- Full blood examination
- Electrolytes
- Coagulation profile
- Blood glucose
- Chest x-ray

Patient-specific tests
- Magnetic resonance imaging/angiography
- Extracranial Doppler ultrasound
- Transcranial Doppler ultrasound
- Transthoracic or transesophageal echocardiography
- Lipids
- Cardiac enzymes
- Blood gases
- Screen for arteritis
- Genetic tests
- Electroencephalography

quickly as possible in the emergency department so that baseline information about the patient can be obtained. A noncontrast CT needs to be performed as soon as possible to exclude cerebral hemorrhage. Early ischemic changes are used in many centres to stratify patients suitable for thrombolysis should they arrive within 3 hours of stroke onset (20) (see below). Because of the significance of cardiac arrhythmia, ischemia, and other heart diseases as the cause of stroke, a 12-lead electrocardiogram should be performed in all patients with acute stroke. Full blood count is needed to determine whether there are any hematologic contributions to the ischemic stroke, such as anemia, malignancies, or polycythemia. Electrolytes including renal function are an essential screen in case contrast agents must be given and as a baseline in case dehydration is present. Blood glucose levels are needed because of the importance of diabetes as a risk factor for stroke and emerging evidence that high blood glucose levels are associated with poorer outcome (21). A chest x-ray film should be obtained to assess cardiac size, presence of calcified valvular disease, and pulmonary edema.

Other more patient-specific tests may be required, depending on history and examination (Table 42-2). More commonly these tests would be performed once the patient has been transferred to the SCU (see later). In many centers, MRI will be performed on all patients although CT remains the imaging "workhorse" of stroke investigation (22). Further imaging using ultrasound of extracranial carotid arteries when artery to artery embolism is suspected as a mechanism and transcranial Doppler ultrasound may be useful as a screen in the posterior circulation for large-vessel disease or to confirm the hemodynamic status of the carotid system by demonstrating the presence or absence of cross-flow from one hemisphere to the other. Using MR angiography or CT angiography if available, occlusion of the main vessels can be reliably detected within a few minutes. This is particularly important in patients suspected of having basilar artery thrombosis, in whom transcranial ultrasound examination may not be able to provide the correct diagnosis. Similarly, if embolism is a suspected mechanism and carotid arteries are essentially normal, transesophageal echocardiography may be indicated to determine the presence or absence of aortic arch atheroma as a potential embolic source (23,24).

Cardiac enzymes and blood gases may provide useful additional information if a cardiac source of embolism is suspected or respiratory compromise is observed. An electroencephalogram (EEG) may be indicated if the nature of the event, particularly in the presence of a preexisting ischemic stroke, is unclear. Todd's paresis may mimic recurrent ischemic stroke and ongoing subclinical ictal activity on EEG may give a clue to this diagnosis (25).

Specific Treatments

The current status of specific treatments for acute ischemic stroke is given in Table 42-3. There is level 1 evidence for use of tissue plasminogen activator (tPA) if it is given within 3 hours of onset of acute ischemic stroke (6), administration of oral aspirin within 48 hours of ischemic stroke onset (11,12), and management within a stroke unit environment (26). Neuroprotectants are still being evaluated, although a large number of trials have reported negative results (27). Approaches that have been subjected to clinical trial in an adequate manner without any evidence of efficacy include the use of heparin or heparinoids (11,28,29), hemodilution (30), and steroids (31).

TABLE 42-3. *Current status of specific treatment for acute ischemic stroke*

Yes[a]
  1. Tissue plasminogen activator within 3 h
  2. Aspirin within 48 h
  3. Management in stroke care unit
Maybe
  1. Neuroprotectants
No?
  1. Heparin, heparanoids
  2. Hemodilution
  3. Steroids

[a]Level 1 evidence of efficacy in improving outcomes.

Thrombolysis with Tissue Plasminogen Activator

Because tPA must be administered within 3 hours of stroke onset, based on current evidence, this usually is done more often the emergency department. The evidence for efficacy now is strong and fulfills level 1 criteria (Fig. 42-2). When the accumulated evidence from all trials of intravenous tPA is considered within the 3-hour time window, relative risk reduction is 44% (32–34), absolute risk reduction is about 13%, and number needed to treat to save one person from death or disability is about seven to eight (35). This is quite a powerful biologic effect and its extent often is underrecognized. To counter this, there is only a modest and nonsignificant increase in mortality (Fig. 42-3) but an approximately three-fold increase in intracranial hemorrhage (Fig. 42-3); however. only about 6% to 7% of all intracranial hemorrhages result in neurologic deterioration (11).

Although thrombolysis has been embraced in many countries as a routine form of management and phase IV data (Table 42-4) are generally in keeping with data from the clinical trials (36–46), this has not been uniform. At the time of this publication, tPA is licensed for acute ischemic stroke treatment within 3 hours in the following countries: United States, Canada, Columbia, Paraguay, Uruguay, Argentina, Germany, Estonia, Lithuania, and Romania. tPA now is administered in most centers using the National Institute of Neurological Disorders and Stroke (NINDS) protocol, an abbreviated form of which is presented in Table 42-5. Because of lingering uncertainty as to the risk-to-benefit ratio in certain patient categories, further trials are being conducted, particularly the International Stroke Trial 3 (IST-3) coordinated from Edinburgh (46).

All randomized studies on thrombolysis for acute stroke were based on CT; therefore, findings from MRI examinations can only be used with great care until larger studies using MRI criteria are available. MRI findings are increasing being used, however, to establish the indication for thrombolysis beyond the time window of 3 hours and up to 6 hours because no controlled studies have been undertaken that unequivocally support this practice.

Aspirin

There is equally strong evidence that the administration of aspirin within 48 hours of onset of acute ischemic stroke improves outcome (11,12). This is well summarized in Fig. 42-4. Again, the general principle that "time is brain" should be adhered to

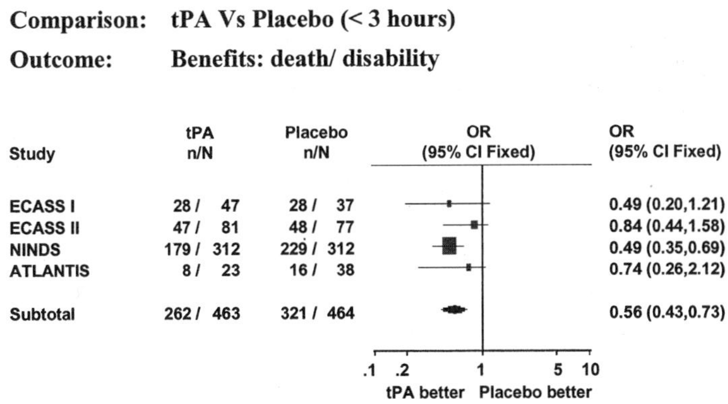

Comparison: tPA Vs Placebo (< 3 hours)

Outcome: Benefits: death/ disability

Study	tPA n/N	Placebo n/N	OR (95% CI Fixed)	OR (95% CI Fixed)
ECASS I	28 / 47	28 / 37		0.49 (0.20,1.21)
ECASS II	47 / 81	48 / 77		0.84 (0.44,1.58)
NINDS	179 / 312	229 / 312		0.49 (0.35,0.69)
ATLANTIS	8 / 23	16 / 38		0.74 (0.26,2.12)
Subtotal	262 / 463	321 / 464		0.56 (0.43,0.73)

.1 .2 1 5 10
tPA better Placebo better

FIG. 42-2. Meta-analysis of thrombolysis within 3 hours using intravenous tissue plasminogen activator: outcome death/disability.

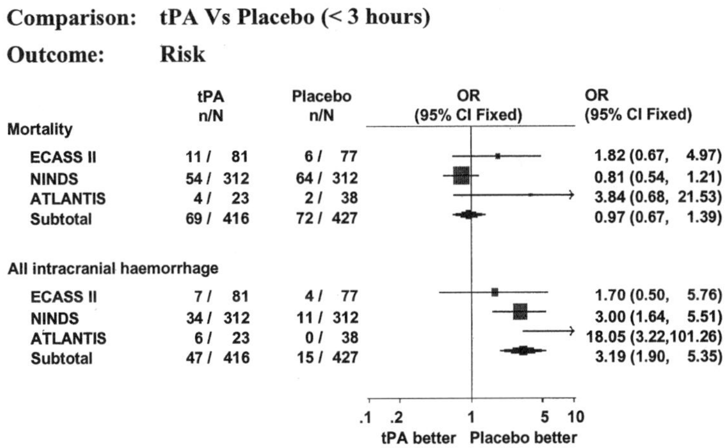

Comparison: tPA Vs Placebo (< 3 hours)

Outcome: Risk

	tPA n/N	Placebo n/N	OR (95% CI Fixed)	OR (95% CI Fixed)
Mortality				
ECASS II	11 / 81	6 / 77		1.82 (0.67, 4.97)
NINDS	54 / 312	64 / 312		0.81 (0.54, 1.21)
ATLANTIS	4 / 23	2 / 38		3.84 (0.68, 21.53)
Subtotal	69 / 416	72 / 427		0.97 (0.67, 1.39)
All intracranial haemorrhage				
ECASS II	7 / 81	4 / 77		1.70 (0.50, 5.76)
NINDS	34 / 312	11 / 312		3.00 (1.64, 5.51)
ATLANTIS	6 / 23	0 / 38		18.05 (3.22,101.26)
Subtotal	47 / 416	15 / 427		3.19 (1.90, 5.35)

.1 .2 1 5 10
tPA better Placebo better

FIG. 42-3. Meta-analysis of thrombolysis within 3 hours using intravenous tissue plasminogen activator: mortality and intracranial hemorrhage.

TABLE 42-4. *NINDS: phase IV tissue plasminogen activator studies*

Study	N	Baseline NIHSS (%)	Protocol variation (%)	Symptomatic ICH (%)
NINDS	312	14	3	6
Grond et al. (Cologne) 1998 (41)	100	12	2	5
Trouilias et al. (Lyon) 1998 (44)	100	?	?	7
Katzan et al. (Cleveland) 2000 (37)	70	?	50	15.7
Chiu et al. (Houston) 1998 (40)	30	14	?	7
Tanne et al. (Multicenter USA) 1999 (38)	189	?	30	6
Chapman et al. (Vancouver) 2000 (45)	46	14	17	2.2
Wang et al. (Preoria) 2000 (43)	57	14	9	5
Albers et al. (STARS) 2000 (36)	389	13	32	3.3
Schmuliing et al. (Cologne) 2000 (42)	150	11	1	4
Lopez-Yunal et al. (Indianapolis) 2001 (39)	50	11	16	5

ICH, intracranial hemorrhage; NIHSS, National Institutes of Health Stroke Scale; NINDS, National Institute of Neurological Disorders and Stroke.

TABLE 42-5. *Tissue plasminogen activator protocol*

NINDS criteria for *tPA in acute ischemic stroke*
  1. Stroke onset ≤3 h
  2. No hemorrhage noted on computed tomography
  3. No previous stroke or trauma ≤3 mo
  4. Blood pressure ≤185 systolic and ≤110 diastolic

NINDS, National Institute of Neurological Disorders and Stroke; tPA, tissue plasminogen activator.
Modified from The National Institute of Neurological Disorders and Stroke Study Group. Tissue plasminogen activator for acute ischemic stroke. *N Engl J Med* 1995;333:1581–1587.

and aspirin administered in the emergency department rather than waiting until the patient is transferred to the SCU. Overall, the benefit is somewhat small: For every 1,000 patients treated, only about nine or 10 are saved from death or disability. However, because the therapy is so inexpensive, is widely available, and is associated with modest risk (an increase of two intracranial hemorrhages per 1,000 patients treated), the approach is well worthwhile and now is part of standard stroke management practice.

Management in a Stroke Unit

Stroke units vary in type, ranging from high-dependency/intensive care models that are more common in Germany and the United States to a lower-impact ward-based model (26,47). Evidence from accumulated trials suggest that the overall risk reduction in mortality is about 20% compared to management on a general medical ward and that this difference is robust, persisting for up to 10 years (48). There is some evidence that a geographically discrete unit within one ward is associated with better outcomes than either management at home or by a mobile stroke service team visiting general wards (Fig. 42-5) (49). The reasons for this improved outcome are not clear but probably are related to better and more aggressive management of general medical complication. Indredavik et al. (50) accurately showed that better management of blood pressure and earlier mobilization may be important.

Although the evidence for better outcomes with stroke unit management is strong, unfortunately the majority of patients in most countries do not have access to stroke units. In Australia, it has been estimated that only about 25% of all incidence strokes are treated in an SCU (51) and in the United Kingdom approximately 50% (52). Because establishing an SCU in many instances involves merely reorganizing existing resources, more centers in more countries should be encouraged to increase the availability of these facilities.

General Treatment

Many patients with acute ischemic stroke have comorbidities such as diabetes, cardiac failure, hypertension, and renal impairment. Management of these conditions forms an important part of the stroke management process and, logically, optimal management is likely to improve outcomes. In the emergency department, only the most pressing conditions need to be addressed, such as cardiac failure, recent

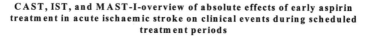

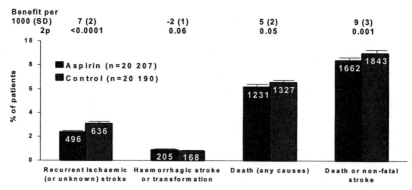

FIG. 42-4. Aspirin therapy in all trials. (From Kalra L, Evans A, Perez I, et al. Alternative strategies for stroke care: a prospective randomised controlled trial. *Lancet* 2000;356:894–899, with permission.)

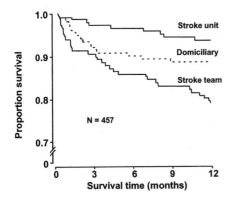

FIG. 42-5. Survival of stroke patients in different treatment units. (From Kalra L, Evans A, Perez I, et al. Alternative strategies for stroke care: a prospective randomised controlled trial. *Lancet* 2000;356:894–899, with permission.)

myocardial infarction, and extreme levels of hyperglycemia. These should be managed in a standard fashion before transfer to the SCU. The remaining issues as outlined in Table 42-2 can be addressed upon arrival at the SCU.

In the emergency department, the decision must be made as to whether a patient is best treated in the stroke unit or critical care unit, if available. Indications for treatment in the critical care unit are (a) significant cardiac or pulmonary dysfunction or cardiac arrhythmia that may reflect medical comorbidity or neurologic changes due to the ischemic stroke; (b) large hemispheric stroke with the risk of subsequent space-occupying brain edema [usually infarcts covering >50% of the middle cerebral artery (MCA) territory]; and (c) extensive brainstem infarcts. Clinical signs of massive hemispheric infarction are dense hemiplegia and forced eye deviation. Decreased consciousness and coma are present only infrequently within the first hours after symptom onset in these patients. Abnormal breathing patterns, decreased level of consciousness, or upper airway obstruction due to decreased muscle tone of the pharynx or relapsing tongue indicate a complicated and potentially life-threatening clinical course in patients with brainstem stroke.

STROKE CARE UNIT: THE FIRST FORTY-EIGHT HOURS

Within the SCU, the same principles of therapy apply as in the emergency department, that is, specific and general therapeutic approaches are addressed.

Specific Therapies

Thrombolysis/Aspirin

If tPA and/or aspirin were not administered in the emergency room, they may be administered within the SCU. In the majority of instances, however, the therapy itself will have been administered earlier and the main role of the SCU staff is to monitor patients after therapy. In the case of tPA, this is particularly important because clinical deterioration may be associated with hemorrhagic transformation, which may need to be addressed using cryoprecipitate or intravenous platelets (53). Occasionally, surgical decompression may be indicated.

Surgery

Occasionally surgical intervention is required in acute ischemic stroke (54). At about 48 hours, the presence of cerebral edema may be maximal in either cerebral or cerebellar hemispheres (55). In the latter case, there is little argument that posterior fossa craniectomy is required and can be a life-saving procedure (56). Patients with large cerebellar infarcts often present initially with relatively mild symptoms but may rapidly develop hydrocephalus and brainstem symptoms over the next subsequent days due to the expanding perifocal edema, leading to obstruction of the fourth ventricle and brainstem compression. Quadriparesis may ensue and mortality rates may be high. Direct posterior fossa craniectomy with or without ventricular shunt is indicated rather than ventricular shunt only (57).

General Treatments

Once the patient is in the SCU, general issues that were not addressed in the emergency department (Table 42-1) may need to be addressed. Particularly, DVT prophylaxis, using either stockings or low-dose heparin, should be introduced for patients who are not able to mobilize early (58). Airway management and swallowing care may need to be addressed after early assessment of both (59). Early use of a nasogastric tube for 48 to 72 hours may be useful to avoid aspiration and chest infection (59). Chest physiotherapy should be introduced early if patients cannot be mobilized. Chest infections may need to be treated with antibiotics and renal impairment monitored. The latter may be particularly important if investigation involving contrast agents is to be considered. Screening tests for arteritis, genetic tests [e.g., cerebral autosomal dominant arteriopathy with subcortical infarcts and leukoencephalopathy (CADASIL)], and serum lipids may be ordered if indicated.

Monitoring Vital Functions

Because of the high prevalence of cardiovascular comorbidity and the neurogenic changes in pulmonary and cardiac functions, the significance of which is increasingly being recognized, continuous ECG monitoring, pulse oximetry, and frequent measurements of blood pressure should be performed during the first days in many causes. Preexisting chronic obstructive lung disease or sleep apnea syndrome frequently may herald serious pulmonary dysfunction after stroke, particularly during sleep; therefore, cardiac and pulmonary function should be closely monitored in most patients. It should be established whether patients with absent gag, coma, or frequent episodes of oxygen desaturation despite supplemental oxygen require endotracheal intubation.

Blood Pressure

In most patients with acute stroke, blood pressure levels are elevated for the first few days and its management remains uncertain during this acute phase. Based upon pathophysiologic considerations and various case reports of patients in whom neurologic deficits significantly worsened after administration of antihypertensive drugs, most recommendations for acute stroke therapy do not advise lowering elevated blood pressure levels. Arterial hypertension should be treated only in patients with extremely high blood pressure levels (>220 mm Hg systolic or >120 mm Hg diastolic) and if tPA therapy is indicated. To date, the question of which antihypertensive drug should be administered has not been addressed in systematic studies. Vasodilatory drugs such as calcium antagonists should be avoided because of the danger of cerebral vasodilation with increased brain edema. In Europe, urapidil, an α-blocking agent, is given frequently. In North America, labetalol and nitroprusside are the antihypertensive drugs of choice in many institutions. In Australia, glycerol trinitrate patch or intravenous hydralazine may be used (60). It probably is more important that if antihypertensive drugs are administered, blood pressure is lowered slowly and not to hypotensive levels. There are insufficient data to generally recommend active elevation of blood pressure in hypotensive patients. Theoretically, induced hypertension may have negative effects in patients with lacunar stroke or in whom an occluded vessel becomes hyperperfused after revascularization. However, induced hypertension using volume substitution and vasopressor drugs might be beneficial in patients with severe hemodynamic stenosis or persistent vascular occlusion with a large ischemic penumbra surrounding the infarct core.

Body Temperature and Infection

There is a convincing body of evidence that fever worsens the prognosis after stroke. Although an improved prognosis after fever-lowering treatment has not yet been proven, body temperature should be closely monitored and fever rigorously treated in these patients. The symptomatic treatment of fever should be accompanied by a search for the origin of fever. Fever of central origin can be diagnosed only after all other causes have been ruled out, particularly systemic infections. The most common source of fever is pulmonary infection, followed by urinary tract infection.

Fluid and Electrolyte Management

Stroke patients should have a balanced fluid and electrolyte status to avoid plasma volume contraction and raised hematocrit levels, which impair rheologic properties of the blood. Cardiac function is compromised in many stroke patients; therefore, uncontrolled volume replacement can rapidly lead to cardiac failure and pulmonary edema. In some centers, the serum electrolytes are monitored on a daily basis. Specifically, hyponatremia must be avoided because it may aggravate postischemic brain edema.

Blood Glucose

As for fever, hyperglycemia after stroke is associated with a poorer prognosis (21,61). Hyperglycemia is a frequent finding after acute stroke. Glucose homeostasis may rapidly become disordered, particularly in patients with diabetes mellitus. It is not clear whether there is a causal relationship between outcome and hyperglycemia or whether hyperglycemia is only an indicator of severe disease with no direct impact on patient prognosis.

Seizure

About 5% of all patients with acute stroke develop epileptic seizure within the first 2 weeks (61). Some physicians would commence antiepileptic treatment immediately after the first seizure, but this approach is not uniform. Carbamazepine is still the first-choice drug for the majority of patients. In patients who develop a series of seizures or status epilepticus, adequate antiepileptic serum levels are reached more rapidly with intravenously administered phenytoin. In Australia, intravenous clonazepam is the drug of choice. Oxcarbazepine, valproate, and gabapentin are effective alternatives, particularly in patients receiving another medication that interacts with carbamazepine metabolism.

Prevention of Deep Venous Thrombosis

Before prophylactic measures for DVT were introduced, venous thrombosis and pulmonary embolism were frequent causes of death in stroke patients. With the routine use of compression stockings and subcutaneous heparin, the incidence of DVT has been greatly reduced. The importance of early mobilization and physical therapy should be emphasized.

Treatment of Brain Edema

Subsequent neurologic deterioration due to increasing brain edema is a common phenomenon in patients who have suffered massive stroke (62,63). Several treatments for postischemic brain edema currently are used. Traditionally, the mainstay of conventional therapy has consisted of ventilation, sedation, blood pressure monitoring, hyperventilation, osmotic agents, and barbiturates. The recommendations for these therapies are based upon small case series, evidence from animal experiments, or theoretical observation. None of them has been evaluated in a randomized study. Whether intracranial pressure monitoring should be included in the routine management of patients with large strokes is still a matter of controversy.

Hypertonic, low-molecular-weight solutions such as mannitol, sorbitol, glycerol, or hypertonic saline are used to reduce brain water content by creating an osmotic gradient between brain and plasma, which draws water into the plasma. The long-term effects of repeated treatments with hypertonic solution are unknown. Repeated infusions of mannitol may aggravate cerebral edema if the osmotic substances migrate through a damaged blood-brain barrier into the brain tissue, reversing the osmotic gradient (64).

Hyperventilation can induce cerebral vasoconstriction, but the effect of hyperventilation is short lived if normoventilation is resumed too rapidly. Hyperventilation may critically reduce cerebral blood flow, leading to additional ischemic damage. Barbiturates can reduce cerebral blood flow and intracranial pressure promptly, but their use is limited because of various side effects and reports from two studies that failed to demonstrate any long-term beneficial effects.

TABLE 42-6. *Proven forms of secondary prevention*

1. Antiplatelet agents
2. Carotid endarterectomy
3. Anticoagluation (in patients with atrial fibrillation)
4. Blood pressure lowering (perindopril-based) agents

Early Secondary Prevention

There are four main categories of treatment where secondary prevention has been of proven benefit, as given in Table 42-6. While the patient is under SCU management, it often is reasonable to commence secondary prevention early so that regimens can be stabilized and patterns of therapy established before the patient enters into the community. In our experience, if this is not done in the stroke unit environment it may be missed during the follow-up phase.

Antiplatelet Therapy

Whereas there is good evidence that aspirin alone (11,12), aspirin plus dipyridamole (66), and clopidogrel (67) alone are useful secondary prevention strategies after ischemic stroke, the timing of their introduction after the acute stroke event is unclear. The strongest evidence that secondary prevention should commence early is with aspirin alone based on the International Stroke Trial (IST) and Chinese Acute Stroke Trial (CAST) data (11,12). Here, where aspirin was given within 48 hours of stroke onset, significant reductions in recurrent stroke and stroke-related death occurred during the follow-up periods. It is possible that most of the aspirin benefit in these trials is due to early secondary prevention, although this is not certain. Regardless, a pragmatic approach is to introduce aspirin within 48 hours of stroke onset and then establish the final antiplatelet regimen within the first 5 days of SCU stay.

Carotid Endarterectomy

This is now well established and of proven benefit for secondary prevention (68,69); however, the timing after acute stroke is less clear. Many surgeons are wary of performing carotid endarterectomy too soon after minor ischemic stroke. The possibility of hemorrhage into a fresh infarct has received a great deal of anecdotal attention. Of interest, when investigators from the NASCET study analyzed patients undergoing early endarterectomy (<1 week) after minor stroke, there was no increased incidence of hemorrhagic complications (70).

Anticoagulation in Patients with Atrial Fibrillation

In the European Atrial Fibrillation Trial, patients were anticoagulated within 3 months of a transient ischemic attack or minor stroke (71). No intracerebral hemorrhages were recorded in this study. However, in IST, subcutaneous administration of high doses of heparin (12,500 International Units BD) were associated with an increased cerebral hemorrhage rate (11). Hence, there is no real consensus on when to start anticoagulants after ischemic stroke because evidence is modest and somewhat conflicting. Our practice is to use intravenous heparin with activated partial thromboplastin time between 60 and 80 seconds when there is evidence of ongoing embolization. Otherwise, warfarin (Coumadin) is introduced gradually within the first 5 days or so.

Agents That Lower Blood Pressure

Perindopril Protection Against Recurrent Stroke Study (PROGRESS) provided clear evidence that lowering blood pressure protects against subsequent stroke and death (72). However, the mean time to commencement of therapy was 6 months, with range up to 5 years after the event. Given that there is no firm evidence on how to manage blood pressure during the acute phase (60) (see earlier), our practice is to introduce perindopril or perindopril plus indapamide during inpatient SCU stay rather than waiting for outpatient review.

EXPERIMENTAL THERAPIES

To provide additional space for the expanding infarcted brain tissue, extended craniectomy with dural augmentation or lobectomy has been used in patients with large supratentorial and cerebellar infarcts. Retrospective case series and uncontrolled studies that involved fewer than 200 patients show surgical treatment improves functional outcome in surviving patients and probably mortality. The ideal candidate for surgery, optimum point of time, and surgical technique are subject of debate.

Animal experiments have shown that induced hypothermia has a neuroprotective effect after focal and global ischemia (73). However, in patients with severe acute head trauma, a recent controlled multicenter study did not show any benefit from hypothermia. Results of pilot studies with mild-to-moderate hypothermia (about 33°C) up to 3 days in patients with complete MCA infarction suggested that hypothermia reduces ischemic brain edema and intracerebral pressure. Larger controlled trials currently are underway to assess the efficacy and appropriate technique of cooling and rewarming.

Intraarterial thrombolysis with prourokinase may be a treatment option for patients arriving in the 3- to 6-hour time window. Several uncontrolled studies showed a high rate of revascularization and probable trend toward reduced mortality. In patients with acute basilar occlusion, the time restriction may be extended to 48 hours after the onset of symptoms given the poor prognosis of these patients.

One randomized study indicated that the snake venom Ancrod, a defibrinogenating enzyme, may improve the outcome after acute stroke if it is used within 3 hours. A second study of Ancrod had to be stopped after an interim analysis of the data for safety reasons.

FUTURE DIRECTIONS

Over the next decade there are likely to be further treatment and management options developed for acute ischemic stroke. One of the most important of these treatments may be the routine use of neuroprotectants to prolong the time window for other therapeutic interventions. Should this occur, neuroprotectants can be administered by ambulance personnel to stroke patients on site. A hypothetical treatment approach then may be undertaken, as shown in Fig. 42-6. The position of the timing of the image can be moved forward as patients are transported more efficiently to hospitals or imaging devices are incorporated into mobile units such as ambulances. If this is the case, then thrombolysis likely will be administered earlier.

Neuroimaging, particularly MRI with DWI and perfusion-weighted imaging, is likely to become useful in stratifying patients who likely will to respond to

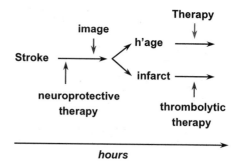

FIG. 42-6. Possible algorithm for stroke therapy in the future.

various forms of therapy, particularly thrombolysis. A number of trials, such as Echoplanar Imaging Thrombolysis Evaluation Trial (EPITHET) (68), are testing this hypothesis. Intravenous thrombolysis beyond the 3-hour window should be performed only in carefully selected patients at stroke centers experienced in such treatment. A typical candidate for thrombolysis beyond the 3-hour time window is a patient with an occluded MCA in whom there is a marked difference between a small ischemic lesion already visible on the diffusion-weighted MR images and a large perfusion deficit on the perfusion-weighted MR images.

Invasive acute neuroradiologic approaches such as angioplasty may become the norm, as is the case with myocardial ischemia.

We are moving from a state of nihilism to active intervention in the treatment of acute ischemic stroke, and this is likely to accelerate further over the next few years. As these therapies become more broadly applicable worldwide, significant reduction in case fatality rates likely will be seen.

REFERENCES

1. Bonita R. Epidemiology of stroke. *Lancet* 1992;339: 342–344.
2. Baron JC, von Kummer R, del Zoppo GJ. Treatment of acute ischemic stroke: challenging the concept of a rigid and universal time window. *Stroke* 1995;26:2219–2221.
3. Read SJ, Hirano T, Abbott DF, et al. The fate of hypoxic tissue on 18F-fluoromisonidazole PET after ischemic stroke. *Ann Neurol* 2000;48:228–235.
4. Heiss WD, Huber M, Fink GR, et al. Progressive derangement of peri-infarct viable tissue in ischemic stroke. *J Cereb Blood Flow Metab* 1992;12:599–606.
5. Heiss WD, Thiel A, Grond M, et al. Which targets are relevant for therapy of acute ischemic stroke? *Stroke* 1999;30:1486–1489.
6. The National Institute of Neurological Disorders and Stroke rt-PA Stroke Study Group. Tissue plasminogen activator for acute ischemic stroke. *N Engl J Med* 1995;333:1581–1587.
7. Kidwell CS, Starkman S, Eckstein M, et al. Identifying stroke in the field. Prospective validation of the Los Angeles Prehospital Stroke Screen (LAPSS). *Stroke* 2000;31:71–76.
8. Kothari R, Pancioli A, Liu T. Cincinnati Prehospital Stroke Scale: reproducibility and validity. *Ann Emerg Med* 1999;33:373–378.
9. McDowell FH, Brott T. The emergency treatment of stroke: the first 6 hours. *J Stroke Cerebrovasc Dis* 1993; 3:133–144.
10. Wahlgren NG, MacMaMahon DG, De Keyser J, et al. Intravenous Nimodipine West European Stroke Trial (INWEST) of nimodipine in the treatment of acute ischaemic stroke. *Cerebrovasc Dis* 1994;4:204–210.
11. International Stroke Trial Collaborative Group. The International Stroke Trial (IST): a randomised trial of aspirin, subcutaneous heparin, both, or neither amount 19435 patients with acute ischaemic stroke. *Lancet* 1997;349:1569–1581.
12. CAST (Chinese Acute Stroke Trial) Collaborative Group. CAST: randomised placebo-controlled trial of early aspirin use in 20000 patients with acute ischaemic stroke. *Lancet* 1997;349:1641–1649.
13. Lacy C, Suh DC, Bueno M, et al., for the S.T.R.O.K.E. Collaborative Study Group. Delay in presentation and evaluation for acute stroke. Stroke Time Registry for Outcomes Knowledge and Epidemiology (S.T.R.O.K.E.). *Stroke* 2001;32:63–69.
14. Kothari R, Jauch E, Broderick JP. Acute stroke: delays to presentation and emergency department evaluation. *Ann Emerg Med* 1999;33:3–8.
15. Toni D, Iweins F, von Kummer R, et al. Identification of lacunar infarcts before thrombolysis in the ECASS I study. *Neurology* 2000;54:648–688.
16. Kothari R, Barsan W, Brott T, et al. Frequency and accuracy of prehospital diagnosis of acute stroke. *Stroke* 1995;26:937–941.
17. Baird AE, Dambrosia J, Janket SK, et al. A three-item scale for the early prediction of stroke recovery. *Lancet* 2001;357:2095–2099.
18. Davis S, Donnan G, Grotta J, et al. *Interventional therapy in acute stroke.* Boston: Blackwell Science, 1998: 14–17.
19. Weir CJ, Murrar GD, Adams FG, et al. Poor accuracy of stroke scoring systems for differential clinical diagnosis of intracranial haemorrhage and infarction. *Lancet* 1994;344:999–1002.
20. von Kummer R, Allen K, Holle R, et al. Acute stroke: usefulness of early CT findings before thrombolytic therapy. *Radiology* 1997;205:327–333.
21. Weir C, Murray G, Dyker A, et al. Is hyperglycaemia an independent predictor of poor outcome after acute stroke? Result of a long term follow up study. *BMJ* 1997;314:1303–1306.
22. Donnan G. Investigation of patients with stroke and transient ischaemic attacks. *Lancet* 1992;339:473–447.
23. Jones EF, Kalman JK, Calafiore P, et al. Proximal aortic atheroma. *Stroke* 1995;26:218–224.
24. Amarenco P, Cohen A, Tzourio C, et al. Atherosclerotic disease of the aortic arch and the risk of ischemic stroke. *N Engl J Med* 1994;331:1474–1479.
25. Bladin C, Alexandrov A, Bellavance A, et al. Seizure after stroke—a prospective multicenter study. *Arch Neurol* 2000;57:1617–1622.
26. Langhorne P, Williams B, Gilchrist W, et al. Do stroke units save lives? *Lancet* 1993;342:395–398.
27. Martinez-Vila E, Sieira P. Current status and perspectives of neuroprotection in ischaemic stroke treatment. *Cerebrovasc Dis* 2001;11[Suppl 1]:60–70.
28. Publication Committee for the Trial of Org 10172 in Acute Stroke Treatment (TOAST) Investigators. Low molecular weight heparinoid, Org 10172 (danaparoid), and outcome after acute ischaemic stroke. A randomized, controlled trial. *JAMA* 1998;279:1265–1272.
29. Bath P, Lindenstrom E, Boysen G, et al. Tinzaparin in acute ischaemic stroke (TAIST): a randomised aspirin-controlled trial. *Lancet* 2001;358:702–710.
30. Asplund K, Israelsson K, Schampi I. Haemodilution for acute ischaemic stroke (Cochrane Review). *Cochrane Library,* Issue 3, 2001, Oxford: Update Software.
31. Qizilbash N, Lewington SL, Lopez-Arrieta JM. Corticosteroids for acute ischaemic stroke (Cochrane

Review). *Cochrane Library,* Issue 3, 2001, Oxford: Update Software.
32. Hacke W, Kaste M, Fieschi C, et al., for the ECASS Study Group. Intravenous thrombolysis with recombinant tissue plasminogen activator for acute hemispheric stroke: the European Cooperative Acute Stroke Study (ECASS). *JAMA* 1995;274:1017–1025.
33. Hacke W, Kaste M, Fieschi C, et al., for the Second European-Australasian Acute Stroke Study Investigators. Randomised double-blind placebo-controlled trial of thrombolytic therapy with intravenous alteplase in acute ischaemic stroke (ECASS II): Second European-Australasian Acute Stroke Study Investigators. *Lancet* 1998;352:1245–1251.
34. Clark WM, Wissman S, Alers GW, et al., for the Alteplase Thrombolysis for Acute Non-interventional Therapy in Ischaemic Stroke Study Group. Recombinant tissue-type plasminogen activator (Alteplase) for ischaemic stroke 3 to 5 hours after symptom onset. The ATLANTIS Study: a randomised controlled trial. *JAMA* 1999;282:2019–2026.
35. Hacke W, Brott T, Caplan L, et al. Thrombolysis in acute ischemic stroke: controlled trials and clinical experience. *Neurology* 1999;53[Suppl 4]:S3–S14.
36. Albers GW, Bates VE, Clark WM, et al. Intravenous tissue-type plasminogen activator for the treatment of acute stroke. The Standard Treatment with Alteplase to Reverse Stroke (STARS) Study. *JAMA* 2000;283: 1145–1150.
37. Katzan IL, Furlan AJ, Lloyd LE, et al. Use of tissue-type plasminogen activator for acute ischemic stroke. The Cleveland experience. *JAMA* 2000;283:1151–1158.
38. Tanne D, Bates VE, Verro P, et al., and t-PA Stroke Survey Group. Initial clinical experience with IV tissue plasminogen activator for acute ischemic stroke: a multicenter survey. *Neurology* 1999;53:424–427.
39. Lopez-Yunez AM, Bruno A, Williams LS, et al. Protocol violations in community-based rTPA stroke treatment are associated with symptomatic intracerebral hemorrhage. Stroke 2001;32:12–16.
40. Chiu D, Krieger D, Villar-Cordova C, et al. Intravenous tissue plasminogen activator for acute ischemic stroke: feasibility, safety, and efficacy in the first year of clinical practice. *Stroke* 1998;29:18–22.
41. Grond M, Stenzel C, Schmulling S, et al. Early intravenous thrombolysis for acute ischemic stroke in a community-based approach. *Stroke* 1998;29: 1544–1549.
42. Schmulling S, Grond M, Rudolf J, et al. One-year follow-up in acute stroke patients treated with rtPA in clinical routine. *Stroke* 2000;31:1552–1554.
43. Wang DZ, Rose JA, Honings DS, et al., for the OSF Stroke Time. Treating acute stroke with intravenous tPA. The OSF Stroke Network Experience. *Stroke* 2000;31:77–81.
44. Trouillas P, Nighoghossian N, Derex L, et al. Thrombolysis with intravenous rtPA in a series of 100 cases of acute carotid territory stroke. Determination of etiological, topographic, and radiological outcome factors. *Stroke* 1998;29:2529–2540.
45. Chapman KM, Woolfenden AR, Graeb D, et al. Intravenous tissue plasminogen activator for acute ischemic stroke. A Canadian hospital's experience. *Stroke* 2000; 31:2920–2924.

46. Lindley RI. Further randomized controlled trials of tissue plasminogen activator within 3 hours are required. *Stroke* 2001;32:2708–2709.
47. Diez-Tejedor E, Fuentes B. Acute care in stroke: do stroke units make the difference? *Cerebrovasc Dis* 2001;11[Suppl 1]:31–39.
48. Indredavik B, Bakke F, Slordahl SA, et al. Stroke unit treatment 10-year follow-up. *Stroke* 1999;30: 1524–1527.
49. Kalra L, Evans A, Perez I, et al. Alternative strategies for stroke care: a prospective randomised controlled trial. *Lancet* 2000;356:894–899.
50. Indredavik B, Bakke F, Slordahl SA, et al. Treatment in a combined acute and rehabilitation stroke unit. Which aspects are most important? *Stroke* 1999;30:917–923.
51. Donnan G, et al., for the Stroke Australia Task Force. National Stroke Strategy. The National Stroke Foundation, 1996.
52. Sudlow CLM, Warlow CP. Comparable studies of the incidence of stroke and its pathological subtypes: results from an international collaboration. *Stroke* 1997;28:491–499.
53. The NINDS t-PA Stroke Study Group. Intracerebral hemorrhage after intravenous t-PA therapy for ischemic stroke. *Stroke* 1997;28:2109–2118.
54. Schwab S, Steiner T, Aschoff A, et al. Early hemicraniectomy in patients with complete middle cerebral artery infarction. *Stroke* 1998;29:1888–1893.
55. Kasner SE, Demchuk AM, Berriuschot J, et al. Predictors of fatal brain edema in massive hemispheric ischemic stroke. *Stroke* 2001;32:2117–2123.
56. Macdonell R, Donnan G, Kalnins R. Cerebellar infarction: natural history prognosis and pathology. *Stroke* 1987;18:849–855.
57. Heros R. Surgical treatment of cerebellar infarction. *Stroke* 1992;23:937–938.
58. Kelly J, Rudd A, Lewis R, et al. Venous thromboembolism after acute stroke. *Stroke* 2001;32:262–267.
59. Mann G, Hankey G, Cameron D. Swallowing function after stroke. Prognosis and prognostic factors at 6 months. *Stroke* 1999;30:744–748.
60. Bath P, Boysen G, Donnan GA, et al. Hypertension in acute stroke: what to do? *Stroke* 2001;32:1697–1698.
61. Kagansky N, Levy S, Knobler H. The role of hyperglycemia in acute stroke. *Arch Neurol* 2000;58: 1209–1212.
62. Labovitz DL, Allen Hauser W, Sacco RL. Prevalence and predictors of early seizure and status epilepticus after first stroke. *Neurology* 2001;57:200–206.
63. Ropper AH, Shafran B. Brain edema after stroke. Clinical syndrome and intracranial pressure. *Arch Neurol* 1984;41:26–29.
64. Frank JI. Large hemispheric infarction, deterioration, and intracranial pressure. *Neurology* 1995;45: 1286–1290.
65. Bereczki D, Liu M, do Prado GF, et al. Mannitol for acute stroke (Cochrane Review). Cochrane Database System Review, 2001;1.
66. Diener HC, Cunha L, Forbes C, et al. European Stroke Prevention Study 2. Dipyridamole and acetylsalicylic acid in the secondary prevention of stroke. *J Neurol Sci* 1996;143:1–13.
67. CAPRIE Steering Committee. A randomised, blinded, trial of clopidogrel versus aspirin in patients at risk of

ischaemic events (CAPRIE). *Lancet* 1996;348: 1329–1339.

68. Ferguson GG, Eliasziw M, Fox AJ, et al., for the North American Symptomatic Carotid Endarterectomy Trial (NASCET) Collaborators. The North American Symptomatic Carotid Endarterectomy Trial: surgical results in 1415 patients. *Stroke* 1999;30:1751–1758.

69. European Carotid Surgery Trialists' Group. Randomised trial of endarterectomy for recently symptomatic carotid stenosis: final results of the MRC European Carotid Surgery Trial (ECST). *Lancet* 1998;351: 1379–1387.

70. Alamowitch S, Eliasziw M, Algra A, et al., for the North American Symptomatic Carotid Endarterectomy Trial (NASCET) Group. Risk, causes, and prevention of ischaemic stroke in elderly patients with symptomatic internal-carotid-artery stenosis. *Lancet* 2001;357: 1154–1160.

71. EAFT (European Atrial Fibrillation Trial) Study Group. Secondary prevention in non-rheumatic atrial fibrillation after transient ischaemic attack or minor stroke. *Lancet* 1993;342:1255–1262.

72. PROGRESS Collaborative Group. Randomised trial of a perindopril-based blood pressure lowering regime among 6105 patients with prior stroke or transient ischemic attack. *Lancet* 2001;358:1033–1041.

73. Ginsberg M, Busto R. Combating hyperthermia in acute stroke. *Stroke* 1998;29:529–534.

Ischemic Stroke: Advances in Neurology, Vol. 92. Edited by
H.J.M. Barnett, Julien Bogousslavsky, and Heather Meldrum.
Lippincott Williams & Wilkins, Philadelphia © 2003.

43

Intensive Care Management of Specific Stroke Treatment

Cenk Ayata and *Allan H. Ropper

*Department of Radiology, Harvard Medical School; Department of Neurology,
Massachusetts General Hospital, Boston, Massachusetts; *Department of Neurology,
St. Elizabeth's Medical Center, Tufts University School of Medicine, Boston, Massachusetts, U.S.A.*

The neuro-intensive care unit (neuro-ICU) offers the ability to detect and react quickly to neurologic changes and to monitor or institute treatments that require a higher level of attention than can be provided on a routine ward. Certain technologic and invasive monitoring techniques are best provided in a unit that is staffed by specially trained nurses who are familiar with the apparatus and the interpretation of its measurements. The types of cerebrovascular cases that most often require critical care attention are listed in Table 43-1.

Most approaches to acute stroke aim to improve cerebral blood flow (CBF) to the ischemic brain. At the moment, from the critical care perspective, the most important aspects of acute stroke management are the prevention and treatment of secondary neurologic complications such as ischemic brain swelling, seizures, and care of coma; and treatment of early medical complications, particularly aspiration pneumonia, fever, and a number of frequently occurring pulmonary, cardiovascular, and infectious events. These problems are encountered more commonly in patients with large hemispheric strokes, but their presence may influence the outcome of infarctions of

all types. Technologic advances have permitted better monitoring of such patients to guide decision-making, particularly choices with regard to intervention and their timing.

As a derivative of the neuro-ICU, organized stroke units appear to reduce stroke mortality and improve functional outcome regardless of patient age, gender, stroke severity, and comorbidities. They also may reduce the length of inpatient stay (1). In particular, stroke units have been found to reduce the relative risk of death within 5 years after stroke by 40% (2). This benefit is apparent early and is long lasting. Whether such units can be encompassed within a neuro-ICU depends on local circumstances, but neuro-ICU beds are used for this purpose in many hospitals.

Among the types of cerebrovascular cases that are likely to require neuro-ICU care, large middle cerebral artery (MCA) infarction with edema and cerebral hemorrhages, which are masses by definition, compress adjacent and distant brain structures and produce coma, the latter at a higher rate than ischemic stroke. All of the comments that follow regarding the management of coma, intracranial hypertension, and

TABLE 43-1. *Types of stroke admitted to a neuro-intensive care unit*

Large middle cerebral artery stroke with edema
Cerebellar infarction or hemorrhage
Basilar artery occlusion or critical stenosis
Hemodynamically sensitive critical stenosis or occlusion of carotid or middle cerebral artery
Large cerebral hemorrhage
Subarachnoid hemorrhage
Observation after thrombolysis and endovascular interventions
Postoperative carotid endarterectomy, craniectomy or decompression of brain edema, or removal of cerebral
    hematoma

medical complications also pertain to expanding strokes and to hematomas. Cerebellar infarcts with even modest edema, and cerebellar hemorrhages have a propensity to produce life-threatening medullary compression as a result of the compact nature of the posterior fossa. Their management is different in that surgical removal of the cerebellar clot or infarcted and edematous tissue has been established to be beneficial. Patients with basilar artery occlusion also are admitted to the neuro-ICU for several reasons, the most obvious being the need to prevent airway obstruction and the care of coma, but also because of the precarious nature of ischemic and vascular lesions, which require close observation.

EVALUATION FOR NEUROLOGIC INTENSIVE CARE ADMISSION

Management of the acutely ill and drowsy or comatose stroke patient appropriately focuses on securing the airway, establishing sufficient breathing, and hemodynamic stabilization (Table 43-2). Overall stroke severity can be determined from the level of consciousness, breathing pattern, extent and distribution of deficit that indicate the size of the infarcted territory, and signs of brainstem compromise. Ancillary data, such as evidence of large infarct, diffusion-perfusion mismatch, arterial dissection, or internal carotid, MCA, or basilar artery occlusion or critical

stenosis on computed tomographic angiogram (CTA) or magnetic resonance angiogram (MRA) often are crucial in decision making. The immediate future implications of the stroke (e.g., depressed level of consciousness, high risk for increased intracranial pressure (ICP), accompanying seizures, thrombolysis), and the need for intubation due to respiratory insufficiency/distress also indicate ICU admission. Patients may be admitted to the neuro-ICU immediately or transferred there if their clinical conditions deteriorate. The distribution of cases depends largely on the directorship, interests, and controlling service that provide physician staff.

CLINICAL DETERIORATION FROM STROKE EDEMA

Mechanisms of Clinical Deterioration

Of the complications that follow large acute strokes, ischemic brain swelling and resultant brain herniation have received the most attention because they are the major causes of death in patients with large infarcts of MCA territory (3–6). These so-called "malignant MCA strokes" have had up to an 80% mortality rate despite medical treatment (6,7). It has been reported that 15% to 20% of all MCA infarcts display this type of delayed and progressive and untreatable edema, but the frequency has been far

TABLE 43-2. *Indications for neuro-intensive care unit admission of stroke patients*

A. Signs and symptoms
    Depressed level of consciousness
    Progressing deficits with large arterial stenosis or occlusion
    Hemodynamic fluctuation of deficits with large arterial stenosis or occlusion
    Crescendo transient ischemic attacks
    Cardiovascular or respiratory insufficiency
    Seizures
B. Radiographic signs
    Infarction of >50% of middle cerebral artery territory or 30% of cerebellum (appropriate for observation
        depending on level of nursing surveillance on general ward)
    Symptomatic high-grade basilar stenosis or occlusion
    Sinus vein thrombosis with large venous stroke, or signs of elevated intracranial pressure
    Large intrainfarct hematoma formation
C. Special causes of progressive stroke
    Fluctuating syndrome from arterial dissection with stroke
    Vasculitis with progressive deficits
    Hematologic disease (e.g., polycythemia, thrombotic thrombocytopenic purpura), coagulopathy, or
        endocarditis with progressive stroke or cerebral hematoma formation
D. Treatment requiring special surveillance
    Following intravenous or intraarterial thrombolysis, with or without intervention (e.g., stenting, angioplasty)
    Therapeutic hypertension
    Hemodilution
    Therapeutic hypothermia
    Ventriculostomy
    Hemicraniectomy

lower in our experience. Although the onset of ischemic brain swelling and its clinical representations are variable, they typically become evident between 2 and 5 days after the stroke (8). In certain cases, deterioration occurs as early as the first 24 hours or as late as the sixth day.

Expansion of any one intracranial compartment [brain, cerebrospinal fluid (CSF), and vasculature] is accommodated at the expense of another. ICP remains relatively normal until the initial accommodative mechanisms that shift intracranial CSF (75–150 mL) to the spinal compartment and that reduce venous blood volume (75–100 mL) are exhausted. Once these shifts have occurred, ICP increases precipitously and, as a parallel but separate phenomenon, brain tissue shifts occur that may result in herniation from one cerebral compartment to an adjacent one. It is desirable to anticipate brain swelling and elevated ICP in order to take action before clinical deterioration arises.

As ICP rises, cerebral perfusion pressure [CPP; the difference between intracranial blood pressure (BP) and ICP] and CBF are reduced. There is an autoregulatory response of cerebral vasodilation that attempts to maintain blood flow. If CPP drops below a critical threshold (generally thought to be ~60 mm Hg), the precapillary arterioles become maximally dilated and autoregulation fails. Beyond this point, experimental models suggest that CBF is further compromised and ischemic edema may be further aggravated, creating a vicious cycle.

Even before any detectable ICP increase, regional edema causes a local increase in tissue pressure, distorting the adjacent brain tissue and interfering with the local microcirculation. For these reasons, treatments that reduce ischemic brain edema and elevated ICP not only potentially diminish tissue shifts and herniation but also may avoid worsening ischemia and secondary cerebral damage .

Signs of Clinical Deterioration

The earliest sign of ischemic brain edema has generally been a reduced level of consciousness (3). Drowsiness alone for 2 to 5 days may be reversible in our experience. In most cases, however, drowsiness is followed by a reduced or absent pupillary light reaction ipsilateral to the stroke and later by the classic signs of an acutely expanding cerebral mass, pupillary enlargement, and finally periodic breathing. Brain tissue shifts usually are accompanied by a Babinski sign ipsilateral to the infarct (Kernohan-Woltman sign attributed to compression of the oppo-

site cerebral peduncle against the tentorium from horizontal brain displacement). Headache, nausea and vomiting, and worsening of the initial neurologic deficits are variably accumulated. In patients who exhibit these signs, further management should be carried out in a specialized environment such as a neuro-ICU.

Predictors of Clinical Deterioration

Patients at risk for ischemic brain edema are those with large hemispheric strokes, generally involving at least 50% of the estimated MCA territory. Involvement of additional territories (e.g., anterior cerebral artery) increases the risk. Smaller cerebellar strokes carry a similar risk due to the compact anatomy of the posterior fossa and the risk of aqueductal or fourth ventricular compression causing obstructive hydrocephalus. The clinical predictors of worsening have been the subject of a number of studies that underscore the importance of timely recognition in high-risk patients. Severe paralysis, gaze deviation (9), systolic BP above 180 mm Hg at 12 hours (10), and a higher serum glucose on admission (11) each have been suggested as early indicators of clinical deterioration based on limited case series. Early mortality, likely an indirect reflection of the same problem, has been associated with a depressed level of alertness, gaze deviation, leg weakness, and older age (12). Among patients who do deteriorate, signs of uncal herniation have occurred more commonly in younger individuals and gradual rostrocaudal deterioration in older individuals (8). Not surprisingly, the need for endotracheal intubation carries a worse prognosis (6).

The presence of low-density infarction and edema on CT scan that occupies more than 50% of the MCA territory (10,13,14,15) has been the most consistent predictive feature of subsequent malignant edema after MCA stroke (6), especially if these changes involved both cortical and subcortical regions (11). Hemorrhagic transformation has been closely associated with ischemic edema and tissue shifts. Whether hemorrhagic transformation by itself contributes to clinical deterioration is uncertain, but our view is that it probably does not (16). Intrainfarct hematoma formation, on the other hand, has been predictive of a worse outcome in the presence of intraventricular or subarachnoid extension (17). A "hyperdense MCA" (i.e., visible clot within the lumen of the stem of the vessel) also has been predictive for edema in some but not all studies and seems to us less relevant than the radiographic signs (8,13,18). Angiographically, siphon or top of the internal carotid artery or MCA stem occlusion, and absence of collateral blood flow were more often associated with severe edema (11).

ACUTE STROKE TREATMENTS AND NEED FOR INTENSIVE CARE UNIT MONITORING

Currently, thrombolytic and interventional treatments require ICU monitoring for at least 24 hours. A common concern regarding these treatment options has been reperfusion injury and its contribution to stroke edema. Although hemorrhagic complications of thrombolysis have been emphasized as the major risk associated with its use, mortality more often has been due to malignant brain edema than to hemorrhage following thrombolysis (19). There is clinical and experimental evidence for deleterious effects of thrombolytic agents on the blood–brain barrier (BBB) and on neurons, suggesting that thrombolysis may aggravate reperfusion injury and ischemic brain edema. Nevertheless, there is more compelling evidence that malignant edema is prone to develop if recirculation is not established (6,20). It appears that the risk for ischemic brain edema and intrainfarct hemorrhage is increased if thrombolysis is delayed to the point that significant infarction has occurred (21).

INTENSIVE CARE UNIT MONITORING OF STROKE PATIENTS

Vital Signs

Tachypnea may be a sign of pulmonary or cardiac insufficiency. In immobilized stroke patients who have not been anticoagulated, it always raises a concern of pulmonary embolism (PE). Hyperpnea (i.e., increased spontaneous tidal volume) along with tachypnea may be an early sign of elevated ICP. Stridor may be due to vocal cord paralysis or poor pharyngeal tone, problems that arise mainly in brainstem strokes. Hence, the ability to cough and clear secretions and to swallow should be assessed in awake patients. Body temperature must be monitored regularly to allow prompt treatment of fever. Cardiac monitoring for the first few days of acute stroke is necessary for prompt recognition and management of arrhythmias. An arterial line provides continuous measurement of BP and allows frequent sampling for arterial blood gas but is not imperative except perhaps in comatose patients with ICP monitors or to induce hypertension. Pulmonary artery catheterization is only necessary to guide treatment in patients with poor cardiac or renal function, or sepsis. Pulmonary artery pressures can guide ICP management indirectly by preventing hypovolemia that results from aggressive

use of osmolar agents or diuretics, but most often hypotension can be precluded by other means.

Intracranial Pressure

There is general agreement that elevated ICP is predictive of a poor prognosis in patients with large strokes (3,6). Controversy still exists, however, regarding the benefit of ICP monitoring to detect elevations in pressure before the development of tissue shifts and thereby predict subsequent deterioration. Our impression has been that this approach is helpful (3,22), but others have not found such an association (23). Recent publications have indicated that clinical deterioration does not always follow ICP elevation, and the benefit of ICP measurement over observation of clinical signs in predicting deterioration has been questioned (22). Substantial horizontal tissue displacement, which is quantitatively related to the level of depressed consciousness, may occur before ICP elevation (3,22,24,25). Similarly uncal herniation can follow middle fossa swelling without a rise in global ICP. At this time, a case cannot be made that ICP monitoring directly improves outcome (26). However, use of ICP monitoring in a heuristic manner to guide the specific timing and dosing of treatment for brain edema has not been tested. As clinical and radiologic predictors of deterioration in large hemispheric strokes have been better defined, antiedema measures have been instituted independently of ICP measurement. In other words, there is no established consensus regarding the initiation and the manner of use of ICP monitoring.

We take the approach of selecting patients for monitoring who already demonstrate marked ischemic brain edema with tissue shifts and a diminished level of consciousness and in whom maximal efforts for lifesaving interventions are justified. The techniques of ICP monitoring are discussed elsewhere (27). Most units have been using miniaturized strain gauges that are coupled to a transducer by fiberoptic cable. The transducer tip is inserted directly into the superficial layers of brain tissue. The main drawback of this class of devices is the inability to "rezero" to atmospheric pressure without withdrawing the device. Directly fluid coupled intraventricular monitors have found less favor in this setting because of the limited ability to drain CSF and the increased infection risk. Raised pressure within the cranium is not homogeneously distributed, and there may be significant differences between the two sides as well as between the supratentorial and infratentorial compartments. Therefore, ICP measurement may not directly reflect the degree of swelling. In general, the monitor is inserted on the side of the edematous brain.

Neuroimaging

Neuroimaging is invaluable in the intensive care of stroke because the majority of problems are due to hemorrhage, edema, hydrocephalus, and herniation. The major contributor to ischemic brain swelling is the vasogenic component secondary to BBB disruption. Vasogenic edema, as visualized by T2-weighted magnetic resonance imaging (MRI), starts within few hours of stroke onset and progressively increases over hours to days (28,29). Early contrast enhancement on either CT or MRI has been predictive of more severe BBB breakdown and ischemic brain swelling. CT scanning may not demonstrate cerebral infarction for up to 1 day; however, it is of great utility to follow the progression of infarcts.

As mentioned earlier, the degree of horizontal displacement of midline structures has been correlated with depressed consciousness. Pineal calcification is a reliable landmark for this purpose. Lateral pineal shift of 2.5 to 4 mm from the midline (anatomic dimension) is associated with drowsiness, 6 to 9 mm with stupor, and more than 9 mm with coma. A shift of ≥4 mm within 48 hours of ischemic stroke was associated with higher mortality (24,25,30). The degree of lateral shift may be more pronounced in older patients with more brain atrophy (8). Any significant change in a patient's clinical state should prompt repeat CT.

Although techniques to measure CBF are not widely available, it has been shown that profoundly reduced CBF (<15–20 mL/100g/min) predicts the development of edema formation and death from herniation. A number of imaging techniques have been used to determine CBF and the severity of ischemia (31–33). Assessment of CBF in patients with large infarcts with or without increased ICP and tissue shifts carries prognostic value and, when properly obtained, may help direct further medical or surgical therapy. However, most methods to measure CBF are not suitable for frequent or continuous bedside assessment. Several alternative bedside techniques are being studied as surrogates, particularly involving cerebral oxygenation (see later).

Transcranial Doppler

Transcranial Doppler (TCD) ultrasonography allows noninvasive assessment of the intracranial vas-

culature that can be performed repeatedly to diagnose and monitor intracranial stenosis or occlusion (34–36), recanalization after thrombolysis and thrombectomy (37), and hemodynamic changes after carotid endarterectomy or stenting, and to determine the effectiveness of induced hypertension. Using these approaches, one potentially could tailor intravenous or intraarterial thrombolysis in a more sensible manner, and hemorrhagic complications perhaps could be minimized (38). The main TCD finding at the stenosis site is elevated flow velocity, unless the stenosis is very tight, to the degree of pseudoocclusion or preocclusion. Overall, TCD is more sensitive in the assessment of anterior compared to posterior circulation; however, changes in vertebral artery waveform can provide important clues suggesting basilar artery occlusion. TCD can be used as an adjunct to other imaging modalities (e.g., diffusion and perfusion MRI, CT angiography) in the decision to initiate hyperdynamic therapy when critical stenosis and limited collateral perfusion are demonstrated in patients with a large ischemic territory. Furthermore, TCD is useful for monitoring the presence of increased ICP, which reduces end-diastolic velocity (i.e., increased pulsatility index), followed by systolic peaks. In addition, brain death can be confirmed by TCD and is reflected by brief systolic forward flow and zero or reverse diastolic flow, and systolic spikes oscillating with respiratory cycle.

Use of TCD in cerebral ischemia has regained popularity as more recanalization options have become available. Despite its strengths, TCD is highly dependent on personal experience and skill. The use of newer Doppler technologies, such as M-mode, color-coded, contrast-enhanced, and power Doppler ultrasound, will improve the sensitivity and specificity, as well as the examination duration in TCD.

Electrophysiologic Monitoring

Electroencephalography (EEG) and evoked potentials, while potentially valuable as noninvasive measures of brain function, have not found wide use in clinical stroke work. Wave V of the brainstem auditory evoked response has been used to follow midbrain shift and compression and may be used serially to follow degree of shift and pressure on the brainstem in cerebellar infarction or brainstem ischemia from basilar thrombosis (39,40).

Brain Temperature Monitoring

Brain temperature differs from core body temperature in stroke patients (41). It is not clear if monitoring temperature improves management and outcome, except if hypothermia will be used. Temperature elevations increase CBF and ICP. In most instances, all that is required is to measure temperature routinely at 8- to 12-hour intervals and to treat fever fairly aggressively. Most episodes of fever will be related to aspiration pneumonia in stroke, but they also may lead to the detection of deep vein thrombosis (DVT).

Brain Tissue Oxygen Measurement

Brain tissue oxygen measurement using electrochemical methods has been studied in a number of circumstances, particularly head trauma. The electrode is placed intraparenchymally, usually through a single bolt that also provides ports for brain tissue temperature and ICP measurement. The electrode measures oxygen availability rather than the real tissue oxygen partial pressure. Therefore, changes in inspired oxygen level, CPP, CBF, brain temperature and oxygen consumption (such as in hypothermia), hematocrit, and hemoglobin dissociation curve all affect the tissue oxygen reading. In other words, relatively normal readings can be observed in metabolically inactive brain tissue, such as complete infarction. Use of parenchymal oxygen electrodes has not found widespread acceptance in ischemic stroke; however, encouraging case series have been reported (42). The potential applications of this type of monitoring in ischemic stroke and its value in patient care remain to be determined.

Cerebral oximetry using near infrared spectroscopy measures cortical hemoglobin oxygen saturation noninvasively. However, like jugular venous oxygen measurement it has not yet found wide use. The degree of hemoglobin oxygen saturation depends on the balance between oxygen supply and demand. Therefore, just like electrochemical methods, measurements may not be reliable in cases where tissue oxygen consumption is significantly reduced. Moreover, extracerebral blood flow is a limiting factor, and it interferes with CBF estimates. More studies are needed to establish guidelines for its use and interpretation.

Jugular bulb venous oxygen measurements provide an indirect assessment of cerebral oxygen extraction (43). Similar to tissue oxygen measurement, jugular venous oxygen saturation ($SjvO_2$) reflects the balance between cerebral oxygen supply and demand. In cerebral ischemia, $SjvO_2$ (normally ~60%) and oxygen content (normally ~4 μmol/mL) are reduced. The threshold $SjvO_2$ and content, below which chemical signs of oxidative metabolic failure emerge, have been 50% and 3 μmol/mL, respectively. Clinically, confusion has been associated with $SjvO_2 < 45\%$ and unconsciousness with $SjvO_2 < 24\%$. Similarly, EEG changes occur when $SjvO_2$ is reduced to less than 40% (44). In case of elevated ICP due to ischemic edema, jugular bulb venous oxygen measurement may provide an indirect assessment of CPP (45). It has been suggested as an adjunct to induced hyperventilation for elevated ICP. The variations in the pattern of cerebral venous return between the two hemispheres, the dilution of venous return from relatively small ischemic regions, and the possibility of extracerebral contamination of internal jugular flow have limited the usefulness of this technique in focal cerebral ischemia.

TREATMENT OF ISCHEMIC STROKE FROM A NEURO-INTENSIVE CARE UNIT PERSPECTIVE

The ICU management of stroke patients is aimed at restoring or improving cerebral circulation, preventing morbidity due to ischemic brain edema, providing adequate respiratory support with or without mechanical ventilation, and preventing early medical complications of acute stroke. In addition, certain neuroprotective modalities theoretically also reduce ischemic brain edema. Although most of the following treatment recommendations have not been unequivocally shown to be beneficial, they constitute the most rational approach based on available data and our own experience.

MANAGEMENT OF ISCHEMIC BRAIN EDEMA WITH ELEVATED INTRACRANIAL PRESSURE OR TISSUE SHIFTS

This requires an integrated approach between the neurointensivist and the neurosurgeon. Clinical factors take precedence but detailed hemodynamic monitoring, neuroimaging, and ICP monitoring are the main tools guiding management. A number of medical treatment options exist, but none are entirely satisfactory. However, medical reduction of ICP is initiated in patients who become drowsy with brain shift from stroke edema. Recently, decompressive craniectomy has been used early in the process, and its benefit in terms of functional improvement is being actively studied.

Hyperosmolar Agents

Hyperosmolar agents increase serum osmolality, and because they do not appreciably cross the BBB under normal conditions, water follows the osmolar gradient and diffuses out of the brain tissue. Therefore, hyperosmolar agents reduce ICP mainly by dehydrating and shrinking undamaged brain tissue. Experimental data suggest that the degree of reduction in ischemic edema and tissue shift is linearly correlated with total body weight as a reflection of whole body dehydration regardless of the treatment used (i.e., furosemide or mannitol), unless intravascular volume was significantly compromised (46). Hemodilution is the natural consequence of the osmolar gradient produced by these agents and contribute significantly to reduced blood viscosity. In areas where BBB is disrupted, the dehydrating effect is reduced because the hyperosmolar substance diffuses into brain tissue and the gradient is reduced. It has even been suggested that the leakage of dehydrating agents in areas of disrupted BBB might worsen tissue shifts (47). This has never been convincingly demonstrated either experimentally or clinically (48,49). Similarly, "rebound" edema in the infarcted brain has been feared after discontinuation of the hyperosmolar therapy (50), but studies of this phenomenon have given conflicting results (51,52). The clinical relevance of potentially worsening shifts and rebound phenomenon is not clear, but in our experience it has been minimal.

Mannitol is the most commonly used hyperosmolar agent. It decreases ICP and ischemic tissue pressure by multiple mechanisms, including decreased tissue water content and increased CSF absorption (53,54). There are changes in the rheology of blood (mainly a transient reduction in viscosity via altered red blood cell deformability and reduced hematocrit, i.e., hemodilution) that increase CBF and tissue oxygenation (42). This, in turn, causes a compensatory vasoconstriction and reduces cerebral blood volume and ICP rapidly but transiently (55). This appears to be the mechanism of improvement in intracranial compliance and reduction in ICP that occurs even before significant dehydration occurs. The effect of mannitol on ICP appears to be more pronounced when CPP is low and the baseline vessel caliber is already enlarged due to autoregulation (56). Because mannitol is rapidly eliminated by renal clearance, it causes osmotic diuresis and concentration hypernatremia that allows for a longer-lasting brain dehydration. Additional effects of mannitol include transient vasodilation and hypotension, particularly at rapid infusion rates, and increased cardiac output. Mannitol-induced ICP reduction is relatively predictable, but its extent and duration may be small and brief (26).

Interestingly, mannitol has reduced cerebral edema, infarct size, and neurologic deficit in experimental stroke when it is given within 6 hours, suggesting a neuroprotective effect (48,57), probably related to improved CBF, and free radical scavenging action. However, these observations have been inconsistent between models (58). Therefore, the use of early mannitol treatment, before the appearance of brain swelling, is not recommended, even if there is radiographic evidence of vasogenic edema (59).

Mannitol (20% solution) is administered as an initial dose of 1 to 1.5 g/kg (infused over 15 minutes) followed by 0.25 to 0.5 g/kg every 4 to 6 hours as required to keep ICP in the desired range (<20 mm Hg, or CPP > 60 mm Hg) or to effect persistent clinical improvement if possible. The onset of action usually is within minutes, peaking within 1 hour. Serum osmolarity can be used as a guide to the dosage and interval of administration, aiming for 290 to 295 mOsm/L initially but not more than 310 mOsm/L after repeated doses. Serum sodium can be used to gauge the dehydrating effect because it approximates half of serum osmolality. In most units, mannitol is used to treat ischemic brain edema with the goal of a serum sodium of approximately 148 mEq/L or an osmolality of 295 mOsm/L. Depending on local practice, ICP measurements are used to guide the dosing of mannitol. An attempt is made to maintain normal central venous pressure and BP. It should be noted that mannitol induces a diuresis that may reach in volume several times that of mannitol itself; therefore, fluid balance should be followed closely and major deficits need to be corrected using normal saline. If serum osmolality is measured, the sample should be taken well after mannitol has been excreted, typically several hours after administration, or just before the next dose, in order to approximate the degree of static dehydration caused by diuresis (i.e., the contribution of mannitol itself to the measurement should be minimized). Renal insufficiency prolongs the elimination half-life of mannitol; therefore, dose interval should be extended. Mannitol usually is discontinued by a slow taper proportional to the duration of use.

Glycerol is another potent osmotic agent that has been advanced as a putative free radical scavenger and antioxidant. It causes vasodilation and inhibits leukocyte adherence, mechanisms that may block inflammatory reaction and improve CBF (60). However, it lacks the favorable hemodynamic effects of rapid infusion of mannitol. Despite strong supportive evidence from experimental studies, data showing improvement of CBF and energy metabolism in ischemic territories in human stroke, and a benefit in terms of mortality, neurologic status, or activities of daily living in a few small studies, controlled clinical trials have not demonstrated a benefit over placebo in stroke outcome (61,62). It is favored more often in Europe and has several side effects, including fluid overload, hemolysis (particularly upon rapid infusion), electrolyte disturbance, hypotension due to dehydration (less than mannitol), and occasionally nausea, vomiting, diarrhea, hemoglobinuria, and bleeding diathesis. Glycerol can be used at 0.25 to 1.5 g/kg every 6 hours enterally (50%) or intravenously via central line (10%). Oral administration often is well tolerated. Glucose intake can be lowered during glycerol treatment.

Hypertonic saline (3%–23.4%) induces a shift of water from extravascular to intravascular compartment. Although there are no conclusive data, it effectively lowers ICP in stroke (63). It probably should be reserved until mannitol proves ineffective. *Hydroxyethylstarch,* an agent favored for its ostensible hemodilution effect when used in conjunction with hypertonic saline, may be more effective and quicker in action compared to mannitol in reducing ICP in patients with large strokes.

Albumin (0.63–2.5 g/kg) has reduced ischemic brain edema, diffusion-weighted imaging (DWI) changes, and infarct size, and improved functional status, in experimental cerebral ischemia (64). It raises the plasma oncotic pressure and simply may act as a hyperosmolar agent. Additional mechanisms of action may partly involve improved CBF to the ischemic brain, possibly as a result of a significant hemodilution (hematocrit around 28%) and due to free radical scavenging action. Albumin has a significantly longer half-life (2–3 weeks) compared to other hyperosmolar agents. In the clinical setting, albumin has reduced edema associated with trauma and intracerebral hemorrhage; however, data supporting its use in stroke are lacking.

Loop Diuretics

Loop diuretics (e.g., furosemide 10–80 mg) can be added to the treatment regimen to potentiate mannitol's dehydrating effect (65). They also can be used independently to achieve hyperosmolality and a degree of brain shrinkage. Their effect may be due in part to reduced CSF formation. In patients with large strokes, fluid and electrolyte status must be monitored closely during mannitol and/or diuretic therapy, because dehydration that is pronounced enough to cause hypotension worsens brain tissue perfusion, whereas fluid overload may predispose to further brain edema or cardiovascular failure. Routine fluid restriction is not used during osmotic or loop diuretic treatment but sources of free water are avoided. A state of euvolemic hyperosmolality is most desirable.

Hyperventilation

Hyperventilation causes cerebral vasoconstriction and reduces ICP. The effect reaches a peak in less than 1 hour and disappears after several hours. Hyperventilation reduces $Sjvo_2$; therefore, theoretically it may exacerbate ischemia through vasoconstriction, but this has not been shown to be a clinically important factor. Nonetheless, its brief duration of action makes it useful only to gain time until a more definitive treatment such as hemicraniectomy is instituted. Reducing Pco_2 to about 30 mm Hg by increasing the minute ventilation reduces the ICP by about 25%, but abrupt discontinuation causes rebound vasodilation (66). Continuous mandatory ventilation mode is suitable. Attempts to prolong its effect by the use of ammonium buffers (tromethamine, THAM) have been variably successful in head injury (67). Because of its potential side effects, which include hypotension, barotrauma, hypokalemia, and short duration of action, hyperventilation should be used judiciously as an emergency approach.

Hypothermia

Just as fever increases cerebral metabolism and ischemic damage, hypothermia may have a protective effect. It increases the resistance of brain to ischemia due to slower metabolism and oxygen consumption, and it prolongs the survival of penumbra until more blood flow is reinstituted either spontaneously via collaterals or by therapeutic measures such as tissue plasminogen activator (tPA) or interventional procedures. Hypothermia reduces cerebral metabolic rate, CBF, and volume. Furthermore, it reduces ICP and prevents BBB disruption and edema formation after ischemia. Moderate hypothermia (33°C) in large MCA strokes has reduced ICP and mortality, but the effect on ischemic edema formation and long-term functional outcome has not been tested. The reduction in CBF is less than that expected from the reduced metabolic rate, so there may actually be luxury perfusion. Hypothermia is protective in elevated ICP due to traumatic brain injury (68) and in experimental stroke; however, its feasibility and benefit in human stroke with brain swelling are being investigated. Experimental data are compelling. Brain cooling, cooling blanket sandwich, gastric ice-cold saline lavage, peritoneal dialysis, extracorporeal circulation, intravascular cooling devices, and pharmacologic manipulation of temperature regulating systems all are available tools to induce hypothermia. Rewarming has been associated with a rebound increase in ICP and should be slow over greater than 12 hours (<0.5°C/h) (69). Brain may be significantly warmer when the body is hypothermic; therefore, brain temperature recording may be needed.

Sedation, Pain Control, and Neuromuscular Blockade

Sedation, pain control, and neuromuscular blockade often are required in patients with impaired communication or altered sensorium. Pain and irritation increase intrathoracic pressure and impede cerebral venous return. Sedation reduces sympathetic overactivation, increases cooperation to procedures and nursing care, provides pain relief, reduces fighting the ventilator, and, when appropriate drugs are chosen, reduces cerebral metabolism and ICP. However, it also masks valuable neurologic examination. Hypotension is a frequent side effect, particularly with barbiturates; therefore, it is important to assess fluid status before using these drugs. If the patient is hypovolemic, serious hypotension may develop. Other undesirable side effects include gastrointestinal hypomotility, delay in tolerating enteral feeding, and reduced respiratory drive. Therefore, before instituting sedation one must rule out treatable causes of agitation (e.g., infection, hypercapnia, hypoxia, heart failure, myocardial ischemia, acidosis, metabolic derangement). Intermittent sedation is better than continuous sedation because it provides a window of opportunity for neurologic assessment. Short-acting drugs such as midazolam (initial 1–5 mg, infusion 0.05–0.1 mg/kg/h), fentanyl (50–100 μg/min), thiopental (initial 25–100 mg, infusion 2–3 mg/kg/h), or propofol (initial 10–20 mg, infusion 0.6–6 mg/kg/h), often are preferred over those with longer duration of action, including lorazepam (1–2 mg), morphine (2–7 mg), and droperidol (1–5 mg).

The process of intubation causes a surge of sympathetic activity and may increase ICP. For this reason, proper sedation and analgesia must be instituted before intubation and care must be taken in the choice of the anesthetic because some also raise ICP. Etomidate (0.3 mg/kg) or propofol (1–3 mg/kg) are commonly used along with neuromuscular blockade to premedicate the patient before intubation. Both drugs cause transient hypotension. The duration of action of propofol is quite short; however, recovery may be delayed in case of prolonged uninterrupted use.

Propofol infusion may be continued after intubation to prevent agitation and "bucking" the ventilator.

Neuromuscular blockade helps prevent the increases in intrathoracic pressure during suctioning and coughing, which prevents subsequent decrease in cerebral venous return and increase in ICP. Succinylcholine (1.2 mg/kg), a depolarizing neuromuscular blocker, or vecuronium (10 μg/h), a nondepolarizing neuromuscular blocker with minimal histamine release or ganglionic blockade, are commonly used. Nondepolarizing agents may be preferred because they do not carry the risk of inducing muscle fasciculations or increasing intrathoracic and ICPs. Short-acting neuromuscular blockers can be used to transiently relax the patient during interventions such as suctioning; however, sufficient sedation must be provided. Long-term use of neuromuscular blockade may increase the risk for critical illness myopathy (69a).

Therapeutic Pharmacologic Central Nervous System Suppression

Barbiturate coma has been used in an attempt to reduce elevated ICP in patients with large ischemic strokes and swelling (70,71). Barbiturates reduce cerebral metabolic rate, blood flow, and blood volume, and have free radical scavenging properties. Although they induce an often unsustained reduction in ICP (70,72), they also cause systemic hypotension; therefore, the effect on CPP is unpredictable. Overall, barbiturates are of limited efficacy and have serious adverse effects, including increased infection rate and reduced cardiac contractility. Pentobarbital is the most commonly used barbiturate. The depth of barbiturate coma should be titrated to achieve the desired ICP reduction, or a burst suppression pattern on continuously monitored EEG. *Propofol* is an ultra-short-acting pure sedative/hypnotic, acting possibly on $GABA_A$ (γ-aminobutyric acid) receptor α-subunit (73). It reduces cerebral metabolic rate, CBF, and ICP; however, it also reduces systemic vascular resistance and causes hypotension.

Indomethacin

Indomethacin (50 mg intravenously) lowers ICP and has been reported to improve CPP in stroke (74). Repeated doses continue to be effective after other medical therapies fail. It also reduces edema after experimental unilateral carotid occlusion (75). Indomethacin, however, is a cerebral vasoconstrictor and may reduce CBF in stroke. It has not been clinically tested beyond case reports.

Corticosteroids

Corticosteroids have not improved outcome in ischemic edema, but they have increased infection rate and the incidence of diabetic hyperglycemia (76).

Decompressive Craniectomy

The relative ineffectiveness of medical management of ischemic brain edema has led to a reconsideration of various forms of decompressive surgery. This subject is covered in other chapters in this book and only a few comments are made here. In the specific cases of large cerebellar infarction with edema and cerebellar hemorrhage, surgical decompression by suboccipital craniectomy has become a standard treatment, especially if there is hydrocephalus and a progressive decline in the level of alertness (77). Ventricular drainage provides a temporary means of reducing ICP in patients who have hydrocephalus and in patients who are not surgical candidates. Early hemicraniectomy in large anterior circulation strokes before the development of clinical or radiologic signs of transtentorial herniation and horizontal shift apparently has been more effective in reducing mortality and improving functional outcome (78). The duration of neuro-ICU stay also was shorter, suggesting that early surgical intervention is advisable. The outcome after hemicraniectomy has been worse in older individuals (79). Younger patients with nondominant hemisphere infarction and higher risk for life-threatening ischemic edema appear to benefit most from early hemicraniectomy. However, the association of younger age with a better outcome holds true even without a hemicraniectomy. There is little question that hemicraniectomy effectively prevents death from malignant MCA stroke; however, the functional outcome has been highly variable. Patients often remain dependent on their families for care, and many have had mood disturbances. Therefore, better definition of patient selection and the timing of surgery is needed (80).

HEMODYNAMIC MANAGEMENT OF THE ACUTE STROKE PATIENT

There is considerable controversy as to whether hypertension should be treated in acute ischemic stroke. Autoregulation is impaired in ischemic brain. Antihypertensive agents can cause more than the degree of desired hypotension and thereby critically compromise penumbral CBF (81), especially in patients with intracranial or extracranial stenoses.

TABLE 43-3. *Approach to induced hypertension, hypervolemia, and hemodilution therapy*

Mean arterial pressure 120–130 mm Hg
Central venous pressure 10–12 mm Hg
Pulmonary capillary wedge pressure 14–18 mm Hg
Cardiac index 3.5–4.5 $L/min/m^2$
Hematocrit 30%–33%
Positive fluid balance, no body weight loss

Conversely, uncontrolled hypertension promotes ischemic brain edema. Some of the therapeutic hemodynamic targets are listed in Table 43-3.

The Hypotensive Patient

Volume replacement is the mainstay with saline, hydroxyethyl starch, or albumin. Most often, stroke patients are dehydrated and benefit from fluid replacement. However, this should be done cautiously in elderly people with potentially low ejection fraction or low creatinine clearance. In patients with good cardiac reserve, hydration can be maintained with isotonic solutions such as 0.9% NaCl. This approach decreases blood viscosity and prevents hypoosmolality. In patients at high risk of developing ischemic cerebral edema, hypotonic solutions and overhydration must be avoided.

The Hypertensive Patient

Most stroke patients are hypertensive in the acute phase, and BP gradually returns to baseline over the next 48 hours (82). The common practice is not to treat hypertension unless mean arterial pressure is above 130 to 140 mm Hg, systolic pressure is more than 200 mm Hg, or diastolic pressure is higher than 110 mm Hg, which itself is a matter of debate (82,83). The optimum BP range seems to be 160–180/90–100 mm Hg; however, these values must be individualized for every patient. For example, if there is no diffusion-perfusion mismatch or there is significant ischemic brain edema or hemorrhage, a lower mean arterial pressure (<100–120 mm Hg) may be targeted; however, care must be given not to critically reduce CPP in patients with concomitant raised ICP. Conversely, in patients with a history of hypertension, higher BP values may be acceptable. Therefore, declaring a general target BP value does little to improve management because most often it is difficult to determine the optimum BP in any given patient. TCD and tissue oxygen monitoring provide valuable information on CBF and may be useful to guide BP management.

In patients who have undergone thrombolysis, systolic BP must be kept below 185 mm Hg based on current protocols (84). The choice of the ideal antihypertensive is not settled (81,83,85). Most units have used labetalol, a potent α_1- and nonselective β-blocker that does not significantly alter ICP (86) (20 mg intravenous bolus repeated every 5–10 minutes up to a total 300 mg/d, changed to oral dosing once desired BP reduction is achieved). Angiotensin-converting enzyme or receptor inhibitors preserve cerebral autoregulation at low BPs (87) and have improved cerebral edema in a number of experimental models (88). Nitrates and their derivatives (e.g., nitroglycerin, sodium nitroprusside) are potent vasodilators that carry the risk of increasing ICP and may precipitate hypotension in untrained hands. They dilate cerebral vessels and peripheral circulation and increase cerebral blood volume, for which reason they are generally avoided if there is stroke edema (89). They also may increase BBB permeability (90).

Some calcium channel blockers exacerbate increased ICP in humans and ischemic brain edema in rats and cats (91). We currently do not include calcium channel blockers in the antihypertensive regimen in acute stroke with brain edema. In Europe, nifedipine, urapidil, and clonidine have been used for isolated systolic hypertension (>220), whereas nitroglycerine and nitroprusside have been spared for more severe hypertension or isolated diastolic hypertension (92).

Therapeutic-Induced Hypertension

Neurologic improvement has been observed with induced hypertension in experimental stroke models (93,94). Preliminary data in humans have been encouraging but not confirmed (95). BP is maintained within the plateau segment of the normal autoregulatory curve; however, autoregulation is impaired in ischemic brain and even moderate hypertension may worsen ischemic brain edema. In acute stroke, higher BPs on admission were associated with higher mortality rates (96). A 20% to 30% drop in BP on the second day after stroke has been associated with better odds of recovery and less brain edema on CT (97). Similarly, a 15% drop in systolic BP within 24 hours of intravenous tPA treatment was not associated with neurologic worsening in the European Cooperative Acute Stroke Study I (ECASS-I) (18). There is some experimental support for a detrimental

effect of elevated BP on ischemic edema formation (98,99). Therefore, induced hypertension in an attempt to improve CBF in acute stroke is controversial. It is only recommended if there is a perfusion-diffusion mismatch on MRI or if there is BP-dependent fluctuation of deficits.

Hemodilution

A reduction in hematocrit lowers blood viscosity, which is an important parameter in cerebrovascular resistance. The oxygen delivery to the normal tissues remains almost constant between a hematocrit of 30% and 40%. Whether this relationship holds true in ischemic brain is not known; therefore, hematocrit goal in hemodilution should be 30% to 33%. In order to improve microcirculation, hemodilution has been used in various settings, but the results of trials have been variable and as yet there is no conclusive evidence that it is helpful (100). The effects of hemodilution on ischemic cerebral edema are not known. Although there are some supportive experimental data, it has not been beneficial in the treatment of stroke overall. When hemodilution is combined with hypertensive hypervolemia, the results, although preliminary, have been more encouraging.

RESPIRATORY MANAGEMENT

Airway management is of utmost importance to prevent respiratory complications in stroke patients with bihemispheric or brainstem strokes, or depressed level of alertness. Aspiration is a major cause of morbidity and mortality. Oral feeding or hydration should be avoided until the patient is awake and cooperative, is able to swallow liquids without coughing or choking, and can cough upon command. Elevating the head of the bed helps reduce aspiration. Pulmonary toilet and chest physical therapy should be part of daily management, unless there are concerns regarding elevated ICP and patient irritation. Aspiration pneumonia should be suspected in those with progressive hypoxemia, fever, productive cough, or increased pulmonary secretions. The details of treatment of aspiration pneumonia can be found elsewhere.

Mechanical Ventilation

Six percent of all acute strokes and 24% of those admitted to a neuro-ICU have required intubation and mechanical ventilation with a latency of about 30 hours after the onset (101,102). About half of the patients were intubated upon presentation (101). The most common indication for intubation was depressed level of consciousness (80%–90%), followed by cardiopulmonary failure and bulbar dysfunction (101,103). Glasgow Coma Scale (GCS) <10 has been suggested as an indication for intubation. This often is due to ischemic brain edema and tissue shifts. Brainstem strokes often are associated with abnormal breathing patterns such as ataxic or apneustic breathing, which carry a high risk of progression to apnea. In this regard, the indications for intubation in patients with stroke differ from other neurologic illnesses, such as neuromuscular failure, where the main culprit is compromised respiratory effort, as opposed to central respiratory drive and the ability to protect airway (Table 43-4). Hyperpnea often is due to the patient's attempt to autohyperventilate as a reflection of increased ICP. Therefore, tachypnea without hyperpnea more likely is a sign of respiratory compromise (mainly pneumonia), exhaustion of respiratory effort, and impending failure.

The synchronized intermittent mandatory ventilation mode is used most often, with a tidal volume of 7–10 mL/kg, inspiratory-to-expiratory ratio 1:3, fraction of inspired oxygen initially 100% then reduced rapidly to maintain a SaO_2 of more than 95%, and respiratory rate adjusted to keep PCO_2 40 to 50 mm Hg (unless there is elevated ICP). It should be pointed out that the need for intubation does not necessarily mean a need for mechanical ventilation, and patients with intact central respiratory drive but poor airway protection often do well with pressure support ventilation alone. Application of positive end-expiratory pressure (PEEP) has been considered to reduce cerebral venous return and increase ICP, although this relationship is inconstant and largely obviated by raising the patient's head to facilitate cerebral venous drainage (104). Weaning the ventilator may begin once a patient regains a sufficient level of consciousness. Tracheostomy is needed in those who are expected to remain intubated (either a prolonged comatose state, or failed weaning) for more than 2 to 3 weeks, particularly in vertebrobasilar occlusion with apnea.

Neurogenic Pulmonary Edema

Neurogenic pulmonary edema deserves mention, although it is not common after stroke. Certain infarcts, such as those in the medulla, may produce this problem. It is thought to be related to a massive sympathetic discharge causing pulmonary vascular endothelial damage and increased leakiness. Myocardial overload and damage due to increased peripheral vascular resistance may contribute (105). It develops rapidly within a few hours and causes diffuse bilateral pulmonary infiltrates. It is differentiated from purely cardiogenic pulmonary edema by low pulmonary capillary wedge pressures. Neurogenic pulmonary edema is rapidly responsive to mechanical ventilation with PEEP usually at 10 cm H_2O.

GENERAL MEDICAL MEASURES AND PRACTICAL ISSUES
Electrolyte Imbalance

Syndrome of inappropriate antidiuretic hormone secretion (SIADH) causing persistent hyponatremia is relatively common, especially after large strokes with edema and tissue shifts. The main therapeutic measure in SIADH is fluid restriction, which may not be well advised in the acute stages of stroke. If there is ischemic brain edema one needs to be more aggressive in correcting the hyponatremia, possibly by hypertonic saline and furosemide therapy. However, generally stated guidelines regarding the rate of correction should be followed strictly in order to avoid

TABLE 43-4. *Indications for mechanical ventilation in stroke*

Depressed level of consciousness with poor airway protection/aspiration (e.g., brain edema and/or seizure)
Absent gag reflex (brainstem ischemia or shift, or reduced level of consciousness)
PO_2 <60, PCO_2 >50–60 (or 10–20 mm Hg above baseline)
Vital capacity <800–1,000 mL, negative inspiratory force <25 cm H_2O
Tachypnea >30/min or accessory respiratory muscle use
Absent respiratory drive (e.g., vertebrobasilar ischemia)
Apneustic, agonal, Cheyne-Stokes breathing seen in large middle cerebral artery or posterior circulation ischemia and strokes
Concurrent severe cardiopulmonary disease
Reduced respiratory muscle strength
Airway obstruction
Extreme agitation or the need for deep sedation, such as for procedures
Induced hyperventilation

central pontine myelinolysis. *Cerebral salt wasting* is seen more often in the setting of subarachnoid hemorrhage and should be differentiated from SIADH.

Magnesium is an *N*-methyl-D-aspartate (NMDA) receptor antagonist and augments vascular smooth muscle relaxation and vasodilation. Hypomagnesemia can be deleterious in acute stroke (106) by reducing the excitability threshold of brain tissue. Routine magnesium supplementation to keep its level above 2.0 to 2.5 carries virtually no risk. It can be recommended as a standard component of treatment although it often is not implemented (107). Hyperglycemia can be a side effect of magnesium treatment.

Fever

Fever within first 7 days has been predictive of larger infarcts and poor outcome in stroke (108). There are many sources of fever in the ICU setting. Atelectasis can be a source of fever and is better avoided by sighs in mechanically ventilated patients, or spirometer exercises in nonintubated cooperative patients. Aspiration pneumonia and sinusitis are common, the latter particularly when a nasogastric tube is placed. Urinary tract infection is very common, especially in patients with an indwelling catheter. Stroke by itself also raises body temperature. Therefore, an underlying source for fever must be investigated and treated if found. Fever must be promptly treated by cooling blankets, wet wraps, antipyretics, and, in resistant cases, by intravascular cooling devices. We use antipyretics around the clock unless temperature is ≤37°C. Chills and shivering can be important causes of ICP elevation by triggering plateau waves.

Deep Vein Thrombosis Prophylaxis

Deep vein thrombosis (DVT) is a common problem in bedridden patients after stroke. Calf tenderness often is associated. PE was a very frequent cause of mortality in the past; however, awareness of complications of immobilization has reduced its incidence. PE often presents with dyspnea, tachypnea, arterial oxygen desaturation, and pleuritic-type chest pain, and it carries a mortality of 50% (109). Heparin (5,000 units subcutaneously two or three times a day), pneumatic boots, elastic stockings, physical therapy, and early ambulation all are helpful in preventing DVT and subsequent PE. Lower-extremity Doppler ultrasonography is useful to rule out DVT and ventilation-perfusion lung scan or contrast-enhanced chest CT to rule out PE. If there is PE then anticoagulation with intravenous heparin is indicated but an inferior vena cava filter can be used if anticoagulation is contraindicated. It is imperative to watch for heparin-induced thrombocytopenia (HIT). All heparin and similar agents should be stopped and HIT antibodies checked if platelet count drops by 25% to 30% from baseline or if the count is less than 100,000. Argatroban or recombinant hirudin, which are direct thrombin inhibitors, can be used safely in these patients.

Hyperglycemia

Hyperglycemia and chronic diabetes are associated with larger infarcts, and fasting hypoglycemia with smaller infarcts in experimental models (110,111). Hyperglycemia on admission or a history of diabetes appears to worsen stroke outcome in humans (112,113). Results of studies have been inconsistent; some showed no effect of admission glucose on outcome (114). Mechanism of worsening may be aggravation of lactic acidosis in ischemic areas. Optimal blood glucose probably is less than 130 mg/dL. It should be pointed out that the adrenergic activation in the acute setting may increase blood sugar level even in nondiabetics. The principles of *feeding and nutrition* are similar to general ICU patients; however, particular care must be taken not to induce hyperglycemia.

Systemic Complications of Stroke

Systemic complications of stroke include infections, myocardial infarction, and atrial or ventricular arrhythmias (115). Repolarization abnormalities are common, and myocardial infarction may be present in up to 10% of stroke patients. It may be the cause of stroke, such as in akinetic thrombogenic wall, or the result of stroke (e.g., increased catecholamine release and hypercoagulable state with increased fibrinogen production) (116).

PROGNOSIS AND END-OF-LIFE ISSUES IN STROKE PATIENTS ADMITTED TO NEURO-INTENSIVE CARE UNIT

Predictive Factors

Stroke size, but not the mechanism, has been predictive of mortality (108). Mortality has been significantly more common in stroke patients with depressed level of consciousness, many of whom become intubated. Male gender and absent pupillary reflexes were predictive of mortality in one study (101). Elevated serum creatinine (1.9 vs. 1 mg/100 mL) has not only been a risk factor for having stroke but also predictive of increased mortality (108). Elevated white blood cell count can be the cause or the result of a larger stroke and poor outcome.

The influence of endotracheal intubation on stroke patients has been the subject of several studies. The short-term mortality among intubated patients had ranged from 50% to 80% and long-term mortality up to 90% (101,102,108,117–119). Patients intubated electively appeared to have better prognosis than those intubated for neurologic deterioration, GCS <10 at the time of intubation, and age older than 65 years have been predictive of mortality within 2 months and poor long-term functional outcome (103,108,119). Patients with GCS ≥12 appeared to have a higher 30-day survival and better outcome measured by the Barthel index (103). The poor prognosis of intubated stroke patients is closely related to the severity of underlying disorder. Whether intubation improves the outcome cannot be stated confidently. In particular, patients with basilar occlusion requiring intubation after apneic episodes carry a grim prognosis (118). A small proportion of patients have been reported to have a good outcome after surviving a large hemispheric stroke and intubation. The decision for intubation and the overall level of care depend on the generally estimated prognosis of a particular patient as well as the patient's, and if this information is not available the family's, wishes. In a previous study, approximately 50% of patients have been labeled "do-not-resuscitate" after stroke, and 50% said they would agree to reintubation if it is necessary (103).

ACKNOWLEDGMENT

The authors thank Dr. M. Akif Topçuoglu for critical review of this manuscript.

REFERENCES

1. Stroke Unit Trialists' Collaboration. Organised inpatient (stroke unit) care for stroke: Stroke Unit Trialists' Collaboration. *Cochrane Database Syst Rev* 2000; issue 4.
2. Jørgensen HS, Kammersgaard LP, Nakayama H, et al. Treatment and rehabilitation on a stroke unit improves 5-year survival: a community-based study. *Stroke* 1999;30:930–933.
3. Ropper AH, Shafran B. Brain edema after stroke. Clinical syndrome and intracranial pressure. *Arch Neurol* 1984;41:26–29.
4. Silver FL, Norris JW, Lewis AJ, et al. Early mortality following stroke: a prospective review. *Stroke* 1984;15: 492–496.
5. Moulin DE, Lo R, Chiang J, et al. Prognosis in middle cerebral artery occlusion. *Stroke* 1985;16:282–284.
6. Hacke W, Schwab S, Horn M, et al. "Malignant" middle cerebral artery territory infarction: clinical course and prognostic signs. *Arch Neurol* 1996;53:309–315.
7. Berrouschot J, Sterker M, Bettin S, et al. Mortality of space-occupying ("malignant") middle cerebral artery infarction under conservative intensive care. *Intensive Care Med* 1998;24:620–623.
8. Wijdicks EFM, Diringer MN. Middle cerebral artery territory infarction and early brain swelling: progression and effect of age on outcome. *Mayo Clin Proc* 1998;73:829–836.
9. Steiger HJ. Outcome of acute supratentorial cerebral infarction in patients under 60. Development of a prognostic grading system. *Acta Neurochir* 1991;111: 73–79.
10. Krieger DW, Demchuk AM, Kasner SE, et al. Early clinical and radiological predictors of fatal brain swelling in ischemic stroke. *Stroke* 1999;30:287–292.
11. Toni D, Fiorelli M, Gentile M, et al. Progressing neurological deficit secondary to acute ischemic stroke. A study on predictability, pathogenesis, and prognosis. *Arch Neurol* 1995;52:670–675.
12. Chambers BR, Norris JW, Shurvell BL, et al. Prognosis of acute stroke. *Neurology* 1987;37:221–225.
13. von Kummer R, Meyding-Lamade U, Forsting M, et al. Sensitivity and prognostic value of early CT in occlusion of the middle cerebral artery trunk. *AJNR Am J Neuroradiol* 1994;15:9–15.
14. Moulin T, Cattin F, Crepin-Leblond T, et al. Early CT signs in acute middle cerebral artery infarction: predictive value for subsequent infarct locations and outcome. *Neurology* 1996;47:366–375.
15. von Kummer R, Bourquain H, Bastianello S, et al. Early prediction of irreversible brain damage after ischemic stroke at CT. *Radiology* 2001;219:95–100.
16. Pessin MS, Estol CJ, Lafranchise F, et al. Safety of anticoagulation after hemorrhagic infarction. *Neurology* 1993;43:1298–1303.
17. Motto C, Ciccone A, Aritzu E, et al. Hemorrhage after an acute ischemic stroke. MAST-I Collaborative Group. *Stroke* 1999;30:761–764.
18. Davalos A, Toni D, Iweins F, et al. Neurological deterioration in acute ischemic stroke: potential predictors and associated factors in the European Cooperative Acute Stroke Study (ECASS) I. *Stroke* 1999;30: 2631–2636.
19. Hacke W, Kaste M, Fieschi C, et al. Intravenous thrombolysis with recombinant tissue plasminogen activator for acute hemispheric stroke. The European Cooperative Acute Stroke Study (ECASS). *JAMA* 1995;274:1017–1025.
20. von Kummer R, Holle R, Rosin L, et al. Does arterial recanalization improve outcome in carotid territory stroke? *Stroke* 1995;26:581–587.
21. Rudolf J, Grond M, Stenzel C, et al. Incidence of space-occupying brain edema following systemic thrombolysis of acute supratentorial ischemia. *Cerebrovasc Dis* 1998;8:166–171.
22. Schwab S, Aschoff A, Spranger M, et al. The value of intracranial pressure monitoring in acute hemispheric stroke. *Neurology* 1996;47:393–398.
23. Frank JI. Large hemispheric infarction, deterioration, and intracranial pressure. *Neurology* 1995;45: 1286–1290.
24. Ropper AH. Lateral displacement of the brain and

level of consciousness in patients with an acute hemispheral mass. *N Engl J Med* 1986;314:953–958.

25. Ropper AH. A preliminary MRI study of the geometry of brain displacement and level of consciousness with acute intracranial masses. *Neurology* 1989;39: 622–627.

26. Schwab S, Schellinger P, Aschoff A, et al. Epidural cerebrospinal fluid pressure measurement and therapy of intracranial hypertension in "malignant" middle cerebral artery infarct. *Nervenarzt* 1996;67: 659–666.

27. Ropper AH. *Neurological and neurosurgical intensive care,* 3rd ed. New York: Raven Press, 1993.

28. Loubinoux I, Volk A, Borredon J, et al. Spreading of vasogenic edema and cytotoxic edema assessed by quantitative diffusion and T2 magnetic resonance imaging. *Stroke* 1997;28:419–426.

29. Neumann-Haefelin T, Moseley ME, et al. New magnetic resonance imaging methods for cerebrovascular disease: emerging clinical applications. *Ann Neurol* 2000;47:559–570.

30. Pullicino PM, Alexandrov AV, Shelton JA, et al. Mass effect and death from severe acute stroke. *Neurology* 1997;49:1090–1095.

31. Hanson SK, Grotta JC, Rhoades H, et al. Value of single-photon emission-computed tomography in acute stroke therapeutic trials. *Stroke* 1993;24:1322–1329.

32. Berrouschot J, Barthel H, von Kummer R, et al. 99m technetium-ethyl-cysteinate-dimer single-photon emission CT can predict fatal ischemic brain edema. *Stroke* 1998;29:2556–2562.

33. Firlik AD, Yonas H, Kaufmann AM, et al. Relationship between cerebral blood flow and the development of swelling and life-threatening herniation in acute ischemic stroke. *J Neurosurg* 1998;89:243–249.

34. Lindegaard KF, Bakke SJ, Aaslid R, et al. Doppler diagnosis of intracranial artery occlusive disorders. *J Neurol Neurosurg Psychiatry* 1986;49:510–518.

35. Alexandrov AV, Demchuk AM, Wein TH, et al. Yield of transcranial Doppler in acute cerebral ischemia. *Stroke* 1999;30:1604–1609.

36. Demchuk AM, Christou I, Wein TH, et al. Specific transcranial Doppler flow findings related to the presence and site of arterial occlusion. *Stroke* 2000:31: 140–146.

37. Demchuk AM, Burgin WS, Christou I, et al. Thrombolysis in brain ischemia (TIBI) transcranial Doppler flow grades predict clinical severity, early recovery, and mortality in patients treated with intravenous tissue plasminogen activator. *Stroke* 2001;32:89–93.

38. Christou I, Alexandrov AV, Burgin WS, et al. Timing of recanalization after tissue plasminogen activator therapy determined by transcranial doppler correlates with clinical recovery from ischemic stroke. *Stroke* 2000; 31:1812–1816.

39. Krieger D, Adams HP, Rieke K, et al. Monitoring therapeutic efficacy of decompressive craniotomy in space occupying cerebellar infarcts using brain-stem auditory evoked potentials. *Electroencephalogr Clin Neurophysiol* 1993;88:261–270.

40. Krieger D, Adams HP, Rieke K, et al. Prospective evaluation of the prognostic significance of evoked potentials in acute basilar occlusion. *Crit Care Med* 1993; 21:1169–1174.

41. Schwab S, Spranger M, Aschoff A, et al. Brain temperature monitoring and modulation in patients with severe MCA infarction. *Neurology* 1997;48:762–767.

42. Steiner T, Pilz J, Schellinger P, et al. Multimodal online monitoring in middle cerebral artery territory stroke. *Stroke* 2001;32:2500–2506.

43. Feldman Z, Robertson CS. Monitoring of cerebral hemodynamics with jugular bulb catheters. *Crit Care Clin* 1997;13:51–77.

44. Meyer JS, Gotoh F, Ebihara S, et al. Effects of anoxia on cerebral metabolism and electrolytes in man. *Neurology* 1965;15:892–901.

45. Cruz J. The first decade of continuous monitoring of jugular bulb oxyhemoglobin saturation: management strategies and clinical outcome. *Crit Care Med* 1998; 26:344–351.

46. Paczynski RP, Venkatesan R, Diringer MN, et al. Effects of fluid management on edema volume and midline shift in a rat model of ischemic stroke. *Stroke* 2000;31:1702–1708.

47. Kaufmann AM, Cardoso ER. Aggravation of vasogenic cerebral edema by multiple-dose mannitol. *J Neurosurg* 1992;77:584–589.

48. Paczynski RP, He YY, Diringer MN, et al. Multiple-dose mannitol reduces brain water content in a rat model of cortical infarction. *Stroke* 1997;28: 1437–1443.

49. Manno EM, Adams RE, Derdeyn CP, et al. The effects of mannitol on cerebral edema after large hemispheric cerebral infarct. *Neurology* 1999;52:583–587.

50. Node Y, Nakazawa S. Clinical study of mannitol and glycerol on raised intracranial pressure and on their rebound phenomenon. *Adv Neurol* 1990;52:359–363.

51. Troupp H, Valtonen S, Vapalahti M. Intraventricular pressure after administration of dehydrating agents to severely brain-injured patients: is there a rebound phenomenon? *Acta Neurochir* 1971;24:89–95.

52. Kofke WA. Mannitol: potential for rebound intracranial hypertension? *J Neurosurg Anesthesiol* 1993;5: 1–3.

53. Cloyd JC, Snyder BD, Cleeremans B, et al. Mannitol pharmacokinetics and serum osmolality in dogs and humans. *J Pharmacol Exp Ther* 1986;236:301–306.

54. Andrews RJ, Bringas JR, Muto RP. Effects of mannitol on cerebral blood flow, blood pressure, blood viscosity, hematocrit, sodium, and potassium. *Surg Neurol* 1993;39:218–222.

55. Muizelaar JP, Wei EP, Kontos HA, et al. Mannitol causes compensatory cerebral vasoconstriction and vasodilation in response to blood viscosity changes. *J Neurosurg* 1983;59:822–828.

56. Rosner MJ, Coley I. Cerebral perfusion pressure: a hemodynamic mechanism of mannitol and the post-mannitol hemogram. *Neurosurgery* 1987;21:147–156.

57. Kobayashi H, Ide H, Kodera T, et al. Effect of mannitol on focal cerebral ischemia evaluated by magnetic resonance imaging. *Acta Neurochir Suppl* 1994;60: 228–230.

58. Pena H, Gaines C, Suess D, et al. Effect of mannitol on experimental focal ischemia in awake monkeys. *Neurosurgery* 1982;11:477–481.

59. Adams HP, Brott TG, Crowell RM, et al. Guidelines for the management of patients with acute ischemic stroke. A statement for healthcare professionals from a special writing group of the Stroke Council, American Heart Association. *Circulation* 1994;90:1588–1601.

60. Frank MS, Nahata MC, Hilty MD. Glycerol: a review of its pharmacology, pharmacokinetics, adverse reactions, and clinical use. *Pharmacotherapy* 1981;1: 147–160.

61. Bayer AJ, Pathy MS, Newcombe R. Double-blind randomised trial of intravenous glycerol in acute stroke. *Lancet* 1987;1:405–408.

62. Yu YL, Kumana CR, Lauder IJ, et al. Treatment of acute cortical infarct with intravenous glycerol. A double-blind, placebo-controlled randomized trial. *Stroke* 1993;24:1119–1124.

63. Schwarz S, Schwab S, Bertram M, et al. Effects of hypertonic saline hydroxyethyl starch solution and mannitol in patients with increased intracranial pressure after stroke. *Stroke* 1998;29:1550–1555.

64. Belayev L, Liu Y, Zhao W, et al. Human albumin therapy of acute ischemic stroke: marked neuroprotective efficacy at moderate doses and with a broad therapeutic window. *Stroke* 2001;32:553–560.

65. Roberts PA, Pollay M, Engles C, et al. Effect on intracranial pressure of furosemide combined with varying doses and administration rates of mannitol. *J Neurosurg* 1987;66:440–446.

66. Muizelaar JP, Marmarou A, Ward JD, et al. Adverse effects of prolonged hyperventilation in patients with severe head injury: a randomized clinical trial. *J Neurosurg* 1991;75:731–739.

67. Wolf AL, Levi L, Marmarou A, et al. Effect of THAM upon outcome in severe head injury: a randomized prospective clinical trial. *J Neurosurg* 1993;78:54–59.

68. Marion DW, Penrod LE, Kelsey SF, et al. Treatment of traumatic brain injury with moderate hypothermia. *N Engl J Med* 1997;336:540–546.

69. Schwab S, Schwarz S, Spranger M, et al. Moderate hypothermia in the treatment of patients with severe middle cerebral artery infarction. *Stroke* 1998;29: 2461–2466.

69a. Lacomis D, Giuliani MJ, van Cott A, Kramer DJ. Acute myopathy of intensive care: clinical, electromyographic, and pathological aspects. *Ann Neurol* 40 (4):645–654, 1996.

70. Woodcock J, Ropper AH, Kennedy SK. High dose barbiturates in non-traumatic brain swelling: ICP reduction and effect on outcome. *Stroke* 1982;13:785–787.

71. Piatt JH, Schiff SJ. High dose barbiturate therapy in neurosurgery and intensive care. *Neurosurgery* 1984; 15:427–444.

72. Schwab S, Spranger M, Schwarz S, et al. Barbiturate coma in severe hemispheric stroke: useful or obsolete? *Neurology* 1997;48:1608–1613.

73. Hara M, Kai Y, Ikemoto Y. Propofol activates GABA$_A$ receptor-chloride ionophore complex in dissociated hippocampal pyramidal neurons of the rat. *Anesthesiology* 1993;79:781–788.

74. Schwarz S, Bertram M, Aschoff A, et al. Indomethacin for brain edema following stroke. *Cerebrovasc Dis* 1999;9:248–250.

75. Iannotti F, Crockard A, Ladds G, et al. Are prostaglandins involved in experimental ischemic edema in gerbils? *Stroke* 1981;12:301–306.

76. Norris JW, Hachinski VC. High dose steroid treatment in cerebral infarction. *BMJ* 1986;292:21–23.

77. Mathew P, Teasdale G, Bannan A, et al. Neurosurgical management of cerebellar haematoma and infarct. *J Neurol Neurosurg Psychiatry* 1995;59:287–292.

78. Schwab S, Steiner T, Aschoff A, et al. Early hemicraniectomy in patients with complete middle cerebral artery infarction. *Stroke* 1998;29:1888–1893.

79. Holtkamp M, Buchheim K, Unterberg A, et al. Hemicraniectomy in elderly patients with space occupying media infarction: improved survival but poor functional outcome. *J Neurol Neurosurg Psychiatry* 2001; 70:226–228.

80. Demchuk AM. Hemicraniectomy is a promising treatment in ischemic stroke. *Can J Neurol Sci* 2000;27: 274–277.

81. Lisk DR, Grotta JC, Lamki LM, et al. Should hypertension be treated after acute stroke? A randomized controlled trial using single photon emission computed tomography. *Arch Neurol* 1993;50:855–862.

82. Britton M, Carlsson A, de Faire U. Blood pressure course in patients with acute stroke and matched controls. *Stroke* 1986;17:861–864.

83. Yatsu FM, Zivin J. Hypertension in acute ischemic strokes. Not to treat. *Arch Neurol* 1985;42:999–1000.

84. Adams HP, Brott TG, Furlan AJ, et al. Guidelines for thrombolytic therapy for acute stroke: a supplement to the guidelines for the management of patients with acute ischemic stroke. A statement for healthcare professionals from a Special Writing Group of the Stroke Council, American Heart Association. *Stroke* 1996;27: 1711–1718.

85. Lavin P. Management of hypertension in patients with acute stroke. *Arch Intern Med* 1986;146:66–68.

86. Puchstein C, van Aken H, Hidding J, et al. Treatment of hypertension with labetalol in neurosurgical practice. Influence of labetalol on cerebral perfusion pressure in dogs without and with intracranial mass lesions. *Acta Neurochir* 1983;67:283–290.

87. Vraamark T, Waldemar G, Strandgaard S, et al. Angiotensin II receptor antagonist CV-11974 and cerebral blood flow autoregulation. *J Hypertens* 1995;13: 755–761.

88. Blezer EL, Nicolay K, Bar D, et al. Enalapril prevents imminent and reduces manifest cerebral edema in stroke-prone hypertensive rats. *Stroke* 1998;29: 1671–1677.

89. Tietjen CS, Hurn PD, Ulatowski JA, et al. Treatment modalities for hypertensive patients with intracranial pathology: options and risks. *Crit Care Med* 1996;24: 311–322.

90. Mayhan WG. Nitric oxide donor-induced increase in permeability of the blood-brain barrier. *Brain Res* 2000;866:101–108.

91. Johshita H, Asano T, Takara T. Effect of a calcium antagonist nicardipine on ischemic brain edema formation. In: Inaba Y, Klatzo I, Spatz M eds. *Brain edema.* New York: Springer-Verlag, 1990:555–559.

92. Hund E, Grau A, Hacke W. Neurocritical care for acute ischemic stroke. *Neurol Clin* 1995;13:511–527.

93. Hayashi S, Nehls DG, Kieck CF, et al. Beneficial effects of induced hypertension on experimental stroke in awake monkeys. *J Neurosurg* 1984;60:151–157.

94. Cole DJ, Drummond JC, Osborne TN, et al. Hypertension and hemodilution during cerebral ischemia reduce brain injury and edema. *Am J Physiol* 1990; 259:H211–H217.

95. Rordorf G, Koroshetz WJ, Ezzeddine MA, et al. A pilot study of drug-induced hypertension for treatment of acute stroke. *Neurology* 2001;56:1210–1213.

96. Carlberg B, Asplund K, Hagg E. The prognostic value of admission blood pressure in patients with acute stroke. *Stroke* 1993;24:1372–1375.

97. Chamorro A, Vila N, Ascaso C, et al. Blood pressure and functional recovery in acute ischemic stroke. *Stroke* 1998;29:1850–1853.

98. Bleyaert AL, Sands PA, Safar P, et al. Augmentation of postischemic brain damage by severe intermittent hypertension. *Crit Care Med* 1980;8:41–47.

99. Kogure K, Busto R, Scheinberg P. The role of hydrostatic pressure in ischemic brain edema. *Ann Neurol* 1981;9:273–282.

100. Asplund K, Israelsson K, Schampi I. Haemodilution for acute ischaemic stroke. *Cochrane Database Syst Rev* 2000;issue 4

101. Gujjar AR, Deibert E, Manno EM, et al. Mechanical ventilation for ischemic stroke and intracerebral hemorrhage: indications, timing, and outcome. *Neurology* 1998;51:447–451.

102. Berrouschot J, Rossler A, Koster J, et al. Mechanical ventilation in patients with hemispheric ischemic stroke. *Crit Care Med* 2000;28:2956–2961.

103. Bushnell CD, Phillips-Bute BG, Laskowitz DT, et al. Survival and outcome after endotracheal intubation for acute stroke. *Neurology* 1999;52:1374–1381.

104. Georgiadis D, Schwarz S, Baumgartner RW, et al. Influence of positive end-expiratory pressure on intracranial pressure and cerebral perfusion pressure in patients with acute stroke. *Stroke* 2001;32:2088–2092.

105. Mayer SA, Fink ME, Homma S, et al. Cardiac injury associated with neurogenic pulmonary edema following subarachnoid hemorrhage. *Neurology* 1994;44:815–820.

106. Muir KW. New experimental and clinical data on the efficacy of pharmacological magnesium infusions in cerebral infarcts. *Magnes Res* 1998;11:43–56.

107. Lampl Y, Gilad R, Geva D, et al. Intravenous administration of magnesium sulfate in acute stroke: a randomized double-blind study. *Clin Neuropharmacol* 2001;24:11–15.

108. Rordorf G, Koroshetz W, Efird JT, et al. Predictors of mortality in stroke patients admitted to an intensive care unit. *Crit Care Med* 2000;28:1301–1305.

109. Wijdicks EFM, Scott JP. Pulmonary embolism associated with acute stroke. *Mayo Clin Proc* 1997;72:297–300.

110. Nedergaard M, Diemer NH. Focal ischemia of the rat brain, with special reference to the influence of plasma glucose concentration. *Acta Neuropathol* 1987;73:131–137.

111. Yip PK, He YY, Hsu CY, et al. Effect of plasma glucose on infarct size in focal cerebral ischemia-reperfusion. *Neurology* 1991;41:899–905,

112. Pulsinelli WA, Levy DE, Sigsbee B, et al. Increased damage after ischemic stroke in patients with hyperglycemia with or without established diabetes mellitus. *Am J Med* 1983;74:540–544.

113. Berger L, Hakim AM. The association of hyperglycemia with cerebral edema in stroke. *Stroke* 1986;17:865–871.

114. Sieber FE, Traystman RJ. Special issues: glucose and the brain. *Crit Care Med* 1992;20:104–114.

115. Oppenheimer SM. Hachinski. VC. The cardiac consequences of stroke. *Neurol Clin* 1992;10:167–76

116. Myers MG, Norris JW, Hachinski VC, et al. Cardiac sequelae of acute stroke. *Stroke* 1982;13:838–842.

117. Grotta J, Pasteur W, Khwaja G, et al. Elective intubation for neurologic deterioration after stroke. *Neurology* 1995;45:640–644.

118. Wijdicks EFM, Scott JP. Outcome in patients with acute basilar artery occlusion requiring mechanical ventilation. *Stroke* 1996;27:1301–1303.

119. Steiner T, Mendoza G, De Georgia M, et al. Prognosis of stroke patients requiring mechanical ventilation in a neurological critical care unit. *Stroke* 1997;28:711–715.

Ischemic Stroke: Advances in Neurology, Vol. 92. Edited by
H.J.M. Barnett, Julien Bogousslavsky, and Heather Meldrum.
Lippincott Williams & Wilkins, Philadelphia © 2003.

44

Hemicraniectomy for Treatment of Middle Cerebral Artery Infarction

Joseph. G. D'Alton

Department of Neurology, Tufts Medical School, Boston, Massachusetts;
Department of Medicine (Neurology), Metrowest Medical Center, Framingham, Massachusetts, U.S.A.

Large hemispheric infarction has a high mortality rate (1) and seems to be poorly responsive to optimal medical management (2). Complete middle cerebral territory involvement, with or without concomitant anterior cerebral and less commonly posterior cerebral artery infarction, has a mortality in excess of 50% (1,2). "Malignant" middle cerebral artery (MCA) territory infarction (2) is associated with focal cerebral edema, initially cytotoxic and later vasogenic (3). Swelling leads to compartmental shifts, with subfalcine or transtentorial herniation, which is the major cause of death (4,5). Compression of the anterior cerebral or posterior cerebral arteries can lead to additional and more extensive infarction. Early neurologic deterioration is not due to a generalized increase in intracranial pressure (6), and therapeutic strategies that focus on lowering intracranial pressure have not been shown to be effective.

Clinically, patients present with a major hemispheric stroke syndrome that includes hemiplegia and forced eye deviation. Drowsiness in the first 2 days is followed by ipsilateral pupillary dilation and death from transtentorial herniation in 2 to 7 days (2). Early hypodensity usually is seen in the affected territory on computed tomographic (CT) scanning. A study that attempted to identify early predictors of fatal brain edema in massive hemispheric ischemic stroke retrospectively looked at 201 patients from seven centers in three countries who had large MCA infarcts (1). In that study, 94 (47%) died of brain swelling, 12 (6%) died of nonneurologic causes, and 95 (47%) survived at day 30. A history of hypertension or heart failure, increased baseline white blood cell count, major early CT hypodensity involving more than 50% of the MCA territory, and involvement of additional vascular territories all were identi-

fied as risk factors. Among the initial clinical factors, level of consciousness, early nausea and vomiting, and stroke severity on presentation were not associated with neurologic death.

SURGERY

Craniectomy to relieve high intracranial pressure is a longstanding neurosurgical concept (7) and initially was used for palliation in patients with tumors that could not be localized with available diagnostic techniques (Fig. 44-1). The technique has been largely abandoned for massive edema due to head trauma because edema usually is diffuse and associated with brainstem injury. Posterior fossa decompression, often with resection of infarcted tissue, has become widely accepted for treatment of life-threatening cerebellar infarction (8). Several studies have shown that early decompressive craniectomy in rats with endovascular induced MCA infarction reduces mortality and significantly improves outcome. If performed early after vessel occlusion, it also significantly reduces infarct size (9,10).

The surgical technique for treatment of large hemispheric infarction requires an extensive craniectomy involving the frontal, parietal, and temporal bones, the latter being resected toward the skull base to allow extracranial herniation of the temporal lobe. After the dura is opened, a duraplasty is performed, and the resected bone can be stored in a bone bank or subcutaneously for later reinsertion. Resection of infarcted brain, "strokectomy," sometimes is performed, although delineation of abnormal tissue may be difficult in early infarcts. The rationale for the procedure is to allow herniation of edematous brain, thus preventing vertical and hori-

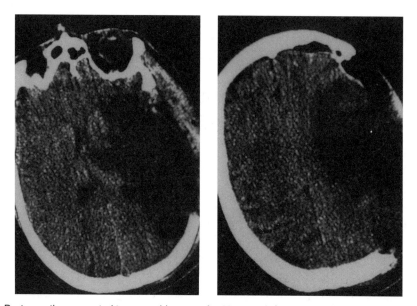

FIG. 44-1. Postoperative computed tomographic scan of a 68-year-old man who had an anterior temporal lobectomy and craniectomy for a large right middle cerebral artery infarct, with clinical evidence of herniation.

zontal intracranial shifts, with improved perfusion pressure and reduced intracranial pressure. Surgical complications include infection, subdural or epidural hematoma, and subdural hygroma.

RESULTS OF SURGERY

All reported series are nonrandomized, and most are simply anecdotal reports of small groups of patients. There is significant variation in patient populations, surgical technique, and outcome assessment (11–21). Most procedures were performed on the nondominant hemisphere. Some series included patients with MCA infarcts caused by diverse etiologies, such as vasospasm complicating aneurysm rupture, carotid cavernous fistula, and carotid balloon occlusion for treatment of nasopharyngeal carcinoma (12,13). One early series reports six patients who had surgery because of suspected brain tumor (16). Sev-

eral authors reported radical resection of infarcted tissue (12,13,18,19).

The largest reported series includes 63 patients. The first 32 patients were reported separately (14) and later compared to another 31 patients who tended to be operated on earlier, usually in fewer than 24 hours (15). For the whole group, mean age was 49.74 ± 10.8 years. Stroke etiology was cardioembolism in 41, carotid dissection with secondary MCA embolism in 19, and unknown in three. The surgical technique involved a wide craniotomy without resection of infarcted tissue. An artificial bone flap was inserted at 6 to 12 weeks. A total of 46 patients (73%) survived. Nondominant hemisphere strokes predominated [52 (82%)]; patients with global aphasia were excluded. Forty-one patients had a compete MCA territory infarct, and 22 had an additional anterior or posterior cerebral artery infarct. Mean time between onset of

TABLE 44-1. *Outcome in recent series*

Author	No. of patients	Mortality	Survivors with Barthel index ≤70
Carter et al. (12)	14	3 (21.4%)	7
Nussbaum (12a)	10	7 (30%)	1
Kalia and Yonas (13)	4	0 (00/0)	?
Delashaw et al. (11)	9	1 (11%)	6
Rieke et al. (14)	32	11 (34.4%)	17
Schwab et al. (15)	31	5 (16%)	9

symptoms and surgery was 39 hours (range 6–112 hours) in the first group versus 21 hours (range 8–42 hours) in the later group. Uncal herniation developed in 24 patients (75%) of the first group but only in four patients (13%) of the later group before surgery. Mortality was 34.4% (11/32) in the first group, 16% (5/31) in the second group, and 78% (43/55) in a group of historic controls. Functional outcome in survivors using the Barthel index showed a mean score of 70, with scores of 80 to 90 in two patients, 70 to 80 in 15 patients, and 60 to 70 in nine patients. There was no statistical difference in functional outcome between the two groups.

CONCLUSION

Hemicraniectomy is a possible treatment for large hemispheric cerebral infarction. Although this condition carries a high mortality and often leads to uncal herniation despite optimal medical management, this surgical approach cannot be recommended for routine clinical practice until a well-designed randomized controlled trial proves efficacy. The evidence suggests that early surgery may be more beneficial, and a trial would optimally randomize high-risk patients, preferentially within 24 or 48 hours of stroke onset. A multicenter approach would require that enrolling sites have extensive neurosurgery skills and high-quality neurointensive care. A key question will be whether morbidity in survivors justifies any potential reduction in mortality. There currently is no evidence that techniques such as diffusion and perfusion magnetic resonance imaging can select patients more appropriately for this treatment (22).

REFERENCES

1. Kasner SE, Demchuk AM, Berrouschot J, et al. Predictors of fatal brain edema in massive hemispheric ischemic stroke. *Stroke* 2001;32:2117–2123.
2. Hacke W, Schwab S, Horn M, et al. "Malignant" middle cerebral artery territory infarction. Clinical course and prognostic signs. *Arch Neurol* 1996;53:309–315.
3. Rosenberg GA. Ischemic brain edema. *Prog Cardiovasc Dis* 1999;42:209–216.
4. Ropper AH, Shafran B. Brain edema after stroke: clinical syndrome and intracranial pressure. *Arch Neurol* 1984;41:26–29.
5. Silver FL, Norris JW Lewis AJ, et al. Early mortality following stroke: a prospective review. *Stroke* 1984;15:492–496.
6. Frank JI. Large hemispheric infarction, deterioration, and intracranial pressure. *Neurology* 1995;45:1286–1290.
7. Cushing H. The establishment of cerebral hernia as a decompressive measure for inaccessible brain tumors: with the description of intermuscular methods of making the bone defect in temporal and occipital regions. *Surg Gynecol Obstet* 1905;1:297–314.
8. Heros RC. Surgical treatment of cerebellar infarction. *Stroke* 1992;23:937–938.
9. Forsting M, Reith W, Schabitz WR, et al. Decompressive craniectomy for cerebral infarction. An experimental study in rats. *Stroke* 1995;26:259–264.
10. Doerfler A, Forsting M, Reith W, et al. Decompressive craniectomy in a rat model of "malignant" cerebral hemispheric stroke: experimental support for an aggressive therapeutic approach. *J Neurosurg* 1996;85:853–859.
11. Delashaw JB, Broaddus WC, Kassell NF, et al. Treatment of right hemispheric cerebral infarction by hemicraniectomy. *Stroke* 1990;21:874–881.
12. Carter BS, Ogilvy CS, Candia GJ, et al. One-year outcome after decompressive surgery for massive nondominant hemispheric infarction. *Neurosugery* 1997;401:168–1176.
12a. Nussbaum ES, Wolf AL, Sebring L, Mirvis S. Complete temporal lobectomy for surgical resuscitation of patients with transtentorial herniation secondary to unilateral hemispheric swelling. *Neurosurgery* 1991;29:62–66.
13. Kalia KK, Yonas H. An aggressive approach to massive middle cerebral artery infarction. *Arch Neurol* 1993;50:1293–1297.
14. Rieke K, Schwab S, Krieger D, et al. Decompressive surgery in space-occupying hemispheric infarction: results of an open prospective trial. *Crit Care Med* 1995;23:1576–1587.
15. Schwab S, Steiner Taschoff A, et al. Early hemicraniectomy in patients with complete middle cerebral artery infarction. *Stroke* 1998;29:1888–1893.
16. Scarcella G. Encephalomalacia simulating the clinical and radiological aspects of brain tumor: a report of six cases. *J Neurosurg* 1956;13:366–380.
17. Young PH, Smith KJ, Dunn RC. Surgical decompression after cerebral hemispheric stroke: indications and surgical selection. *South Med J* 1982;75:473–475.
18. Greenwood JJ. Acute brain infarctions with high intracranial pressure: surgical indications. *John Hopkins Med J* 1968;122:254–260.
19. Ivamato H, Numato M, Donaghy R. Surgical decompression for cerebral and cerebellar infarcts. *Stroke* 1974;5:365–370.
20. Kondziolka D, Fazl M. Functional recovery after decompressive craniotomy for cerebral infarction. *J Neurosurg* 1988;23:143–147.
21. Rengachary SS, Batnitzky S, Morantz RA, et al. Hemicraniectomy for acute massive cerebral infarction. *Neurosurgery* 1981;8:321–328.
22. Schellinger PD, Fiebach JB, Jansen O, et al. Stroke magnetic resonance imaging within 6 hours after onset of hyperacute cerebral ischemia. *Ann Neurol* 2001;49:460–469.

Ischemic Stroke: Advances in Neurology, Vol. 92. Edited by
H.J.M. Barnett, Julien Bogousslavsky, and Heather Meldrum.
Lippincott Williams & Wilkins, Philadelphia © 2003.

45

Intraarterial Thrombolysis for Acute Ischemic Stroke

Reza Jahan and *Fernando Vinuela

*Division of Interventional Neuroradiology and *Department of Radiological Sciences,
UCLA School of Medicine, Los Angeles, California, U.S.A.*

Stroke is the third most common cause of death in the United States, with approximately 750,000 cases leading to more than 50,000 deaths annually (1–5). The yearly cost of stroke is more than $30 billion in medical costs, rehabilitation, and loss of employment (6,7). The majority of strokes are ischemic strokes, including thrombotic, cardioembolic, and lacunar strokes (4,8). Most ischemic strokes are caused by blockage of a cerebral blood vessel by a clot. Angiographic studies performed in stroke patients within 8 hours of symptom onset show arterial occlusions corresponding to the symptoms in more than 80% of cases (9–11). An arterial occlusion in a cerebral vessel rapidly produces a core of infarcted brain tissue surrounded by hypoxic but potentially salvageable tissue, that is, the ischemic penumbra (12–14). The underlying rationale for administering a thrombolytic agent is rapid restoration of blood flow and preservation of the ischemic penumbra.

The role of thrombus in stroke combined with the success of thrombolysis in acute myocardial infarction has generated great interest in cerebral fibrinolysis. Intravenous (IV) recombinant tissue plasminogen activator (tPA) currently is approved by the United States Food and Drug Administration (FDA) for treatment of acute ischemic stroke within 3 hours of symptom onset (15). Previous chapters discussed IV thrombolysis in some detail. More recently, intraarterial (IA) thrombolysis has been shown to improve neurologic outcome in patients with acute ischemic stroke (11). In this chapter, we review the clinical trials in IA therapy of acute ischemic stroke.

INTRAARTERIAL THROMBOLYSIS

The benefit of thrombolytic drugs is lysis of acute thromboemboli. IV therapy has several advantages,

including ease and rapidity of administration. However, to lyse the clot, a sufficient amount of the thrombolytic drug must reach its target. If major arteries are blocked, too little of the IV administered drug reaches intracranial thrombi; therefore, much interest has developed in IA delivery of thrombolytic agents. Compared to IV therapy, localized IA thrombolysis has the theoretical advantage of achieving faster, more complete recanalization with less fibrinolytic drug. This presumably is due to the fact that the microcatheter is placed adjacent to the clot for drug delivery, thus achieving the highest concentration of fibrinolytic agent at the site of the clot while minimizing the systemic dose to the patient. In addition, the microcatheter can be used to traverse the clot with mechanical disruption of the clot. Other advantages include the fact that, during administration of the thrombolytic drug, clot lysis can be assessed with follow-up angiograms. Drug infusion can be stopped when clot lysis is achieved, leading to potentially less thrombolytic drug being used. Finally, with IA thrombolysis, treatment can be initiated up to 6 hours after symptom onset. This greatly expands the time window, which increases the number of patients who potentially can benefit from this treatment.

The first reports of IA thrombolysis were in 1983 when five patients with vertebrobasilar occlusion were treated with local IA fibrinolysis (16). Successful recanalization was achieved in three patients, all of whom had subsequent neurologic improvement. Since that time a large number of case series have been reported (17–31). Neurologic improvement was variable in these studies, with minimal or no neurologic deficit reported in 15% to 75% of patients. Several factors likely contribute to this wide variation in outcome: (a) grading system used for assessing outcome; (b) dose of thrombolytic agent used; (c) differences in baseline patient demographics, such as age and baseline neurologic status; and (d) site of arterial occlusion. Complete recanalization is seen on average in approximately 40% of patients and partial recanalization in 35% (17–30). These rates of recanalization are higher than those reported with IV thrombolysis (32–34). To date, however, there have been no randomized trials comparing IA and IV thrombolysis.

As with IV thrombolysis, only randomized trials can answer questions regarding the safety and efficacy of IA therapy. Two such trials have been performed in IA thrombolysis: Prolyse in Acute Cerebral Thromboembolism Trial (PROACT) and PROACT II (10,11).

PROACT (10) was a randomized phase II trial of recombinant prourokinase (rpro-UK) versus placebo in patients with angiographically documented proximal middle cerebral artery occlusion. Angiography was performed after intracranial hemorrhage (ICH) was excluded by computed tomography. Patients displaying occlusion of the M1 or M2 segment of the middle cerebral artery were randomized 2:1 to receive rpro-UK (6 mg) or placebo over 120 minutes into the proximal thrombus face. Mechanical disruption of the clot was not attempted. Recanalization efficacy was assessed at the end of the 2-hour infusion and symptomatic ICH at 24 hours. A total of 105 patients underwent angiography for evaluation for entry into the study. Of these patients, 65 were excluded for various reasons: 25 had no occlusion; 36 had no M1 or M2 occlusion; two were beyond the 6-hour time limit; and two had complications. Among the 40 treated patients, 26 received rpro-UK and 14 received placebo at a median of 5.5 hours from symptom onset. Recanalization was significantly associated with rpro-UK ($p = 0.0085$). Complete recanalization was achieved in five rpro-UK patients as opposed to none of the placebo patients. ICH occurred in 15.4% of the rpro-UK–treated patients and 7.1% of the placebo-treated patients (nonsignificant). All patients with rpro-UK and early computed tomographic signs of greater than 33% suffered ICH. There was a trend toward lower mortality in the rpro-UK group.

The success of PROACT led to PROACT II, which was a larger randomized trial (11). This trial included patients with onset of symptoms within 6 hours and angiographic occlusion of the middle cerebral artery (M1 or M2 occlusion). The primary outcome of the trial was the ability to live independently at 3 months after the stroke. Randomization was 2:1 for treatment to placebo. Four hundred seventy-four patients underwent angiography and 180 were enrolled, with 121 receiving IA prourokinase and low-dose IV heparin. In the control group, 59 received low-dose IV heparin. At 2 hours, 67% of treated patients had complete or partial recanalization compared to 18% in the heparin only group ($p < 0.001$) (Table 45-1). The primary outcome of the study was attained by 40% of the patients treated with prourokinase compared to 25% in the heparin only group ($p = 0.04$). Symptomatic ICH was seen in 10% of patients undergoing thrombolysis compared to 2% in the heparin group ($p = 0.06$). IA thrombolysis initiated within 6 hours of symptom onset was shown to have a benefit in patients with occlusion of the middle cerebral artery.

There have been no randomized trials of IA thrombolysis in the posterior circulation. Vertebrobasilar stroke differs in several respects from anterior circulation ischemic stroke. Compared to anterior circulation stroke, clinical outcome of patients with vertebrobasilar occlusion is less favorable, with death in the majority of patients and severe deficit in most survivors (23,35,36). In addition, patients with posterior circulation infarcts have a high frequency of severe intracranial large-artery disease (37). This is rarely the case in anterior circulation strokes and presents a unique problem in posterior circulation thrombolysis in that reocclusion can be a potential complication (16,23,27). Thrombolysis in the anterior circulation is not performed beyond 6 hours because of higher rates of hemorrhagic transformation and poor outcome (38) (see Chapter 15). No such conclusive data exist

TABLE 45-1. *PROACT II results*

	rpro-UK	Control	*p* Value
Successful recanalization	66%	18%	<0.001
Symptomatic hemorrhage	10%	2%	0.06
Outcome 90 days (RS ≤2)	40%	25%	0.04
Mortality	25%	27%	0.80

PROACT, Prolyse in Acute Cerebral Thromboembolism Trial; rpro-UK, recombinant pro-urokinase.

indicating increased risk beyond 6 hours in posterior circulation strokes, and reported series have included patients up to 24 hours after symptom onset (16,17,27). This extension beyond 6 hours in the posterior circulation has yet to be justified.

A pilot study evaluating the safety and efficacy of IA urokinase in patients with brainstem stroke was reported by Mitchell et al. (39). Sixteen patients with vertebrobasilar occlusion were treated within 24 hours of symptom onset. Urokinase was administered until clot lysis was achieved up to a maximum dose of one million units. Successful recanalization initially was achieved in 13 (82%) of 16 patients. Of these patients, two reoccluded within 24 hours with a final recanalization rate of 69%. Six-month functional status was assessed by a neurologist using the Barthel index. A good outcome was defined as Barthel index of 60 or more. Eleven (69%) patients survived and nine (56%) had a good outcome, but two (13%) were left severely disabled. The authors concluded that IA thrombolysis in the posterior circulation is safe and feasible, capable of achieving recanalization in a significant number of patients. Interestingly, time between symptoms and thrombolysis was not predictive of outcome. Recanalization correlated with survival ($p = 0.02$).

COMBINED INTRAVENOUS AND INTRAARTERIAL TREATMENT

One major disadvantage of IA thrombolysis is the delay to treatment because of the waiting period for initiation and performance of the cerebral angiography and interventional procedure. The Emergency Management of Stroke (EMS) Study and the Interventional Management of Stroke (IMS) Trial are the only reported trials of combined IV and IA thrombolysis (40). This approach combines the advantages of the two treatment strategies. IV therapy is initiated without delay but at a lower dose, which allows some of the tPA to be given intraarterially for the higher recanalization rates that potentially can be achieved with IA treatment. The EMS Study was a double blind randomized study with a total of 35 patients enrolled within 3 hours of symptom onset. Of these patients, 17 were randomized to receive IV tPA at a dose of 0.6 mg/kg (maximum dose 60 mg); 18 patients in the second arm of the study received IV placebo. These patients then underwent immediate angiography. If no clot was visualized, the angiogram was stopped. If a clot was visualized, then IA treatment with tPA was initiated, with 20 mg of the drug given over 2 hours or until recanalization was achieved.

The study demonstrated higher successful recanalization rates in the combined IV/IA group (55% vs. 10%). There was no difference in 7-day or 3-month outcomes, and there were more deaths in the treated group of patients. The numbers of symptomatic hemorrhage in the two groups were similar.

The IMS Trial was supported by the National Institutes of Health and involved 14 centers in North America. Patients with National Institute of Health Stroke Scale (NIHSS) greater than 10 within 3 hours of deficit onset were offered treatment with IV tPA at 0.6 mg/kg, followed by neuroangiography. If an arterial occlusive lesion was present, up to 22 mg IA tPA was given over 2 hours.

Successful recanalization with partial or complete reperfusion was seen in 57% of patients. Symptomatic ICH was seen in 6% of patients, with 16% mortality at 3 months. Good outcome at 3 months (Rankin score 0–1) was seen in 30% of treated patients.

Interestingly, several advantages of the combined approach over pure IV thrombolysis were demonstrated in this study. The average total dose of tPA used in the IMS Study was 59 mg (46 mg IV and 17 mg IA). In the National Institute of Neurological Disorders and Stroke II (NINDS II) Study, the average total IV dose was 69 mg. The need to adjust the IA dose to achieve recanalization accounts for the lower dose in the IMS Study. Thus, although a maximum IA dose of 22 mg could have been given, less than that was used. This is an advantage of IA strategies over pure IV therapy, where in the latter the dose cannot be adjusted to achieve recanalization with minimum drug.

The combined strategy has advantages over the pure IA approach as well. In the IMS Trial, the time to initiation of IV therapy was 140 minutes and the time to onset of IA therapy was 212 minutes. There was a 72-minute delay after initiation of IV therapy before initiation of IA therapy. This points out the potential advantage of IV therapy in which the fibrinolytic drug can be given sooner after onset of symptoms. Had this been a pure IA trial, there would have been a delay in the initiation of fibrinolysis.

The EMS and IMS Trials demonstrate that the combined approach is feasible, reasonably safe, and worthy of further study. A randomized trial comparing combined IV/IA tPA to standard IV tPA may be warranted at this time.

MECHANICAL STRATEGIES

The experience of cardiology in acute myocardial infarction (MI) has served as a road map of what may work in the setting of acute ischemic stroke. Randomized studies in the setting of acute MI have demonstrated the superiority of mechanical strategies in improving outcome compared with IV thrombolytic agents alone (41). Use of angioplasty to reopen cerebral vessels has been reported (42). The potential disadvantage of this strategy is forcing the clot into the deep penetrating arteries, with worsening ischemia and the potential risk of rupturing the blood vessel.

The Angiojet catheter has been used to fragment and suck in the clot (43). Other means of delivering energy to fragment the clot are being developed, including the use of ultrasound and laser devices. The current limitation of these mechanical devices is their relatively larger catheter size and less flexibility, which limit access to the tortuous vessels of the intracranial circulation.

The Mechanical Embolus Removal in Cerebral Ischemia (MERCI) Trial is underway to evaluate the safety of the MERCI Retriever System (Concentric Medical, Mountain View, CA, U.S.A.). The MERCI Retriever System consists of a unique nitinol wire (Retriever) and a guide catheter with a silicone balloon. The Retriever device consists of a flexible, tapered core wire with a soft, helically shaped distal tip. A microcatheter is navigated to the clot in the middle cerebral artery using conventional catheterization techniques. The microguidewire is removed and the Retriever introduced into the lumen of the microcatheter. The shape memory properties of nitinol allow the helix to straighten, which allows the Retriever to be delivered through the lumen of the microcatheter. The Retriever has a hydrophilic coating that facilitates movement within the catheter lumen. The hydrophilic coating coupled with the low-profile design allows the Retriever to be easily positioned within the distal tortuous vasculature. When the distal tip of the Retriever exits the tip of the microcatheter, the helical loops return to their original shape. These helical loops may be used to engage and retrieve thrombus from the neurovasculature. Before retraction of the Retriever and thrombus, the balloon on the guide catheter is inflated to control blood flow. Five centers in the United States are participating in the trial, with planned recruitment of 30 patients.

CONCLUSIONS

IA delivery of thrombolytic agent seems to lyse clots more effectively compared to IV tPA and has extended the time window to intervention up to 6 hours. The disadvantage is that IA delivery takes longer, and thus far no head-to-head comparison of the two methods of treatment has been reported. The approach of combining IA and IV thrombolysis has the theoretical advantage of combining the benefits of the two methods of treatment. The IMS Trial has shown the safety and feasibility of this combined approach, and a phase III trial comparing pure IV thrombolysis to combined IV and IA may be warranted at this time.

Mechanical approaches to ischemic stroke are attractive because they may obviate the need for thrombolytic drugs that increase the risk of reperfusion hemorrhage. As this strategy is proving to be effective in treatment of acute MI, it is predicted that it will serve a major role in treatment of acute ischemic stroke. Advances in catheter technology are required to meet the special needs of clot lysis in the cerebral circulation.

The future treatment of acute ischemic stroke likely will include a combination of mechanical strategies and thrombolytic agents that minimize risk of ICH and maximize recanalization rates.

REFERENCES

1. Wolf PA, Kannel WB, McGee DL. Epidemiology of strokes in North America. In: Barnett HJM, Stein BM, Mohr JP, et al., eds. *Stroke: pathophysiology, diagnosis and management.* New York: Churchill Livingstone, 1986:19–29.
2. Chambers BR, Norris JW, Shurvell BL, et al. Prognosis of acute stroke. *Neurology* 1987;37:221–225.
3. Broderick J, Brott T, Kothari R, et al. The Greater Cincinnati/Northern Kentucky Stroke Study: preliminary first-ever and total incidence rates of stroke among blacks. *Stroke* 1998;29:415–421.
4. Feussner JR, Matchar DB. When and how to study the carotids. *Ann Intern Med* 1988;109:805–818.
5. Thorvaldsen P, Kuulasmaa K, Rajakangas AM, et al. Stroke trends in the WHO MONICA project. *Stroke* 1997;28:500–506.
6. Barnaby W. Stroke intervention. *Emerg Med Clin North Am* 1990;8:267–281.
7. Dobbin B. The economic impact of stroke. *Neurology* 1995;45[Suppl 1]:S10–S14.
8. Zeumer H, Freitag HJ, Knospe V. Intravascular thrombolysis in central nervous system cerebrovascular disease. *Neurol Clin N Am* 1992;2:359–369.
9. del Zoppo GJ, Poeck K, Pessin M, et al. Recombinant tissue plasminogen activator in acute thrombotic and embolic stroke. *Ann Neurol* 1992;32:78–86.
10. del Zoppo G, Higashida RT, Furlan AJ, et al. PROACT: a phase II randomized trial of recombinant pro-urokinase by direct arterial delivery in acute middle cerebral artery stroke. PROACT Investigators. Prolyse in Acute Cerebral Thromboembolism. *Stroke* 1998;29:4–11.
11. Furlan A, Higashida R, Wechsler L, et al. Intra-arterial

prourokinase for acute ischemic stroke. The PROACT II study: a randomized controlled trial. Prolyse in Acute Cerebral Thromboembolism. *JAMA* 1999;282: 2003–2011.

12. Baron J. Mapping the ischaemic penumbra with PET: implications for acute stroke treatment. *Cerebrovasc Dis* 1999;9:193–201.

13. Heiss WD, Thiel A, Grond M, et al. Which targets are relevant for therapy of acute ischemic stroke? *Stroke* 1999;30:1486–1489.

14. Nagesh V, Welch KM, Windham JP, et al. Time course of ADCw changes in ischemic stroke: beyond the human eye! *Stroke* 1998;29:1778–1782.

15. The National Institute of Neurological Disorders and Stroke rt-PA Stroke Study Group. Tissue plasminogen activator for acute ischemic stroke. *N Engl J Med* 1995; 333:1581–1587.

16. Zeumer H, Hacke W, Ringelstein EF. Local intraarterial thrombolysis in vertebrobasilar thromboembolic disease. *AJNR Am J Neuroradiol* 1983;4:401–404.

17. Zeumer H, Freitag HJ, Zanella F, et al. Local intra-arterial fibrinolytic therapy in patients with stroke: urokinase versus recombinant tissue plasminogen activator (r-TPA). *Neuroradiology* 1993;35:159–162.

18. Jansen O, von Kummer R, Forsting M, et al. Thrombolytic therapy in acute occlusion of the intracranial internal carotid artery bifurcation. *AJNR Am N Neuroradiol* 1995;16:1977–1986.

19. Theron J, Courtheoux P, Casasco A, et al. Local intraarterial fibrinolysis in the carotid territory. *AJNR Am J Neuroradiol* 1989;10:753–765.

20. Barr JD, Mathis JM, Wildenhain SL, et al. Acute stroke intervention with intraarterial urokinase infusion. *J Vasc Interv Radiol* 1994;5:705–713.

21. del Zoppo GJ, Ferbert A, Otis S, et al. Local intra-arterial fibrinolytic therapy in acute carotid territory stroke. A pilot study. *Stroke* 1988;19:307–313.

22. Mori E, Tabuchi M, Yoshida T, et al. Intracarotid urokinase with thromboembolic occlusion of the middle cerebral artery. *Stroke* 1988;19:802–812.

23. Hacke W, Zeumer H, Ferbert A, et al. Intraarterial therapy improves outcome in patients with acute vertebrobasilar disease. *Stroke* 1988;19:1216–1222.

24. Ezura M, Kagawa S. Selective and superselective infusion of urokinase for embolic stroke. *Surg Neurol* 1992; 38:353–358.

25. Barnwell SL, Clark WM, Nguyen TT, et al. Safety and efficacy of delayed intraarterial urokinase therapy with mechanical clot disruption for thromboembolic stroke. *AJNR Am J Neuroradiol* 1994;15:1817–1822.

26. Brandt T, von Kummer R, Müller-Küppers M, et al. Thrombolytic therapy of acute basilar artery occlusion. Variables affecting recanalization and outcome. *Stroke* 1996;27:875–881.

27. Becker KJ, Monsein LH, Ulatowski J, et al. Intraarterial thrombolysis in vertebrobasilar occlusion. *AJNR Am J Neuroradiol* 1996;17:255–262.

28. Ueda T, Sakaki S, Kumon Y, et al. Multivariable analysis of predictive factors related to outcome at 6 months

after intra-arterial thrombolysis for acute ischemic stroke. *Stroke* 1999;30:2360–2365.

29. Jahan R, Duckwiler GR, Kidwell CS, et al. Intraarterial thrombolysis for treatment of acute stroke: experience in 26 patients with long-term follow-up. *AJNR Am J Neuroradiol* 1999;20:1291–1299.

30. Suarez JI, Sunshine JL, Tarr R, et al. Predictors of clinical improvement, angiographic recanalization, and intracranial hemorrhage after intra-arterial thrombolysis for acute ischemic stroke. *Stroke* 1999;30: 2094–2100.

31. Zeumer H, Hundgen R, Ferbert A, et al. Local intraarterial fibrinolytic therapy in inaccessible internal carotid occlusion. *Neuroradiology* 1984;26:315–317.

32. Yamaguchi T, Hayakawa T, Kiuchi H. Intravenous tissue plasminogen activator ameliorates the outcome of hyperacute embolic stroke. *Cerebrovasc Dis* 1993;3: 269–272.

33. Wolpert SM, Bruckmann H, Greenlee R, et al. Neuroradiologic evaluation of patients with acute stroke treated with recombinant tissue plasminogen activator. *AJNR Am J Neuroradiol* 1993;14:3–13.

34. Mori E, Yoneda Y, Tabuchi M, et al. Intravenous recombinant tissue plasminogen activator in acute carotid artery territory stroke. *Neurology* 1992;42:976–982.

35. Bruckmann H, Ferbert A, del Zoppo GJ, et al. Acute basilar thrombosis: angiologic-clinical comparison and therapeutic implications. *Acta Radiol* 1987;369[Suppl]: 38–42.

36. Archer CR, Horenstein S. Basilar artery occlusion: clinical and radiographic correlation. *Stroke* 1977;8:383–391.

37. Bogousslavsky J, Regli F, Maeder P, et al. The etiology of posterior circulation infarcts: a prospective study using magnetic resonance imaging and magnetic resonance angiography. *Neurology* 1993;43:1528–1533.

38. Del Zoppo GJ, Zeumer H, Harker LA. Thrombolytic therapy in stroke: possibilities and hazards. *Stroke* 1986;17:595–607.

39. Mitchell PJ, Gerraty RP, Donnan GA, et al. Thrombolysis in the vertebrobasilar circulation: the Australian Urokinase Stroke Trial: a pilot study. *Cerebrovasc Dis* 1997;7:94–99.

40. Lewandowski CA, Frankel M, Tomsick TA, et al. Combined intravenous and intra-arterial r-TPA versus intra-arterial therapy of acute ischemic stroke: Emergency Management of Stroke (EMS) Bridging Trial. *Stroke* 1999;30:2598–2605.

41. Weaver WD, Simes RJ, Betriu A, et al. Comparison of primary coronary angioplasty and intravenous thrombolytic therapy for acute myocardial infarction: a quantitative review. *JAMA* 1997;278:2093–2098.

42. Balousek PA, Knowles HJ, Higashida RT, et al. New interventions in cerebrovascular disease: the role of thrombolytic therapy and balloon angioplasty. *Curr Opin Cardiol* 1996;11:550–557.

43. Bücker A, Schmitz-Rode T, Vorwerk D, et al. Comparative in vitro study of two percutaneous hydrodynamic thrombectomy systems. *J Vasc Interv Radiol* 1996;7: 445–449.

Ischemic Stroke: Advances in Neurology, Vol. 92. Edited by
H.J.M. Barnett, Julien Bogousslavsky, and Heather Meldrum.
Lippincott Williams & Wilkins, Philadelphia © 2003.

46

Investigation by Perfusion CT and Diffusion-Weighted MR Imaging

Reto Meuli, *Julien Bogousslavsky, and Max Wintermark

*Department of Diagnostic and Interventional Radiology and *Department of Neurology,
University Hospital, Centre Hospitalier Universitaire Vaudois, Lausanne, Switzerland*

Cerebral perfusion warrants the viability of the cerebral parenchyma. It supplies the brain with glucose, the oxidation of which is its main source of energy. The high metabolic needs of the brain, combined with the absence of cerebral glucose storage, requires a high and constant cerebral blood flow (CBF), which averages about 50 mL/100 g per minute. Gray matter is perfused two or three times as much as white matter. Cerebral activity changes induce CBF modifications, which may reach up to 40% in extreme conditions such as convulsions or coma (1). Complex autoregulation processes ensure CBF stability despite arterial pressure modifications, as well as CBF adjustment to the local metabolic activity of neurons (2). Brain perfusion is altered in a variety of cerebrovascular pathologies, among which ischemic stroke is the most frequent. Diagnostic imaging methods recently developed for ischemic stroke are intended to map CBF quantitatively and precisely. This goal can be achieved by a highly quantitative, newly developed technique called perfusion computed tomography (CT) or by the more qualitative data obtained by perfusion magnetic resonance imaging (MRI).

Acute ischemic stroke is a dynamic process where the core of the ischemic lesion with neuronal death gradually replaces the penumbral area formed by no functional cerebral tissue. At the time of therapeutic decision making, precise measurement of the size and ratio of cerebral infarction and penumbra may be a selection criterion for use of thrombolytic agents. Patients with a large penumbral area and a small infarct core will be good candidates for thrombolysis. Patients who present with a large infarct without penumbra will not benefit from thrombolysis and will have a high risk of cerebral bleeding. MR diffusion-weighted imaging (DWI) is the best accepted imaging method that can depict the size of the infarcted cerebral tissue. In conjunction with perfusion MR, MRI is able to show brain infract and penumbra (3). From the most recent literature, it appears that perfusion CT also is able to separate and map brain infarct and penumbra in the hyperacute stage of ischemic stroke because of its highly quantitative capability of measuring CBF and cerebral blood volume (CBV) (4). In the last decade, stroke therapeutic trials used only native CT as a diagnostic imaging test, mainly to rule out cerebral bleeding (5). The capability of MRI to map cerebral infarct and perfusion was difficult to integrate on a large scale into this type of multicenter clinical study, probably because of limited access to MR scanners 24 hours a day in many centers and the long period of time needed to obtained the data in situations where even minutes are important. Given that CT scanners are present in many emergency departments and CT currently is obtained upon admission of any stroke patient, perfusion CT can be obtained in an additional 5 minutes and thus provide essential data on brain infarction and penumbra before therapeutic decision making (4). This chapter describes perfusion CT and DWI as applied to ischemic strokes from a technical and clinical point of view.

MAPPING OF CEREBRAL BLOOD SUPPLY BY PERFUSION COMPUTED TOMOGRAPHY

Perfusion CT is a simple and accurate imaging technique that allows quantitative assessment of brain perfusion. It involves dynamic acquisition of sequential CT slices in a cine mode during intravenous administration of nonionic iodinated contrast material. Data acquisition is achieved in less than 5 minutes. Perfusion CT studies can be performed easily and quickly in emergency settings as part of the admission cerebral imaging survey. The studies are well tolerated, even by acute patients. Perfusion CT can be achieved in all hospital institutions equipped with CT units, which usually are available 24 hours a day, 7 days a week. It does not require specialized technologists or extra material, only dedicated postprocessing software.

Perfusion CT fundamentals were developed about 20 years ago (6–11). However, its implementation was limited by the slowness of CT data acquisition and the limited coverage of the brain parenchyma by single-slice CT units. MR techniques benefitted from these drawbacks and were developed preferentially. Today, CT is getting a new lease of life with the advent of subsecond slice acquisition and multislice CT (MSCT) units. With two successive acquisitions, MSCT allows assessment of a total 40-mm thickness of cerebral parenchyma, and the radiation dose to the patient remains acceptable.

At our institution, perfusion CT studies are performed with a MSCT unit. Studies consist of two series obtained within a 5-minute interval. Each series consists of 40 successive CT slices obtained every second in a stationary mode, with acquisition parameters of 80 kVp and 100 mA. For each series, acquisition begins 5 seconds after starting intravenous administration of 50-mL nonionic iodinated contrast material. The intravenous material is administered via an antecubital vein with a power injector at a rate of 5 mL/s. The four 10-mm CT slices, which can be examined by this protocol with MSCT technology, are chosen immediately above the orbits to protect lenses, going through the basal nuclei and toward the vertex. Perfusion CT series are performed after a native cerebral CT is obtained and sometimes completed by cervical and cerebral angio-CT, the latter involving an additional dose of 40 mL of nonionic iodinated contrast material.

Iodine included in the contrast material having a 33 keV K-edge and use of 80 kVp provide benefit from an increased photoelectric effect compared to the Compton effect and leads to a statistically significant increase in enhancement after contrast material administration. Moreover, it lowers the radiation dose by a factor 2.8 (12). On the other hand, it does not result in a statistically significant increase in noise, so 80-kVp images can be used in perfusion CT analysis.

Finally, the choice of a 4- or 5-mL/s injection rate is justified by reports that, in the setting of intravenous administration of iodinated contrast material, use of injection rates greater than 5 to 10 mL/s did not induce significant changes in the time-concentration curves in the pulmonary veins and aorta, and thus in cerebral arteries (13,14). Moreover, a computerized simulation demonstrated that increasing the injection rate to greater than 5 mL/s did not significantly change the quantitative CBF map, whereas lowering the rate to less than 4 mL/s induced significant overestimation of blood flow values.

THEORETICAL BASIS OF PERFUSION COMPUTED TOMOGRAPHY

Perfusion CT data are related to contrast enhancement curves registered in each pixel of cerebral CT slices. Contrast enhancement in each of these curves is directly proportional to iodinated contrast material plasmatic concentration. To extract quantitative blood flow values from these data, a theoretical model, which consists of a few source assumptions giving a simplified version of the reality, is mandatory to state and solve the equations giving access to regional cerebral blood flow (rCBF) from the acquired images. The best model for perfusion CT performed at low injection rates of iodinated contrast material is the central volume principle, because its source hypotheses are few and well fulfilled by iodinated contrast material. It considers regional vascular networks as isolated volumes, each with an arterial input and a venous output. It also assumes that the entire amount of contrast material introduced at some time in the isolated volume eventually will be removed. The output time-concentration curve can be described as a convolution between the input time-concentration curve and an impulse function, convolution designating a "memory" mathematical operation. The key of the central volume principle lies in solving the inverse operation, that is, the deconvolution of the measured parenchymal and arterial time-concentration profiles (15–19).

The mean transit time (MTT) (Fig. 46-1) is the average time delay necessary for an instantaneous bolus of iodinated contrast material to cross the cerebral capillary network. In each pixel of the CT slice, it can be calculated by a deconvolution of the parenchymal time-concentration curves by a reference arterial curve.

In the central volume principle (6–8), the regional cerebral blood volume (rCBV), which is related to the relative volume occupied by blood in a pixel, is inferred from a quantitative evaluation of a partial volume averaging effect (PVAE). Time-concentration curves measured during perfusion CT studies do not have the same areas: the latter are larger in pure vascular pixels than in parenchymal pixels, including blood within capillaries, but also neurons, axonal tubes, and myelin sheaths. In these parenchymal pixels, the vascular volume only represents a few percentages of the total tissue volume, thus leading to PVAE. As such, PVAE is completely absent in a reference pixel in the middle of the large superior longitudinal sinus, and the following equation ensues:

$$rCBV = \frac{\text{Area under the curve in a parenchymal pixel}}{\text{Area under the curve in the reference pixel}}$$

Correction factor, which is related to the microhematocrit in the cerebral microvascularization, must be introduced to account for the restriction of iodinated contrast material to the plasma phase of the blood. Normal values of rCBV are about 6 mL/100 g in the gray matter and 2 mL/100 g in the white matter (1).

Finally, the combination of rCBV designating a blood volume and MTT related to the time delay necessary for the blood to cross the local capillary network leads to rCBF:

$$rCBF = \frac{rCBV}{MTT} .$$

Normal values of rCBF are 80 mL/100 g per minute in the gray matter and 20 mL/100 g per minute in the

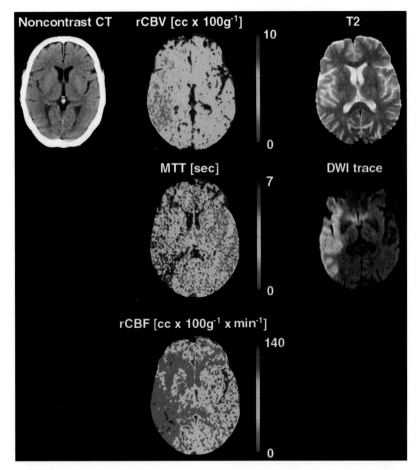

FIG. 46-1. A 75-year-old male patient admitted to our institution after sudden onset of a left face-arm-leg sensorimotor hemisyndrome. Physical examination revealed left hemianopsia, rightward gaze deviation, dysarthria, and left hemineglect. The patient underwent cerebral computed tomography (CT) and magnetic resonance examinations 2 and 3 hours after admission, respectively. Perfusion CT [regional cerebral blood volume (rCBV), mean transit time (MTT), regional cerebral blood flow (rCBF)] and diffusion-weighted image trace clearly depict an acute stroke extending to the superficial right middle cerebral artery territory, whereas the latter is much more subtle on T2-weighted image and especially on noncontrast cerebral CT, where it features a "cortical ribbon loss" sign.

white matter, with variations related to local cerebral activity changes (1).

Other searchers have attempted to apply another model to perfusion CT studies: the maximal slope model. The maximal slope model initially was developed for microspheres, such as radiolabeled spheres. These microspheres are completely "extracted at first pass": They are trapped in the capillary networks, with the measured activity growing up to a plateau and then remaining constant. The perfusion in a given area is linearly related to the total amount of microspheres accumulated in this area, as well as to the accumulation rate of microspheres, that is, the maximal slope of the accumulation curve (20). The maximal slope model applied to perfusion CT studies

(21,22) underestimates rCBF values and does not outline the contrast between gray and white matter perfusion (18). This is true with low injection rates of iodinated contrast material, even in the case of adequate perfusion CT data postprocessing (rebuilding of an accumulation curve by adding successive measurements of contrast material along with time) (16) and with very short injection times allowed by very high injection rates for intravenous administration of contrast material. Injection rates as high as 20 mL/s have been reported (22), but we have never used those high rates in our patients. The 5 mL/s rate is the maximal injection rate that can be tolerated by patients in the setting of intravenous administration of iodinated contrast material through a small peripheral vein.

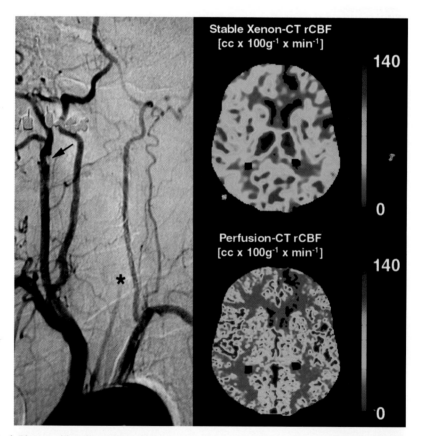

FIG. 46-2. A 50-year-old male smoker with severe cerebral artery atherosclerosis. Posteroanterior angiographic view displays complete occlusion of the left common carotid artery *(star)* and right internal carotid artery *(arrow)*, as well as atherosclerotic changes of the brachiocephalic artery, right external carotid artery, and right subclavian artery. The left subclavian artery had been stented, but endothelial hyperplasia within this stent explained the recurrence of a subclavian steal syndrome in this patient. Stable xenon computed tomography (CT) was obtained after angioplasty within the stent in order to evaluate brain perfusion. The stable xenon CT regional cerebral blood flow (rCBF) map demonstrates an anterior and left superficial sylvian hypoperfusion, related to previous strokes. The perfusion CT rCBF map according the central volume principle is closely related to the corresponding reference stable xenon CT map in both the gray and the white matter.

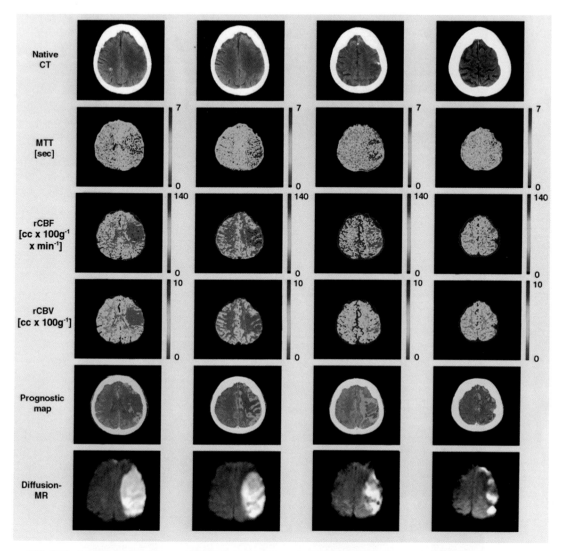

FIG. 46-3. A hypertensive 43-year-old female patient was admitted to our institution 3.5 hours after sudden onset of a right face-arm-leg hemisyndrome, associated with a right homonymous hemianopsia and a global aphasia. Thrombolysis was not performed because it was contraindicated. The native cerebral computed tomogram (CT) obtained 30 minutes after admission *(first line)* demonstrates a subtle loss of the cortical ribbon in the left sylvian territory, whereas the more sensitive perfusion CT prognostic map *(fifth line)* clearly identifies a posterior left middle cerebral artery (MCA) infarct *(red)* with a limited rim of penumbra *(green)*. Mean transit time (MTT) *(second line)* and regional cerebral blood flow (rCBF) *(third line)* are increased and decreased, respectively, in both the infarct and the penumbra, whereas regional cerebral blood volume (rCBV) *(fourth line)* is decreased in the infarct and preserved or increased in the penumbra because of self-regulation processes. Due to persistent occlusion of the left MCA (demonstrated by angio-CT and angio-magnetic resonance), the penumbra noted on admission perfusion CT evolved toward infarct and was completely replaced by it, as demonstrated by the close correlation of the entire ischemic area (penumbra + infarct) as seen on perfusion CT with the infarct displayed on the delayed diffusion-weighted MR *(sixth line)* obtained 2 days after admission.

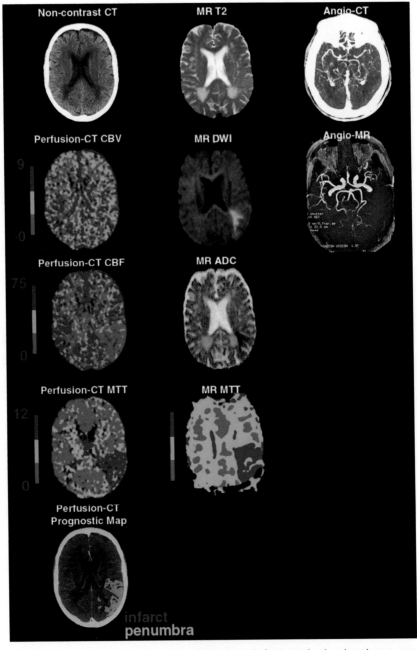

FIG. 46-4. A 71-year-old male patient with sudden onset of a right face-arm-leg hemisyndrome, associated with nonfluent aphasia. Noncontrast cerebral computed tomography (CT)/perfusion CT and diffusion-weighted/perfusion-weighted magnetic resonance imaging (DW/PW MRI) were performed 2 and 2.3 hours after symptomatology onset, respectively. Noncontrast cerebral CT demonstrates left insula ribbon sign and left parietal hypodensity. Cerebral infarct and cerebral blood volume abnormality on perfusion CT (mL × 100 g^{-1}) show similar sizes to DWI MR abnormality. Cerebral ischemic lesion and cerebral blood flow/mean transit time (CBF/MTT) abnormality on perfusion CT [(mL × 100 g^{-1} × min^{-1})/s] and MR MTT abnormality involve the entire left middle cerebral artery territory, related to an M1 occlusion on both angio-CT and angio-MR. The patient underwent unsuccessful thrombolysis.

VALIDATION OF QUANTITATIVE CEREBRAL BLOOD FLOW OF MEASUREMENT BY PERFUSION COMPUTED TOMOGRAPHY

Quantitative assessment of CBF can be obtained by imaging techniques other than perfusion CT. Among them is stable xenon CT. Stable xenon CT is related to dynamic CT acquisition during inhalation of stable xenon by the patient. Stable xenon is an inert gas that freely diffuses from alveolar air into the blood and then into all tissues, and notably into the cerebral parenchyma, until a steady state is established. The brain concentration of stable xenon is evaluated on sequential CT data because of its radiopacity. Stable xenon CT studies require specialized and expensive equipment, as well as excellent collaboration from patient that may be acutely affected. Side effects, such as respiratory rate decrease, headaches, nausea and vomiting, and convulsions, are observed in 4.4% of patients (23). Because of these side effects, stable xenon CT studies are difficult to use in the emergency settings. Stable xenon CT results were proved to be quantitatively accurate by comparison with radiolabeled microspheres studies; thus, stable xenon CT studies constitute an adequate gold standard for rCBF quantitative assessment.

Perfusion CT results have been quantitatively validated against those of stable xenon CT (24). A strong correlation was demonstrated between perfusion CT and stable xenon CT results, both in healthy cerebral regions and pathologic cerebral regions with low rCBF (Fig. 46-2, see page 392). This accurate correlation in cerebral areas with lowered blood flows confers an adequate reliability to perfusion CT studies in the evaluation of ischemic cerebral parenchyma (24).

IMPACT OF PERFUSION COMPUTED TOMOGRAPHY ON MANAGEMENT OF ACUTE STROKE

rCBF lowering is responsible for progressive inhibition of the various electric and metabolic activities of the neurons, which are related to as many thresholds. This inhibition, first reversible and called "penumbra," becomes significant as soon as rCBF decreases to less than 20 mL/100 g per minute. Below 10-to 15 mL/100 g per minute, alteration of adenosine triphosphate (ATP) synthesis leads to disturbance of membrane ion pumping. If the latter persists for more than 3 minutes, irretrievable cerebral infarct occurs. Early after a cerebral arterial occlusion, penumbra occurs in the territory of cerebral parenchyma perfused by this artery. With time, infarct progressively replaces the penumbra from the center to the periphery of the arterial territory, with the replacing rate varying according to the collateral circulation level (25–28).

The aim of thrombolysis is to rescue the penumbra (29). However, thrombolysis is associated with a significant increase in cerebral bleeding, up to 15% (30). This explains why strict criteria have been defined to include acute middle cerebral artery (MCA) stroke patients in intravenous thrombolysis protocols, as follows:

Delay from the symptomatology onset is less than 3 hours

Extent of abnormality noted on the admission native CT is less than to one third of the MCA territory

Absence of contraindications constituting risk factors for intracranial hemorrhage (31–33)

Evaluation of brain perfusion before thrombolysis has been suggested as a possible selection criterion for treatment (34,35) because extensive oligemia in the territory of an occluded MCA seems to be related to an unfavorable risk-to-benefit ratio. Thrombolysis achieved in patients with extended cerebral infarcts having limited penumbra not only would have little benefit but also increases the risk of intracranial bleeding (32,36).

Perfusion CT, as already reported, can be performed easily in the emergency settings, even in acute stroke patients. Moreover, nonionic iodinated contrast material is not toxic for ischemic neurons (37). Perfusion CT permits rCBF and rCBV maps. It also can make a differentiation of penumbra and infarct by persistence or disappearance of vascular autoregulation reflexes. In both penumbra and infarct, rCBF is lowered to less than 15 to 20 mL/100 g per minute. However, in penumbra, rCBV is increased in an attempt to compensate for rCBF lowering by autoregulation processes, which are responsible for local vasodilation. In infarct, autoregulation reflexes are compromised and rCBV is lowered (2,3). A prognostic map can be created from perfusion CT, representing location and extension of both penumbra and infarct (Fig. 46-3, see page 393).

The accuracy of prognostic maps extracted from admission perfusion CT results was demonstrated by comparison with delayed MR (4). In patients with persistent arterial occlusion on delayed angio-MR, the ischemic area (penumbra + infarct) on the admission perfusion CT gradually evolves toward infarct because of prolongation of the arterial occlusion. In patients with arterial repermeabilization, either spontaneous or as a result of thrombolysis, most of the penumbra recovers. From a clinical point of view, the initial severity of the clinical condition is proportional to the size of the ischemic area on admission perfusion CT (penumbra + infarct). Last but not least, in case of arterial recanalization, the observed clinical improvement is linearly correlated with the potential recuperation ratio (PRR), which is defined as the relative extent of penumbra compared to the whole ischemic area (penumbra + infarct) on the admission perfusion CT. This indicates that the clinical prognosis is better with a high PRR, that is, when the penumbra predominates over the infarct with regard to size (4).

Perfusion CT allows for quantitative assessment of rCBF and rCBV, as well as accurate prognosis of final cerebral infarct size in acute stroke patients, and this can be done as early as upon admission. It affords precise delineation of salvageable penumbra. Perfusion CT results correlate with the patient's clinical condition, and the severity of the clinical condition on admission is directly related to the size of the ischemic cerebral area on admission perfusion CT. Perfusion CT allows for definition of PRR, which is related to improvement of the National Institutes of Health Stroke Scale (NIHSS) with time. Thus, perfusion CT may constitute an additional worthy criterion used to decide whether to perform thrombolysis in acute stroke patients.

DIFFUSION-WEIGHTED MAGNETIC RESONANCE IMAGING

DWI is an MRI technique that assesses random brownian motion of water molecules. Diffusion of water molecules alters conventional T1- and T2-weighted MRI because it induces signal dephasing and signal loss. This signal change can be turned into specific information that constitutes the basis of DWI. Acute stroke is the clinical situation where DWI shows its most spectacular application, because alteration of the diffusion coefficient (characterizing the brownian motion of water molecules) of the cerebral tissue is the first change that can be observed by MRI after an ischemic event (38–41). Alteration of the diffusion coefficient is sufficient to create a large contrast between infarcted and normal brain tissue in DWI.

In practice, two types of diffusion-related images are available on state-of-the-art MR scanners. The first is the *DWI trace image,* and the second is the *apparent diffusion coefficient (ADC) map.*

Information carried by DWI traces and ADC maps are complementary. The DWI trace provides sharp delineation of pathologic processes by the removal of anisotropy of myelin fibers and the absence of contrast between gray and white matter, whereas ADC maps allow elimination of "T2 shine-through" (42).

TIME EVOLUTION OF DIFFUSION-WEIGHTED IMAGING AFTER ACUTE STROKE

The volume and diffusion characteristics of ischemic lesions evolve during the first weeks after stroke (Fig. 46-5). CT or T2-weighted MR images become positive only several hours, usually 5 or 6, after stroke onset. DWI provides valuable information not available on standard T1- and T2-weighted MR images, particularly by showing hyperacute brain ischemia within minutes after stroke onset. In a rodent model, sensitivity of DWI for detection of acute infarction was 60% within 50 minutes and 100% within 2 hours after symptom onset (43–47).

The volume of the ischemic lesion markedly increases until 24 to 36 hours after stroke onset and reaches its maximum at 2 to 5 days. The relative contribution of further infarction to lesion growth depends on the persistence or resolution of perfusion abnormality. The lesion volume then shows a limited decrease in size between 7 to 10 days and 3 months after stroke onset, which is related to edema resolution and possibly early atrophy (48–57).

Hyperacute cerebral ischemia is characterized by decreased diffusion coefficients, featuring hyperintensity on DWI trace and hypointensity on ADC maps. Decrease in diffusion persists until 2 to 7 days after stroke onset. As the infarct ages, variability in ADC decrease can be seen throughout the infarct, with some subregions having decreased ADC and other ones increased ADC compared with normal brain tissue, even though the lesion appears homogeneous on T2-weighted images. Between 7 and 14 days after infarct, a transition to normal ("pseudonormalization") and then to increased ADC values occurs, even though increased signal intensity is seen within this tissue on T2-weighted MRI. During the late subacute and chronic phases, ADC values increase further as encephalomalacia and gliosis occur. Because of T2 shine-through, infarct may remain hyperintense on DWI trace even in the late subacute stage, and increased ADC values permit distinction of the acute stage (44).

The exact cause of ADC decrease in ischemic cerebral parenchyma remains controversial. Several

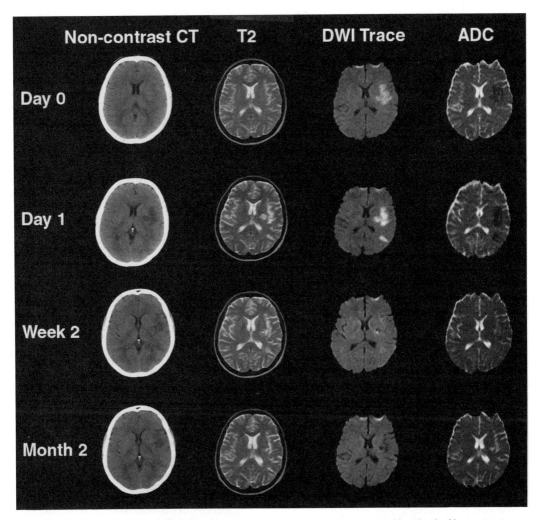

FIG. 46-5. A 51-year-old female patient was admitted for a right hemisyndrome with aphasia. Noncontrast computed tomography (CT) and T2-weighted magnetic resonance (MR) examinations obtained 4 and 5 hours after symptomatology onset, respectively, are normal. Only a slight left cortical ribbon erasing can be suspected on noncontrast CT. On the other hand, diffusion-weighted imaging (DWI) clearly identifies low diffusion coefficients in the deep left sylvian territory. This patient did not undergo thrombolysis; however, this clinical condition evolved favorably. Twenty-four hours later, a sequelar DWI abnormality persists in the left lenticular nucleus and external capsula, with additional lesion at the left parietooccipital junction. On follow-up examination, apparent diffusion coefficient (ADC) values first undergo "pseudonormalization." During the late subacute and chronic phases, ADC values increase further as encephalomalacia and gliosis occur. Lesion size decreases because of edema resolution and early atrophy.

mechanisms have been proposed. Among them, cytotoxic edema currently is the most frequently advocated mechanism. However, changes in intracellular and/or extracellular diffusion coefficients and changes in cell membrane permeability also have been postulated. Cytotoxic edema involves water redistribution from the extracellular to the intracellular compartment. In healthy cerebral parenchyma, the intracellular-to-extracellular volume ratio is about 80%:20% (58). In case of stroke, the intracellular compartment swells from 80% of the overall volume to 95% (59). Because this intracellular compartment is characterized by reduced diffusion coefficients due to macromolecular content (60), an increase in its volume might explain the observed lowering in ADC values. However, some believe that a 15% movement of water is insufficient to cause the ADC decrease of up to 50% usually seen in infarcts. Alternatively, shrinking of the extracellular volume, and subsequent increased tortuosity of diffusion pathways around cells, might lead to decreased ADC values (43,61). More experimental work is needed to obtain a better understanding of the physiopathologic processes at the origin of DWI contrast.

The potential reversibility of restricted diffusion seen on DWI is of major concern when therapeutic strategy selection relies on distinction between irretrievable infarct and salvageable penumbra. Experimental animal studies have demonstrated reversible DWI abnormalities within the first minutes or hours of cerebral ischemia. These reversible changes occurred in the periphery of the infarct core, in regions with mild perfusion deficit, and not in regions of severely decreased perfusion (62,63). Note that the pathophysiologic significance of these reversible abnormalities has been discussed and its correlation with penumbra questioned (64). Reversible changes have been reported occasionally in humans (65–67).

DIFFUSION-WEIGHTED IMAGING AND PERFUSION-WEIGHTED IMAGING IN CLINICAL MANAGEMENT OF STROKE

Several studies were dedicated to using potential existing thresholds in ADC values to distinguish between infarct and penumbra (68–70). Perfusion-weighted imaging (PWI) by bolus tracking demonstrates hemodynamic abnormalities and may provide additional information to DWI for early characterization of hyperacute cerebral ischemia. The initial PWI abnormality usually is larger than the initial DWI abnormality. It has been postulated that the DWI/PWI mismatch may identify cerebral regions of salvageable penumbra and represent a potential target for thrombolytic therapy (Fig. 46-4, see page 394). By following the progression of the lesion and determining the factors that influence its development, DWI and PWI have the potential to be prognostic tools and predict neurologic outcome (46–49,71–77).

Patients with cerebrovascular diseases often have multiple ischemic lesions seen on conventional MR examination at the time of their first symptomatic event. In our registry, among 1,000 consecutive patients with first-ever stroke, 3% showed infarcts in multiple territories supplied by carotid arteries, 2% multiple infarcts in the vertebrobasilar territory, and 2% multiple infarcts in both territories (78). Among patients with multiple cerebral ischemic lesions, 30% showed multiple acute infarcts, 56% single acute infarct and multiple old infarcts, and 14% multiple acute and multiple old infarcts (79). One limitation of conventional MRI is that acute and old infarcts appear very similar. T2-weighted images do not allow differentiation of acute versus chronic infarcts, and T1-weighted images with gadolinium enhancement are helpful in only 12% of patients (79). This can cause diagnostic confusion with regard to determining which lesions are acute and symptomatic, even with the help of neurologic findings, especially in elderly patients whose conventional MR examination demonstrates a large number of high-signal foci in the corona radiata, basal ganglia, and brainstem on T2-weighted images. Moreover, in such patients it may be difficult to determine whether new neurologic symptoms represent a new ischemic event or just the unmasking of a prior deficit due to a concurrent illness. DWI can easily distinguish between new and old ischemic brain injuries, which show hyposignal and hypersignal on ADC maps, respectively. In 77% to 100% of patients with multiple cerebral infarcts, DWI not only delineates early ischemic brain injury better than conventional MR but it also successfully identifies the acute lesion responsible for the clinical deficit (79,80).

REFERENCES

1. Lassen NA. Cerebral blood flow and oxygen consumption in man. *Physiol Rev* 1959;39:183–238.
2. Harper AM. Autoregulation of cerebral blood flow: influence of the arterial blood pressure on the blood flow through the cerebral cortex, *J Neurol Neurosurg Psychiatry* 1966;29:398–403.
3. Sorensen AG, Copen WA, Ostergaard L, et al. Hyperacute stroke: simultaneous measurement of relative cerebral blood volume, relative cerebral blood flow, and mean tissue transit time. *Radiology* 1999;210:519–527.
4. Wintermark M, Reichhart M, Thiran J-Ph, et al. Prognostic accuracy of admission cerebral blood flow measurement by perfusion-computed tomography, at the time of emergency room admission, in acute stroke patients. *Ann Neurol* 2002; 51(4):417–432.
5. National Institute of Neurological Disorders and Stroke (NINDS) rt-PA Stroke Study Group. Tissue plasminogen activator for acute ischaemic stroke. *N Engl J Med* 1995;33:1581–1587.
6. Axel L. Cerebral blood flow determination by rapid-sequence computed tomography. *Radiology* 1980;137: 679–686.
7. Axel L. A method of calculating brain blood flow with a CT dynamic scanner. *Adv Neurol* 1981;30:67–71.
8. Axel L. Tissue mean transit time from dynamic computed tomography by a simple deconvolution technique. *Invest Radiol* 1983;18:94–99.
9. Ladurner G, Zilkha E, Iliff LD, et al. Measurement of regional cerebral blood volume by computerized axial

tomography. *J Neurol Neurosurg Psychiatry* 1976;39: 152–155.

10. Ladurner G, Zikha E, Sager WD, et al. Measurement of regional cerebral blood volume using the EMI 1010 scanner. *Br J Radiol* 1979;52:371–374.

11. Zilkha E, Ladurner G, Linette D, et al. Computer subtraction in regional cerebral blood-volume measurements using the EMI-scanner. *Br J Radiol* 1976;49: 330–334.

12. Wintermark M, Maeder P, Verdun FR, et al. Using 80 kVp versus 120 kVp in perfusion CT measurement of regional cerebral blood flows. *AJNR Am J Neuroradiol* 2000;21:1881–1884.

13. Claussen CD, Banzer D, Pfretzschner C, et al. Bolus geometry and dynamics after intravenous contrast medium injection. *Radiology* 1984;153:365–368.

14. Reiser UJ. Study of bolus geometry after intravenous contrast medium injection: dynamic and quantitative measurements (chronogram) using an X-ray CT device. *J Comput Assist Tomogr* 1984;8:251–262.

15. Meier P, Zierler KL. On the theory of the indicator-dilution method for measurement of blood flow and volume. *J Appl Physiol* 1954;12:731–744.

16. Zierler KL. Theoretical basis of indicator-dilution methods for measuring flow and volume. *Circ Res* 1962;10: 393–407.

17. Zierler KL. Equations for measuring blood flow by external monitoring of radioisotopes. *Circ Res* 1965;16: 309–321.

18. Wintermark M, Maeder P, Thiran J-P, et al. Quantitative assessment of regional cerebral blood flows by perfusion CT studies at low injection rates: a critical review of the underlying theoretical models. *Eur Radiol* 2001; 11:1220–1230.

19. Ostergaard L, Sorensen AG, Kwong KK, et al. High resolution measurement of cerebral blood flow using intravascular tracer bolus passages. Part I: mathematical approach and statistical analysis. *Magn Res Med* 1996; 36:715–725.

20. Peters AM, Gunasekera RD, Henderson BL, et al. Noninvasive measurements of blood flow and extraction fraction. *Nucl Med Commun* 1987;8:823–837.

21. Miles KA. Measurement of tissue perfusion by dynamic computed tomography. *Br J Radiol* 1991;64:409–412.

22. König M, Kraus M, Theek C et al. Quantitative assessment of the ischemic brain by means of perfusion-related parameters derived from perfusion CT. *Stroke* 2001;32:431–437.

23. Latchaw RE, Yonas H, Pentheny SL, et al. Adverse reactions to xenon-enhanced CT cerebral blood flow determination. *Radiology* 1987;163:251–254.

24. Wintermark M, Maeder P, Thiran J-P, et al. Simultaneous measurements of regional cerebral blood flows by perfusion-CT and stable xenon-CT: a validation study. *AJNR Am J Neuroradiol* 2001 22:905–914.

25. Bogousslavsky J, Van Melle G, Regli F. The Lausanne stroke registry: analysis of 1,000 consecutive patients with first stroke. *Stroke* 1988;19:1083–1092.

26. Symon L, Branston NM, Strong AJ, et al. The concepts of thresholds of ischaemia in relation to brain structure and function. *J Clin Pathol* 1977;30[Suppl]:149–154.

27. Hossmann KA. Viability thresholds and the penumbra of focal ischemia. *Ann Neurol* 1994;36:557–565.

28. Heiss WD. Ischemic penumbra: evidence from functional imaging in man. *J Cereb Blood Flow Metab* 2000;20:1276–93.

29. Heiss WD, Grond M, Thiel A, et al. Ischemic brain tissue salvaged from infarction with alteplase. *Lancet* 1997;349:1599–1600.

30. Katzan IL, Furlan AJ, Lloyd LE, et al. Use of tissue-type plasminogen activator for acute ischemic stroke: the Cleveland area experience. *JAMA* 2000;283: 1151–1158.

31. Hacke W, Kaste M, Fieschi C, et al. Intravenous thrombolysis with recombinant tissue plasminogen activator for acute hemispheric stroke. The European Cooperative Acute Stroke Study (ECASS). *JAMA* 1995;274: 1017–1025.

32. Hacke W, Kaste M, Fieschi C. Randomised double-blind trial placebo-controlled trial of thrombolytic therapy with intravenous therapy with intravenous alteplase in acute ischaemic stroke (ECASS II). *Lancet* 1998; 352:1245–1251.

33. Hennerici M. Improving the outcome of acute stroke management. *Hosp Med* 1999;60:44–49.

34. Rubin G, Firlik AD, Levy EI, et al. Relationship between cerebral blood flow and clinical outcome in acute stroke. *Cerebrovasc Dis* 2000;10:298–306.

35. Ezura M, Takahashi A, Yoshimoto T. Evaluation of regional cerebral blood flow using single photon emission tomography for the selection of patients for local fibrinolytic therapy of acute cerebral embolism. *Neurosurg Rev* 1996;19:231–236.

36. Oppenheim C, Samson Y, Manai R, et al. Prediction of malignant middle cerebral artery infarction by diffusion-weighted imaging. *Stroke* 2000;31:2175–2185.

37. Doerfler A, Engelhorn T, von Kummer R, et al. Are iodinated contrast agents detrimental in acute cerebral ischemia? An experimental study in rats. *Radiology* 1998;206:211–217.

38. Le Bihan D, Breton E, Lallemand D, et al. MR imaging of intravoxel incoherent motions: application to diffusion and perfusion in neurologic disorders. *Radiology* 1986;161:401–407.

39. Moseley ME, Sevick R, Wendland MF, et al. Ultrafast magnetic resonance imaging: diffusion and perfusion. *Can Assoc Radiol J* 1991;42:31–38.

40. Warach S, Gaa J, Siewert B, et al. Acute human stroke studied by whole brain echo planar diffusion-weighted magnetic resonance imaging. *Ann Neurol* 1995;37: 231–241.

41. Warach S, Boska M, Welch KM. Pitfalls and potential clinical diffusion-weighted MR imaging in acute stroke. *Stroke* 1997;28:481–82.

42. Provenzale JR, Engelter ST, Petrella JR, et al. Use of MR exponential diffusion-weighted images to eradicate T2 shine-through effect. *AJR Am J Roentgenol* 1999; 172:537–539.

43. Moseley M, Kucharczyk J, Mintorovirch J, et al. Diffusion-weighted MR imaging of acute stroke: correlation with T2-weighted and magnetic susceptibility enhanced MR imaging in cats. *AJNR Am J Neuroradiol* 1990;11: 423–429.

44. Jones SC, Perez-Trepichio AD, Xue M, et al. Magnetic resonance diffusion-weighted imaging: sensitivity and apparent diffusion constant in stroke. *Acta Neurochir* 1994;60:207–210.

45. Baird A, Warach S. Magnetic resonance imaging of acute stroke. *J Cereb Blood Flow Metab* 1998;18: 583–609.

46. Beaulieu C, de Crespigny A, Tong DC, et al. Longitudinal magnetic resonance imaging study of perfusion and

diffusion in stroke: evolution of lesion volume and correlation with clinical outcome. *Ann Neurol* 1999;46: 568–578.

47. Gonzalez RG, Schaefer PW, Buonanno F, et al. Diffusion-weighted MR imaging: diagnostic accuracy in patients imaged within 6 hours of stroke symptom onset. *Radiology* 1999;210:155–162.

48. Baird A, Benfield A, Schlaug G, et al. Enlargement of human cerebral ischemic lesion volumes measured by diffusion-weighted magnetic resonance imaging. *Ann Neurol* 1997;41:581–589.

49. Barber P, Darby D, Desmond PM, et al. Prediction of stroke outcome with echoplanar perfusion- and diffusion-weighted MRI. *Neurology* 1998;51:418–426.

50. Sorensen A, Buonanno F, Gonzalez R, et al. Hyperacute stroke: evaluation with combined multisection diffusion-weighted and hemodynamically weighted echoplanar MR imaging. *Radiology* 1996;199:391–401.

51. Schwamm L, Koroshetz W, Sorensen A, et al. Time course lesion development in patients with acute stroke: serial diffusion- and hemodynamic-weighted magnetic resonance in aging. *Stroke* 1998;29:2268–2276.

52. van Everdingen K, van der Grond J, Kappelle L, et al. Diffusion-weighted magnetic resonance imaging in acute stroke. *Stroke* 1998;29:1783–1790.

53. Chien D, Kwong KK, Gress DR, et al. MR diffusion imaging of cerebral infarction in humans. *AJNR Am J Neuroradiol* 1992;13:1097–1102.

54. Moseley ME, Buns K, Yenari MA, et al. Clinical aspects of DW imaging. *NMR Biomed* 1995;8:387–396.

55. Schlaug G, Siewert B, Benfield BS, et al. Time course of the apparent diffusion coefficient (ADC) abnormality in human stroke. *Neurology* 1997;49:113–119.

56. Lutsep HL, Albers GW, de Crespigny A, et al. Clinical utility of diffusion-weighted magnetic resonance imaging in the assessment of ischemic stroke. *Ann Neurol* 1997;41:575–580.

57. Nagesh V, Welch KMA, Windham JP, et al. Time course of ADC changes in ischemic stroke: beyond the human eye! *Stroke* 1998;29:1778–1782.

58. Fenstermacher JD, Li CL, Levin VA. Extracellular space of the cerebral cortex of normal thermic and hypothermic cats. *Exp Neurol* 1970;27:101–104.

59. Kempski O, Staub F, van Rosen F, et al. Molecular mechanisms of glial swelling in vitro. *Neurochem Pathol* 1988;9:109–125.

60. Herbst RH, Goldstein JH. A review of water diffusion measurement by NMR in human red blood cells. *Am J Physiol* 1989;256:C1097–C1104.

61. Latour LL, Svoboda K, Mitra PP, et al. Time-dependent diffusion of water in a biological model system. *Proc Natl Acad Sci USA* 1994;91:1229–1233.

62. Pierpaoli C, Alger JR, Righini A, et al. High-temporal resolution diffusion MRI of global cerebral ischemia and reperfusion. *J Cereb Blood Flow Metab* 1996;16: 892–905.

63. Minematsu K, Li L, Sotak CH, et al. Reversible focal ischemic injury demonstrated by diffusion-weighted magnetic resonance imaging in rats. *Stroke* 1992;23: 1310–1311.

64. Ringer TM, Neumann-Haefelin T, Sobel RA, et al. Reversal of early diffusion-weighted magnetic resonance imaging abnormalities does not necessarily reflect tissue salvage in experimental cerebral ischemia. *Stroke* 2001;32:2362–2369.

65. Krueger K, Kugel H, Grond M, et al. Late resolution of diffusion-weighted MRI changes in a patient with prolonged reversible ischemic neurological deficit after thrombolytic therapy. *Stroke* 2000;31:2715–2718.

66. Doege CA, Kerskens CM, Romero BI, et al. MRI of small human stroke shows reversible diffusion changes in subcortical gray matter. *NeuroReport* 2000;11:2021–2024.

67. Kidwell CS, Saver JL, Mattiello J, et al. Thrombolytic reversal of acute human cerebral ischemic injury shown by diffusion/perfusion magnetic resonance imaging. *Ann Neurol* 2000;47:462–469.

68. Hasegawa Y, Fisher M, Latour LL, et al. MRI diffusion mapping of reversible and irreversible ischemic injury in focal brain ischemia. *Neurology* 1994;44:1484–1490.

69. Desmond PM, Lovell AC, Rawlinson AA, et al. The value of apparent diffusion coefficient maps in early cerebral ischemia. *AJNR Am J Neuroradiol* 2001;22: 1260–1267.

70. Lutsep HL, Nesbit GM, Berger RM, et al. Does reversal of ischemia on diffusion-weighted imaging reflect higher apparent diffusion coefficient values? *J Neuroimaging* 2001;11:313–316.

71. Rordorf G, Koroshetz W, Copen W, et al. Regional ischemia and ischemic injury in patients with acute middle cerebral artery stroke as defined by early diffusion-weighted and perfusion-weighted MRI. *Stroke* 1998;29:939–943.

72. Sorensen A, Buonanno F, Gonzalez R, et al. Hyperacute stroke: evaluation with combined multisection diffusion-weighted and hemodynamically weighted echoplanar MR imaging. *Radiology* 1996;199:391–401.

73. Sorensen AG, Copen WA, Ostergaard L, et al. Hyperacute stroke: simultaneous measurement of relative cerebral blood volume, relative cerebral blood flow, and mean tissue transit time. *Radiology* 1999; 210: 51–527.

74. Baron J, von Kummer R, del Zoppo G. Treatment of acute ischemic stroke: challenging the concept of a rigid and universal time window. *Stroke* 1995;26:2219–2221.

75. Wu O, Koroshetz WJ, Ostergaard L, et al. Predicting tissue outcome in acute human cerebral ischemia using combined diffusion- and perfusion-weighted MR imaging. *Stroke* 2001;32:933–942.

76. Warach S. New imaging strategies for patient selection for thrombolytic and neuroprotective therapies. *Neurology* 2001;57:S48–S52.

77. Rohl L, Ostergaard L, Simonsen CZ, et al. Viability thresholds of ischemic penumbra of hyperacute stroke defined by perfusion-weighted MRI and apparent diffusion coefficient. *Stroke* 2001;32:1140–1146.

78. Bogousslavsky J, Van Melle G, Regli F. The Lausanne Stroke Registry: analysis of 1,000 consecutive patients with first ever stroke. *Stroke* 1988;19:1083–1092.

79. Altieri M, Metz RJ, Müller C, et al. Multiple brain infarcts: clinical and neuroimaging patterns using diffusion-weighted magnetic resonance. *Eur Neurol* 1999; 42:76–82.

80. Kumon Y, Zenke K, Kusunoki K, et al. Diagnostic use of isotropic diffusion-weighted MRI in patients with ischaemic stroke: detection of the lesion responsible for the clinical deficit. *Neuroradiology* 1999;41:777–784.

Ischemic Stroke: Advances in Neurology, Vol. 92. Edited by
H.J.M. Barnett, Julien Bogousslavsky, and Heather Meldrum.
Lippincott Williams & Wilkins, Philadelphia © 2003.

47

Ongoing Trials and Future Directions for Acute Ischemic Stroke Treatment

Marc Fisher

*Department of Neurology, University of Massachusetts Medical School, Worcester,
Massachusetts, U.S.A.*

Currently, the only approved therapy for acute ischemic stroke in some countries is intravenous recombinant tissue plasminogen activator (rtPA) within 3 hours of stroke onset based upon the favorable results of the National Institute of Neurological Disorders and Stroke (NINDS) rt-PA Trial (1). The only other phase III acute stroke therapy trials to achieve a favorable response of the prespecified primary outcome measure were the 3-hour time window trial of the fibrinogen-lowering agent Ancrod and the 6-hour window trial of intraarterial prourokinase (2,3). Neither of these two drugs currently is approved or available for use in acute stroke patients. Ancrod failed to show benefit in a 6-hour window trial and further development has been discontinued. The prourokinase trial included only 180 patients randomized in a 2:1 manner to active treatment or placebo. Regulatory authorities apparently required additional proof of efficacy before granting approval, and it remains uncertain if an additional pivotal trial will be performed. These few successful trials are far outweighed by many other acute stroke therapy trials where no statistically significant difference was determined for the experimental therapeutic agent in comparison to placebo (Table 47-1). These negative trials include all of the purported neuroprotective drugs that have been investigated to date (4). A wide variety of different approaches and drug platforms were studied in phase III trials, including voltage-regulated calcium channel antagonists, competitive and noncompetitive N-methyl-D-aspartate (NMDA) antagonists, glycine site antagonist, polyamine site antagonist, γ-aminobutyric acid (GABA) agonist, glutamate release inhibitor, free radical scavenger, monoclonal antibody directed against the intracellular adhesion molecule-1 (ICAM-1) receptor, growth factor, promoter of membrane repair, and nootropic agent. This list is not complete and does not include other neuroprotective drugs that were not studied beyond phase II trials because of safety concerns, inability to achieve presumed neuroprotective plasma levels, or other reasons.

TABLE 47-1. *Negative large neuroprotective trials*

1. Voltage-regulated calcium channel antagonist: nimodipine
2. NMDA antagonist: aptiganel (Cerestat)
3. Glycine antagonist: GV150526
4. Polyaminesite antagonist: eliprodil
5. Sodium channel blockers: lubeluzole
6. GABA agonist: clomethiazole
7. Free-radical scavengers: tirilazad
8. Anti-adhesion molecule: enlimolab
9. Maxi-K channel agonist: Maxi-post
10. Growth factor: basic fibroblast growth factor
11. Membrane repair agent: citicoline
12. Norotropic agent: piracetam

GABA, α-aminobutyric acid; NMDA, N-methyl-D-aspartate.

Currently, there are few ongoing phase II or phase III trials of new therapeutic agents for acute ischemic stroke. Many challenges confront physicians and the pharmaceutical industry interested in developing effective new therapies for acute ischemic stroke. These efforts can be helped by appreciating the lessons contained within the preclinical assessment of previously tested drugs and the data from prior trials. Issues to consider for new acute stroke therapy trials include why did prior trials fail, how the therapeutic time window can be extended, what basic science advances in determining the mechanisms of focal ischemic brain injury can contribute to enhancing acute stroke therapy, and most importantly how the important endeavor to increase the availability and effectiveness of acute stroke therapy can be reenergized.

WHY DO ACUTE STROKE THERAPY TRIALS FAIL?

There are many potential reasons why a drug will not demonstrate efficacy for improving outcome after ischemic stroke. For thrombolytic drugs, there appear to be two primary reasons. Streptokinase appears to cause an excessive rate of hemorrhagic side effects that would mask potential beneficial treatment effects (5). The negative intravenous rtPA trials enrolled patients beyond the 3-hour time window, and at this later time point treatment efficacy likely will be more difficult to detect unless patients more likely to respond to the treatment and less likely to bleed are identified a priori (6–8). The second European Cooperative Acute Stroke Study (ECASS) Trial did attempt to reduce the hemorrhagic risk by careful pretreatment computed tomographic (CT) evaluation (7). The trial did not achieve a statistically significant benefit for the prespecified outcome measure of a Rankin score of 0 or 1, but post hoc analysis with a Rankin cutoff of 0 to 2 did show a statistically significant treatment effect

with intravenous rtPA initiated within 6 hours of stroke onset. These results were not replicated in the 3- to 5-hour time window Alteplase Thrombolysis for Acute Noninterventional Therapy in Ischemic Stroke (ATLANTIS) trial of intravenous rtPA (8). It is possible that intravenous rtPA can be shown to significantly improve outcome when given more than 3 hours after stroke onset if hemorrhagic risk is reduced and enrollment of patients with a greater chance to improve with reperfusion is enriched. Potential strategies to enhance the enrollment of stroke patients more likely to respond to therapy will be discussed in detail later.

The many negative neuroprotective trials have not succeeded for a variety of reasons. The first possible explanation for lack of efficacy of a neuroprotective drug in clinical trials is that the drug does not have neuroprotective effects. If the animal testing of a neuroprotective drug does not demonstrate efficacy that is robust and reproducible, then it is unlikely that the drug has a substantial likelihood of reducing infarct size and improving outcome in patients. For neuroprotective drugs to improve functional and/or neurologic outcome, infarct size must be reduced. The adequacy of preclinical testing for some neuroprotective drugs subsequently studied in clinical trials has been questioned, as has the breadth of testing that would provide reassurance that the drug has potent neuroprotective effects. A group of academic investigators and pharmaceutical industry representatives reported recommendations for preclinical testing of purported neuroprotective drugs (9). The recommendations are summarized in Table 47-2. The main features of the recommendations are that the neuroprotective drug should reduce infarct size and improve functional outcome in a variety of animal stroke models at multiple investigative sites with a reasonable dose and time window range. Many pharmaceutical companies are using these recommendations while new neuroprotective drugs are being developed.

TABLE 47-2. *STAIR-1 recommendations for preclinical assessment of neuroprotective drugs*

1. Evaluate most drugs initially in rodent permanent occlusion models
2. Provide an adequate dose–response curve
3. Explore the time window of therapeutic benefit in well-characterized models
4. All preclinical studies should be performed in a blinded randomized manner with adequate physiologic monitoring
5. Outcome measures should include infarct volume and functional measures both within a few days after stroke and at later time points
6. For drugs primarily directed at reperfusion injury, initial studies can be done in temporary occlusion models, and such models can be used secondarily for standard neuroprotective drugs
7. Consideration for evaluating novel, first-in-class drugs in gyrencephalic species is strongly recommended

STAIR, Stroke Therapy Academic Industry Roundtable.

Another important problem in neuroprotective drug development has been toxicity and side effects. These complications limited the doses of drug that could be given safely to humans and in some cases precluded achieving plasma drug levels that were needed to achieve neuroprotection in preclinical studies (10). Thus, the efficacy of the drug could not be tested because only inadequate doses could be safely given. Additionally, if the therapeutic range was not well defined in animals, then the doses used in humans may have not been adequate or at the wrong place in the dose–response curve. Trial design issues also have hampered many neuroprotective trials. It now is clear that patients with mild initial neurologic deficits have a favorable outcome without intervention, so if many placebo-treated patients included in the trial improve spontaneously the power to detect a treatment effect will be compromised (11). Conversely, patients with a severe initial neurologic deficit have little chance to recover with any intervention (12). It is apparent that moderate to moderately severe stroke patients are the most appropriate patients to include in initial trials. The mechanism of action of the drug to be tested is an important consideration for designing clinical trials and for deciding what stroke subtypes to include. The likely mechanisms of ischemic injury appear to be somewhat different in gray and white matter (13). If the drug to be tested has a mechanism of action not amenable to impeding white matter injury, then patients with predominantly white matter ischemic strokes (i.e. lacunes) should not be included in the trial. In most early ischemic stroke trials, stroke subtype and mechanism of injury/protection were not considered. This lack of subtyping could have masked potential treatment benefits in appropriately targeted patients. Consideration of the time window of drug activity is another area of concern (14). For many neuroprotective drugs, the time window for tissue salvage is short, yet essentially all neuroprotective clinical trials have had a time window for enrollment of 6 hours or longer. In most trials, a large percentage of patients are randomized in the last hour of the enrollment window. It is possible that one or more of the previously tested neuroprotective drugs might have demonstrated efficacy if the time window for enrollment had been shorter or time to enrollment had been stratified to mandate a shorter mean enrollment time. No neuroprotective drug has ever been tested in a manner comparable to rtPA in the NINDS trial, which had a 3-hour enrollment window and mandated that half of the enrolled patients be included within 90 minutes of stroke onset. Measurement of treatment effect is problematic. As mentioned, in ECASS-2 the prespecified primary outcome measure of Rankin score 0 to 1 was not statistically significantly different between the rtPA and placebo groups, yet a Rankin dichotomization of 0 to 2 did demonstrate a significant treatment effect (7). For the neuroprotective and recovery-enhancing drug citicoline, a similar problem with outcome assessment also occurred. In none of the citicoline trials has a significant treatment effect been demonstrated on the prespecified primary outcome measure, but meta-analysis of the citicoline trials using a global assessment of the Rankin score, Barthel index, and change of National Institutes of Health Stroke Scale (NIHSS) score from baseline does reveal a statistically significant effect in favor of citicoline (15,16) (B. Sandage, *personal communication*, 2002). Another problem with many trials has been the lack of adequate power to detect a small but potentially meaningful treatment effect (17). Trying to observe a 10% or greater absolute difference between the active treatment group and the placebo group may be overly optimistic. Powering trials to detect a 5% difference may be more realistic. Concerns about all of these issues led to the organization of a second Stroke Therapy Academic Industry Roundtable (STAIR) conference that provided recommendations about clinical trial design for neuroprotective and thrombolytic drugs, as well as combination drug trials (18). Hopefully, these recommendations, along with the prior preclinical recommendations, will improve the chances for future success in stroke trials.

EXPANDING THE THERAPEUTIC TIME WINDOW

As noted, the only drug approved for treatment of acute ischemic stroke is rtPA within 3 hours of stroke onset. This 3-hour window is the main reason treatment with rtPA is limited, with fewer than 5% of acute stroke patients receiving this treatment (19). It is not surprising that intravenous rtPA was shown to be effective with very early initiation of treatment, but it has not been conclusively proven to be effective beyond this time point. The earlier the treatment is begun, the more potentially salvageable ischemic tissue exists in individual stroke patients (14). Therefore, reperfusing early after stroke onset affords the opportunity to salvage ischemic tissue from irreversible injury, and this tissue salvage should translate into improved clinical outcome. The current challenge for both thrombolytic and neuroprotective therapy is to expand the therapeutic time window beyond 3 hours, if possible.

The first question concerning expanding the therapeutic time window is whether any therapy can improve outcome if initiated beyond the 3-hour time window. The results of the intraarterial thrombolytic therapy trial of prourokinase imply that therapy initiated after 3 hours can be effective in selected patients. In PROACT II, intraarterial prourokinase was started at a mean time of 5.2 hours after stroke onset in patients with an angiographically documented occlusion of the proximal middle cerebral artery (2). The patients included in this trial were in severe condition, with a mcdian baseline NIHSS score of 17. Despite the delayed initiation of therapy in a severely affected stroke patient cohort, intraarterial prourokinase demonstrated an absolute 15% rate of improving patients to mild or no disability (Rankin score 0–2) compared to placebo. This clinical improvement was accompanied by a markedly increased rate of documented reperfusion. The PROACT II study documents that delayed thrombolytic therapy with a high rate of reperfusion can improve outcome in carefully selected patients. Selecting patients by angiographic criteria is not practical in most clinical settings. Additionally, angiographic documentation of a vascular occlusion does not provide information about the viability status of ischemic tissue distal to the occlusion to provide reassurance that reperfusion can lead to tissue salvage.

A substantial amount of information now is available from positron emission tomography (PET) and diffusion-perfusion magnetic resonance imaging (MRI) studies that potentially salvageable ischemic tissue exists in some patients for many hours after stroke onset (20). PET studies use various definitions of ischemic tissue that is potentially viable, but several studies clearly demonstrated the persistence of such tissue for many hours after stroke onset. PET availability is limited and the technique is time consuming, so it likely will remain an imaging tool restricted to a small number of research centers. Diffusion-perfusion MRI is an imaging modality now widely available at many clinical facilities. Diffusion-weighted imaging (DWI) rapidly demonstrates the presence of ischemic regions where failure of energy metabolism has occurred (21,22). These abnormal regions on DWI are not synonymous with infarction, however, as early reperfusion can reverse DWI changes in animals and stroke patients (23,24). Perfusion-weighted imaging (PWI) evaluates tissue perfusion in the brain microvasculature and can rapidly determine the presence of hypoperfused regions. Combining the results of PWI and DWI provides valuable information about the location, extent, and severity of focal ischemic brain injury (25). In most stroke patients studied early after the start of their event, the PWI volume of abnormality is noticeably greater than the DWI volume of abnormality (26,27). This discrepancy of PWI and DWI volumes is called the diffusion-perfusion mismatch and appears to identify potentially salvageable ischemic tissue, that is, the ischemic penumbra. The presence of a mismatch is much more likely in stroke patients imaged very early after onset and becomes less likely later on. Left untreated, much of the PWI-DWI mismatch will evolve into infarction, whereas early reperfusion will reduce the amount of the mismatch that progresses onto infarction (28). The PWI-DWI mismatch thus provides a readily identifiable imaging marker of potentially salvageable ischemic tissue that can be widely used to identify potentially treatable ischemic stroke patients irrespective of time from onset (29). Clinical trials now are underway that are using the presence or absence of PWI-DWI mismatch as a criterion for inclusion or exclusion in the trial. Hopefully, using this approach to identify patients with the presumed target of therapy will move patient selection to a pathophysiologically based assessment and away from rigid time windows. This presumably will help expand the therapeutic time window for both thrombolysis and neuroprotection.

One caveat to remember is that the PWI-DWI mismatch is only a rough approximation of the ischemic penumbra because some of the PWI region of abnormality is oligemic and will not go on to infarction because the level of blood flow compromise is too mild. Additionally, as previously mentioned, a portion of the DWI abnormality is potentially reversible with early treatment. In the future, perfusion and diffusion absolute value maps likely will be generated and estimations provided as to what percentage of ischemic tissue is highly likely to be irreversibly injured, what percentage is not at risk of infarction, and what percentage is at risk for infarction but can be salvaged with appropriate treatment. The availability of such a three-compartment assessment of ischemic tissue will require many additional clinical treatment experiments but likely will move acute stroke treatment into a new era of time-independent decision making (30). MRI has great promise to improve patient selection for future clinical trials, expand the therapeutic time window for appropriate patients, and revolutionize clinical management of acute ischemic stroke.

BASIC SCIENCE ADVANCES THAT MAY ENHANCE STROKE THERAPY

The basic premise underlying acute stroke therapy is that reperfusion and/or neuroprotection will prevent ischemic brain tissue that is not yet irreversibly injured from progressing onto infarction (14). The principle of reperfusion therapy is inherently simple.

Early and rapid reestablishment of adequate blood flow by lysing thrombi can provide nourishing reperfusion and amelioration of the tissue consequences of ischemia. This concept was validated in part by the PROACT II study because the clinical improvement observed with prourokinase was associated with a much higher rate of angiographically documented restoration of flow at 2 hours after the start of therapy (2). In the NINDS rt-PA Trial, no confirmation of reperfusion was obtained to correlate with improved clinical outcome, but it is estimated that intravenous rtPA will successfully lyse approximately 50% of thrombi in the cerebrovascular circulation (31). Although it is highly likely that timely reperfusion can prevent infarction in ischemic, potentially salvageable brain tissue, neither the NINDS trial nor PROACT II directly confirmed this hypothesis. Several nonrandomized studies of intravenous rtPA did provide evidence that thrombolytic treatment can reduce the development of infarction in hypoperfused ischemic tissue (28,32).

Thrombolysis clearly can benefit ischemic stroke, but associated deleterious effects may partly temper the benefits. Animal and initial human studies document that delayed tissue injury can occur after successful reperfusion (23,24). This delayed reperfusion related injury is presumed to occur secondary to a variety of mechanisms, but likely important contributors include activation of programmed cell death pathways, free radical production, and inflammation. The clinical significance of reperfusion injury remains to be confirmed, but the observation with diffusion MRI of reperfusion injury suggests an additional therapeutic target after successful thrombolysis. Animal studies also suggest that the rtPA molecule itself may be harmful to ischemic brain tissue (33). Although, not all animal studies confirmed that

rtPA is neurotoxic (34). It appears that rtPA increases infarct volume in mice when given at higher doses at the time of reperfusion, but not at low doses or when given prior to the onset of ischemia (35). Interestingly, concomitant use of heparin ameliorated the neurotoxic effect of rtPA. The precise mechanism of rtPA induced tissue injury remains uncertain, but preliminary investigations demonstrated that rtPA can enhance NMDA receptor mediated signaling and also cause delayed hypoperfusion (36). Elucidation of the mechanisms associated with rtPA related deleterious effects, might suggest additional therapies that could be given conjointly with rtPA to reduce rtPA related enhancement of ischemic injury and maximize the clinical benefits of thrombolytic therapy.

Enhanced comprehension of the cellular and molecular mechanisms associated with cell death after focal brain ischemia has occurred with increasing alacrity over the past decade. Initial depictions of the ischemic injury cascade were relatively simplistic, with the primary focus on mechanisms controlling calcium influx and the intracellular consequences of calcium accumulation (37). The ischemic injury cascade has been greatly expanded as an ever-increasing number of pathways leading to cell death are elucidated. These pathways of cell injury can be divided into two major categories: those requiring protein synthesis for activation and those not requiring protein synthesis (Table 47-3). The mechanisms of cell death not requiring protein synthesis can occur in ischemic tissue where cerebral blood flow (CBF) is below the threshold required for maintenance of protein synthesis, that is, in ischemic regions where CBF is below approximately 25 mL/100 g per minute (38). Likely important mechanisms of cell death not requiring protein synthesis include excitotoxicity related to activation of receptor-mediated calcium

TABLE 47-3. *Mechanisms of ischemic cell death*

Nonprotein synthesis-dependent pathways
1. Adenosine triphosphate depletion, disrupted glutamate homeostasis, and glutamate receptor hyperactivation
2. Cytosoloic and mitochondrial calcium overload, endoplasmic reticulum calcium depletion
3. Free-radical overload (nitric oxide, superoxide, and hydrogen peroxide)
4. Phospholipase activation, increased oxidized fatty acids and lipids
5. Protease activation: calpain and caspases
6. Posttranslation activation of pro-death factors
Protein synthesis-dependent pathways
1. Increased expression of proinflammatory molecules: cytokines, inducible nitric oxide synthase, and cyclooxygenase
2. Increased expression of pro-apoptotic proteins
3. Increased expression of cell proteins
4. Increased activity of pro-apoptotic transcription factors
5. Increased expression of matrix metalloproteinases

channels, nitric oxide-mediated injury, activation of proteases and phospholipases, and mitochondrial disruption (39). Activation of these mechanisms traditionally was associated with a necrotic type of cell death, characterized pathologically by swelling of cytoplasmic organelles and the nucleus with disruption of mitochondrial and plasma membranes (40). Protein-synthesis–dependent mechanisms of cell death include cytochrome C release, leading to activation of the caspase-mediated pathway of deoxyribonucleic acid (DNA) damage, activation of transcription factors leading to induction of inflammatory mediators and other mediators of neuronal and blood–brain barrier injury, and activation of the extrinsic apoptotic pathway mediated by activation of caspase-8 (41). These protein-synthesis–dependent mechanisms related to the cell death pathway are termed programmed cell death and are characterized morphologically by nuclear condensation and fragmentation with development of cytoplasmic appendages (42). Such changes may not be observed in mature neurons. The requirement for protein synthesis implies that CBF levels must be greater than 25 mL/100 g per minute, and these levels are maintained only in regions of relatively mild ischemia or after reperfusion (43).

This concept of protein-synthesis–independent and protein-synthesis–dependent mechanisms relates the level of CBF decline in ischemic tissue to the predominant pathway of cell death. Moderately severe to severely compromised CBF levels are associated with a necrotic-type of cell death, whereas mild-to-moderate levels of CBF decline are associated with programmed cell death. This dichotomization of the mechanism of cell death and ultimately tissue infarction is simplistic. It is well known that massive glutamate release and activation of the excitotoxic injury cascade occurs in regions with very low residual CBF, leading to necrotic (protein synthesis independent) cell death (44). In cell culture systems, exposure to low concentrations of NMDA causes cell death with the characteristics of programmed cell death (45). Additionally, it was observed that the amount of glutamate release after the onset of ischemia is dependent upon both the time and the level of CBF decline (46). Thus, at later time points after the onset of focal ischemia a particular level of CBF decline that earlier may not have induced the release of much glutamate now may be associated with much more glutamate release, likely in a graded fashion. Another confounding issue that makes characterization of the precise mechanism of cell death difficult is that there appears to be at least one apoptotic pathway that does not require de novo protein synthesis. Energy-depleted mitochondria release apoptosis-inducing factor (AIF), which is a proapoptotic molecule that can directly induce many of the features of apoptotic cell death (47).

It is becoming increasingly apparent that precise determination of the most important mechanism of cell death after focal brain ischemia may be difficult, if not impossible. It is likely that individual stroke patients have multiple mechanisms of cell injury and death in different regions of the ischemic zone actively participating in the evolution of tissue injury at the same time. Reperfusion will only complicate the complex process of cell injury. It is only logical to assume that targeting one mechanism of cell injury will be of limited value. A more comprehensive approach to the multiple mechanisms of cell injury likely will be more effective. This can be accomplished by at least two approaches. The first would be to use a cocktail of several different drugs, each working predominantly on one aspect of the ischemic cascade and therefore in aggregate impeding multiple aspects of the ischemic cascade (48). This may cause difficulties in clinical drug development because of drug–drug interactions, confluence of toxic effects, and regulatory concerns. Another approach would be to use a single agent with multiple treatment effects that could simultaneously impact upon different aspects of the ischemic cascade.

FUTURE DIRECTIONS

The future development of acute stroke therapies will be a difficult but vital task. There remains a large unmet need to develop additional acute stroke treatments, especially beyond the 3-hour time period. To successfully develop new acute stroke treatments beyond 3 hours will require a confluence of efforts. Imaging technology that better identifies patients appropriate for inclusion in clinical trials and then in clinical practice are needed. Neuroprotective therapies with robust preclinical effects now can be tested more effectively in clinical trials and then are more likely to demonstrate treatment efficacy in appropriately targeted patients. This will especially true with neuroprotective drugs having a broad spectrum of activity. Ultimately, combining neuroprotection with thrombolysis will afford the best opportunity to maximally improve outcome and extend the therapeutic time window. Therefore, despite previous failures with neuroprotection and difficulties demonstrating efficacy of thrombolysis beyond 3 hours, the future of acute stroke therapy must be viewed with cautious optimism.

REFERENCES

1. The National Institute of Neurological Disorders and Stroke rt-PA Stroke Study Group. Tissue plasminogen activator for acute ischemic stroke. *N Engl J Med* 1995; 333:1581–1587.
2. Furlan A, Higashida R, Wechsler LA, et al. Intraarterial prourokinase for acute ischemic stroke. The PROACT II Study: a randomized controlled trial. *JAMA* 1999;282: 2003–2011.
3. Sherman DG, Atkinson RP, Chippendale T, et al. Intravenous Ancrod for treatment of acute ischemic stroke. *JAMA* 2000;283:2395–2403.
4. Fisher M, Schaebitz W. An overview of acute stroke therapy. *Arch Intern Med* 2000;160:3196–3200.
5. Multicenter Acute Stroke Trial—Italy (MAST-1) Group. Randomized, controlled trial of streptokinase, aspirin and combination of both in treatment of acute ischemic stroke. *Lancet* 1995;346:1509–1514.
6. Hacke W, Kaste M, Fieschi C, et al. Intravenous thrombolysis with recombinant tissue plasminogen activator for acute hemispheric stroke. The European Cooperative Acute Stroke Study (ECASS). *JAMA* 1995;274: 1017–1025.
7. Hacke W, Kaste M, Fieschi C, et al. Randomized double-blind placebo-controlled trial of thrombolytic therapy with intravenous alteplase in acute ischaemic stroke (ECASS II). Second European-Australasian Acute Stroke Study Investigators. *Lancet* 1998;352:1245–1251.
8. Clark WM, Wissman S, Albers GW, et al. Recombinant tissue-type plasminogen activator (Alteplase) for ischemic stroke 3 to 5 hours after symptom onset. The ATLANTIS trial: a randomized controlled trial. *JAMA* 1999;282:2019–2026.
9. Stroke Therapy Academic Industry Roundtable (Fisher M, Chair). Recommendations for standards regarding preclinical neuroprotective and restorative drug development. *Stroke* 1999;30:2752–2758.
10. Albers GW, Atkinson RP, Kelley RE, et al. Safety, tolerability, and pharmacokinetics of the N-methyl-D-aspartate antagonist dextrorphan in patients with acute stroke. Dextrorphan Study Group. *Stroke* 1995;26: 254–258.
11. Adams HP, Davis PH, Leira EC, et al. Baseline NIH stroke scale score strongly predicts outcome after stroke. *Neurology* 1999;53:126–131.
12. Frankel MR, Morgenstern LB, Kwiatkowski T, et al. Predicting prognosis after stroke. *Neurology* 2000;55: 952–959.
13. Schabitz WR, Li F, Fisher M. The NMDA antagonist CNS-1102 protects cerebral gray and white matter from ischemia following temporary focal ischemia in the rat. *Stroke* 2000;31:1709–1714.
14. Fisher M. Characterizing the target of acute stroke treatment. *Stroke* 1997;28:866–872.
15. Gammans RE, Sherman DG, ECCO 2000 Investigators. ECCO study of citicoline for treatment of acute ischemic stroke. *Stroke* 2000;31:278(abst).
16. Clark WM, Wechsler LA, Sabonjian LA, et al., for the Citicoline Stroke Group. A phase III randomized efficacy trial of 2000 mg citicoline in acute ischemic stroke. *Neurology* 2001;57:1595–1602.
17. Samsa GP, Matchar DB. Have controlled trials of neuroprotective drugs been underpowered? *Stroke* 2000;32: 669–674.
18. Stroke Therapy Academic Industry Roundtable (Fisher M, Chair). Recommendations for clinical trial evaluation of acute stroke therapies. *Stroke* 2001:32;1598–1606.
19. Hacke W, Brott T, Caplan LR, et al. Thrombolysis in acute ischemic stroke: controlled trials and clinical experience. *Neurology* 1999;53[Suppl]:S3–S14.
20. Baron JC. Mapping the ischemic penumbra with PET: implications for acute stroke treatment. *Cerebrovasc Dis* 1999;9:193–201.
21. Lansberg MG, Albers GW, Beaulieu C, et al. Comparison of diffusion-weighted MRI and CT in acute stroke. *Neurology* 2000;54:1557–1561.
22. Gonzalez B, Schaefer PW, Buananno FS, et al. Diffusion-weighted MRI imaging: diagnostic accuracy in patients imaged within 6 hours of stroke symptom onset. *Radiology* 1999;210:155–162.
23. Li F, Liu KF, Silva, et al. Secondary decline in apparent diffusion coefficient and neurological outcome after a short period of focal brain ischemia in rats. *Ann Neurol* 2000;48:236–244.
24. Kidwell CS, Saver JL, Mattiello J, et al. Thrombolytic reversal of acute human cerebral ischemic injury shown by diffusion/perfusion magnetic resonance imaging. *Ann Neurol* 2000;47:462–469.
25. Neumann-Haefelin T, Moseley ME, Albers GW, et al. New magnetic resonance imaging methods for cerebrovascular disease: emerging clinical applications. *Ann Neurol* 2000;31:559–570.
26. Schellinger PD, Fiebach JB, Jansen O, et al. Stroke magnetic resonance imaging within 6 hours after onset of hyperacute cerebral ischemia. *Ann Neurol* 2001;49: 460–469.
27. Parsons Muu, Yang Q, Barbar A, et al. Perfusion magnetic resonance imaging maps in hyperacute stroke. *Stroke* 2001;32:1581–1587.
28. Schellinger FD, Jansen O, Fiebach JB, et al. Monitoring intravenous recombinant tissue plasminogen activator thrombolysis for acute ischemic stroke with diffusion and perfusion MRI. *Stroke* 2000;31:1318–1328.
29. Wu O, Koroschetz WJ, Ostergaard L, et al. Predicting tissue outcome in acute human cerebral ischemia using combined diffusion-and perfusion-weighted MR imaging. *Stroke* 2001;32:933–942.
30. Baird AE, Dambrosia J, Janket SJ, et al. A three item scale for the early prediction of stroke recovery. *Lancet* 2001;357:2095–2099.
31. del Zoppo GJ, Hamann G, Hosoni N. Thrombolytic therapy. In: Fisher M, ed. *Stroke therapy.* Boston: Butterworth-Heinemann, 2001:261–274.
32. Marks MP, Tong DC, Beaulieu C, et al. Evaluation of early reperfusion and I.V. tPA therapy using diffusion and perfusion-weighted MRI. *Neurology* 1999;52: 1792–1798.
33. Wang YF, Tsirka SE, Strickland V, et al. Tissue plasminogen activator (tPA) increases neuronal damage after focal cerebral ischemia in wild-type and tPA deficient mice. *Nat Med* 1998;4:228–231.
34. Kilic E, Hermann DM, Hessmann KA. Recombinant tissue plasminogen activator reduces infarct size after reversible thread occlusion of middle cerebral artery in mice. *NeuroReport* 1999;10:107–111.
35. Kilic E, Bahr M, Hermann DM. Effects of recombinant tissue plasminogen activator after intraluminal thread occlusion in mice. *Stroke* 2001;32:2641–2647.
36. Nicole O, Docagne F, Ali C, et al. The proteolytic activ-

ity of tissue-plasminogen activator enhances NMDA receptor-mediated signaling. *Nat Med* 2001;7:59–64.

37. Kristian T, Siesjo BK. Calcium in ischemic cell death. *Stroke* 1998;29:705–18.

38. Hossmann KA. Viability thresholds and the penumbra of focal ischemia. *Ann Neurol* 1994; 36:557–565.

39. Nietera P, Lipton SA. Excitotoxins in neuronal apoptosis and necrosis. *J Cereb Blood Flow Metab* 1999;19: 583–591.

40. Majno G, Joris I. Apoptosis, oncosis and necrosis—an overview of cell death. *Am J Pathol* 1995;146:3–15.

41. Graham SG, Chen J. Programmed cell death in cerebral ischemia. *J Cereb Blood Flow Metab* 2001;21:99–109.

42. Burek MJ, Oppenheim RW. Programmed cell death in the developing nervous system. *Brain* Pathol 1996;6: 427–446.

43. Mier G, Ishimaru S, Xie Y, et al. Ischemic thresholds of cerebral protein synthesis and energy state following middle cerebral artery occlusion in rat. *J Cereb Blood Flow Metab* 1991;22:753–761.

44. Lipton SA, Rosenberg PA. Mechanisms of disease: excitatory amino acids as a final common pathway for neurological disorders. *N Engl J Med* 1994;330: 613–622.

45. Ankarcena M, Dypbukt JM, et al. Glutamate-induced neuronal death: a succession of necrosis or apoptosis depending on mitochondrial function. *Neuron* 1995;15: 961–973.

46. Matsumoto K, Graf R, Rosner G, et al. Evaluation of neuroactive substances in the cortex of cats during prolonged focal ischemia. *J Cereb Blood Flow Metab* 1993;13:586–594.

47. Susis SA, Daugar E, Ravagnan L, et al. Two distinct pathways leading to nuclear apoptosis. *J Exp Med* 2000; 192:571–580.

48. Maynard KI, Quinones-Minojosa A, Matek JM. Neuroprotection against ischemia by metabolic inhibition revisited: a comparison of hypothermia, a pharmacologic cocktail and magnesium plus mexiletine. *Ann NY Acad Sci* 1999;890:240–254.

Ischemic Stroke: Advances in Neurology, Vol. 92. Edited by
H.J.M. Barnett, Julien Bogousslavsky, and Heather Meldrum.
Lippincott Williams & Wilkins, Philadelphia © 2003.

48

Medical Complications During Stroke Rehabilitation

Alexander W. Dromerick and Syed Ahmed Abdul Khader

Department of Neurology, Washington University School of Medicine;
Department of Neurology/Rehabilitation, Barnes-Jewish Hospital, St. Louis, Missouri, U.S.A.

The major goal of medical management during the rehabilitation period is to provide the stroke patient the best possible physiologic environment for recovery. The time pressures placed on the inpatient rehabilitation period call for judicious prophylaxis of complications and mandate treatment choices that minimize any effects on the patient's ability to cooperate. Complications after stroke usually are predictable, and their prevention and management constitute a major component of the care delivered by physicians to their patients with stroke.

Several studies have examined the complications that occur during stroke rehabilitation (Table 48-1). Death rates for the overall stroke population are 10%

TABLE 48-1. *Medical complications during stroke rehabilitation*

	Dobkin 1987 (2)	Dromerick and Reding 1994 (3)	Kalra et al. 1995 (4)	Davenport et al 1996 (1)	Roth et al. 2001 (5)
Subjects	200	100	124	613	1,029
Setting	Specialty stroke rehabilitation (US)	Specialty stroke rehabilitation (US)	Specialty stroke rehabilitation (UK)	All hospitalized stroke (UK)	Specialty stroke rehabilitation (US)
Death (%)	NR	1	5.6	22.4	2.9
Acute care transfer (%)	NR	13	NA	NA	19
Urinary infection (%)	14	44	17	16	30.5
Depression (%)	20	33	34	5	13
Musculoskeletal pain (%)	12	31	38	12	14.2
Falls/fractures (%)	NR	25/0	NR	22/3	10.5/NR
Hypotension (%)	NR	19	NR	NR	2
Hypertension (%)	12	15	NR	NR	9
Encephalopathy (%)	NR	8	NR	5	NR
Arrhythmia (%)	9	8	NR	3	3.2
Pneumonia (%)	3	7	8	12	4
Heart failure (%)	NR	6	NR	2	2
Agitation (%)	NR	4	5	NR	8
Deep venous thrombosis (%)	NR	4	3	3	4.1
Angina (%)	4	4	NR	NR	2.9
Seizure (%)	3	3	4	4	1.5
Stroke progression/transient ischemic attack (%)	9	3	5	2	1.6
Pulmonary embolus (%)	3	0	2	1	1.1
Myocardial infarction (%)	NR	0	NR	1	NR
Gastrointestinal bleed (%)	1	NR	NR	3	3.1

NA, not applicable; NR, not reported.

to 20% (1), but mortality rates in rehabilitation patients is surprisingly low, typically 2% to 4% (2–5). Transfers back to the acute care setting occurred in 13% to 20% of patients in the US studies, mostly related to cardiopulmonary complications. Strikingly, the complications of rehabilitation stereotypes (pneumonia, venous thromboembolism, recurrent stroke) were uncommon, and most management issues centered on pain, bladder function, and cognition. Because rehabilitation focuses on return to independence, patients often are pushed to their limits in an effort to improve their mobility. Reassuringly, fractures have been rare, although falls have been common.

VENOUS THROMBOEMBOLISM

The data presented in Table 48-1 may underestimate the frequency of subclinical deep vein thrombosis (DVT) because patients were not systematically screened with ultrasonography or other diagnostic modalities. Stroke rehabilitation populations screened with labeled fibrinogen scans have DVT rates around 50%, the majority involving the leg on the affected side. DVT risk increases with increasing weakness, neglect, atrial fibrillation, and reduced ambulatory capacity (6). DVT incidence is reported to peak between days 2 and 7, and most fatal pulmonary emboli (PE) occur between weeks 2 and 4 after stroke. One plethysmography study found that 14% of persons admitted to a stroke rehabilitation unit had DVT and another 5.5% developed DVT during the rehabilitation stay (7). Detection of DVT and PE on physical examination can be confounded by cognitive or sensory impairment, but the diagnostic evaluation algorithms for DVT and PE are no different for persons with stroke.

The optimal DVT prophylaxis regimen after ischemic stroke has not yet been clearly defined, particularly in the rehabilitation setting. Most data are from studies evaluating all stroke patients, not the subset undergoing rehabilitation, and the intervention tested usually lasts only 14 or 28 days. Aspirin alone did not significantly reduce fatal or nonfatal PE in either the International Stroke Trial (IST) or the Chinese Acute Stroke Trial (CAST), but pooled analyses of these data in combination with others found a statistically significant reduction in PE (8). Large-scale randomized trials have demonstrated the effectiveness of low-dose fractionated heparin, enoxaparin, and danaparoid in reducing PE; however, low-dose unfractionated heparin may be less effective in preventing DVT. Graded elastic stockings (thromboem-

bolic disease stockings) are widely used, but their effectiveness in stroke patients is unproved (6). Sequential pneumatic compression stockings often are impractical in the rehabilitation setting, where the patient is engaged in several hours per day of mobility and transfer training.

Several issues regarding venous thromboembolism prevention and management in persons with hemorrhagic stroke are unresolved. In the absence of evidence-based data, use of graded elastic stockings plus nighttime sequential pneumatic compression stockings, pulsatile pneumatic foot pumps, or low-dose fractionated heparin may be reasonable choices. The optimal duration of venous thromboembolism prophylaxis is unknown. We typically discontinue prophylaxis when the patient reliably ambulates 150 feet or at least 28 days have passed. In the spinal cord injury literature, the rate of venous thromboembolism decreases dramatically by 3 months after injury, and such data could serve as a guide for the upper limit of prophylaxis duration in stroke patients.

POSTSTROKE DEPRESSION

As shown in Table 48-1, poststroke depression (PSD) may affect 34% of stroke rehabilitation inpatients. Studies in other stroke populations report an incidence upward of 60%. Differences in study populations and timing of evaluations can account for at least some of the variability in results. Considerable controversy remains regarding the diagnosis and taxonomy of PSD. The relationship between lesion location and frequency of stroke remains controversial. The work of Robinson et al. (9) suggested that involvement of anterior portions of the brain, particularly in the left hemisphere, is associated with a higher frequency of depression. However, this finding has been questioned, and several subsequent studies of more population-based cohorts of stroke patients found no such relationship (10).

Most investigators differentiate in some way between a syndrome that resembles a traditional major depression and a milder syndrome termed *dysphoria* or a *minor depression*. Many manifestations of PSD will be identical to persons without stroke, but they can be confounded by aphasia, neglect, or other stroke-related impairments. Family and staff may attribute a multitude of complaints and behaviors to depression, but these behaviors actually may be related to inattention, apraxia, aprosody, deconditioning, cardiac failure, or a variety of other conditions. In such cases, it is helpful to evaluate for the presence of vegetative signs of depression (insomnia, anorexia, fatigue out of proportion to physical condition) and to evaluate whether the patient is cooperating with therapy procedures with an effort compatible to his or her physical and cognitive impairments.

Treatment of PSD is similar to depression treatment in other medical settings. Grieving for the loss associated with stroke is necessary and appropriate, and the physician cannot bypass this process with medication. Emotional support and encouragement from staff, family, and support groups can be effective; concrete problem-based strategies often are more effective than formal psychotherapy. The choice of antidepressant medications often is driven by medical comorbidities. Only a few antidepressants have been formally tested in PSD: citalopram, nortriptyline, fluoxetine, and trazodone. Treatment will improve mood, but improvements in depression scale scores are not clearly related to improvements in activities of daily living function or independence.

PAINFUL HEMIPLEGIC SHOULDER

Pain in the hemiplegic shoulder has been reported in up to 84% of stroke rehabilitation patients. Most cases of hemiplegic shoulder pain are caused by local pain generators, such as adhesive capsulitis, subacromial bursitis, bicipital tendonitis, and spastic muscles. A thorough musculoskeletal examination usually can isolate the cause in these cases (11). Less common are distant causes of pain, including central pain syndrome or brachial plexus injury. There is a "shoulder-hand" syndrome, which is said to be a variant of reflex sympathetic dystrophy. Features include poorly localized pain, trophic changes in the skin and hair of the affected arm, and reddening over the knuckles. However, similar trophic changes and dependent edema can occur with chronic disuse, and no studies have addressed the specificity of the diagnosis of the shoulder-hand syndrome.

There are no large-scale trials of treatments, but treatment must address any local pain generators. Patients with dependent edema should elevate the arm on a pillow whenever they are seated. Daily range of motion exercises are essential in any treatment plan and should be overseen by a therapist to prevent further injury. Standing regimens of acetaminophen (2,000–3,000 mg/day) or a nonsteroidal antiinflammatory agent will supplement the pain relief of stretching. Hemiplegia often results in a downward subluxation of the humeral head out of the glenoid fossa, and many clinicians go to great lengths to correct this deformity. However, several studies have failed to find a clear relationship between shoulder pain and subluxation, and there is no convincing evidence that reversal of subluxation with slings reduces pain or improves arm function. Localized bursitis or tendonitis can be treated with corticosteroid injections, but indiscriminate injection of all painful hemiplegic shoulders is not indicated (12).

CARDIAC AND NEUROVASCULAR DECONDITIONING

Deconditioning is a general term for the deleterious physiologic effects of prolonged immobility. The prevention and reversal of deconditioning offer an important means of improving the status of persons with stroke, even in the absence of improvement in neurologic impairment. The frequency of cardiac disease in stroke patients is as high as 75%, and the presence of hemiparesis can double the demands on the cardiovascular system during ambulation and other physical activities (13). Thus, although weakness and incoordination obviously hamper ambulation, it may be the patient's overall cardiovascular status that is a rate-limiting factor in effective walking after stroke.

Prolonged bed rest causes an increased resting heart rate, an abnormally high heart rate on submaximal exercise, a decreased stroke volume, and a decrease in cardiac size. The diastolic filling period is shortened with decreased myocardial perfusion, and angina may be precipitated in patients with previously asymptomatic coronary artery disease if the myocardial hypoperfusion continues. Vo_2max, an indicator of general aerobic fitness, is reduced, and it takes a longer period of time for the heart rate to return to a resting state after a period of exercise.

Deconditioning also affects the postural reflexes that prevent orthostasis. These neurovascular deconditioning effects occur in as few as 3 days of immobilization and are thought to be more severe in elderly patients in whom stroke is common.

Avoidance of prolonged bed rest and immobility is essential. The clinical rule of thumb is that it takes twice as long to recover as it took to deteriorate, and it can several weeks to reverse the orthostasis associated with a prolonged intensive care unit or hospital stay. Seating the patient in a chair for a few hours a day reduces loss of Vo_2max and reduces orthostasis. Exercises done in the supine position help to maintain Vo_2max but do not prevent orthostatic intolerance. Isometric exercises (voluntary muscle contraction without movement of the limb) reduce loss of Vo_2max but fail to preserve positional reflexes (14).

For patients in whom neurovascular deconditioning is firmly established, reversal requires progressively increasing activity and regaining the upright posture. A tilt table can be used to gradually increase tolerance of the upright position. A standing frame then can be used to increase the amount of time in the standing position. A seating schedule, in which progressively more time each day is spent in a chair, will quickly improve postural reflexes in milder cases.

Chronically, cardiovascular deconditioning is treatable despite the motor and balance limitations associated with hemiparesis. Small-scale randomized controlled trials in persons with chronic stroke demonstrate clinically significant improvements in aerobic capacity with cycle ergometer or motorized treadmill training (15). These improvements should enhance not only walking but also tolerance to ordinary activities of daily living because these tasks can be performed at a lower percentage of Vo_2max.

SPASTICITY

The clinical syndrome of spasticity is the clinical manifestation of the upper motor neuron syndrome. The "positive" signs of spasticity include velocity-dependent increase in muscle tone, flexor spasms, hyperreflexia, painful muscle spasms, and clonus. The "negative" signs include weakness, slowness and incoordination of movement, and cocontraction, which is the simultaneous activation of agonist and antagonist muscles during the attempted execution of movements.

The physician and patient should come to a clear understanding and agreement on the goals of treatment. For patients whose goals are improvement of positive symptoms of spasticity, such as flexor spasms, hypertonia, and clonus, the available treatments can provide considerable relief with relatively few side effects. However, for patients who seek relief for negative symptoms such as incoordination and weakness, the available treatments are much less successful. One misconception about the weakness and incoordination seen with the upper motor neuron syndrome is that much of it is due to hypertonia and that if the hypertonia were reduced the patient would gain improved function. At best, this notion is controversial; most data suggest that weakness is due to poor activation of motor units, not resistance of muscle to movement caused by hyperactivity of the stretch reflex.

Management of spasticity is best approached in a methodical and stepwise fashion. The first step is to remove factors that exacerbate spasticity, including pain, infection, fatigue, and intraabdominal processes. Common sources of pain in physically disabled persons are contractures, decubiti, pressure points from failure to regularly change position, poorly fitting braces, and central pain syndromes.

Intraabdominal processes such as gallbladder disease, urolithiasis, and bowel or bladder distention may present as exacerbations in spasticity.

The second step is to use interventions such as stretching and positioning devices. Stretching prevents contractures and reduces edema, and it is said to reduce tone for at least several hours. Positioning devices such as splints maintain gains in range of motion, protect the splinted areas from mechanical injury, and maintain limbs in functional positions. Careful positioning in a chair or bed minimizes pain, thus minimizing muscle tone.

Systemic medications are used in the management of hypertonia and flexor spasms when nonpharmacologic treatments fail. Most of the commonly used systemic drugs, which include baclofen, diazepam, and tizanidine, act centrally. Baclofen is the most widely used medication for all forms of spasticity; its ability to reduce flexor spasms is particularly well documented. Diazepam also is widely used, but it has the drawback of sedation in patients with cerebral injuries such as stroke. Tizanidine is less sedating and has the advantage of not worsening muscle weakness in clinical trials to date. Dantrolene, which works at the muscle level to prevent calcium release from the sarcoplasmic reticulum, can cause weakness, but it is said to be particularly effective for "cerebral" spasticity. Most other drugs previously used for management of spasticity (clonidine, antiarrhythmics, anticonvulsants) have been superseded in large part by newer treatment methods such as intramuscular botulinum toxin and intrathecal baclofen.

Intramuscular botulinum toxin is used when conservative treatments do not produce the desired effect. It also may be used to achieve functional goals that might be achieved by weakening small muscle groups. One example would be improving grasp by weakening spastic finger flexors, so that finger extensors can act against less resistance, improving grasp and release in a spastic hand. Systemic medications are less expensive and more appropriate when treating generalized hypertonia involving multiple large muscle groups. Beyond botulinum toxin, interventions can include intrathecal baclofen, phenol neurolysis, and surgical procedures.

SLEEP DISORDERED BREATHING AFTER STROKE

Several reports have documented clinically significant sleep disordered breathing in persons with stroke (16). These sleep disorders are clinically important because the excessive daytime sleepiness associated with sleep disordered breathing may impair the ability to cooperate with rehabilitation therapies and worsen cognitive deficits already present from stroke, dementia, or other conditions (17). Sleep apnea is associated with nocturnal enuresis in children, and it can be speculated that a similar mechanism might worsen nocturnal incontinence in persons with stroke. The changes in personality, memory, and occupational performance seen in persons with sleep apnea can exacerbate the disability and reduce quality of life in many persons with stroke.

Whether obstructive, central, or mixed type, sleep apnea is associated with transient and repetitive oxygen desaturation and hypercapnia. Hypoxia can result in pulmonary vasoconstriction, which may evolve into pulmonary hypertension and cor pulmonale, especially in patients with chronic obstructive airway disease. Other cardiovascular complications include systemic hypertension, increased left ventricular afterload, decreased cardiac output, and arrhythmias. All of these conditions can further aggravate cardiovascular deconditioning, but the clinical significance is unknown at this time.

The clinical history usually reports some disorder of breathing during sleep, particularly snoring and pauses in breathing. The caretaker or bed partner may report excessive restlessness or nocturia. The diagnosis rests on the results of a polysomnogram, although the use of an "intelligent" continuous positive airway pressure (CPAP) machine may be useful in screening. Simple oximetry is insensitive to many cases of sleep-disordered breathing and will not detect a large number of persons who go on to meet polysomnographic criteria for sleep disordered breathing.

Treatment during stroke rehabilitation and in chronic stroke can be challenging. Removal of sedating drugs can improve central sleep apnea. CPAP is the mainstay of treatment, but it can be poorly tolerated even in otherwise neurologically normal persons. Many persons with stroke become confused or disinhibited, and they may not be willing to accept the inconvenience of a CPAP mask. In persons with stroke, facial weakness can add to the difficulty in fitting a facemask. If excessive daytime sleepiness occurs during the first month after stroke, it may lessen as neurologic recovery occurs. In such cases, a trial of a daytime stimulant such as modafinil or dextroamphetamine may be helpful to improve coopera-

tion with therapies until the natural recovery process improves the sleep apnea.

REFERENCES

1. Davenport RJ, Dennis MS, Warlow CP. Complications after acute stroke. *Stroke* 1996;27:425–420.
2. Dobkin BH. Neuromedical complications in stroke patients transferred for rehabilitation before and after diagnostic related groups. *J Neurol Rehabil* 1987;1:3–7.
3. Dromerick AW, Reding M. Medical and neurological complications during stroke rehabilitation. *Stroke* 1994;25:358–361.
4. Kalra L, Yu G, Wislon K, Roots P. Medical complications during stroke rehabilitation. *Stroke* 1995;26: 990–994.
5. Roth EJ, Lovell L, Harvey RL, et al. Incidence and risk factors for medical complications during stroke rehabilitation. *Stroke* 2001;32:523–529.
6. Kelley J, Rudd A, Lewis R, et al. Venous thromboembolism after stroke. *Stroke* 2001;32:262–267.
7. Pambianco G, Orchard T, Landau P. Deep vein thrombosis: prevention in stroke patients during rehabilitation. *Arch Phys Med Rehabil* 1995;76:324–330.
8. Gubitz G, Sandercock P, Counsell C. Antiplatelet therapy for acute ischemic stroke (Cochrane review). *Cochrane Rev* 2000;4.
9. Robinson RG, Kubos KL, Starr LB, et al. Mood disorders in stroke patients. Importance of lesion locations. *Brain* 1984;107:81–93.
10. Steffens DC, Krishnan KRR, Crump C, et al. Cerebrovascular disease and evolution of depressive symptoms in the Cardiovascular Health Study. *Stroke* 2002; 33:1636–1644.
11. Kumar A, Virtucio ALC, Edwards D, et al. Hemiplegic shoulder pain syndrome in acute rehabilitation: utility and interrater reliability of associated abnormal physical signs. *Arch Phys Med Rehabil* 1998;79:1170.
12. Snels IAK, Beckerman H, Twisk JWR, et al. Effect of triamcinolone acetonide injections on hemiplegic shoulder pain. *Stroke* 2000;31:2396–2401.
13. Corcoran PJ, Jebson RH, Brengleman GL, et al. Effects of plastic and metal braces on speed and energy cost of hemiparetic ambulation. *Arch Phys Med Rehabil* 1970; 51:69–77.
14. Greenleaf JE. Intensive exercise training during bed rest attenuates deconditioning. *Med Sci Sports Exerc* 1997; 29:207–215.
15. Macko RF, Smith GV, Dobrovolny CL, et al. Treadmill training improves fitness reserve in chronic stroke patients. *Arch Phys Med Rehabil* 2002;82:879–884.
16. Iranzo A, Santamaria J, Berenguer J, et al. Prevalence and clinical importance of sleep apnea in the first night after cerebral infarction. *Neurology* 2002;58:911–916.
17. Sandberg O, Gelber D, Franklin KA, et al. Sleep apnea, delirium, depressed mood, cognition, and ADL ability after stroke. *J Am Geriatr Soc* 2001;49:391–397.

Ischemic Stroke: Advances in Neurology, Vol. 92. Edited by
H.J.M. Barnett, Julien Bogousslavsky, and Heather Meldrum.
Lippincott Williams & Wilkins, Philadelphia © 2003.

49

Cognitive Rehabilitation of Memory Following Stroke

Theory, Practice, and Outcome

George Michael Cuesta

Department of Neurology and Neuroscience,
Joan and Sanford I. Weill Medical College of Cornell University, New York, New York;
Department of Rehabilitation Psychology and Neuropsychology, Burke Rehabilitation Hospital,
White Plains, New York, U.S.A.

OVERVIEW

There has been a rapid progression in the development of cognitive rehabilitation techniques over the last three decades. This chapter summarizes these techniques and applications as they relate particularly to memory or more globally to cognitive psychology, neuropsychology, speech/language therapy, and occupational therapy (1–4). References cited offer a more detailed discussion of the subject, particularly Sohlberg and Mateer's book entitled *Cognitive rehabilitation: an integrative neuropsychological approach* (5).

The effectiveness of cognitive rehabilitation is supported by a number of reviews over the past 20 years (5–18). Cicerone et al. (19) conducted an evidence-based analysis of existing studies and reached similar conclusions.

Critics of cognitive rehabilitation argue that most of the studies supporting its efficacy have been either small case studies or poorly controlled treatment trials. Consequently, conclusions regarding effectiveness must be approached with caution.

MEMORY THEORY

Cognitive rehabilitation is a developing field, the most clearly defined area of which is focused on memory. Most researchers hypothesize that there are at least four stages of memory: *attention, encoding,* *storage,* and *retrieval* (5,20–23). These stages are closely linked and interact with each other.

Attention

At its most fundamental level, the *attention* stage includes alertness and arousal. At higher levels, maintaining concentration over time (i.e., *sustained attention*), resisting interference (i.e., *selective attention*), and being able to allocate one's attention resources (i.e., *alternating and divided attention*) are important components of effective functioning (5). Working memory, or the ability to temporarily hold on to information in order to complete a task, is an integral part of the attention process. According to Sohlberg and Mateer (5), attention is a logical component of any memory model because it is this capacity that initially allows the system to access and ultimately use incoming data in a meaningful way.

Encoding

Encoding is the second stage of memory, which occurs after one has placed attention to particular stimuli. Encoding is the registration of material to be recalled and used later to complete a task. Recalling verbal information depends upon encoding its phonologic characteristics, and recalling visual information depends upon encoding its graphic representation. Craik and Lockhart (24) advanced the levels-of-processing hypothesis, suggesting that information that is deeply processed will have a higher likelihood of being recalled than information that is shallowly processed. Encoding has been shown to be enhanced by a number of strategies that result in deeper processing. For example, chunking or categorizing information is a more effective rehearsal strategy than simply repeating the information to be recalled (5).

Storage

Storage of memory is defined as the transfer of a transient memory to a form or location in the brain for permanent retention or access (5). The mechanisms whereby new learning interacts with old learning are not well understood. However, we know that storage can be disrupted when there is interference in the learning process. *Retroactive interference* refers to interference in learning new information due to the presentation of subsequent learning material. *Proactive interference* refers to disruption in memory due to the presentation of learning material before the new learning.

Retrieval

Retrieval of memory is defined as searching for or activating existing memory traces (5). Retrieval requires that the individuals monitor the accuracy and appropriateness of memories pulled from storage. Tulving (25) conducted a classic experiment that examined retrieval mechanisms. Essentially, he demonstrated that simply attempting to recall a previously presented word list facilitated learning. He found that recall improved with successive administration of lists. Retrieval often is evaluated by comparing recognition ability with recall ability. Recognition of previously presented information typically is better than free recall of that information, implying that memory storage has occurred but that retrieval mechanisms have not yet developed. Cueing strategies used in memory rehabilitation are based on this principle.

TYPES OF MEMORY

There are at least four different types of memory: (a) time-dependent forms of memory, (b) content-dependent forms of memory, (c) everyday memory, and (d) amnesia (5).

Time-Dependent Forms of Memory

Time-dependent forms of memory include *short-term (or working) memory* and *long-term memory.*

Short-term or working memory refers to the storage of limited amounts of information (3–4 items) for short periods of time (up to a few minutes). An example of short-term or working memory is holding a four-digit telephone extension number in your head until you completed dialing it. Long-term memory refers to unlimited memory with no decay. Examples of long-term memory are recalling events from your high school graduation day, the grade and high schools you attended, the teachers you had, and the names of friends you had when you were in high school and what they meant to you.

Content-Dependent Forms of Memory

Content-dependent forms of memory (all involving long-term memory) include declarative memory, episodic memory, semantic memory, nondeclarative memory, procedural memory, and priming. *Declarative memory* refers to a person's explicit knowledge base. All that you know about neurology and neuropsychology are examples of declarative memory. *Episodic memory,* a type of declarative memory, refers to storage of events that are tagged in time and place. Where you went to dinner and what movie you saw last weekend are examples of episodic memory. *Semantic memory,* another type of declarative memory, has to do with the storage of facts. It refers to a broad domain of cognition composed of knowledge acquired about the world, including word meanings, classes of information, facts, and ideas (5). Recalling all of the signs and symptoms of major depression or dementia of the Alzheimer's type are examples of semantic memory. *Nondeclarative memory* refers to implicit memory and does not require episodic memory. *Procedural memory,* a type of nondeclarative memory, has to do with the acquisition of perceptuomotor skills and the learning of rules and sequences. Memory for how to tie your shoe, procedures for starting your car, and operating a computer are examples of procedural memory. *Priming,* another type of nondeclarative memory, refers to increased chance of retrieval when previously exposed to information without explicit learning. It has to do with the phenomenon that cues or partial bits of information can prompt an accurate recall without an individual being aware of or recalling that the information was previously presented. Stem completion activities are an example of priming (26).

Everyday Memory

Everyday memory refers to functional memory constructs. Prospective memory and metamemory fit into this category. *Prospective memory* has to do with remembering to carry out our intentions. *Metamemory* refers to awareness about our own memory functioning.

Amnesia

Amnesia may be anterograde, retrograde, or global. *Anterograde amnesia* is the inability to acquire new information following brain damage. *Retrograde amnesia* is the inability to retrieve information stored prior to damage to the brain. *Global amnesia,* also called *posttraumatic amnesia,* refers to a period of confusion with inability to remember events moment-to-moment and often accompanies decreased consciousness from any cause.

REHABILITATION OF MEMORY

Techniques to manage memory impairments can be divided into two categories: (a) *generalizable methods* that have the goal of restoring or improving memory ability across a variety of tasks and contexts and (b) *domain-specific methods* that have the goal of teaching a particular skill or body of information (5). Some examples of techniques that are designed to restore memory ability are memory practice skills, mnemonic strategy training, prospective memory training, and metamemory training. Some examples of domain-specific memory intervention approaches include mnemonic strategy training for specific information, expanded rehearsal time (spaced retrieval methods), use of preserved priming ability (method of vanishing cues), and creating a personal history for managing retrograde amnesia.

External memory aids can be used to help with reminding a person to do specific tasks or recall specific information. This technique does not fit neatly into the two approaches mentioned earlier, but it has been shown to be helpful to patients who are able to learn how to properly and consistently use the aids. There is no expectation of generalization of improved memory functioning to other contexts. This technique is essentially a compensatory strategy for managing memory impairment.

Once clinicians know the level and extent of memory impairment, the next step is to select the most appropriate and effective memory management technique from the available options. Memory tasks usually are composed of a variety of cognitive operations, and it is not possible to isolate memory as an independent task. Most patients with ischemic stroke who have memory problems also have other cognitive impairments. A good cognitive rehabilitation treatment plan may use more than one memory intervention approach, as well as other techniques.

Regardless of the approach selected, the following guidelines are suggested for clinicians working with patients who have memory problems (27): (a) *simplify* information, that is, be clear, concise, and to the point with instructions; (b) *reduce* the amount of information to be recalled; (c) *check* to see that the patient understands what has been said; (d) help the patient to *link* information to existing information, that is make associations; (e) set up practice regimens with *distributed practice*, for example, it may be better to work at learning something a few minutes several times a day than for 1 hour once a day; (f) help the patient to *organize* the information that needs to be recalled; and (g) *train* the patient to use communication techniques that encourage processing meaning, such as paraphrasing, rehearsal, and asking questions (5).

Generalizable Methods

There are four types of restorative memory interventions: (a) memory practice drills, (b) mnemonic strategy training, (c) metamemory training, and (d) prospective memory training, as delineated by Sohlberg and Mateer (5).

Memory Practice Drills

The use of memory drills to improve impaired recall suggests that memory can be strengthened as if it were a cognitive muscle. Yet about 15 years ago, researchers failed to demonstrate improvement in memory functioning after memory exercises were administered (28). Although there is little objective support for the efficacy of this approach, it remains the most widely used memory rehabilitation technique in clinical practice. If there is improvement in patient performance after memory exercises, Sohlberg and Mateer (5) suggest that it is most likely due to improvement in attention.

Two studies have suggested that isolated components of attention can be selectively improved with drill-oriented attention exercises (29,30). Sohlberg and Mateer (16) have treated clients whose memory impairments abated after attention process training. The organization of attention processes in the brain, along with the fact that relevant discrete components of attention (e.g., selective attention) have been isolated, may account for why attention exercises have been more successful than other memory exercises (5).

Mnemonic Strategy Training

Examples of this type of training include visual imagery; verbal organization strategies, such as forming acronyms; making paired associations with target words; and semantic elaboration, such as linking target words or ideas in a story. Visual imagery is by far the most popular and has been well researched (31). A therapist can teach patients to construct visual images or provide them with associated images for information that must be recalled. This technique has been beneficial to some but not all patients with memory impairments (32–35). They appear to work best in artificial laboratory situations, but they do not work very well in real-life contexts (36). Patients with significant memory impairments have difficulty learning and implementing the strategies spontaneously and reliably. These patients have difficulty maintaining or generalizing the technique beyond the training context (32–36).

Mnemonic strategy training is most useful for patients with mild cognitive impairment. This population of patients appears better able to learn and generalize the strategies than patients with severe memory impairments (37).

Prospective Memory Training

This training is an intervention paradigm in which ischemic stroke patients are administered repetitive prospective memory tasks. Sohlberg et al. (38) developed the prospective memory process training (PROMPT) module to assist with this type of intervention. With the PROMPT, the clinician asks the patient to remember to carry out a target task in a specified number of minutes. The time lapse interval is increased after the patient is reliably successful. Prospective memory training can be coupled with the use of external aids, such as an appointment book or a hand-held computer. The patient is simply trained to consult their external memory aid at specified times.

Metamemory Training

Some patients with memory impairments can benefit from a better understanding of the nature and effects of their memory problems (5). Therapists can increase a patient's awareness about memory disturbances by taking an educational approach to learning about their memory impairments. Other patients with decreased insight or denial of impairments might benefit more from assistance with experiencing the effects of their preserved and damaged memory.

One training method that can improve metamemory is the use of prediction exercises. With this method, patients compare predictions with their actual performance on memory tasks and tests. Rebmann and Hannon (39) reinforced patients for the accuracy of their predictions on memory tasks. They found that differences between predicted performance on memory tests and actual test scores decreased over time. Schlund (40) found that providing feedback to patients on the accuracy of predicted recall of personal information reduced the variability between self-reports and recall performance.

Another aspect of metamemory training is to teach patients self-instructional or self-monitoring routines that will assist them in improving their memory functioning. These are executive strategies that can be used to help them review material to be recalled in such a way that will increase the likelihood of successful recall (5).

Domain-Specific Methods

Researchers have demonstrated that patients with severe memory impairments can learn new information and show transfer of this learning (8,41). This learning has been most successful for the acquisition of domain-specific knowledge. Glisky and Schacter (8) described three defining characteristics of domain-specific training: (a) the goal is to alleviate specific problems associated with memory impairment rather than restore memory processes or improve general memory functioning; (b) the information learned using these instructional techniques has practical value to the patient; and (c) the purpose of the acquisition of domain-specific knowledge is to teach clients information or procedures that they can access or implement independently.

Sohlberg and Mateer (5) provide examples of tasks that may be considered domain-specific: (a) transfer to and from a wheelchair; (b) operation of a walker; (c) operation of a computer; (d) medication schedule; (e) names of people or objects; and (f) swallowing procedures. Mnemonic strategies have been shown to be most effective when teaching domain-specific knowledge. Other domain-specific memory approaches for addressing memory impairments are expanded rehearsal techniques, use of priming, and formation of personal history.

Expanded Rehearsal

Spaced retrieval is an example of an intervention strategy that uses expanded rehearsal. The patient practices successful recall of information over progressively longer intervals of time. Bjork (42) demonstrated the effectiveness of the technique in which name-face associations were taught by presenting photographs in a spaced interval sequence. The research demonstrated that the longer the distracting interval from the first to the second successful recall attempt, the greater the likelihood of recall at a third recall attempt.

Brush and Camp (43,44) suggested the following checklist for clinicians to follow when using spaced retrieval techniques to teach a patient information or procedures (5): (a) learning should be effortless; (b) the information or procedures taught should be concrete; (c) errors should be limited; (d) one piece of information should be taught at a time; (e) data sheets should be used to track intervals, but the length of intervals does not have to be exact; and (f) if patients cannot recall target information longer than 6 minutes after six sessions, chances for retention are limited.

Sohlberg and Mateer (5) have delineated the following examples of behaviors that have been targeted using spaced retrieval techniques: (a) learning key names (43); (b) swallowing techniques (44); (c) learning name-face associations (45); (d) procedures for using external memory aids (46); and (e) learning names of objects (47).

Use of Priming

Patients with severe memory impairments exhibit normal repetition priming effects (5). This means that they have the same likelihood of recalling previously encountered information when given partial cues as individuals who do not have memory impairments. They fail, however, to recall the event itself in which they first encountered the information. Glisky et al. (48) capitalized on this preserved learning and developed a memory technique called the *method of vanishing cues*. It is a faded cueing technique that can be used to teach complex knowledge or behaviors that might be used in daily life. The patient initially is provided with enough information to make a correct response and then parts of the information are gradually withdrawn across learning trials so that the patient receives fewer and fewer cues. Glisky and Schacter (49) and Glisky et al. (48,50) evaluated the technique by attempting to teach subjects computer vocabulary and procedures. The studies demonstrated that patients with memory impairments could learn. The tasks in all of the studies were highly specific and

did not require problem solving. Subjects, however, were consistently slow to acquire the information.

Creation of a Personal History

Ischemic stroke patients with retrograde amnesia have a loss of memory for life events that occurred before the stroke. Learning of new information often is impaired as well. Either priming or expanded rehearsal techniques can be used to teach discrete facts about a patient's personal history. It also can be helpful to create an autobiography. It can take the form of a photographic life essay that is assembled and composed by family members. It could be a written life history, a video composition of important people in the patient's life, or simple orientation pages in a memory book. Involvement of family and friends in the project can be therapeutic for them as well and can give them a sense of active participation in the patient's rehabilitation. When developing a personal history, it is critical to consider the following factors (5): (a) match the format to the patient's abilities and disabilities; (b) the patient should have easy access to the history whenever he or she wants to review it; and (c) use the interests, ideas, and strengths of the individuals (family members, friends, and the patient) producing the history.

Sohlberg and Mateer (5) reported that they facilitated the development of personal histories that clients have reviewed many times for months and years after it was developed. They reported being comforted by having critical personal history that had been compiled in a manner to which they can easily refer.

SUMMARY AND CONCLUSIONS

Impaired memory is a common consequence of ischemic stroke. Cognitive rehabilitation of memory is an essential component of any comprehensive rehabilitation program for these patients. Generalizable methods and methods to teach domain-specific knowledge are two principal means whereby impaired memory can be improved. Compensatory strategies can be taught to patients whose memory is not likely to improve. Cognitive remediation using these methods has been shown to be an effective intervention to treat memory deficits. More well-controlled, randomized studies are needed to further investigate the efficacy of the various interventions available.

ACKNOWLEDGMENTS

Special thanks to Michael Reding, M.D., medical director of the Stroke Recovery Unit at the Burke Rehabilitation Hospital, White Plains, New York, U.S.A. for his kind invitation to write this chapter and for the generous support he provided from start to completion of the work. The author is grateful for the valuable assistance of Lauren M. Greiner, M.A., and Karina Ortega-Verdejo, M.A., with the tedious task of compiling the references and word processing for this work.

REFERENCES

1. Ellis HC, Hunt RR *Fundamentals of cognitive psychology.* Madison, WI: Brown and Benchmark, 1993.
2. Luria AR *Restoration of function after brain injury.* New York: Macmillan, 1963.
3. Luria AR *Higher cortical functions in man.* New York: Basic Books, 1980.
4. Miller E . Psychological intervention in the management and rehabilitation of neuropsychological impairments. *Behavioral Research and Therapy* 1980;18:527–535.
5. Sohlberg MM, Mateer CA *Cognitive rehabilitation: an integrative neuropsychological approach.* New York: Guilford, 2001.
6. Gianutsos R. Cognitive rehabilitation: a neuropsychological specialty comes of age. *Brain Injury* 1991;5: 353–368.
7. Butler RW, Namerow NS. Cognitive retraining in brain-injury rehabilitation: a critical review. *J Neurol Rehabil* 1988;2:97–101.
8. Glisky EL, Schacter DL. Models and methods of memory rehabilitation. In: Boller F, Grafman J, eds. *Handbook of neuropsychology.* Amsterdam: Elsevier, 1989: 233–246.
9. Godfrey HP, Knight RG. Interventions for amnesics: a review. *Br J Clin Psychology* 1987;26:83–91.
10. Gordon WA, Hibbard MR. The theory and practice of cognitive remediation. In: Kreutzer JS, Wehman PH, eds. *Cognitive rehabilitation for persons with traumatic brain injury.* Baltimore: Paul H. Brookes, 1991:12–22.
11. Gouvier WD Assessment and treatment of cognitive deficits in brain damaged individuals. *Behav Modif* 1987;11:312–328.
12. Hayden ME. Rehabilitation of cognitive and behavioral dysfunction in head injury. *Adv Psychosom Med* 1986; 16:194–229.
13. Parente R, Anderson-Parente J. *Retraining memory: techniques and applications.* Houston, TX: CSY, 1991.
14. Prigatano G, Fordyce D. Neuropsychological rehabilitation program: Presbyterian Hospital, Oklahoma City, Oklahoma. In: Caplan B, ed. *Rehabilitation psychology desk reference.* Gaithersburg, MD: Aspen, 1987: 281–298.
15. Seron X, Deloche G, eds. *Cognitive approaches in neuropsychological rehabilitation.* Hillsdale, NJ Lawrence Erlbaum, 1989.
16. Sohlberg MM, Mateer CA. *Introduction to cognitive rehabilitation.* New York: Guilford, 1989.
17. Wehman P, Kreutzer J, Sale P, et al. Cognitive impairment and remediation: implications for employment following traumatic brain injury. *J Head Trauma Rehabil* 1989;4:66–75.
18. Wood RL, Fussey L. *Cognitive rehabilitation in perspective.* London: Taylor & Francis, 1990.
19. Cicerone KD, Dahlberg C, Kalmar K, et al. et al. Evidence-based cognitive rehabilitation: recommendations for clinical practice. *Arch Phys Med Rehabil* 2000;81: 1596–1615.
20. Baddeley AD, Wilson BA, Watts FN, eds. *Handbook of memory disorders.* Chichester, England: Wiley, 1995.
21. Huppert F, Piercy M. In search of the functional locus of amnesic syndromes. In: Cermak LS, ed. *Human memory and amnesia.* Hillsdale, NJ: Erlbaum, 1982: 123–137.
22. McDowall J. Processing capacity and recall in amnesic and control subjects. In: Squire LR, Butters N, eds. *Neuropsychology of memory.* New York: Guilford Press, 1984:63–66.
23. Posner M, Petersen SE. The attention system of the human brain. *Annu Rev Neurosci* 1990;13:25–42.
24. Craik F, Lockhart R. Levels of processing: a framework for memory research. *J Verbal Learn Verbal Behav* 1972;11:671–684.
25. Tulving E. Subjective organization and effects of repetition in multi-trial free-recall learning. *J Verbal Learn Verbal Behav* 1966;5:193–197.
26. Tulving E, Schacter DL. Priming and human memory systems. *Science* 1990;247:301–306.
27. Wilson BA, Moffat N. *Clinical management of memory problems.* London: Chapman & Hall, 1992
28. Schacter D, Glisky E. Memory remediation, restoration, alleviation, and the acquisition of domain specific knowledge. In: Uzzell B, Gross Y, eds. *Clinical neuropsychology of intervention.* Boston: Martinus Nijhoff, 1986:257–282.
29. Sohlberg MM, McLaughlin K, Pavese A, et al. Evaluation of attention process training and brain injury education in persons with acquired brain injury. *J Clin Exp Neuropsychol* 2000; 22(5):656–676.
30. Sturm W, Willmes K, Orgass B, et al. Do specific attention deficits need specific training? *Neuropsychol Rehabil* 1997;7:81–103.
31. Wilson BA. *Rehabilitation of memory.* New York: Guilford Press, 1986.
32. Cermak LS. Imagery as an aid to retrieval for Korsakoff patients. *Cortex* 1975;11:163–169.
33. Wilson BA. Success and failure in memory training following a cerebral vascular accident. *Cortex* 1982;18: 581–594.
34. Baddeley AD, Warrington EK. Memory coding and amnesia. *Neuropsychologia* 1973;11:159–165.
35. Crovitz HF, Harvey MT, Horn RW. Problems in the acquisition of imagery mnemonics: three brain damaged cases. *Cortex,* 1979;15:225–234.
36. Miller E. Psychological approaches to the management of memory impairments. *Br J Psychiatry* 1992;160:1–6.
37. Glisky EL, Schacter DL. Remediation of organic memory disorders: current status and future prospects. *Head Trauma Rehabil* 1986;1:54–63.
38. Sohlberg MM, Mateer CA, Geyer S. *Prospective Memory Screening (PROMS) and Prospective Memory Process Training (PROMPT).* Puyallup, WA: Associa-

tion for Neuropsychological Research and Development, 1985.

39. Rebmann MJ, Hannon R. Treatment of unawareness of memory deficits in adults with brain injury: three case studies. *Rehabil Psychology* 1995;40:279–287.

40. Schlund MW. Self-awareness: Effects of feedback and review on verbal self-reports and remembering following brain injury. *Brain Injury* 1999;13:375–380.

41. Evans JJ, Wilson BA, Schuri U, et al. A comparison of "errorless" and "trial-and-error" learning methods for teaching individuals with acquired memory deficits. *Neuropsychol Rehabil* 2000;10:67–101.

42. Bjork RA. Retrieval practice and the maintenance of knowledge. In: Gruneberg MM, Morris PE, Sykes RN, eds. *Practical aspects of memory: current research and issues.* Chichester, England: Wiley, 1988:283–288.

43. Brush JA, Camp CJ. Using spaced retrieval as an intervention during speech-language therapy. *Clin Gerontol* 1998;19:51–64.

44. Brush JA, Camp CJ. Spaced retrieval during dysphagia therapy: a case study. *Clin Gerontol* 1998;19:96–99.

45. Carruth EK. The effects of singing and the spaced retrieval technique on improving face-name recognition in nursing home residents with memory loss. *J Music Ther* 1997;34:165–186.

46. Stevens AB, O'Hanlon AM, Camp C J. Strategy training in Alzheimer's disease: a case study. *Clin Gerontol* 1993;13:106–109.

47. Moffat, MJ. Home-based cognitive rehabilitation with the elderly. In: Poor LW, Rubin DC, Wilson BA, eds. *Everyday cognition in adulthood and late life.* Cambridge, UK: Cambridge University Press, 1989: 659–680.

48. Glisky EL, Schacter DL, Tulving E. Learning and retention of computer-related vocabulary in amnesic patients: method of vanishing cues. *J Clin Exp Neuropsychol* 1986;8:292–312.

49. Glisky EL, Schacter DL. Long-term retention of computer learning by patients with memory disorders. *Neuropsychologia* 1998;26:173–178.

50. Glisky EL, Schacter DL, Tulving E. Computer learning by memory-impaired patients: acquisition and retention of complex knowledge. *Neuropsychologia* 1986;24: 313–328.

Ischemic Stroke: Advances in Neurology, Vol. 92. Edited by
H.J.M. Barnett, Julien Bogousslavsky, and Heather Meldrum.
Lippincott Williams & Wilkins, Philadelphia © 2003.

50

Partial Body Weight Supported Treadmill Training for Gait Recovery Following Stroke

Stefan Hesse and Cordula Werner

Department of Neurological Rehabilitation, Free University Berlin, Klinik Berlin, Berlin, Germany

Gait training is a major goal of neurologic rehabilitation after stroke. This chapter discusses new developments in locomotor therapy. Partial body weight supported treadmill training (PBWSTT) enables severely affected stroke patients to rehearse complex gait cycles using a task-specific approach to motor recovery. Several controlled studies have documented its potential for enhancing gait recovery during both the acute and chronic phases after stroke. Automated PBWSTT and robot-assisted gait training are recent alternatives to PBWSTT. They are an attempt to reduce the burden on the therapist assisting the patient with weight shifting and leg positioning during PBWSTT.

Stroke is a leading cause of disability and handicap. Each year in the United States, 750,000 individuals suffer a stroke. Its prevalence is 200 to 300 patients per 100,000 inhabitants (1). Approximately 90% of these patients suffer from persisting motor deficits leading to disability and handicap, namely dependence in their daily activities, impaired arm and hand function, and impaired walking ability.

Restoration of gait is a major goal for both patients and therapists in neurologic rehabilitation after stroke. Conventional gait therapy can be described as following one of four approaches: (a) aggressive mobilization using brace, walking assist device, and physical assistance by the therapist; (b) Brunnstrom technique, which encourages the use of synergistic movements; (c), proprioceptive neuromuscular facilitation technique, which encourages the use of spiral and diagonal movements; and (d) neurodevelopmental therapy (NDT, Bobath), which uses reflex inhibitory movements. Although different, none of these techniques has proved to be superior to the others (2–4). Proponents of the NDT approach, however, argue that such studies have not adequately assessed quality and symmetry of movement.

We previously assessed gait velocity, endurance, and symmetry in 156 chronic hemiparetic patients before and after a 4-week comprehensive NDT rehabilitation program (5). Gait symmetry reflecting gait quality served as the primary outcome variable. The mean time interval after stroke was 12.8 weeks. Surprisingly, neither gait function nor gait symmetry improved substantially. We noted that tone-inhibiting maneuvers and gait preparatory tasks during sitting and standing were the primary focus of the NDT program. Gait itself was practiced very little.

MODERN CONCEPTS OF MOTOR REHABILITATION

Modern concepts of motor learning favor task-specific training (6). For instance, Winstein et al. (7) reported that balance training while standing improved balance but not gait symmetry in hemiparetic patients. In another study, Dean and Shepherd (8) instructed hemiparetic patients to train balance while sitting. At the end of the study, weight distribution between both lower limbs when sitting had improved, whereas symmetry of force distribution while standing remained unchanged. A recent large Norwegian outcome study compared the Bobath program and a task-specific motor relearning program (MRP), as advocated by Carr and Shepherd, in 61 acute stroke patients (9). The MRP group stayed in the hospital for fewer days and their improvement in general motor functions was significantly better than in the Bobath group, confirming the benefit of a task-specific repetitive approach. Modern upper extremity rehabilitation follows the same principles. The reader is referred to the work of Bütefisch et al. on repetitive wrist dorsiflexion versus Bobath treatment and to the concept of constraint-induced movement therapy (10,11).

PARTIAL BODY WEIGHT SUPPORTED TREADMILL TRAINING

The task-specific approach to walking is simply stated: "The best way to improve walking is to walk." Our group has used PBWSTT (Fig. 50-1) in stroke rehabilitation since 1992 (5). Our application of this technique to stroke victims followed reports that it had shown promise in treating paraparetic subjects (12,13).

PBWSTT enables otherwise nonambulatory hemiparetic subjects to repetitively practice complex gait cycles.

Patients wear a modified parachute harness to substitute for deficient equilibrium reflexes. The moving treadmill elicits and reinforces complex stepping movements (Fig. 50-1). The harness supports a proportion of their body weight so that subjects can carry their remaining body weight adequately, that is, without knee collapse or excessive hip flexion during single-stance phase on the affected leg.

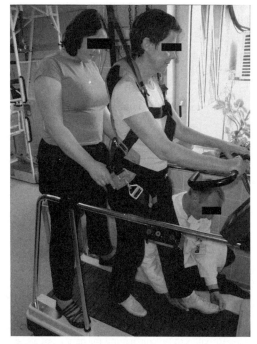

FIG. 50-1. Left hemiparetic stroke patient practicing on the treadmill with partial body weight support assisted by two therapists.

The theoretical background of locomotor therapy is based on experiments in adult spinalized cats and incompletely lesioned primates. These studies show activation of presumed spinal and supraspinal gait pattern generators by locomotor therapy (14). Adult spinalized cats, which do not regain locomotor ability spontaneously, relearn weight-bearing steps with their hind limbs after a several-month training period on the treadmill. Lateral support still is required for balance.

Patients should be able to sit at the edge of the bed independently. Standing ability is not required. Cardiac risk factors, a history of recent deep vein thrombosis of the lower limbs, lower limb joint contractures. and arthrosis can be limiting factors. Pusher syndrome (i.e., pushing toward the affected side while standing and walking) is not an exclusion criterion.

Initially, two (or even three) therapists are required to assist the subjects' movements on the treadmill. Patients should practice stepping not only repetitively but also in as smooth and normal a pattern as possible. One therapist, sitting alongside the patient, helps control the paretic foot and leg during the swing phase of gait and ensures that initial contact is made with the heel during the stance phase. The therapist also prevents hyperextension of the knee and controls the symmetry of steps. A second therapist, who is standing behind the subject, assists weight shift onto the stance limb and promotes hip and trunk extension by applying firm pressure with the thumb on the rear of the pelvis or a flat hand on the chest. Patients are not allowed to sit in the harness because this prevents leg loading and results in continuous hip flexion. Based on animal experiments, alternating loading and unloading of the lower limbs and hip extension during stance are the main peripheral drives needed to activate the gait pattern generator (15). Treadmill velocities of approximately 0.25 m/s and body weight support (BWS) of no more than 30% body weight are initially recommended. During therapy, treadmill speed should be increased and BWS reduced as soon as possible (see later) to facilitate activation of weight-bearing muscles, economize gait, and enhance cardiovascular fitness.

CLINICAL EVALUATION OF TREADMILL THERAPY

Initial studies [a baseline-treatment study (n = 9) and two single case control studies following an A-B-A design (n = 14)] in chronic nonambulatory hemiparetic subjects revealed that PBWSTT was superior to conventional physiotherapy with regard to restoration of gait and improvement of ground walking velocity (3,16). During the A phases, treadmill therapy was applied alone or in combination with functional electrical stimulation (FES). Patients did not receive any additional conventional physiotherapy. During the B phases, patients received conventional physiotherapy but no treadmill therapy. Each of the phases lasted 3 weeks. FES helped to facilitate movement on the treadmill. For instance, stimulation of the N. peroneus during the swing phase assisted with dorsiflexion of the foot. The results showed that patients improved their gait ability and overground walking velocity considerably during the first 3-week A phase (A1) of daily treadmill training. During the subsequent period of 3 weeks of conventional physiotherapy (B) gait ability did not change, whereas the second A phase further enhanced walking ability (Fig. 50-2). All subjects who had been wheelchair bound before therapy became ambulatory at least with verbal support by the end of the study. During one 30-minute session of treadmill training with PBWSTT, patients could practice up to 1,000 gait cycles compared with a median of less than 50 gait cycles during one regular physiotherapy session.

A large Canadian study of 100 acute stroke patients compared treadmill therapy with and without BWS (17). After randomization, 50 patients were trained to walk with up to 40% of their body weight supported (BWS group) and the other 50 subjects were trained to walk with full weight bearing on their lower limbs (no-BWS group). After a 6-week training period, the BWS group scored significantly higher than the no-BWS group for functional balance ($p = 0.001$), motor recovery ($p = 0.001$), overground walking speed ($p = 0.029$), and overground walking endurance ($p = 0.018$) (Fig. 50-3). Follow-up evaluation 3 months later revealed that the BWS group continued to have significantly higher scores for overground walking speed ($p = 0.006$) and motor recovery ($p = 0.039$).

Kosak and Reding (18) conducted the first randomized study in 56 acute stroke patients who needed at least moderate assistance for walking. The experimental group received treadmill therapy with PBW-STT following the principles mentioned. The control treatment consisted of aggressive early therapist-assisted ambulation using knee-ankle combination bracing and hemibar if needed, that is, it did not follow conventional treatment concepts but stressed gait practice. Treatment session of up to 45 minutes per day, 5 days a week, were given as tolerated for the duration of inpatient stay or until the patients could walk overground unassisted. The outcome of the two groups as a whole did not differ. However, a subgroup with major hemispheric stroke (defined by the presence of hemiparesis, hemianopic visual deficit, and hemihypesthesia) who received more than 12 treatment sessions showed significantly better overground endurance and speed scores favoring PBWSTT (Fig. 50-3). The authors concluded that both approaches were equally effective, except in a subset of severely disabled patients who were difficult to mobilize using physiotherapy alone.

Da Cunha et al. (19) conducted a pilot study on 12 acute stroke patients allocated to either treadmill therapy or regular rehabilitation for 2 to 3 weeks. Dependent variables were cardiovascular performance on a bicycle exercise test and the locomotor subscore of the functional independence measure (FIM-L). After intervention, the treadmill group performed better on the bicycle exercise test but the FIM-L did not differ.

Nilsson et al. (20) presented a multicenter trial in hemiparetic patients at an early stage after stroke. Three rehabilitation departments randomly allocated 73 patients to two groups who either received daily 30-minute treadmill therapy or 30-minute walking training overground according to the MRP program of Carr and Shepherd. During their time in the rehabilitation departments (about 2 months), all patients in the study received professional stroke rehabilitation in addition to walking training. There were no statistically significant differences between the groups at discharge or at 10-month follow-up with regard to FIM, walking velocity, Fugl-Meyer Stroke

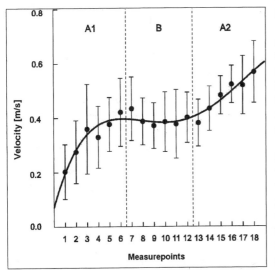

FIG. 50-2. Line graph shows mean (SD) walking velocity over time. Treadmill training applied exclusively during the A1 and A2 phases was more effective than physiotherapy applied during the B period ($p < 0.05$)

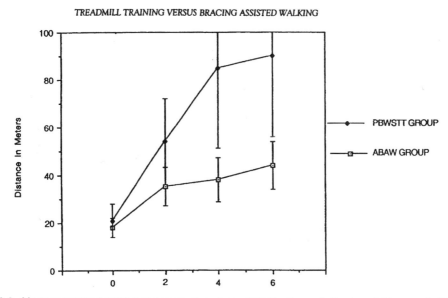

FIG. 50-3. Mean overground walking endurance in meters ± SEM for the partial body weight supported treadmill training (PBWSTT; n = 8) versus aggressive bracing assisted walking (ABAW; n = 14) subgroups with hemiparesis-hemisensory-hemianopic visual deficits and 12 or more treatment sessions. The PBWSTT group showed significantly better overground endurance (90 ± 34 vs. 44 ± 10 m). (From Kosak MC, Reding MJ. Comparison of partial body weight-supported treadmill gait training versus aggressive bracing assisted walking post stroke. *Neurorehabil Neural Repair* 2000;14:13–19, with permission.)

Assessment, or balance scores. The authors concluded that treadmill training with BWS at an early stage after stroke was a comparable choice to walking training overground.

Biomechanical studies document that increasing BWS decreases the muscle activity of relevant weight-bearing muscles in hemiparetic subjects (21). Data suggest that BWS should not exceed 30% BW in order to optimize weight-bearing ability after stroke. Correspondingly, BWS should be reduced as soon as patients are able to carry their weight on the paretic limb without abnormal postures. BWS can be reduced when patients are able to sustain their body weight during single stance on the paretic limb, that is, without knee buckling or "sitting" in the harness.

When PBWSTT with a mean of 15% BWS is compared with floor walking, hemiparetic patients randomized to PBWSTT walk more symmetrically, more dynamically, and with better motor control. The dynamic electromyogram of shank muscles showed less premature activation of the gastrocnemius and more physiologic activation of the tibialis anterior. These results do not support the often-expressed fear of therapists that PBWSTT enforces repetition of an abnormal gait. On the contrary, patients walked more symmetrically with less spasticity during PBWSTT. Danielsson and Sunnerhagen (22) compared oxygen

consumption during treadmill walking with 30% BWS and without BWS in stroke patients. The 30% BWS condition required less oxygen consumption than full weight bearing. The authors concluded that patients with cardiovascular problems could tolerate treadmill therapy with BWS.

A previous study assessed the influence of walking velocity on gait, muscle activation, and energy consumption of 25 hemiparetic subjects walking on the treadmill slowly, at self-adopted speed, and at maximum speed (23). Higher gait velocity on the treadmill correlated with facilitation of relevant antigravity muscles without accompanying cocontraction of antagonist muscles. Furthermore, patients walked more efficient at higher velocities, that is, they consumed less energy per distance covered. These results support faster treadmill speeds to facilitate activation of antigravity muscles, economize the patients' gait, and train cardiovascular fitness. Cardiovascular risk factors, of course, should be considered.

Macko et al. (24) investigated the effects of treadmill aerobic exercise training in 23 ambulatory chronic stroke patients. They had shown that 6 months of low-intensity treadmill endurance training (three 40-minute sessions per week walking at 50% to 60% of heart rate reserve) produced substantial and progressive reductions in the energy expenditure and cardiovascular demands of their study population, thus improving the functional mobility of their patients.

AUTOMATED GAIT TRAINING

The major disadvantage of PBWSTT is the need for two or three therapists to assist with gait training of severely affected subjects. Therefore, an electromechanical gait trainer (Fig. 50-4) was designed and constructed (25). The harness-secured subject is positioned on two footplates whose movements simulate stance and swing in a symmetric manner with a ratio of 60%:40% between stance and swing. The cadence and stride length can be adjusted within a speed range of 0.1 to 2.8 km/h according to individual needs. A servocontrolled drive mechanism assists gait movements. Vertical and horizontal movements of the trunk are controlled in a phase-dependent manner. Phase-dependent electrical stimulation of the quadriceps muscle during the stance phase helps to stabilize the knee; alternatively a therapist sitting in front of the patient can control knee movement.

Sagittal joint kinematics and dynamic electromyography of selected lower limb muscles in control subjects have been shown to closely mimic normal gait. Compared to overground walking, ankle dorsiflexion during the swing phase was less on the gait trainer (due to constructional constraints); correspondingly, patients hit the ground not with their heel but with the entire foot. Severely affected hemiparetic subjects need less help on the gait trainer than on conventional PBWSTT systems. Movement is more symmetric, and the single-stance phase of the paretic limb lasts longer on the gait trainer than on conventional PBWSTT systems. Dynamic electromyography of the lower limbs shows comparable activation of the trunk and thigh muscles. Plantar flexor activity is less on the gait trainer. Activation of the tibialis anterior muscle is, however, diminished on the gait trainer as the weight of the foot is partially carried by the footplate during the "swing phase."

Subsequent clinical results show marked gait improvements for severely affected hemiparetic subjects. An initial treatment study (3 weeks of conventional therapy followed by 4 weeks of additional therapy on the gait trainer) with 14 nonambulatory hemiparetic patients (mean stroke interval 11.2 weeks) confirms the potential of this novel approach. Four weeks of physiotherapy plus use of the gait trainer resulted in significant improvement in gait velocity, cadence, and stride length. The kinesiologic electromyogram of selected lower limb muscles revealed a more physiologic pattern of thigh and shank muscle activation. The confounding influence of spontaneous recovery, the lack of a control group, and the double amount of therapy were limiting factors. Further studies are planned.

Colombo et al. (26) from Zürich, Switzerland, devised another alternative to current PBWSTT. They use a hybrid system consisting of a motor-driven treadmill (to promote weight-bearing during stance phase) and a powered exoskeleton with drives flexing the hip and knee during the swing phase. Currently, the system is purely passive. A force control that can sense the patient's effort is planned as the next step in clinical development. Others have suggested developing robotic arms that control limb movements during the swing and stance phases of gait. Dr. Edgerton at the University of California has used such devices successfully to study gait recovery in spinalized rats.

SUMMARY

PBWSTT has emerged from an interesting idea to a well-accepted and scientifically supported treatment modality for gait training after stroke. PBWSTT offers a task-specific approach to functional gait

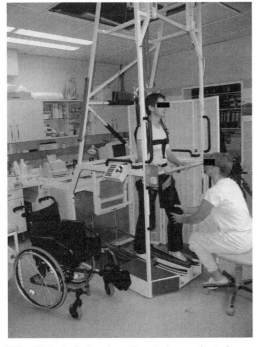

FIG. 50-4. Left hemiparetic stroke patient (same patient shown in Fig. 50-1) practicing on the gait trainer with partial body weight support assisted by one therapist.

retraining that is based on rehearsal of repetitive controlled gait cycles. Newer devices are being developed that will provide better mechanical control of the patient and reduce therapist effort.

REFERENCES

1. Williams GR, Jingo JG, Matchar DB, et al. Incidence and occurrence of total (first-ever and recurrent) stroke. *Stroke* 1999;30:2523–2528.
2. Jorgensen HS, Nakayma H, Raaschou HO, et al. Recovery of walking function in stroke patients: the Copenhagen stroke study. *Arch Phys Med Rehabil* 1995;76: 27–32.
3. Hesse S, Bertelt C, Schaffrin A, et al. Restoration of gait in nonambulatory hemiparetic patients by treadmill training with partial body-weight support. *Arch Phys Med Rehabil* 1994;75:1087– 1093.
4. Ernst E. A review of stroke rehabilitation and physiotherapy. *Stroke* 1990;21:1081–1085.
5. Hesse S, Jahnke MT, Bertelt C, et al. Gait outcome in ambulatory hemiparetic patients after a 4-week comprehensive rehabilitation program and prognostic factors. *Stroke* 1994;25:999–1004.
6. Asanuma H, Keller A. Neurobiological basis of motor learning and memory. *Concepts Neurosci* 1991;2:1–30.
7. Winstein CJ, Gradner ER, McNeal DR, et al. Standing balance training: effects on balance and locomotion in hemiparetic adults. *Arch Phys Med Rehabil* 1989;70: 755–762.
8. Dean C, Shepherd R. Task-related training improves the performance of seated reaching tasks following stroke: a randomised controlled trial. *Stroke* 1997;28:722–728.
9. Langhammer B, Stanghelle JK. Bobath or motor relearning programme? A comparison of two different approaches of physiotherapy in stroke rehabilitation: a randomized controlled study. *Clin Rehabil* 2000;14: 361–369.
10. Bütefisch C, Hummelsheim H, Denzler P, et al. Repetitive training of isolated movements improves the outcome of the centrally paretic hand. *J Neurol Sci* 1995; 130:59–68.
11. Taub E, Miller NE, Novak TA, et al. Technique to improve chronic motor deficit after stroke. *Arch Phys Med Rehabil* 1993;74:347–354.
12. Barbeau H, Wainberg W, Finch L. Description and application of a system for locomotor rehabilitation. *Med Biol Eng Comput* 1987;25:341–344.
13. Wernig A, Müller S. Laufband locomotion with body weight support in persons with severe spinal cord injuries. *Paraplegia* 1992;30:229–238.
14. Lovely RG, Gregor RJ, Roy RR, et al. Effects of training on the recovery of full-weight bearing stepping in the adult spinal cat. *Exp Neurol* 1986;92:421–435.
15. Duysens J, Pearson KG. Inhibition of flexor burst generation by loading ankle extensor muscles in walking cats. *Brain Res* 1980;187:321–332.
16. Hesse S, Bertelt C, Jahnke MT, et al. Treadmill training with partial body weight support as compared to physiotherapy in non-ambulatory hemiparetic patients. *Stroke* 1995;26:976–981.
17. Visintin M, Barbeau H, Korner-Bitensky N, et al. A new approach to retrain gait in stroke patients through body weight support and treadmill stimulation. *Stroke* 1998; 29:1122–1128.
18. Kosak MC, Reding MJ. Comparison of partial body weight-supported treadmill gait training versus aggressive bracing assisted walking post stroke. *Neurorehabil Neural Repair* 2000;14:13–19.
19. da Cunha Filho IT, Lim PAC, Qureshy H, et al. A comparison of regular rehabilitation and regular rehabilitation with supported treadmill ambulation training for acute stroke patients. *J Rehabil Res Dev* 2001;38: 37–47.
20. Nilsson L, Carlsson J, Daniellson A, et al. Walking training of patients with hemiparesis at an early stage after stroke: a comparison of walking training on a treadmill with body weight support and walking training on the ground. *Clin Rehabil* 2001;15: 515–527.
21. Hesse S, Konrad M, Uhlenbrock D. Treadmill walking with partial body weight support versus floor walking in hemiparetic subjects. *Arch Phys Med Rehabil* 1999;80: 421–427.
22. Danielsson A, Sunnerhagen KS. Oxygen consumption during treadmill walking with and without body weight support in patients with hemiparesis after stroke and in healthy subjects. *Arch Phys Med Rehabil* 2000;81: 953–957.
23. Hesse S, Werner C, Paul T, Bardeleben A, et al. The influence of walking speed on lower limb muscle activity and energy consumption during treadmill walking of hemiparetic patients. *Arch Phys Med Rehabil* 2001;82: 71–77.
24. Macko RF, Smith GV, Dobrovolny CL, et al. Treadmill training improves fitness reserve in chronic stroke patients. *Arch Phys Med Rehabil* 2001;82:879–885.
25. Hesse S, Uhlenbrock D, Werner C, et al. A mechanized gait trainer for restoring gait in non-ambulatory subjects. *Arch Phys Med Rehabil* 2000;81:1158–1161.
26. Colombo G, Wirz M, Dietz V. Driven gait orthosis for improvement of locomotor training in paraplegic patients. *Spinal Cord* 2001;39:252–255.

Ischemic Stroke: Advances in Neurology, Vol. 92. Edited by
H.J.M. Barnett, Julien Bogousslavsky, and Heather Meldrum.
Lippincott Williams & Wilkins, Philadelphia © 2003.

51

Robot-Aided Sensorimotor Training in Stroke Rehabilitation

*†Bruce T. Volpe, *‡Hermano Igo Krebs, and ‡Neville Hogan

*Burke Medical Research Institute, White Plains, New York; †Department of Neurology and
Neuroscience, Weill Medical College of Cornell University, New York, New York; ‡Mechanical
Engineering Department, Massachusetts Institute of Technology, Cambridge, Massachusetts, U.S.A.

Reducing the degree of permanent disability remains the goal of poststroke neurorehabilitation programs, and new approaches to impairment reduction through systematic enhancement of the sensorimotor experience may contribute to further altering disability. Recent reports from a number of laboratories using robotic devices have registered significant impairment reductions and increased motor power (MP) in the exercised limb of patients with stroke compared to controls. Equipping the therapist with new tools to treat impairment may be a realistic approach to modern interdisciplinary rehabilitation, especially in view of current standards that shorten the length of treatment.

STROKE IS THE LEADING CAUSE OF PERMANENT DISABILITY

Recent studies suggest that the incidence of stroke has been underestimated (1). In the United States, the ranks of the more than four million survivors of stroke alive today are likely to swell considerably because of increasing life expectancy and the coincidence of the "baby boom" generation growing older, coupled with improved medical treatment of the complications caused by acute stroke (2). Stroke will continue to be the leading cause of disability because nearly 90% of stroke survivors have significant residual physical, cognitive, and psychological impairments. A patient's impairment or neurologic deficit is defined by the specific loss or abnormality of psychological, physiologic, or anatomic structure. Impairment after stroke depends on the lesion size and location in the brain. Disability is a broader term that captures any restriction or lack of ability to perform an activity in the manner or within the range considered normal.

POSTSTROKE TREATMENT PROGRAMS STRESS DISABILITY REDUCTION

Current interdisciplinary treatment programs for patients with stroke attend to both impairment and disability reduction. Functional improvement is the cornerstone of the rehabilitation experience, because if patients with stroke are to regain independence they must successfully readjust to the environment (3). However, the rush to discharge the patient from the rehabilitation hospital has prompted a shift toward encouraging functional improvement by learning compensatory techniques. Recent evidence demonstrated that patients with the most severe strokes who had little or no change in impairment after a rehabilitation effort nevertheless learned to compensate and reduced their disability (4). Some investigators who demonstrated reduction of impairment after additional training for patients with either the acute or chronic phase of stroke recovery have suggested that the emphasis on disability reduction may occur at the expense of potential impairment reduction (5,6).

NOVEL TECHNOLOGIES AND TRAINING PROTOCOLS FOCUS ON IMPAIRMENT REDUCTION

A number of innovative training protocols for impairment reduction have demonstrated that focused additional sensorimotor training for the paralyzed limbs improved outcome (7–12). However, both enhanced protocols and current standard interdisciplinary stroke rehabilitation treatment depend on the labor-intensive, one-on-one, manual interaction with therapists that occurs daily over weeks. For standard poststroke programs, because the therapy that promotes the best recovery is unknown, most therapists use a combination of traditional techniques. Patient evaluation usually is done subjectively, which makes it difficult to monitor treatment effects. This situation presents an opportunity to create new technologic solutions to the problems of neurorecovery. Devices that provide safe, quantifiable, and reproducible physical activity would clearly assist health care delivery experts.

For example, the Massachusetts Institute of Technology (MIT) group has pioneered the design of devices that turn the old man–machine interaction on end (13–16). Rather than test whether robotic technology can serve the brain-injured patient, this group, in collaboration with clinicians from the Burke Medical Research Institute, White Plains, New York, U.S.A. has been testing whether they can improve motor outcome by equipping therapists with robotic devices to enhance the sensorimotor experience (17). The MIT-MANUS robot has been designed with low intrinsic endpoint impedance and with a low and nearly isotropic inertia and friction that translates into a machine with a handle that can be moved easily or, if necessary, is strong enough to move a patient's par-

alyzed arm. A brief review of other approaches to applying robotic technology to exercise the proximal arm has been outlined (17–20). Initial experiments from each of these groups have demonstrated proof of principle. New challenges now ask whether training on these devices is efficacious and produces added value; particularly, can the improved motor performance reflected in reduced impairment compared to controls lead to disability reduction, and are there cost efficiencies that obtain as a result?

EXPERIMENTAL RESULTS ON RECOVERY OF PROXIMAL UPPER LIMB FUNCTION AFTER STROKE WITH ROBOTIC-ENHANCED TRAINING TECHNIQUES

The Burke–MIT group has forged new ground by using robotic training in prospective, randomized, double-blinded studies to begin to test the efficacy of adding these protocols to the standard interdisciplinary rehabilitation program for stroke recovery (Fig. 51-1) (21–25) Results to date have shown an advantage for the robot-trained patients, extending the proof of principle and suggesting that it is an effective technique to enhance motor outcome of the paralyzed upper limb. For each of these studies, consecutive patients were randomly assigned to a robot treatment (sensorimotor) or control (sensory) group. Patients

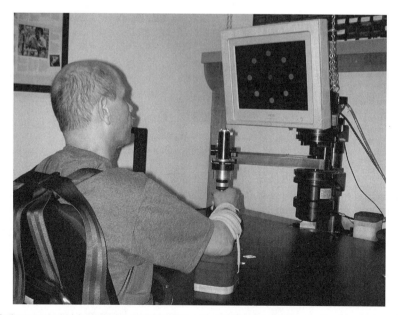

FIG. 51-1. Patient seated in front of the MIT-MANUS with his shoulders strapped to the chair and moving the manipulandum. The patient's hand is strapped to a wrist carrier attached to the manipulandum. The video screen is above the training table.

TABLE 51-1. *Results of treating 96 patients with stroke and upper limb paralysis with robot training sensorimotor protocols or control sensory exposure*

Group	FM S/E (max = 42)	MSS S/E (max = 40)	MP (max = 20)
Robot-trained (n = 56)	6.6 ± 1.0	8.6 ± 0.9	4.1 ± 0.4
Control (n = 40)	4.9 ± 0.8	3.4 ± 0.5	2.2 ± 0.3
p Value	NS	<0.001	<0.005

FM S/E, Fugl-Meyer shoulder and elbow measure; max, maximum; MP, motor power; MSS S/E, motor status score shoulder and elbow measure.

The robot-trained group demonstrated significant improvement compared to controls. The impairment measurements depict interval change (mean ± SEM). Timing of stroke to rehabilitation (around 2.5 weeks), duration of rehabilitation experience (around 3.5 weeks), and all admission impairments measures were comparable between groups.

and clinicians, especially the "measuring" therapist who recorded all assessment procedures, were masked to the group assignments. The robot-trained (sensorimotor) group received an additional hour per weekday of robot-aided therapy, whereas the control (sensory) group had an hour of weekly robot exposure with the robot providing visual feedback but no assistance from the motors. Sensorimotor and sensory training lasted on average 3.5 weeks. If the patient had any power in the proximal upper extremity, he or she easily drove the robot arm while it measured speed, force, and position. If the patient could not move the device the robot guided the limb to the target. Other essential design features included admission to the rehabilitation hospital within 3 weeks of a first stroke, some upper limb weakness, and an ability to follow a few simple instructions. Robot training, which took place in a standard therapy suite and was supervised by a research therapist, lasted 45 minutes (about 10 minutes without setup). The training required that the patient perform 1,024 flexion and extension movements of the arm, with gravity eliminated in eight directions represented by the points of a compass.

Table 51-1 lists the interval change from rehabilitation admission to discharge in the combined group of 96 patients (21–25). Details of the new adaptive training protocols and the various temporal sequences will be elaborated in other work. The robot-trained group demonstrated increased Fugl-Meyer shoulder and elbow measure (FM S/E; maximum = 42) scores, but the difference was not significant. The measure of upper limb motor impairment (MP, standard muscle testing; maximum = 20) and the expanded mixed measure of upper limb impairment and disability [motor status score for shoulder and elbow (MSS S/E); maximum = 40) were significantly improved in the robot-trained group compared to the control. In data not shown (but reviewed in reference 24), the motor improvement was confined to the exercised proximal limb, movements around the shoulder and elbow. There was no advantage conferred by robotic training on sensorimotor activity of the wrist and fingers. Motor performance of lower limb activity, especially gait, was comparable between groups.

Gains that were registered by the sensorimotor-trained group after the acute rehabilitation experience and robot training persisted through the follow-up evaluation more than 2 years later. Table 51-2 lists the clinical assessment of 31 patients studied to date (21 sensorimotor/robot trained; 10 sensory trained/controls). Although the robot-trained group demonstrated sustained impairment gains in the upper limb, compared to the controls the difference was not significant, indicating that improvement continues, albeit to a modest degree, for both groups many months after

TABLE 51-2. *Follow-up evaluation of 31 patients with stroke who had robot sensorimotor training or control over 2.5 years after initial stroke and rehabilitation hospital discharge*

Group	FM S/E (max = 42)	MSS S/E (max = 40)	MP (max = 20)
Robot-trained (n = 21)	14.5 ± 2.9	14.2 ± 2.1	7.0 ± 0.8
Control (n = 10)	17.5 ± 6.3	10.2 ± 3.5	5.8 ± 1.5

FM S/E, Fugl-Meyer shoulder and elbow measure; max, maximum; MP, motor power; MSS S/E, motor status score shoulder and elbow measure.

The impairment measurements depict interval change (mean ± SEM) from admission to follow-up evaluation. As before, the timing of stroke to rehabilitation (around 2.5 weeks), duration of rehabilitation experience (around 3.5 weeks), exact duration of follow-up examination, and all admission impairments measures were comparable between groups. In this follow-up group, a subset of the total group, the robot-trained (sensorimotor) group maintains the impairment gains that had been registered by discharge, but both groups continue to improve.

stroke. These results require greater patient numbers, as the standard error of the mean increased for all groups in follow-up.

For these 96 patients, the interval change in the functional independence measure (FIM) was comparable across groups. The FIM has reliability and validity, but many of the activities measured in the self-care subsection that depend on upper limb motor control can be performed with one limb. Because these scores were not obtained with the restriction of using only the paralyzed or unaffected limb, a definitive conclusion about the link between decreased upper limb motor impairment (increased motor function) and decreased disability currently is not possible.

EXPERIMENTAL RESULTS USING ROBOTIC TRAINING TECHNIQUES TO ENHANCE RECOVERY OF PROXIMAL UPPER LIMB FUNCTION IN PATIENTS WITH CHRONIC STROKE

The Palo Alto VA–Stanford group has been using a different robotic training for patients with chronic stroke (19,20,26,27). Using a robotic device called MIME (mirror image motion enabler, a PUMA 260 machine), these treatment programs focused on more than two dozen patients, 6 months to 2 years after stroke. Subjects were randomly assigned to robot treatment or control. All patients were in a treatment program for the same amount of time. Robot-treated subjects had their upper extremity manipulated by the robot as well as the therapist; controls had only the therapist manipulate their affected upper limb. Therapists determined the stage and the application of the individually tailored robot treatment protocol. The results demonstrate that the robot-treated patients had significantly greater interval change in the FM S/E and not for wrist and hand activity. (26,27). The robot-trained patients also demonstrated significantly improved percentage change in mean strength of shoulder and elbow movements compared to controls. Consistent with the Burke–MIT results in patients treated within weeks of stroke, these experiments suggest that recovery may be induced months to years after the acute stroke.

The RIC–UC Irvine group has reported the training results of adding a therapy with a robotic-controlled reaching device [assistive rehabilitation and measurement (ARM) guide] to a standard program (18,28–30). They trained more than a dozen patients with chronic stroke (some >5 years after stroke) on a reaching paradigm. Initial results demonstrated that trained subjects had improved kinematics of reach, velocity, and better control of tone; patients produced smoother movements (29). If smoothness or quality of movement acquired in recovery matters to outcome, and for normal movement smoothness matters, then it appears that detailed measurements obtained only by technologic instrumentation could add another clinically important dimension. A randomized study demonstrated that patients treated with an equal number of movements as administered or directed by a therapist compared to patients treated by the ARM device robot-delivered training had comparable motor improvement (29,30). However, using a disability measure of bimanual functional activity and a measurement of movement smoothness, they found trends that favored the robotic-treated group (30).

SUMMARY

The first groups to use robotic devices to enhance the sensorimotor experience of patients recovering from upper limb paralysis after stroke have generated encouraging information. Patient acceptance and staff enthusiasm for robot training at Burke–MIT is consistently high. Robot training data are consistent with other controlled studies showing that more activity leads to more motor improvement and decreased impairment. Therapists equipped with a robotic device can increase the amount and intensity of movement of the paralyzed limb without sacrificing time spent training complex functionally appropriate kinematics.

ACKNOWLEDGMENTS

The authors acknowledge support from the Burke Medical Research Institute; the United States Public Health Service (NIH, HD 37397 and 36827); and the Langeloth Foundation.

REFERENCES

1. Broderick J, Brott T, Kothari R, et al. The Greater Cincinnati/Northern Kentucky Stroke Study: preliminary first-ever and total incidence rates of stroke among blacks. *Stroke* 1998;29:415–421.
2. American Heart Disease, 2001 Heart and Stroke Statistical Update, p. 16.
3. Volpe BT. Palliative treatment for stroke. *Neurol Clin* 2001;19:903–920.
4. Shelton FD, Volpe BT, Reding M. Motor impairment as a predictor of functional recovery and guide to rehabilitation treatment after stroke. *Neurorehabil Neural Repair* 2001;15(3):229–237.
5. Taub E, Miller NE, Novack TA, et al. Technique to improve chronic motor deficit after stroke. *Arch Phys Med Rehabil* 1993;74:347–354.

6. Dromerick AW, Edwards DF, Hahn M. Does the application of constraint-induced movement therapy during acute rehabilitation reduce arm impairment after ischemic stroke? *Stroke* 2000;31:2984-2988.

7. Miltner WH, Bauder H, Sommer M, et al. Effects of constraint induced movement therapy on patients with chronic motor deficits after stroke: a replication. *Stroke* 1999;30:586–92.

8. Liepert J, Bauder H, Wolfgang HR, et al. Treatment-induced cortical reorganization after stroke in humans. *Stroke* 2000;31:1210-1216.

9. Kwakkel G, Wagenaar RC, Twisk JWR, et al. Intensity of leg and arm training after primary middle cerebral artery stroke: a randomized trial. *Lancet* 1999;354: 191–196.

10. Feys HM, De Weerdt WJ, Selz BE, et al. Effect of a therapeutic intervention for the hemiplegic upper limb in the acute phase after stroke: a single-blind, randomized, controlled multicenter trial. *Stroke* 1998;29:785–792.

11. Sunderland A, Fletcher D, Bradley L, et al. Enhanced physical therapy for arm function after stroke: a one year follow up study. *J Neurol Neurosurg Psychiatry* 1994;57:856–858.

12. Sunderland A, Tinson DJ, Bradley L, et al. Enhanced physical therapy improves recovery of arm function after stroke. A randomized clinical trial. *J Neurol Neurosurg Psychiatry* 1992;55:530–535.

13. Hogan N. Adaptive control of mechanical impedance by coactivation of antagonist muscles. *IEEE Trans Automatic Control* 1984;AC-29:681–690.

14. Hogan N, Krebs HI, Sharon A, et al. Interactive robot therapist. US patent no. 5,466,213, MIT, November 14, 1995.

15. Hogan N. Impedance control: an approach to manipulation. Part 1, 2, 3. *ASME J Dynam Syst Measurement Control* 1985;107:1–24.

16. Hogan N, Krebs HI, Charnnarong J, et al. MIT-MANUS: a workstation for manual therapy and training. MIT-MANUS: a workstation for manual therapy and training. *SPIE The International Society for Optical Engineering Telemanipulator Technology* 1992;1833: 28–34.

17. Volpe BT, Krebs HI, Hogan N. Is robot-aided sensorimotor training in stroke rehabilitation a realistic option? *Curr Opin Neurol* 2001;14:745–752.

18. Reinkensmeyer DJ, Dewald JPA, Rymer WZ. Robotic devices for physical rehabilitation of stroke patients: fundamental requirements, target therapeutic techniques and preliminary designs. *Technol Disability* 1996;5:205–215.

19. Lum PS, Reinkensmeyer DJ, Lehman SH. Robotic assist devices for bimanual physical therapy: preliminary experiments. *IEEE Trans Rehabil Eng* 1993;1: 185–191.

20. Lum PS, Burgar CG, Kenney DE, et al. Quantification of force abnormalities during passive and active-assisted upper-limb reaching movements in post-stroke hemiparesis. *IEEE Trans Biomed Eng* 1999;46: 652–662.

21. Aisen ML, Krebs HI, Hogan N, et al. The effect of robot assisted therapy and rehabilitative training on motor recovery following stroke. *Arch Neurol* 1997;54: 443–446.

22. Volpe BT, Krebs HI, Hogan N, et al. Robot training enhanced motor outcome in patients with stroke maintained in three year follow-up. *Neurology* 1999;53: 1874–1876.

23. Krebs HI, Aisen M, Volpe BT, et al. Quantization of continuous arm motion in humans with brain injury. *Proc Natl Acad Sci U S A* 1999;96:4645–4649.

24. Volpe BT, Krebs HI, Hogan N, et al. A novel approach to stroke rehabilitation: robot aided sensorimotor stimulation. *Neurology* 2000;54:1938–1944.

25. Krebs HI, Volpe BT, Aisen ML, et al. Increasing productivity and quality of care: robot-aided neurorehabilitation. *VA J Rehabil Res Dev* 2000;37:639–652.

26. Burgar CG, Lum PS, Shor PC, et al. Development of robots for rehabilitation therapy: the Palo Alto VA/Stanford experience. *J Rehabil Res Dev* 2000;37:663–673.

27. Shor PC, Lum PS, Burgar CG, et al. In: Mokhtari M, ed. *The effect of robot aided therapy on upper extremity joint passive range of motion and pain.* Amsterdam, The Netherlands: IOS Press, 2001:79–83.

28. Reinkensmeyer DJ, Kahn LE, Averbuch M, et al. Understanding and treating arm movement impairment after chronic brain injury: progress with the ARM guide. *J Rehabil Res Dev* 2000;37:653–662.

29. Kahn L, Averbuch M, Rymer WZ, et al. Comparison of robot assisted reaching to free reaching in promoting recovery from chronic stroke. In: Mokhtari M, ed. *Integration of assistive technology in the information age.* Amsterdam, The Netherlands: IOS Press, 2001:39–44.

30. Kahn LE, Zygman ML, Rymer WZ, et al. Effect of robot-assisted exercise on functional reaching in chronic hemiparesis. IEEE 23rd Engineering in Medicine and Biology Society, EMBS-1136, October 2001.

Ischemic Stroke: Advances in Neurology, Vol. 92. Edited by
H.J.M. Barnett, Julien Bogousslavsky, and Heather Meldrum.
Lippincott Williams & Wilkins, Philadelphia © 2003.

52

Poststroke Depression

Antonio Carota and Julien Bogousslavsky

Department of Neurology, University Hospital, Centre Hospitalier Universitaire Vaudois,
Lausanne, Switzerland

Poststroke depression (PSD) has high prevalence. Symptoms or signs of depression occur at any time after stroke in about 20% to 60% of patients, have a negative impact on functional outcome, and increase the high cost of disability.

DIAGNOSIS OF POSTSTROKE DEPRESSION

The diagnosis of depression associated with stroke and/or other chronic medical conditions is largely based on *Diagnostic and Statistical Manual of Mental Disorders, Fourth Edition (DSM-IV)* diagnostic criteria (American Psychiatric Association, 1994) (Table 52-1).

It is still a subject of controversy whether PSD and *endogenous depression* (ED) are clinically comparable. In ED, the "*nonreactive*" or "*unmotivated*" (possibly biologically determined) aspects (e.g., feelings of worthlessness, guilt, and suicidal ideation) and morning aggravation prevail, whereas in PSD anxiety, diurnal mood fluctuation, and the "*motivated*" or "*reactive*" (possibly psychological) aspects (e.g., low mood, reduced appetite, and anergia) are more frequent (1).

The *DSM-IV* diagnosis of a "*major depressive-like episode*" is based on the existence of five or more depressive symptoms, two of which must be a depressed mood and a loss of interest and pleasure

TABLE 52-1. *DSM-IV diagnostic criteria*

Mood disorder due to a general medical condition, mood-incongruent delusions or hallucinations, or disorganized speech. The essential feature is a prominent persistent mood judged to be due to the direct physiologic effects of a general medical condition.
Subtypes
I. With depressive features: the predominant mood is depressed, but not all criteria for a major depressive episode are met
II. With major depressivelike episodes
   A. At least five of the following symptoms are present over at least a 2-week period; at least one of the symptoms is either (a) a depressed mood or (b) loss of interest or pleasure
      1. Depressed mood most of the day
      2. Markedly decreased interest or pleasure
      3. Significant weight loss or weight gain
      4. Insomnia or hypersomnia
      5. Psychomotor agitation or retardation
      6. Fatigue or loss of energy
      7. Feelings of worthlessness or excessive or inappropriate guilt
      8. Diminished ability to think or concentrate
      9. Recurrent thoughts of death
   B. Distress or impairment of social, occupational, or other functioning
   C. No bereavement
III. With manic features: the predominant mood is elevated, euphoric, or irritable
IV. With mixed features: symptoms of both mania and depression are present, but neither predominates

DSM-IV, *Diagnostic and Statistical Manual of Mental Disorders, Fourth Edition.*

in almost all activities. *"Minor depression"* is a less severe form of depression with the presence of two, but fewer than five, of the symptoms and includes either a depressed mood or the loss of interest. The *"continuum hypothesis"* considers that, in stroke patients, major and minor depression are two expressions of the same disease, and that they are differentiated by the severity of symptoms on a continuous gradient (2). This continuity may correspond to a psychological reaction to the handicap, variable in its intensity. The *"categorical hypothesis"* considers that the major and minor forms of PSD have different etiologies, different outcomes, and different implications for therapeutical interventions (3). This hypothesis supports a localizationist model for major PSD and a psychodynamic etiology for minor PSD.

SCALES AND QUESTIONNAIRES

In the absence of biologic markers, scales and questionnaires are used for reproducible diagnosis (Table 52-2)

DIAGNOSIS OF MOOD DISORDERS IN PATIENTS WITH APHASIA AND OTHER NEUROLOGIC CONDITIONS

The neurobehavioral sequelae of stroke compromise the validity of patients' answers to scales and questionnaires. Even when language and attention are not impaired, patients still may fail to respond in a reliable fashion (4). Tests to check the validity of replies in interviews are rarely performed. Caution in the use of rating scales is required, because patients might be more sensitive to the stressor event of stroke than being affected by depression and anxiety. The presence of misleading neurologic and neurocognitive conditions (Table 52-3) should be carefully evaluated.

Most studies on PSD have excluded patients with language disturbances because mood changes cannot be reliably tested without verbal examination. The *Stroke Aphasic Depression Questionnaire* (5) and a modified *Analogue Dysphoria Scale* (6) report, together with verbal items, vegetative and other symptoms independently of language ability (i.e., eating and sleep disturbances) and show a good validity compared to the Hamilton Depression Rating Scale (HRDS).

Observational methods should diagnose depression in patients who deny depression but who have correspondent behaviors and signs (*"nonstandard depression"*). However, vegetative symptoms alone may not distinguish minor depression from nonde-pression. Another limitation is that, for a valid report, the informant must be in frequent contact with the patient and that, even then, he or she could not have a complete understanding of the patient's internal state of mood. The neurophysiologic basis of vegetative symptoms remains not completely understood. They are frequently reported by patients with other chronic illness (e.g., chronic heart or renal failure).

Patients with anosognosia can express behavioral correlates of depression although they might deny mood changes. Specific scales and questionnaires should be used to assess mood disorders in patients with right hemispheric lesions.

While talking, patients with affective dysprosody give the impression of a lack of affection and often are considered depressed, even when they are not. The caregiver's and patient's replies to interviews should be evaluated carefully to determine whether dysprosody is the main feature rather than depression.

Apathy after stroke and depression are related dimensions of behavior and probably share neural circuitries (frontosubcortical pathways), but they can be distinguished. Structured interviews, such as the *Apathy Scale* (7) and the *Apathy Evaluation Scale* (8) can help in differentiating apathy from depression.

Fatigue is reported by up to 70% of stroke patients, even at a considerable time after stroke (9), and often is unexplained by depressive feelings, neurologic deficits, and lesion location. The Fatigue Impact Scale can be a useful tool in characterizing this symptom and its causes (9). The recognition of fatigue and its differentiation from PSD may be critical for therapeutic interventions.

In contrast to depression, *loss of self-autopsychic activation* (or *athymhormia*) is reversible under repeated stimulation. Athymhormia can be assessed by special interviews (10) and is generally consequent to ischemic focal lesions involving, often bilaterally, the rostral part of the caudate nucleus, the pallidum, putamen, thalamus, and gyrus cinguli.

Emotionalism or *emotional incontinence* is one manifestation of a more general disorder of emotional control and often is associated with PSD (11), although most people with emotionalism are not depressed. The scale developed by Robinson et al. (12) is useful for characterizing pathologic crying and laughing. Various locations have been reported, such as anterior or frontal and temporal lesions, but a specific link with the emergence of emotionalism has not yet been demonstrated. The underlying abnormality may be serotoninergic and symptoms improve with serotonin reuptake inhibitors (SSRIs) (13).

TABLE 52-2. *Scales and questionnaires for assessment of mood disorders*

Questionnaire	Scoring	Comments
Hamilton Depression Rating Scales (HDRS): 17- or 21-item versions	>25: severe depression 18–24: moderate depression 7–17: mild depression 0–6: no depression	Most widely used Self-rating In stroke patients, cutoff of 8 or 10
Beck Depression Inventory: 21 items (BDI-II)	0–13: minimal, or no, depression 14–19: mild depression 20–28: moderate depression 29–63: severe depression	Most widely used Self-rating Symptoms of sadness, loss of pleasure, guilty feelings, vegetative signs; good correlation with HDRS (0.7); could be implemented by HDRS for somatic items
Hospital Anxiety and Depression (HAD) Scales: 14 items	Depression: 8–10 doubtful cases, ≥11: depression Anxiety: 8–10 doubtful cases, ≥11: anxiety	Self-rating Easy for patients Excellent validity compared to HDRS
General Health Questionnaire: 28 items (GHQ-28)	Score >12: presence of a psychiatric disorder Four subscales: (1) somatic symptoms, (2) anxiety and insomnia, (3) social dysfunction, (4) severe depression No specific for syndromic diagnostic	No significant differences between GHQ-30 and the HAD Scale in identifying depression or anxiety disorders poststroke Cutoff level could be suboptimal
Geriatric Depression Scale (GDS): 30 items	11–30: depression	More useful in geriatric populations; deemphasizes somatic symtpoms
Zung Self-Rating Depression Scale (ZSRDS)	Self-rating	Useful in patients with neurologic disordes; smilar to BDI and CES-D
Post-Stroke Depression Scale (PSDS)	No cutoff scores, but symptomatic profile	Detects depressed mood, feelings of guilt, thoughts of death and suicide, vegetative disorders, apathy, anxiety, catastrophic reactions, emotionalism, anhedonia, and diurnal mood variations
Center for Epidemiologic Studies Depression Scale (CES-D): 20 items	Score >16: depression	Self-rating Correlation with HDRS: 0.44–0.69 No influence of sex, age, race, education Difficulty to discriminate major depression from generalized anxiety
Goldberg Anxiety and Depression Scales (GADS)	Nine questions	Useful as screening measures in medical setting for anxiety or depression, but lacks specificity for each disorder
Montgomery-Asberg Depression Rating Scale (MADRS): 10 items	Cutoff of 35 to separate moderate from severe depression	Significant correlation with HRDS; its capacity to differentiate between responders and nonresponders to antidepressant treatment may be better than HDRS, showing a greater sensitivity to change
Neurobehavioral Cognitive Status Examination (NCSE): 10 scales	Score between 10 and 40; cutoff of 13 for discriminating between patients with organic mental disorder and those without the disorder	Useful as screening tool

(continued)

TABLE 52-2. *Continued.*

Questionnaire	Scoring	Comments
Visual Analogic Mood Scales (VAMS)	No cutoff scores: continous variables	Vertical lines version to avoid bias due to hemineglect; especially constructed for patients with language disturbancies
Stroke Aphasic Depression Questionnaire (SADQ): 10 items	Specific for aphasic patients	Validity: 0.32–0.67 with HDRS
Modified Analogue Dysphoria Scale (MADS)	Specific for patients with severe language disturbances	Sleep and eating disturbances measured by using both self-report and nursing assessments
Neurobehavioral Rating Scale: 27 subscales	Subscales: cognition/energy, metacognition (self-appraisal, planning, disinhibition), somatic concern/anxiety, depression, language, orientation, memory, reasoning, attention	Self-report Used in closed head injury
Neuropsychology Behavior and Affect Profile: 106 statements	Five scales: inappropriateness, indifference, depression, pragnosia (defect in communicative style), mania; it has questions to break the tendency of the patient among the scales	Structured informant interview; useful for stroke and patients with dementia

TABLE 52-3. *Diagnostic confounders of depressive syndromes after stroke*

1. Indirect
   Common to many severely ill hospitalized patients
     Controlled appetite (e.g., NPO and tube feeding)
     Frequently awakened
     Confined to bed
     Delirium (acute confusional states)
   Of special concern in stroke patients
     Immobility (potential confusion with apathy)
     Dysphagia (interferes with eating habits)
     Slurred speech (and resultant miscommunication)
2. Direct
   Aphasia
   Amnesia and cognitive impairment
   Anosognosia and denial of depressive signs
   Aprosody
   Neurologic apathy syndromes
     Isolated abulia/apathy
     Loss of psychic autoactivation
     Frontal lobe syndrome
     Klüver-Bucy syndrome
     Korsakoff's syndrome
     Poststroke fatigue
   Special behavioral syndromes
     Emotional lability or emotionalism
     Catastrophic reaction
   Dementia
   Pseudobulbar syndrome

NPO, nothing by mouth.

INCIDENCE, PREVALENCE, AND DEMOGRAPHIC DATA

In the vast literature, PSD prevalence varies between 6% and 22% in the first 2 weeks, 22% to 53% at 3 to 4 months, 16% to 47% at 1 year, 19% at 2 years, 9% to 41% at 3 years, 35% at 4.9 years, and 19% at 7 years. Similar prevalences are reported in community-based (27%–47%), outpatient (40%), and rehabilitation unit (27.4%–55%) studies.

Major depression accounts for 6% to 56% of stroke patients, whereas minor depression has a prevalence of about 15%. These large variations are due to the use of different structured interviews, the different size and selection criteria, and different times of investigations after the stroke onset.

The incidence of PSD varies slightly with age (14) and gender. In women, major depression correlates with a high level of education, cognitive impairment, and previous psychiatric antecedents, whereas in men, it is more dependent on physical impairment (15). Minor depression could occur more frequently in men and be associated with inadequate spousal social support (16).

To our knowledge, there are no neuroanatomic, functional, and genetic models that can explain sexual differences according to cerebral localization. Psychological factors probably are more relevant.

PSD incidence and prevalence are high, risk factors are not yet clearly understood, and stroke patients should be investigated for PSD even when several years have elapsed since the initial event.

LESION LOCATION IN ENDOGENOUS DEPRESSION

In ED, computed tomography and magnetic resonance imaging studies showed a trend toward orbitofrontal atrophy and a reduction in volume of the basal ganglia, hippocampus, and amygdala. Positron emission tomographic (PET) studies showed reduced metabolism with normalization after therapy in the left frontosubcortical and paralimbic circuits, left anterior cingulate, superior temporal and parietal cortex, and caudate (17,18).

The presence of dysexecutive signs and memory deficits (recall) in patients with ED further supports the association of ED with dysfunction of frontostriatal, frontolimbic, and frontosubcortical pathways.

The role of subcortical lesions is suggested by retrospective magnetic resonance imaging studies (19,20), which showed a relationship between major unipolar depression and silent cerebral infarctions. In these patients, the severity of depression can be greater and the response to pharmacologic treatment less prompt. The majority of cases with senile-onset major depression might correspond to PSD.

ATTEMPTS AT LOCALIZATION IN POSTSTROKE DEPRESSION

Most clinical studies in stroke attempted to identify the cerebral regions whose dysfunction causes PSD, with the underlying hypothesis that the same cerebral regions are involved in ED and that the main abnormality in ED is biochemical.

These regions should be part of, or connected to, the limbic and temporal lobes and be involved in the processing of emotions and mood states to enhance or inhibit oriented-goal behaviors.

Temporal lobe hypoperfusion was found in a group of depressed patients with subcortical lesions but not in a group with similar lesion location but without depression, suggesting that the temporal lobe may be critical for the occurrence of PSD (21). The basal ganglia also are part of the neural pathways underlying behavioral responses. Their major role in emotion and mood state is in highly dynamic modulation, execution, spontaneity, and basic motor processing of

behaviors with emotional content. Several studies (22,23), but not all (24), suggested the role of the limbic connected areas and basal ganglia in the development of PSD

Beblo et al. (25) attempted to reduce methodologic bias by selecting 20 PSD patients without severe physical impairment, psychiatric antecedents, concomitant morbidity, and aphasia and then performing detailed neuropsychologic measurements. Their findings point out to dysfunction of (cortico-) striato-pallido-thalamic-cortical projections that modulate cortico-thalamo-cortical loop systems. Kim and Choi-Kwon (26) found similar evidence in patients with PSD and emotional incontinence. The low incidence of depression with vertebrobasilar stroke (brainstem and cerebellar lesion) further supports the role of anterior brain regions (ACA and ACM vascular territories).

LESION LOCALIZATION AND OTHER NEUROLOGIC DISEASES WITH DEPRESSION

Patients with *Parkinson's disease* often present a depressive syndrome similar to PSD (apathy, psychomotor slowing, frontoamnesic deficits). PET studies showed reduced regional blood flow in the frontal cortex, but the role of dopaminergic circuitries remain unclear (27,28). Severe depression, euphoria, emotional lability, and loss of spontaneity also are reported in patients with *cerebral autosomal dominant arteriopathy with subcortical infarcts and leukoencephalopathy (CADASIL)*.

Depressive symptoms are an early clinical manifestation of *human immunodeficiency virus encephalopathy,* where lesions are diffuse in white matter and basal ganglia. In patients with *multiple sclerosis,* severity of depression correlates with cortico-subcortical atrophy and the amount of demyelinating lesions in the semiovale centers (29) and has been related to an increased lesion load of the projection areas of the basal limbic system (30).

The presence of left dorsolateral frontal lesions and/or left basal ganglia lesions is associated with an increased probability of developing major depression with traumatic brain injury (31).

POSTSTROKE DEPRESSION LOCALIZATIONIST THEORIES

A large number of clinical studies by Robinson and colleagues [reviewed in Robertson (32)] support the role of frontal, subcortical, and basal ganglia lesions in PSD.

The central hypothesis is as follows: left hemisphere location and the proximity of the anterior border of the lesion to the frontal pole are determinant factors for developing the major form of PSD. The neuroanatomy of the biogenic amine-containing pathways, which have a more anterior cortical distribution, might explain the linear correlation between anterior location and PSD severity.

This localizationist model has been the subject of great criticism. Diffuse lesions in the middle cerebral artery (MCA) territory are proximal to both poles. Small samples of patients were analyzed (30–45 subjects) and the major hypothesis linking PSD to lesion site appears statistically weak. The exclusion of patients with severe aphasia or cognitive impairment probably determined a selection bias. The confounding role of amnesia, apathy, fatigue, and loss of psychic autoactivation has not been completely evaluated, and these symptoms are neurobehavioral correlates of basal ganglia and anterior lesions. The depressive symptoms also can be the result of metabolic dysfunction of distant cerebral areas connected with the lesions. Several other clinical studies that used similar methods failed to find any lateralization or any anteroposterior gradient (33), whereas others found that right, rather than left, lesions were significantly associated with PSD (34). It also is possible that, when depression and anxiety coexist, they may be associated with different patterns of asymmetric hemispheric function. It has been suggested that although a clinical syndrome similar to ED is seen in patients with right lesions, symptoms in patients with left lesions more closely resemble those of neurotic depression, even though both conditions respond to antidepressants. The Baltimore group was unable to confirm these data at different delays after stroke. In their later studies they suggested that during the *acute phase* PSD is associated with left anterior and basal ganglia lesions, is a function of the volume of the lesion, and is independent of language dominance, but during *short-term follow-up* (several months) lesion volume and the proximity of the lesion to the frontal pole of both hemispheres are the major determinants. After 1 to 2 years, PSD is consequent to dysfunction of the right hemisphere and to lesion volume and its proximity to the occipital pole. Furthermore, these findings are valid only in patients with typical occipital asymmetry, whereas a reversal pattern is seen in cases of atypical asymmetry. Gender could play a role, because in the case of left lesions women might have a greater risk of depression than men. According to Robinson et al., poststroke delay, occipital asymmetry but not cerebral dominance for language, and gender are the principal factors explaining interstudy differences in PSD anatomic correlates.

Rigorous meta-analysis indicated the methodologic limitations of localizationist findings and concluded that lesion location may contribute only slightly to PSD development (35).

COGNITIVE IMPAIRMENT

A significant association between PSD and cognitive deficits has been reported in several studies, even though stroke itself may be followed by a significant decline in cognitive performance when prestroke and poststroke measurements are compared (36).

The main question is whether depression negatively influences the outcome of cognitive impairment (*"dementia of depression"*) or cognitive impairment leads to depression (*"depression of dementia"*). The link probably is bidirectional.

Frontoamnesic deficits due to disruption of cortical projections to the caudate nucleus have been suggested as an explanation for progressive deterioration of patients with PSD and lesions of the caudate nucleus (37). Working with a group of 53 patients with single stroke lesions, Bolla-Wilson et al. (38) found that patients with left hemispheric lesions and major depression were more impaired in terms of orientation, language (naming), verbal learning, visuoperceptual and visuoconstructional tasks, and executive functions (attention, concentration, nonverbal problem solving, and psychomotor speed) than nondepressed patients with left lesions. The same neuropsychologic profile applies to elderly patients with ED. The presence of dysphasia also increases the risk of major depression (39). Improvement of cognitive impairment after antidepressant therapy is a further argument for dementia of depression (40).

In other community studies, using Mini-Mental State Exam (MMSE) (34,41) or other measurements (42), no evidence was found to support a correlation between cognitive impairment and major depression 1 year after a first-ever stroke or during a 13-year period since stroke onset. The issue remains open to further research.

DISABILITY AND OUTCOME

The development and intensity of depressive symptoms correlate strongly with the grade of functional impairment (14,39) during the acute phase and the first 6 months after stroke. This result has not been confirmed in all the studies, but the real impact of physical impairment to individual patients according to their own system of values and lifestyle has not been taken in account.

A low National Institute of Health Stroke Scale (NIHSS) score on admission is a significant predictor for return to work, absence of PSD, and good quality of life (14). Functional measurements correlate temporally with the progress of PSD and are better longitudinal predictors of depressive symptoms than lesion location (43). Prevalence of depression is comparable in patients with stroke and patients with similar disability due to other medical illness (44). Whether functional impairment leads to depression or the depression itself compromises the recovery of neurologic deficits is an unresolved issue. Again, the link probably is bidirectional. Several studies report that depressive feelings negatively influence the outcome of patients with stroke at short- and long-term follow-up (45,46). Physical functioning, bodily pain, somatic symptoms, and social functioning are worse in patients with affective disorders. There is a negative correlation between physical impairment, reduced autonomy, and the feeling of self-esteem that induces patients to perceive themselves as useless and hopeless. Self-esteem is significantly correlated to functional independence (47). PSD patients may not have the energy or motivation to participate in rehabilitation therapy.

Other authors found that the minor form of depression correlates with greater physical disability and, therefore, only this form corresponds to an adjustment reaction (3).

Depressive feelings before or at the time of stroke result in a greater than three-fold risk of subsequent mortality (over the following 10 years) in patients with PSD compared to stroke patients without depression (48,49). This risk is independent of other cardiovascular risk factors, age, sex, social class, type of stroke, and lesion location, but it is associated with social isolation (50). Patients who are depressed may return to detrimental habits (smoking, alcohol) and may not comply with treatment recommendations or health-promoting behavior. PSD patients are at increased risk of falling (51). Increasing mortality probably is mediated by modifications of the cardiovascular system. Patients with ED experience a higher grade of arterial hypertension, especially the systolic value (52), and myocardial infarction (53). Another possible explanation is enhanced platelet aggregation, which has been reported in patients with ED.

PSYCHIATRIC ANTECEDENTS AND PSYCHOSOCIAL FACTORS

It is important to have an understanding of the patient's baseline characteristics (e.g., previous history of depression) to ensure that a current disorder represents a meaningful change from a premorbid level of function. The process of adjustment to serious physical illness is strongly influenced by personal vulnerability, low self-esteem, conflicts within close relationships (particularly marital), and negative experiences in the developmental history.

An increased incidence of familial history of psychiatric disorders in patients with PSD suggests a genetic predisposition (34).

An impaired relationship with the patient's spouse or closest other relative before the stroke and limited social activities both are associated with depression immediately after stroke and depression at long-term follow-up (54). Other factors are loss of job satisfaction, lack of social contact, financial security, decreased social activity, and adequacy of living arrangements.

After stroke, individuals may settle for a restricted future because their expectations of life with a disability are low. These patients do not search for psychiatric care and are less motivated to intensive physical or cognitive rehabilitation. Clinicians need to be completely aware of stroke effects on each aspect of the patient's life in order to maximize therapy and rehabilitation. The "*Social Functioning Examination*" is a useful tool for determining the causes of impairment in social functioning (55).

SUICIDE

Suicide among stroke patients is extremely rare (56). Suicide rates are 6% in the acute phase and 6% to 12% in the following 2 years. Risk factors include depression, severe insomnia, chronic illness, and organic brain syndrome. The degree of physical impairment, history of alcohol abuse, poor social support, brooding, and self-blame are determinant. Other risk factors are younger age, presence of a sensory deficit, and impaired cognitive functions. Suicidal ideation is frequent (25%) in patients with stroke or other acute life-threatening physical illness (57).

TREATMENT OF POSTSTROKE DEPRESSION

Several pharmacologic treatments have been evaluated for patients with PSD. Significant recovery from PSD is generally considered a reduction equivalent or superior to 50% of HDRS or Beck Depression Inventory (BDI) scores. Pharmacologic treatment for depression related to medical illness (i.e., stroke and other diseases) has evidence-based validation (58).

Tricyclic antidepressants are no longer the treatment of first choice because of the severity and elevated frequency of adverse effects (orthostatic hypotension, atrioventricular block, delirium or confusion, drowsiness, agitation, life-threatening cardiac arrhythmias, heart block, urinary outlet obstruction, and narrow angle glaucoma).

The first-choice drugs are the SSRIs, which have been shown to be more effective than placebo and tricyclic drugs and have fewer side effects.

Side effects of SSRIs are similar in frequency and expression in patients with PSD and ED. They consist of gastrointestinal symptoms (particularly nausea), headache, and "stimulant" effects, such as agitation, anxiety, and insomnia. Fluoxetine-induced mania has been reported in patients with stroke (59). Male sexual dysfunction is rare but must be taken into account when proposing treatment.

Only a few studies have compared the effects of two or more SSRIs, and these studies generally involved only a small sample of patients (60). *Fluoxetine* may not be the first-choice SSRI if a rapid onset is required because steady-state concentrations are not reached until after 4 to 5 weeks. *Sertraline* and *citalopram* require less than 1 week.

The longer half-life of fluoxetine allows less frequent administration in noncompliant patients and results in less severe discontinuation effects. Fluoxetine is helpful when depression is associated with bulimia or diabetes because it increases basal metabolism, enhances weight loss, and reduces glycemic values. For this reason, interaction with oral antidiabetics should be closely monitored. Fluoxetine inhibits P-450 isoenzymes and should not be used in stroke patients receiving anticoagulant therapy.

Sertraline and citalopram seem to be more efficacious in the treatment of stroke-associated lability of mood. Compared to fluoxetine, sertraline and citalopram are better tolerated, have lesser risk of agitation, weight loss, and dermatologic adverse effects, and fewer interactions with drugs influencing P-450 enzymes.

There are no valid guidelines for the choice of specific drugs in the SSRI category. This choice should be considered in individual patients on a clinical basis.

Trazodone and lisuride maleate probably are good alternative to SSRIs.

SSRIs improve the cognitive functions related to depression but probably not those directly consequent to cerebral damage.

Some studies have demonstrated that improvement of PSD induced by SSRIs enhances recovery of neurologic and cognitive deficits (46) and performances in activity of daily living (61). This effect can be large (30% of functional recovery) (62), but a close relationship between appropriate early PSD treatment and functional recovery has not been found in all studies (60,63,64). Nonpharmacotherapeutic mechanisms may be related to recovery from PSD. Prophylactic treatment in all patients with first-ever stroke does not affect outcome (65).

As generally accepted, a placebo effect may account for 35% of the therapeutic response in trials of antidepressants. Spontaneous remissions might be frequent.

Major PSD has been suggested to have a natural course of less than 1 year, whereas minor depression often is more persistent (32). Natural course of PSD, recurrence rate, and effect of pharmacologic therapy remain essentially undetermined.

The use of psychostimulant drugs (methylphenidate, dextroamphetamine) is an interesting option; their beneficial effects probably are due to their ability to overcome the fatigue and apathy components of depression. PSD patients show a rapid response, usually within the first 1 to 2 days of treatment Unfortunately, adverse reactions necessitating the interruption of therapy are not rare and consist of adrenergic-like symptoms (tachycardia and hypertension). Anorexia is infrequent at the doses normally used for PSD. Psychostimulants probably should be encouraged in the acute phase despite the possible cardiovascular side effects, in order to increase arousal and attention and improve the maximal extent of physical and cognitive rehabilitation.

Cognitive and behavioral therapy could be appropriate treatments, especially if all factors contributing to depression are clearly defined. Patients reporting only verbal distress might respond better to cognitive therapy alone, whereas patients with vegetative symptoms might be best treated with an antidepressant drug. Patients with combined symptoms may require cognitive, behavioral, psychological, social, and pharmacologic interventions.

A report of an improved emotional outcome after acute stroke as a result of *informational methods* consisting of workbook-based intervention is particularly interesting (66). The intervention groups exhibited lower levels of anxiety and depression 1 month after discharge. Mood improvement was not explained by differences in age, gender distribution, or initial neurologic impairment. The group of patients who received information were more knowledgeable about, and compliant with, treatment and showed the best response.

CONCLUSIONS

A vast amount of scientific literature failed to define the link between PSD and brain dysfunction, but some notions are worthy of attention.

Lesion location in other neurologic diseases with a depressive syndrome similar to PSD, low incidence of PSD with vertebrobasilar stroke, and the specific neuropsychological PSD profile (executive functions and recall deficits) suggest the role of frontosubcortical, temporolimbic, and basal ganglia areas. It will be interesting to apply the voxel-based morphometry methodology to large stroke populations to investigate lesion location. PET studies and response to pharmacologic therapy indicate a serotonin imbalance. Vascular changes probably contribute to the occurrence of major depression with senile onset. Strategies aimed at preventing vascular diseases (e.g., diet, physical activity/exercise, smoking cessation, and cardiovascular medication compliance) probably may lessen elderly depressive vulnerability.

Planning clinical studies and protocols for investigating PSD is a difficult task. Many factors and variables are involved, and the neurocognitive approach (i.e., the study of specific cognitive functions by means of double dissociation) is impracticable. The marked interpatient variation in clinical expression limits the use of protocol paradigms in functional neuroimaging. There are no biologic or electrophysiologic markers for diagnosis. Univocal diagnostic criteria have been adopted, but the possibility of subgroups of PSD (major and minor, standard/non standard, reactive or nonreactive) makes it problematic not only to carry out clinical investigations on large population samples but also to maximize treatment of individual patients. A major reworking of criteria for case definition is necessary, placing great emphasis on cognitive, behavioral, and vegetative changes. Criteria of causation should be clearly established (strength of the association, consistency, specificity, temporal sequence, biologic gradient, biologic rationale, coherence, experimental evidence, and analogous evidence).

The other concern is to obtain a complete evaluation of the impact of other cognitive, behavioral, physiologic, and psychological changes due to the stroke itself. Extensive neurobehavioral testing is necessary for PSD patients. For example, it is understandable that patients with visual field deficits are prone to anxiety when they are away from home because of the tendency for moving people and vehicles to suddenly appear in their central vision, and that aphasic patients experience frustration and sad-ness when they cannot communicate with their spouses.

All psychosocial factors that possibly interfere with mood changes should be evaluated. The stroke patient is coping with a serious physical illness that reduces his or her self-integrity in terms of personal vulnerability and low self-esteem and generates possible conflicts with close relationships. Strategies to increase social activity, support, contacts, financial security, job satisfaction, adequacy of living arrangements, and psychiatric care are required. Extensive neurobehavioral evaluation can permit the choice of more specific and individual therapies, such as a cognitive approach, a pharmacologic approach, or a combination of the two.

When the diagnosis of PSD is clear, an appropriate therapy can greatly improve not only the quality of life but also recovery from neurologic and cognitive disability.

REFERENCES

1. Gainotti G, Azzoni A, Marra C. Frequency, phenomenology and anatomical-clinical correlates of major post-stroke depression. *Br J Psychiatry* 1999;175: 163–167.
2. Gainotti G, Azzoni A, Razzano C, et al. The Post-Stroke Depression Rating Scale: a test specifically devised to investigate affective disorders of stroke patients. *J Clin Exp Neuropsychol* 1997;19:340–356.
3. Morris PL, Shields RB, Hopwood MJ, et al. Are there two depressive syndromes after stroke? *J Nerv Ment Dis* 1994;182:230–234.
4. Price CI, Curless RH, Rodgers H. Can stroke patients use visual analogue scales? *Stroke* 1999;30:1357–1361.
5. Sutcliffe LM, Lincoln NB. The assessment of depression in aphasic stroke patients: the development of the Stroke Aphasic Depression Questionnaire. *Clin Rehabil* 1998;12:506–513.
6. Stern RA, Bachman DL. Depressive symptoms following stroke. *Am J Psychiatry* 1992;148:351–356.
7. Starkstein SE, Fedoroff JP, Price TR, et al. Apathy following cerebrovascular lesions. *Stroke* 1993;24: 1625–1630.
8. Marin RS, Biedrzycki RC, Firinciogullari S. Reliability and validity of the Apathy Evaluation Scale. *Psychiatry Res* 1992;38:143–162.
9. Ingles JL, Eskes GA, Phillips SJ. Fatigue after stroke. *Arch Phys Med Rehabil* 1999;80:173–178.
10. Habib M. Activity and motivational disorders in neurology: proposal for an evaluation scale. *Encephale* 1995; 21:563–570.
11. Calvert T, Knapp P, House A. Psychological associations with emotionalism after stroke. *J Neurol Neurosurg Psychiatry* 1998;65:928–929.
12. Robinson RG, Parikh RM, Lipsey JR, et al. Pathological laughing and crying following stroke: validation of a measurement scale and a double-blind treatment study. *Am J Psychiatry* 1993;150:286–293.
13. Burns A, Russell E, Stratton-Powell H, et al. Sertraline

in stroke-associated lability of mood. *Int J Geriatr Psychiatry* 1999;14:681–685.

14. Neau JP, Ingrand P, Mouille-Brachet C, et al. Functional recovery and social outcome after cerebral infarction in young adults. *Cerebrovasc Dis* 1998;8:296–302.

15. Paradiso S, Robinson RG. Gender differences in poststroke depression. *J Neuropsychiatry Clin Neurosci* 1998;10:41–47.

16. Morris PL, Robinson RG, Raphael B, et al. The relationship between risk factors for affective disorder and poststroke depression in hospitalised stroke patients. *Aust N Z J Psychiatry* 1992; 26:208–217.

17. Meltzer CC, Price JC, Mathis CA, et al. PET imaging of serotonin type 2A receptors in late-life neuropsychiatric disorders. *Am J Psychiatry* 1999;156:1871–1878.

18. Drevets WC, Frank E, Price JC, et al. PET imaging of serotonin 1A receptor binding in depression. *Biol Psychiatry* 1999;46:1375–1387.

19. Yanai I, Fujikawa T, Horiguchi J, et al. The 3-year course and outcome of patients with major depression and silent cerebral infarction. *J Affect Disord* 1998;47: 25–30.

20. Ballard C, McKeith I, O'Brien J, et al. Neuropathological substrates of dementia and depression in vascular dementia, with a particular focus on cases with small infarct volumes. *Dement Geriatr Cogn Disord* 2000;11: 59–65.

21. Grasso MG, Pantano P, Ricci M, et al. Mesial temporal cortex hypoperfusion is associated with depression in subcortical stroke. *Stroke* 1994;25:980–985.

22. Herrmann M, Bartels C, Schumacher M, et al. Poststroke depression. Is there a pathoanatomic correlate for depression in the postacute stage of stroke? *Stroke* 1995;26:850–856.

23. Lauterbach EC, Jackson JG, Wilson AN, et al. Major depression after left posterior globus pallidus lesions. *Neuropsychiatry Neuropsychol Behav Neurol* 1997;10: 9–16.

24. Sato R, Bryan RN, Fried LP. Neuroanatomic and functional correlates of depressed mood: the Cardiovascular Health Study. *Am J Epidemiol* 1999;150:919–929.

25. Beblo T, Wallesch CW, Herrmann M. The crucial role of frontostriatal circuits for depressive disorders in the postacute stage after stroke. *Neuropsychiatry Neuropsychol Behav Neurol* 1999;12:236–246.

26. Kim JS, Choi-Kwon S. Poststroke depression and emotional incontinence: correlation with lesion location. *Neurology* 2000;54:1805–1810.

27. Paulus W, Trenkwalder C. Imaging of nonmotor symptoms in Parkinson syndromes. *Clin Neurosci* 1998;5: 115–120.

28. Broussolle E, Dentresangle C, Landais P, et al. The relation of putamen and caudate nucleus 18F-Dopa uptake to motor and cognitive performances in Parkinson's disease. *J Neurol Sci* 1999;166:141–151.

29. Bakshi R, Czarnecki D, Shaikh ZA, et al. Brain MRI lesions and atrophy are related to depression in multiple sclerosis. *Neuroreport* 2000;11:1153–1158.

30. Berg D, Supprian T, Thomae J, et al. Lesion pattern in patients with multiple sclerosis and depression. *Mult Scler* 2000;6:156–62.

31. Fedoroff JP, Starkstein SE, Forrester AW, et al. Depression in patients with acute traumatic brain injury. Am J Psychiatry 1992; 149:918–23.

32. Robinson RG. *The clinical neuropsychiatry of stroke.* New York: Cambridge University Press, 1998.

33. House A, Dennis M, Warlow C, et al. Mood disorders after stroke and their relation to lesion location. A CT scan study. *Brain* 1990;113[Pt 4]:1113–1129.

34. Morris PL, Robinson RG, Raphael B. Prevalence and course of depressive disorders in hospitalized stroke patients. *Int J Psychiatry Med* 1990;20:349–364.

35. Carson AJ, MacHale S, Allen K, et al. Depression after stroke and lesion location: a systematic review. *Lancet* 2000;356:122–126.

36. Hénon H, Durieu I, Guerouaou D, et al. Poststroke dementia. Incidence and relationship to prestroke cognitive decline. *Neurology* 2002;57:1216–1222.

37. Bokura H, Kobayashi S, Yamaguchi S, et al. Significance of periventricular hyper-intensity in T2 weighted MRI on memory dysfunction and depression after stroke. *Rinsho Shinkeigaku* 1994;34:438–442.

38. Bolla-Wilson K, Robinson RG, Starkstein SE, et al. Lateralization of dementia of depression in stroke patients. *Am J Psychiatry* 1989;146:627–634.

39. Kauhanen M, Korpelainen JT, Hiltunen P, et al. Poststroke depression correlates with cognitive impairment and neurological deficits. *Stroke* 1999;30:1875–1880.

40. Kimura M, Robinson RG, Kosier JT. Treatment of cognitive impairment after poststroke depression: a double-blind treatment trial. *Stroke* 2000;31:1482–1486.

41. House A, Dennis M, Warlow C, et al. The relationship between intellectual impairment and mood disorder in the first year after stroke. *Psychol Med* 1990;20: 805–814.

42. Kase CS, Wolf PA, Kelly-Hayes M, et al. Intellectual decline after stroke: the Framingham Study. *Stroke* 1998;29:805–812.

43. Singh A, Black SE, Herrmann N, et al. Functional and neuroanatomic correlations in poststroke depression: the Sunnybrook Stroke Study. *Stroke* 2000;31:637–644.

44. Fruhwald S, Loffler H, Eher R, et al. Relationship between depression, anxiety and quality of life: a study of stroke patients compared to chronic low back pain and myocardial ischemia patients. *Psychopathology* 2002;34:50–56.

45. Kotila M, Numminen H, Waltimo O, et al. Post-stroke depression and functional recovery in a population-based stroke register. The Finnstroke study. *Eur J Neurol* 1999;6:309–312.

46. Gainotti G, Antonucci G, Marra C, et al. Relation between depression after stroke, antidepressant therapy, and functional recovery. *J Neurol Neurosurg Psychiatry* 2002;71:258–261.

47. Carson AJ, Ringbauer B, MacKenzie L, et al. Neurological disease, emotional disorder, and disability: they are related: a study of 300 consecutive new referrals to a neurology outpatient department. *J Neurol Neurosurg Psychiatry* 2000;68:202–206.

48. Everson SA, Roberts RE, Goldberg DE, et al. Depressive symptoms and increased risk of stroke mortality over a 29-year period. *Arch Intern Med* 1998;158: 1133–1138.

49. House A, Knapp P, Bamford J, et al. Mortality at 12 and 24 months after stroke may be associated with depressive symptoms at 1 month. *Stroke* 2002;32:669–701.

50. Morris PL, Robinson RG, Andrzejewski P, et al. Association of depression with 10-year poststroke mortality. *Am J Psychiatry* 1993;150:124–129.

51. Ugur C, Gucuyener D, Uzuner N, et al. Characteristics of falling in patients with stroke. *J Neurol Neurosurg Psychiatry* 2000;69:649–651.

52. Jonas BS, Franks P, Ingram DD. Are symptoms of anxiety and depression risk factors for hypertension? Longitudinal evidence from the National Health and Nutrition Examination Survey I Epidemiologic Follow-up Study. *Arch Fam Med* 1997;6:43–49.

53. Hippisley-Cox J, Fielding K, Pringle M. Depression as a risk factor for ischaemic heart disease in men: population based case-control study. *BMJ* 1998;316:1714–1719.

54. Robinson RG, Murata Y, Shimoda K. Dimensions of social impairment and their effect on depression and recovery following stroke. *Int Psychogeriatr* 1999;11:375–384.

55. Starr LB, Robinson RG, Price TR. Reliability, validity, and clinical utility of the social functioning exam in the assessment of stroke patients. *Exp Aging Res* 1983;9:101–106.

56. Kishi Y, Robinson RG, Kosier JT. Suicidal plans in patients with stroke: comparison between acute-onset and delayed-onset suicidal plans. *Int Psychogeriatr* 1996;8:623–634.

57. Kishi Y, Robinson RG, Kosier JT. Suicidal ideation among patients during the rehabilitation period after life-threatening physical illness. *J Nerv Ment Dis* 2002;189:623–628.

58. Gill D, Hatcher S. Antidepressants for depression in medical illness. *Cochrane Database Syst Rev* 2000;CD001312.

59. Berthier ML, Kulisevsky J. Fluoxetine-induced mania in a patient with post-stroke depression. *Br J Psychiatry* 193;163:698–699.

60. Robinson RG, Schultz SK, Castillo C, et al. Nortriptyline versus fluoxetine in the treatment of depression and in short-term recovery after stroke: a placebo-controlled, double-blind study. *Am J Psychiatry* 2000;157:351–359.

61. Chemerinski E, Robinson RG, Kosier JT. Improved recovery in activities of daily living associated with remission of poststroke depression. *Stroke* 2002;32:113–117.

62. van de Weg FB, Kuik DJ, Lankhorst GJ. Post-stroke depression and functional outcome: a cohort study investigating the influence of depression on functional recovery from stroke. *Clin Rehabil* 1999;13:268–272.

63. Wiart L, Petit H, Joseph PA, et al. Fluoxetine in early poststroke depression: a double-blind placebo-controlled study. *Stroke* 2000;31:1829–1832.

64. Paolucci S, Antonucci G, Grasso MG, et al. Post-stroke depression, antidepressant treatment and rehabilitation results. a case-control study. *Cerebrovasc Dis* 2002;12:264–271.

65. Palomaki H, Kaste M, Berg A, et al. Prevention of poststroke depression: 1 year randomised placebo controlled double blind trial of mianserin with 6 month follow up after therapy. *J Neurol Neurosurg Psychiatry* 1999;66:490–494.

66. Morrison VL, Johnston M, MacWalter RS, et al. Improving emotional outcomes following acute stroke: a preliminary evaluation of work-book based intervention. *Scott Med J* 1998;43:52–53.

Ischemic Stroke: Advances in Neurology, Vol. 92. Edited by
H.J.M. Barnett, Julien Bogousslavsky, and Heather Meldrum.
Lippincott Williams & Wilkins, Philadelphia © 2003.

53

Pharmacotherapy in Stroke Rehabilitation

Larry B. Goldstein

*Center for Cerebrovascular Disease, Duke University Medical Center,
Durham, North Carolina, U.S.A.*

A series of laboratory experiments carried out over the last two decades have demonstrated that drugs affecting specific central neurotransmitters can affect behavioral recovery after focal injury to the cerebral cortex (1,2). For example, the administration of D-amphetamine facilitates motor recovery after cortex injury in rats (3) and cats (4). Phentermine (5), phenylpropanolamine (6), and methylphenidate (7) also accelerate motor recovery after experimental focal brain injury. Centrally acting α_2-adrenergic receptor antagonists (yohimbine, idazoxan) are beneficial (8), whereas an α_2-adrenergic receptor agonist (clonidine) impairs motor recovery when it is given soon after brain injury (9) and reinstates motor deficits in recovered animals (10). In addition, administration of an α_1-adrenergic receptor antagonist (prazosin) may be harmful if it is given during the recovery process (11). Coadministration of haloperidol blocks amphetamine-promoted recovery, and haloperidol impairs recovery when given alone (3,12). Other butyrophenones (fluanisone, droperidol) transiently reinstate functional deficits in rats that had recovered motor function after cortex injury (13). Apomorphine, a dopamine agonist, reduces the severity of experimentally induced neglect (14), and spiroperidol, a dopamine receptor antagonist, reinstates neglect in recovered animals (15). Intracortical infusion of the inhibitory neurotransmitter γ-aminobutyric acid (GABA) increases the hemiparesis produced by a small motor cortex lesion in rats (16), and this effect is accentuated by systemic administration of phenytoin (17). Phenobarbital administration to a rat recovering from cortical injury is detrimental (18). Anxiolytics that do not act through the GABA/benzodiazepine receptor complex, such as gepirone, do not appear to impair recovery (19), whereas the short-term administration of diazepam permanently impedes recovery from the sensory asymmetry caused by anteromedial neocortex damage in the rat (20). Drugs affecting acetylcholine and glutamate may affect recovery after brain injury.

The clear implication of these laboratory studies is that specific classes of drugs may affect poststroke recovery in humans. Several general principles arising from animal models of recovery are critical when designing studies to evaluate their effects after stroke. First, the drug effects are dose dependent. For example, the dose–effect curve for amphetamine-promoted motor recovery in rats forms an inverted "U"; the drug is ineffective at low and high doses (21). Second, the timing of drug administration may be critical. Some drugs may have opposite effects on an animal's ultimate behavioral deficit, depending on when it is given in relationship to the injury. For example, immediate postischemic administration of a benzodiazepine is neuroprotective after transient global ischemia (22). Other drugs that presumably act through a GABA-ergic mechanism, such as barbiturates (23), phenytoin (24), and muscimol (25), also have acute neuroprotective properties. In contrast, the experimental studies cited show that benzodiazepines, barbiturates, and phenytoin are harmful when they are given during the recovery period. Third, the window for therapy may be limited. Amphetamine results in reinstatement of binocular depth perception in visually decorticated cats when the drug is given beginning 10 days after injury, but there is no behavioral improvement if administration is delayed for 3 months (26). Fourth, the effects of drugs such as amphetamine on motor recovery are dependent on the behavioral experience of the animal. Amphetamine's effect on motor recovery is blocked if rats are restrained rather than given motor practice after drug administration (3). A smaller independent positive effect of the drug is found in rats that are allowed to freely ambulate but are not given specific training (27). Amphetamine-facilitated recovery of stereoscopic vision in visually decorticated cats also depends on visual experience after the drug is given (26,28). Thus, the combination of drug administration with specific training (i.e., physical therapy) may be critical. The interval between therapy sessions and the duration of therapy are potentially important variables to consider in the design of clinical studies. Finally, drugs given to treat concomitant medical conditions may have an unanticipated detrimental impact on recovery (Table 53-1).

Are the potential detrimental effects of drugs such as α_2-adrenergic receptor agonists, α_1-adrenergic receptor antagonists, dopamine receptor antagonists, benzodiazepines, phenytoin, and phenobarbital clinically relevant? The question is important because these classes of drugs are prescribed for recovering stroke patients for treatment of coincident medical problems (29). In one study, the motor recovery of stroke patients who received one or a combination of the antihypertensives clonidine and prazosin, dopamine receptor antagonists, benzodiazepines, and phenytoin were compared with the recovery of a similar group of patients who were not given any of these medications (30). Patients who received these drugs had poorer recoveries than controls. Multivariate analysis indicated a significant effect of receiving at least one of the hypothesized detrimental drugs even after correcting for the contributions of other variables, including the initial severity of the deficit. Supporting the findings of this study, similar results were found in a separate cohort of patients with anterior circulation ischemic stroke who were control subjects in a prospective acute interventional stroke trial (31). Multivariate analysis again indicated that patients who received at least one drug belonging to these classes had poorer outcomes independent of the degree of initial motor impairment, comorbid conditions, or other patient characteristics. Although these analyses were retrospective, in combination with evidence from laboratory studies, the results suggest that caution should be used when prescribing these classes of drugs to recovering stroke patients.

Are the beneficial effects of drugs on functional recovery after brain injury found in laboratory animal experiments also found in humans recovering from stroke? The first study of amphetamine's effects on poststroke motor recovery was designed to closely follow the paradigm used in laboratory experiments (32). Eight patients with stable motor deficits were randomized to receive either 10 mg of D-amphetamine or placebo coupled with intensive physical therapy within 10 days of ischemic stroke. Assessed the following day (i.e., long after the drug had been metabolized), amphetamine-treated patients were found to have a significant improvement in motor performance, whereas there was little change in the placebo-treated group. However, only this short-term effect was measured, and its clinical significance was not addressed.

A second double-blind, placebo-controlled trial compared the motor recoveries after 30 days of 12 patients who were given 10 mg of D-amphetamine daily for 14 days, followed by 5 mg for 3 days with the recoveries of 12 patients who received placebo (33). There was no benefit of the intervention; however, in contrast to the previous study, treatment began more than 1 month after stroke and the administration of the drug/placebo was not tightly linked with physical therapy.

A third double-blind, placebo-controlled trial compared the motor recoveries of five D-amphetamine–treated and five placebo-treated patients with treatments given once every 4 days for 10 sessions beginning 15 to 30 days after stroke (34). Amphetamine-treated patients had significantly greater improvements in motor function compared to placebo-treated patients 1 year later. Taken together with the laboratory studies, these results suggest that dosing regimen, timing of interventions, and concomitant training (e.g., physiotherapy) are critical.

Using a treatment paradigm similar to that described, six aphasic stroke patients were treated with D-amphetamine in an open pilot study beginning between 10 and 30 days after stroke (35). As measured with the Porch Index of Communicative Ability, five of the six patients met or exceeded their 6-month projected recovery by 3 months after stroke. A subsequent double blind, controlled trial randomized 21 aphasic stroke patients to 10 mg of D-amphetamine or placebo in combination with speech/language therapy (36). Sessions were separated by 3 or 4 days for a total of ten sessions beginning 16 to 45

TABLE 53-1. *Classes of centrally acting drugs that potentially impair poststroke recovery*

α_1-Adrenergic receptor antagonists
α_2-Adrenergic receptor agonists
Dopamine receptor antagonists (butyrophenones)
Benzodiazepines
Certain anticonvulsants
    Phenytoin
    Phenobarbital

days after stroke. Patients given amphetamine had significantly greater gains when assessed 1 week after cessation of therapy. The difference in gain scores between the groups was also present 6 months later, but the difference between the groups was no longer statistically significant.

The effects of the norepinephrine precursor levodopa have been investigated in a prospective, placebo-controlled, double blind study (37). A group of 53 stroke patients were randomized to receive 100 mg of levodopa or placebo daily in combination with physiotherapy for 3 weeks, followed by 3 weeks of physiotherapy alone. Patients given levodopa improved significantly more than those given placebo. The study suggests that drugs having effects similar to D-amphetamine on central norepinephrine levels may facilitate recovery.

Methylphenidate has been used in depressed, brain-injured patients who are not optimally participating in physical therapy (38,39). Experimental studies suggest a complex relationship between methylphenidate dose and training (7). A small placebo-controlled trial found similar improvements in motor function between methylphenidate- and placebo-treated patients (39). Given the laboratory data, methylphenidate dosing needs to be explored in a large number of patients to determine whether a specific regimen might be associated with a clinically meaningful benefit.

Tricyclic antidepressants are commonly used to treat mood disorders in stroke patients. In one study, trazodone treatment was associated with improvement in the activities of daily living when given to depressed stroke patients (40). Other clinical studies found a beneficial effect of the serotonin reuptake blocker fluoxetine (41) and no significant effect of the norepinephrine reuptake blockers maprotiline (41) and nortriptyline (42).

Considered together, these various studies evaluating the potential benefit of D-amphetamine or similar drugs on poststroke recovery are encouraging, but much additional research needs to be completed before clinical efficacy can be established. It is reasonable to avoid drugs that may impair recovery unless they are otherwise necessary for the patient's care.

REFERENCES

1. Goldstein LB. Effects of amphetamines and small related molecules on recovery after stroke in animals and man. *Neuropharmacology* 2000;39:852–859.
2. Feeney DM. From laboratory to clinic: noradrenergic enhancement of physical therapy for stroke or trauma patients. In: Freund H-J, Sabel BA, Witte OW, eds. *Brain plasticity. Advances in neurology.* Philadelphia Lippincott-Raven Publishers, 1997:383–394.
3. Feeney DM, Gonzalez A, Law WA. Amphetamine, haloperidol, and experience interact to affect the rate of recovery after motor cortex injury. *Science* 1982;217: 855–857.
4. Hovda DA, Feeney DM. Amphetamine with experience promotes recovery of locomotor function after unilateral frontal cortex injury in the cat. *Brain Res* 1984;298: 358–361.
5. Hovda DA, Bailey B, Montoya S, et al. Phentermine accelerates recovery of function after motor cortex injury in rats and cats. *Fed Am Soc Exp Biol* 1983;42: 1157(abst).
6. Feeney DM, Sutton RL. Pharmacotherapy for recovery of function after brain injury. *CRC Crit Rev Neurobiol* 1987;3:135–197.
7. Kline AE, Chen MJ, Tso-Olivas DY, et al. Methylphenidate treatment following ablation-induced hemiplegia in rat: experience during drug action alters effects on recovery of function. *Pharmacol Biochem Behav* 1994; 48:773–779.
8. Feeney DM, Sutton RL. Catecholamines and recovery of function after brain damage. In: Stein DG, Sabel BA, eds. *Pharmacological approaches to the treatment of brain and spinal cord injury.* New York: Plenum Publishing, 1988:121–142.
9. Goldstein LB, Davis JN. Clonidine impairs recovery of beam-walking in rats. *Brain Res* 1990;508:305–309.
10. Sutton RL, Feeney DM. α-Noradrenergic agonists and antagonists affect recovery and maintenance of beam-walking ability after sensorimotor cortex ablation in the rat. *Restor Neurol Neurosci* 1992;4:1–11.
11. Feeney DM, Westerberg VS. Norepinephrine and brain damage: alpha noradrenergic pharmacology alters functional recovery after cortical trauma. *Can J Psychol* 1990;44:233–252.
12. Hovda DA, Feeney DM. Haloperidol blocks amphetamine induced recovery of binocular depth perception after bilateral visual cortex ablation in the cat. *Proc West Pharmacol Soc* 1985;28:209–211.
13. Van Hasselt P. Effect of butyrophenones on motor function in rats after recovery from brain damage. *Neuropharmacology* 1973;12:245–247.
14. Corwin JV, Kanter S, Watson RT, et al. Apomorphine has a therapeutic effect on neglect produced by unilateral dorsomedial prefrontal cortex lesions in rats. *Exp Neurol* 1986;94:683–689.
15. Vargo JM, Richard-Smith M, Corwin JV. Spiroperidol reinstates asymmetries in neglect in rats recovered from left or right dorsomedial prefrontal cortex lesions. *Behav Neurosci* 1989;103:1017–1027.
16. Brailowsky S, Knight RT, Blood K. γ-Aminobutyric acid-induced potentiation of cortical hemiplegia. *Brain Res* 1986;362:322–330.
17. Brailowsky S, Knight RT, Efron R. Phenytoin increases the severity of cortical hemiplegia in rats. *Brain Res* 1986;376:71–77.
18. Hernandez TD, Holling LC. Disruption of behavioral recovery by the anti-convulsant phenobarbital. *Brain Res* 1994;635:300–306.
19. Schallert T, Jones TA, Weaver MS, et al. Pharmacologic and anatomic considerations in recovery of function. *Phys Med Rehab* 1992;6:375–393.

20. Schallert T, Hernandez TD, Barth TM. Recovery of function after brain damage: severe and chronic disruption by diazepam. *Brain Res* 1986;379:104–111.
21. Goldstein LB. Pharmacology of recovery after stroke. *Stroke* 1990;21[Suppl III]:III-139–III-142.
22. Schwartz RD, Huff RA, Yu X, et al. Postischemic diazepam is neuroprotective in the gerbil hippocampus. *Brain Res* 1994;647:153–160.
23. Sternau LL, Lust WD, Ricci AJ, et al. Role for γ-aminobutyric acid in selective vulnerability in gerbils. *Stroke* 1989;20:281–287.
24. Boxer PA, Cordon JJ, Mann ME, et al. Comparison of phenytoin with noncompetitive N-methyl-D-aspartate antagonists in a model of focal brain ischemia in the rat. *Stroke* 1990;21[Suppl III]:III-47–III-51.
25. Lyden P, Lonzo L, Nunez S. Combination chemotherapy extends the therapeutic window to 60 minutes after stroke. *J Neurotrauma* 1995;12:223–230.
26. Feeney DM, Hovda DA. Reinstatement of binocular depth perception by amphetamine and visual experience after visual cortex ablation. *Brain Res* 1985;342:352–356.
27. Goldstein LB, Davis JN. Post-lesion practice and amphetamine-facilitated recovery of beam-walking in the rat. *Restor Neurol Neurosci* 1990;1:311–314.
28. Hovda DA, Sutton RL, Feeney DM. Amphetamine-induced recovery of visual cliff performance after bilateral visual cortex ablation in cats: measurements of depth perception thresholds. *Behav Neurosci* 1989;103:574–584.
29. Goldstein LB, Davis JN. Physician prescribing patterns following hospital admission for ischemic cerebrovascular disease. *Neurology* 1988;38:1806–1809.
30. Goldstein LB, Matchar DB, Morgenlander JC, et al. Influence of drugs on the recovery of sensorimotor function after stroke. *J Neurol Rehabil* 1990;4:137–144.
31. Goldstein LB, Sygen in Acute Stroke Study Investigators. Common drugs may influence motor recovery after stroke. *Neurology* 1995;45:865–871.
32. Crisostomo EA, Duncan PW, Propst MA, et al. Evi-
dence that amphetamine with physical therapy promotes recovery of motor function in stroke patients. *Ann Neurol* 1988;23:94–97.
33. Reding MJ, Solomon B, Borucki SJ. Effect of dextroamphetamine on motor recovery after stroke. *Neurology* 1995;45[Suppl 4]:A222(abst).
34. Walker-Batson D, Smith P, Curtis S, et al. Amphetamine paired with physical therapy accelerates motor recovery after stroke: further evidence. *Stroke* 1995;26:2254–2259.
35. Walker-Batson D, Unwin H, Curtis S, et al. Use of amphetamine in the treatment of aphasia. *Restor Neurol Neurosci* 1992;4:47–50.
36. Walker-Batson D, Curtis S, Natarajan R, et al. A double-blind, placebo-controlled study of the use of amphetamine in the treatment of aphasia. *Stroke* 2001;32:2093–2098.
37. Scheidtmann K, Fries W, Muller F, et al. Effect of levodopa in combination with physiotherapy on functional motor recovery after stroke: a prospective, randomized, double-blind study. *Lancet* 2001;358:787–790.
38. Larsson M, Ervik M, Lundborg P, et al. Comparison between methylphenidate and placebo as adjuvant in care and rehabilitation of geriatric patients. *Comp Gerontol* 1988;2:53–59.
39. Grade C, Redford B, Chrostowski J, et al. Methylphenidate in early poststroke recovery: a double-blind, placebo-controlled study. *Arch Phys Med Rehabil* 1998;79:1047–1050.
40. Reding MJ, Orto LA, Winter SW, et al. Antidepressant therapy after stroke. A double-blind trial. *Arch Neurol* 1986;43:763–765.
41. Dam M, Tonin P, De Boni A, et al. Effects of fluoxetine and maprotiline on functional recovery in poststroke hemiplegic patients undergoing rehabilitation therapy. *Stroke* 1996;27:1211–1214.
42. Lipsey JR, Pearlson GD, Robinson RG, et al. Nortriptyline treatment of post-stroke depression: a double-blind study. *Lancet* 1984;1:297–300.

Subject Index

Page numbers in italics denote figures; those followed by "t" denote tables